Design Engineering and Science

Nam Pyo Suh • Miguel Cavique •
Joseph Timothy Foley
Editors

Design Engineering and Science

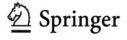 Springer

Editors
Nam Pyo Suh
M.I.T.
Cambridge, MA, USA

Miguel Cavique ⓘ
Department of Sciences and Technology
Portuguese Naval Academy
Almada, Portugal

Joseph Timothy Foley ⓘ
Department of Engineering
Reykjavík University
Reykjavik, Iceland

ISBN 978-3-030-49234-2   ISBN 978-3-030-49232-8   (eBook)
https://doi.org/10.1007/978-3-030-49232-8

This Springer imprint is published by the registered company Springer Nature Switzerland AG
The registered company address is: Gewerbestrasse 11, 6330 Cham, Switzerland

Preface

Many engineers chose their profession because they like to design and create artifacts using their imagination—even the writers of fiction design their stories and their presentation scheme early in their endeavor. People in business must design their business plan well to succeed. Even government policy-makers must design new policies and implementation plans to get the support of the public and benefit their constituents. Design is the first step in creating something new. This book is for those who are interested in learning a systematic and rational way of designing artifacts to fulfill their goals.

An international group of professors, scholars, and practitioners of a design prepared this book for students of all ages, especially for those college students who want to design, innovate, and create. They have taught design in several universities located throughout the world and practiced the design in diverse fields. This book is a manifestation of their desire to improve the design education of the upcoming generations and the practice of the designers and others in the field who must design to satisfy new needs and aspirations.

The synthesis of a variety of systems is an integral part of education, especially in engineering. This book reflects the authors' belief that design education can and should be done more effectively, since it teaches the basics of synthesis, i.e., how to conceive, create, and deliver new solutions to complex problems of all kinds, transcending specific disciplines. To be a leader in any field, it will be of immense help to know the fundamental of the design field to be effective in delivering solutions of all kinds. The ability to design is essential to everyone who wants to improve societal functions, to create new imaginative products and processes, to formulate enlightened policies, to improve organizational effectiveness, and to deliver creative solutions to problems of all kinds.

The artifacts created through designs have changed the course of human history. Indeed, various designed systems, combined with scientific advances in natural and biological sciences, constitute the essence of recent human history. Newton's pioneering scientific work in 1686 and the Industrial Revolution that began with the invention of the steam engine by James Watt in 1782 helped to create a modern era with unprecedented improvements in the quality of human life as well as significant economic advances. Overall, humanity has done well during the past four centuries through their ingenuity. They created designed systems that have laid the foundation for all aspects of human lives. Most of all, they initiated the movement for knowledge-based technological, scientific, and innovative cultural era for humanity. In the future, the design thinking that has partly led to these advances will contribute much more to advance worthy human causes and avoid anthropogenic disasters we face in the twenty-first century. We, humanity, know what logical thinking can do in the creation of new solutions to deal with challenging problems.

The contents of this book are primarily based on Axiomatic Design (AD). It has been applied to a variety of different problems in many fields. The common goal in writing this book is to improve the capability of the student and industrial practitioners in designing and implementing a variety of different systems, both technical and non-technical. Through proper teaching of design, we hope that the costly mistakes—both financially and humans—made in the past because of poor designs can be minimized or ultimately eliminated in the future. Mistakes made out of ignorance or the misunderstanding of the existing knowledge that could have saved a calamity are difficult to be excused or justified.

We are fortunate to be living in this enlightened era of the twenty-first century, where logical and rational reasoning power of humans is guiding the thought processes and behavior of people across many continents. As a result, the economic development of the world is at an unprecedented level of advance; scientific discoveries are taking humanity into unchartered, and often exciting, territories. Technologies have transformed many countries to new heights of prosperity, and healthcare has extended the longevity of people by decades. Overall, people enjoy a higher quality of life in the twenty-first century than ever before in human history. Many in many fields have contributed to these advances: scientists, technologists, humanists, and societal leaders. Design thinking has been one of the final steps in harnessing the advances in human knowledge to create practical and realizable solutions for society.

Human history dates back several thousands of years. During most of this period, many people lived under the dictates of a few tyrants who ruled the people within their territory with iron fists under a class system that used most people as power sources (with intellect) in such fields as farming, construction, transportation, and others. Farmers—tenant farmers, hired hands, and slaves—tilted grounds that were owned by landlords; laborers forged metal parts, transported goods, constructed dwellings, and even gave up their lives fighting for their masters. Most people, except those in privileged positions, toiled without the time, freedom, and mental capacity to think and contemplate about improving their lots and plan for a better future for their posterity. Their daily subsistence was the critical issue that preoccupied their minds. Poverty can be most cruel to those without independent means. These systems lasted for centuries until relatively recently.

Starting about 350 years ago, the life of people began to change because of the emergence of science and technology. The "new science" of the seventeenth century rejected the Aristotelian idea of seeking the essence of four causes. The new paradigm of science accepts that there are laws for physical phenomena, opening the doors for modern science and technology. This birth of a new era was initiated because humanity was blessed with bright people with exceptional minds (e.g., Isaac Newton) who changed the relationship between humanity and nature through discoveries and inventions. New power sources that were introduced with the invention of the steam engine by James Watt enabled people to replace human power with machine power. It also increased their productivity, and allowed people to use their minds to conceive, discover, and invent many artifacts that improved the quality of life as well as productivity. Scientific theories were advanced to explain the invisible as well as observable causality of various natural phenomena. Also, the advances made in human-designed systems amplified the efficiency and productivity of human efforts. In three short centuries, people with exceptional minds have transformed the world and humanity, creating an enlightened modern era.

The table below is a partial and arbitrary list of the significant events that changed or might change the world. They are theories, inventions, and innovations, some of which have transformed or had the potential of changing the future of humanity through technological advances. These advances in science and technology began to occur only about ten generations ago, a short time relative to preceding tens of thousands of years of human existence.

A partial and random list of science and technology that created or may change the basis of human society in the future.

1686: Newton's laws.
1767: Electricity by Ben Franklin and others.
1782: Steam Engine by James Watt.
1854: Thermodynamics (Lord Kelvin).
1861: Electromagnetism, Maxwell's Equations.
1876: Telephone, A. G. Bell.
1903: Airplane (Wilbur and Orville Wright).
1905: Einstein's Special theory of relativity.
1906: Digital Computer (Alan Turing, John Astanoff in 1939).
1911: IBM mainframe.
1917: Moving automobile assembly line by Henry Ford.
1928: Penicillin by Fleming.
1936: Turing machine by Alan Turing.
1946: Transistor.
1948: Information theory by C. Shannon.
1950: NC machine tools by John D. Parson and MIT.
1950: Jet airliner.
1953: DNA by Watson and Crick.
1956 Artificial Intelligence (AI) by Newell, Simon, et al.
1960: FDA approval of the contraceptive pill.
1960: Packet Switching (Internet) by Donald W., Davis and Paul Baran.
1960: Global Positioning Device by Roger L. Easton, Ivan A. Getting, and Bradford Parkinson.
1964: IBM Mainframe 360.

1964: Medical IT software by A. N. Pappalardo.
1973: First mobile telephone.
1975: Microsoft by Bill Gates.
1976: Apple by Steve Jobs.
1976: Axiomatic Design Theory.
1980: Microcellular Plastic.
1993: 3D Printing.
1998: Google by Larry Page and Sergey Brin.
2004: Facebook by Marc Zuckerberg.
2011: On-Line Electric Vehicle (OLEV).

The modern scientific and technological era that began with the Industrial Revolution, thanks to the invention of the steam engine by James Watt, and scientific contributions by Newton and others, established the foundation for the democracy that we enjoy today in many parts of the world. However, even today, it will take constant vigilance to be sure that scientific and technological advances are employed to further democracy because there is always a tendency by a few to attempt to assume dictatorial power.

People used three different paths for the development of scientific theories and technologies. First is the technological invention such as the steam engine by James Watt. The second path was through scientific discoveries (such as the DNA structure) based on observable experimental evidence. Many of them were readily accepted as soon as they were published. The third is based on fundamental scientific postulates and axioms, e.g., thermodynamics had gone through years of debate and discussions before they were finally accepted. Even today, the second law of thermodynamics is still being debated after more than a century. That must be the nature of axioms that make people skeptical because of their simplicity and yet capture profound thoughts and principles. It is remarkable that even Newton's laws, which were partly axiomatic at the time they were advanced, were disputed by some of Newton's contemporaries.

The field of Axiomatic Design is still in its early phase of replacing the old practice of making design decisions based on experience and empiricism through long recursive design/build/test cycles. Establishing Axiomatic Design as the basis for decision-making in the design of systems has been challenging. Many people in charge of development projects throughout the world depend primarily on their experience, notwithstanding numerous failures of highly publicized projects, attesting to the limiting nature of this practice. Universities must lead to the transformation of design practice by generating people who are better rooted in design science and practice. Education is the ultimate means of changing engineering practice for the better.

The purpose of this book is to teach the theory and practice of Axiomatic Design (AD) to students. AD provides a logical framework and the scientific basis for design, which can generate better and creative solutions in many fields of design and synthesis, including engineering, materials, information, systems, and organizations. Major development projects demonstrated that Axiomatic Design could effectively replace lengthy trial-and-error processes often used in developing new solutions and artifacts. AD enables the designer to organize one's thoughts quickly and correctly in dealing with large systems. The organized methods of AD can enhance creativity. People can improve their design practice and advance the field of design by learning the basics of AD.

Our hope in writing this book is modest. The reader of this book acquires the basics of how to design "systems" in a rational way.

The student who masters the subjects presented in this book should be able to execute the following:

1. design uncoupled or decoupled systems of many different kinds;
2. manage large projects to create imaginative design solutions and satisfy customer needs;
3. become a system architect who can lead the development of large systems projects;
4. manage projects without incurring cost overruns and missed schedules;
5. lead significant projects by making the right decisions that do not lead to coupled designs;
6. avoid introducing complexity to designed systems;
7. lead and manage large organizations to achieve the intended goals of the organization.

The abilities listed above, once internalized, should give the student the in-depth systematic knowledge on the design and operation of many different systems. The knowledge they acquire should prepare them for diverse career paths. It should also complement the experience-based expertise gained in the industry by practicing engineers. Ultimately, their success in creating imaginative and rational solutions should enhance the quality of life of humanity that began with the invention of the Watt engine and scientific advancements made during the past three centuries. The intellectual challenges related to the discipline of design will always be there, the latest being the design of cybersecurity systems for the information stored in computer systems throughout the world.

On the Role of Computers and Software in the Field of Design

In this preface, only design theories in dealing with the real problems of the world were discussed. However, the computational power of computers and the application of artificial intelligence (AI) in design to augment human design capability deserve much attention. All of these developments will benefit from the theoretical foundation laid down by design theories such as Axiomatic Design.

The attempt to use computers in design began in the mid-1950s with the effort to replace human drafting, graphics, and sketches with computer-generated tools under the heading of computer-aided design (CAD). Then, it quickly moved into the 3D rendering of complicated mechanical designs. In the 1970s, solid geometric modeling became the fashion of the day, replacing many draftsmen and mechanical part designers. It is soon followed by the 3D representation of complicated parts. Now, these are the commonly used tools.

Several related developments have driven the use of computers in design: low cost of memory, fast computational speed, ability to reduce the memory size, the high quality of graphics, and advances in telecommunications that also depend on the use of computers. Because of the low cost, high speed of computation, and advances in AI, many things, even very inefficient systems, have been attempted to advance the design field. Such an effort will continue, but ultimately, they will increasingly be based on issues and advances discussed in this book. Probably, the industry will drive this transformation because of their urgent need and demand for efficiency, accuracy, and reliability. Most of all, there is the driving need to prevent such spectacular failures as Boeing 737MAX.

The use of computers in design will continue to expand in many dimensions, some of which we cannot even fathom today. However, one thing is clear—a firm theoretical foundation for decision-making in design will be of immense importance in the future development of design engineering and science, regardless of which tools are used to improve the design efficiency.

In Conclusion

The idea of writing this book was agreed on at the 2017 International Conference on Axiomatic Design (ICAD), which was held at Gheorghe Asachi Technical University in Iaşi-România between September 13 and 15, 2017, kindly hosted by Professor Laurentiu Slatineanu. It was a great deliberation. Since then, many people worked hard to deliver what they promised.

Many outstanding people toiled and worked hard, revising their chapters many times. In many ways, it has been a gratifying experience to work together so well, notwithstanding the geographical distances, language barriers, and differences in educational systems and engineering practice. It was a labor of love—a salute to all of them.

Cambridge, USA   Nam Pyo Suh
November 2019   for the Editorial Committee

Acknowledgments

Design is the third leg of the proverbial three-legged stool of engineering, science, and nearly all other fields, including economics. The ingenuity of people created many amazing things that have been designed over many decades and centuries to raise the quality of life of people everywhere. Yet, the field of design has never gained academic and disciplinary rigor because of the view of some people that "everyone can design through the acquisition of experience," albeit intuitively. Humanity has paid the price for this attitude—planes that fell out of the sky, nuclear power plant accidents with substantial human costs, cars that killed many because of malfunctioning car keys, cost overruns in building airports, and hundreds of other unfortunate incidents. We also have many organizations that cannot fulfill their missions because they are so poorly designed. In 2020, the world is facing a historical calamity due to the spread of coronavirus (COVID-19), for which we need to design enlightened and wise policies as well as medication (i.e., vaccine and others) and medical treatments. All of these problems in so many diverse fields require rational, logical, and thoughtful designs. These challenges require better design education in our schools, colleges, universities, and even in industrial firms.

At the 2017 International Conference on Axiomatic Design (ICAD), which was held in Gheorghe Asachi Technical University in Iaşi-România, the idea of improving design education was discussed. A solution was to write a comprehensive textbook on design for students throughout the world. We thus formed the Editorial Committee. We produced a tentative Table of Contents for the book, and sample chapters were written as a general reference and to promote consistency of style of presentation. Professor Miguel Cavique of Portugal assumed the chairmanship of the Editorial Committee. He performed the difficult task of coordinating and reviewing all the chapters through a confidential review process to be sure that the quality of writing is on par with our goal of producing a world-class textbook. The results of his effort are proof of his energy and leadership.

This book is a result of a labor of love and the spirit of cooperation. It reflects the shared belief that design education can be done more effectively to improve the quality of all designed things, ranging from organizations to products and processes. Without the dedication of the authors, we would not have this book. The chapters they produced were thoroughly reviewed and commented by the reviewers and by the members of the Editorial Committee. The challenge of writing this book was higher than usual because authors represented diverse cultures, nationalities, educational backgrounds, various languages, religions, and ethnicity. These different backgrounds enriched our deliberations and increased the zeal to produce a genuinely world-class textbook. All the authors should be complimented for their contributions, hard work, and dedication. They deserve much credit for their effort to improve the quality of design education worldwide.

Many enabled the completion of this book project. Oliver Jackson of Springer promptly accepted our offer to write this book; some of the students at the New South Wales University read the early chapters of the book and offered their candid evaluations. Professor Evelyn Wang, Head of the MIT Department of Mechanical Engineering, rendered her support for this project. Galia Stoyanova of MIT was an able Editorial Assistant throughout the editing process. Emily Welsh provided her expertise with a few figures in the book.

The members of the Editorial Committee provided valuable inputs to the review of the contributed chapters as well as in providing editorial guidance. The members of the Editorial Committee were (in alphabetical order) as follows:

Gabriele Arcidiacono of Italy,
Christopher A. Brown of USA,
Miguel Cavique of Portugal,
Amro Farid of USA,
Joseph Timothy Foley of Iceland and USA,
Inas Khayal of USA,
Ang Liu of Australia,
Dominik Matt of Italy,
Masayuki Nakao of Japan,
Gyung Jin Park of Korea,
Erik Puik of Netherlands,
Laurenţiu Slătineanu of Romania, and
Nam Pyo Suh of USA.

In addition to the members of the Editorial Committee, a distinguished group of professors and scholars reviewed the manuscript. They made specific suggestions to improve the quality of writing, including the delivery of intellectual contents of various topics. The task of the Chairman of the Editorial Committee, Professor Miguel Cavique, was made so much easier because of the expert support and advice he received from many reviewers, including the Editorial Committee members. The rigorous reviews performed by the following professors and scholars have become an integral part of this book:

António Gonçalves-Coelho,
Hilario Oh,
António Mourão,
Petra Foith-Förster,
Taesik Lee,
Erwin Rauch,

João Fradinho,
Paolo Citti,
Gheorghe Nagît,
Oana Dodun,
Marianna Marchesi,
Alessandro Giorgetti,
Rajesh Jugulum,
Vladimir Modrak, and
Efrén Benavides.

The Chairman of the Editorial Committee is particularly grateful to Professor António Gonçalves-Coelho for his guidance and consultation throughout his academic career.

All the chapters were reviewed—sometimes several times—to be sure that the book can serve the need of the readers of the book. Mr. Oliver Jackson of Springer had the book proposal reviewed based on a table of contents and a few sample chapters. Three reviewers positively supported this book project, while one reviewer did not feel that there is any reason to change the design education. The Editorial Committee is grateful for their reviews.

Education has become global—the faculty and students at most leading universities of the world are multi-racial, representing many ethnicities and religions, and are gender-neutral. Leading universities are no longer competing and cooperating only with other institutions within the same country. They operate on a global stage to spread knowledge and produce future leaders who can deal with the needs and problems of the future, such as global warming. The young graduates of these universities will be operating on a worldwide stage—no longer confined to any national boundaries or narrow confines of disciplines—just as many other human affairs have indeed become global. In the future, all inhabitants of Earth must share knowledge for the common good of humanity and the mutual prosperity of all nations. The era of one group of people living better at the expense of others, especially those downtrodden as a consequence of historical accidents, should be replaced by a more enlightened approach for the common good of all people. It is the hope of the authors of this book that our effort will help in elevating the level of knowledge of all people in our global village.

Finally, it is our great personal pleasure to acknowledge many decades of support given to our research on AD and complexity by Dr. and Mrs. Byung-Jun (BJ) Park. With their latest gift, our community has established the Axiomatic Design Research Foundation (ADRF) to give awards to researchers who have made outstanding research contributions to the field of Axiomatic Design and complexity. They have been the lifelong friends of the Suh family and supporters of our vision for better tomorrow at MIT, KAIST, and elsewhere. Young and Nam have been most fortunate to have them as their dear friends.

Any significant tasks such as this undertaking would be impossible without the support and sacrifice of the spouses of the Editorial Committee members. We thank them all. It is our special privilege to acknowledge the support and encouragement of Mrs. Young Ja Surh, Mrs. Cristina Cavique, and Mrs. Markéta Foley. Without their support and encouragement, we would not have completed this book.

Sudbury, Massachusetts, USA   Nam Pyo Suh
Almada, Portugal   Miguel Cavique
Reykjavík, Iceland   Joseph Timothy Foley
March 2020

Contents

4   Design Representations 117

Paolo Citti, Alessandro Giorgetti, Filippo Ceccanti, Fernando Rolli,
Petra Foith-Förster, and Christopher A. Brown

Introduction to Design

Nam Pyo Suh

Abstract

The human ability to design and invent has changed the world in a relatively short time—less than ten generations since the invention of the Watt steam engine in the eighteenth century, which led to the Industrial Revolution. Since then, the number of inventions and design artifacts has exploded to create the current technology-based world and the overall much higher standard of living for a population of about 7–8 billion in the twenty-first century that is about ten times larger than that of the pre-Industrial Revolution!

In the late nineteenth century and the twentieth century, the design of internal combustion engines created the automotive industry and the oil industry that dominated the world's economy for more than a century. The jet engines introduced in the mid-twentieth century shrunk the world—people can travel anywhere in the world in about 24 h. In the twenty-first century, semiconductors and advances in telecommunications have revolutionized all aspects of human lives. The advances in biotechnology are also improving the quality of life of many and are likely to create a new era of human history. All this progress has been possible because of the human ability to design, inspired by challenging goals and promising ideas.

Our ability to design creatively is likely to determine humanity's future. There are many challenges. We need to grow the economy, producing goods and services, to improve the quality of life, all while improving the environment. We also have to combat various old and new diseases through the design of better drugs and healthcare systems. The advances that have enriched and improved the quality of life have also created new challenges for humanity in the form of global warming and others, which must be addressed during the next few decades. The animal husbandry that has satisfied the human need for protein

N. P. Suh (✉)
M.I.T., Cambridge, MA, USA
e-mail: npsuh@mit.edu

© Springer Nature Switzerland AG 2021
N. P. Suh et al. (eds.), *Design Engineering and Science*,
https://doi.org/10.1007/978-3-030-49232-8_1

intakes of people is likely to be replaced by proteins derived from vegetables, partly related to human attempt to solve global warming problems and health issues. Solutions to all these issues depend on our ability to design.

What is design? Design refers to a set of creative activities to satisfy human and societal needs and goals through synthesis. Design is motivated and driven by three basic elements of human nature: inspiration, curiosity, and necessity to improve the quality of life through creation of something new and better. Sometimes, these three factors reinforce each other. Regardless of the motivating factor that initiates the design thinking and activity, the first thing the designer must do is to "establish goals" of the design task. Then, the designer must identify the problem(s) that must be overcome to reach the design goals. Finally, the designer must create useful and meaningful solutions to the problem identified.

Design and creativity have a symbiotic relationship. The ability to design generates creative solutions. Conversely, creative minds yield unique and appropriate designs. Axiomatic Design theory enhances the probability of strengthening this symbiotic relationship to create solutions that are better than random trial-and-error processes. Axiomatic Design (AD) provides a theoretical foundation for the creation of imaginative and optimum designs that satisfy the desired functional requirements (FRs) that the design must fulfill to solve the identified problem. The ability to state the FRs is a foundation for modern technologies and various non-technological systems.

The design is a series of transformational processes. It could be a routine process or an inspirational process of creating new ideas and solutions. Briefly, it begins with "design goals." In the customer domain, we define the "problem" we must address to achieve the design goals. After the problem is established, we create a set of FRs that we must satisfy to solve the problem identified. Then, we transform the FRs to design parameters (DPs), followed by the transformation of DPs to process variables (PVs). Depending on the nature of the system to be developed, DPs and PVs take on specific physical, informational, biological, and organizational entities.

The transformational process of going from problem definition to FRs, DPs, and PVs follows the same methods regardless of the specific nature of the design task. All of them must satisfy the Independence Axiom and the Information Axiom. When we complete the design, the resulting embodiment is a collection of DPs that constitute a system or product. We must check for physical compatibility, information flow, biological functions, and safe operations, among others, to assemble the final system.

To find an appropriate DP for a given FR or the right PV for the chosen DP, we must depend on the fundamental laws, principles, and known phenomena of science, engineering, and other relevant fields. The quality of design thinking and ideas depends on the designer's understanding of natural laws and principles as well as human aspirations, needs, and limitations. In scientific and technological fields, the relationship between FRs and DPs is often governed by natural laws, which may require mathematical modeling to predict the outcome. In general, the **uncoupled design** simplifies and enables the fulfillment of design goals. We can make right design decisions based on our understanding of design principles, natural laws, and the human needs.

Throughout the design process, we must seek inspirations to generate designs that are most imaginative, appropriate, and creative for the task identified or defined. Ultimately, through creative and rational designs, we advance the lot of humanity and even the natural world.

1.1 Human Creativity and Design

"Through design, human beings satisfy their curiosity, create solutions to satisfy the perceived needs, and fulfill human aspirations. Inspiration, logical reasoning, perspiration, and persistence enhances this creative process. The design axioms guide the creative thought process."

What sets humans apart from other creatures is "creativity" and their ability to conceive and create solutions through design, i.e., generation of solutions that have not existed hitherto through synthesis. It has taken many centuries to cultivate this human creativity. Until about 6,000 to 8,000 years ago, human beings lived in the Stone Age. Eventually, the Stone Age ended, not because humans ran out of stones, but they had found something better, i.e., iron. Thus, the new Iron Age was born. However, the subsequent advances in technology and science were slow. They had to wait many tens of centuries for science and modern technologies to emerge. In the mid-seventeenth century, people like Isaac Newton began to lay the foundation for science, and another 100 years later, inventors like James Watt started to create new technologies that led to the Industrial Revolution. Then, a new era for humanity has begun, accelerating the transformation of the world through the use of human brains. What humans have created in basic knowledge and technologies during the past three centuries is most impressive. Furthermore, the rate of new advances and innovation has been accelerating ever since, which has challenged many aspects of human and societal assumptions and practices.

"Design" is an intrinsic human activity, which enables people to develop solutions to the problem that they need to solve through synthesis, analysis, and discovery. Curiosity plays a major role in initiating and deriving these creative activities. Curiosity has its roots in human thought processes that culminate in raising the question: "WHY, WHY NOT, and WHAT IF?" In some fields that do not require manufacturing, materials, and long-term testing to answer these questions, such as the information technology industry, the transition from curiosity to implementation has occurred relatively quickly, as attested by rapid development of IT industry, accelerating the pace of innovation.

The design used to be done and is still practiced in many organizations, based on experience and trial-and-error processes, including extensive prototyping, building, and testing. Many companies depend on their expertise and accumulated database to design and manufacture their products. Good experience and know-how are invaluable in these processes, often generating a reservoir of knowledge and "trade secrets." People have also designed and created public organizations such as universities and governments, often through trial-and-error processes. It is simply amazing how much humanity has improved the quality of life and advanced technologies through these trial-and-error processes of creating new products, solutions, and, eventually, wealth. Humanity has generated many amazing products and processes through these empirical approaches. The human ability to design and create has culminated through such achievement as Apollo 11 that took human beings to the moon in 1969.

Notwithstanding the amazing human achievements of the past three centuries, depending only on experience and adopting the "design-build-test" process of creating new products or systems have their limitations. Such a process is slow and expensive because it requires extensive trial-and-error procedures, costly experiments, and testing of prototypes. In some cases, these purely experience-based approaches to design have resulted in unanticipated failures of the newly created system that resulted in the loss of human lives and extensive cost overruns. Strictly experience-based design approaches have led to failures due to the mistakes and inappropriate decisions made, especially when the new set of requirements deviates from the old ones. There are many well-known examples of failed designs due to these "design-build-test" practices in product and system development. Famous examples are airplanes that fell out of the sky, nuclear power plants that exploded, newly constructed airports that have incurred significant cost overruns and delays, and many costly failures of consumer products such as automobiles due to faulty ignition switches.

Design based on fundamental principles of design should augment experienced-based know-hows, which should assure the creation of successfully designed systems and products that work the first time around without repetitive redesigns and incremental changes to overcome design errors. Rationally designed products and systems based on design principles also simplify analysis and testing, reducing the time and cost associated with innovations of new technologies, products, and systems of all kinds, including organizations, software, and hardware.

Some people believe that design is an "experiential subject," which cannot be taught well at universities. They claimed that design could be learned only through experience. This "experiential school of design" has dominated the design field until fairly recently. As a result, many people engaged in the creation of new design solutions, including engineers, depended on repeated trial-and-error processes and their experience in creating new systems and products. They use the repetitious cycle of "design-build-test" and "redesign-build-test" in developing new products and systems, including organizations. This experience-based design practice is equivalent to attempting to improve the efficiency of jet engines without knowing the fundamental laws of thermodynamics. Similarly, design cannot be done rationally, minimizing mistakes, in the absence of fundamental design principles.

Axiomatic Design (AD) was advanced about 40 years ago to overcome and eliminate the costly trial-and-error processes of design. The goal was to enable us to make the right design decisions and avoid making mistakes and wrong solutions in the development of new products and systems. Since the advent of AD, many innovative products, processes, and organizations have been created quickly and reliably. Many people have become much more creative after learning AD. These results are not surprising, because the design axioms are distillations of common features found in rational designs. The axioms were discovered through the examination of past design decisions that had generated good designs and often, highly creative products. The purpose of this book is to teach AD to students in all fields of intellectual endeavor, who are interested in the synthesis of innovative systems and products.

To learn AD, students must acquire the "language of AD," i.e., definitions of keywords, axioms, mapping, domains, the Independence Axiom, and the Information Axiom. They are not difficult concepts to understand but must be able to follow the logical reasoning used in AD.

1.2 Design: A Basic Human Intellectual Instinct

The need to design exists in most fields of human endeavor. We encounter "design" in many different contexts and situations. Sometimes it is driven by human *curiosity* and by problems that must be solved. Design principles discussed in this book help in both of these situations. Curiosity arises when "something" violates the design principles. These principles also guide the process of creating solutions to the perceived problem.

The design is done to achieve a set of goals. In other words, without a clear set of goals, we cannot commence design. Once we define the goal, we can identify the problem that must be solved to achieve the goal. Based on the identified problem, the designer can establish FRs that must be satisfied to solve the problem. Then, the designer must look for design ideas and the corresponding DPs that can satisfy the FRs of the design. It is a creative process that could be lots of fun because the process of conceiving something new that no one else thought about in the past is a challenging and exciting endeavor. There can be many equally acceptable design solutions, but often, there is a superior design. The joy that follows when we come up with creative ideas can be intoxicating. Furthermore, the same design thinking that leads to innovative design applies to many different problems in many diverse fields!

This book presents the process and the principles that will lead to the creation of designs after we identify the problem—creatively, effectively, and efficiently— regardless of the specific field of application. AD leads to rational and useful design solutions in all areas of synthesis. By being able to identify weak or bad designs early, it prevents the creation of a design that is not acceptable, thus improving the efficiency of the design process. In practical terms, it means that a person who is good at dealing with design issues can be useful in many other fields where synthesis is essential.

The following are real design stories that illustrate how important it is to establish the goals and identify the problem that must be overcome to achieve the goal, leading to new design solutions:

Design Story 1.1:

An aspiring engineering student had to earn enough money to pay for his living expenses while attending a university in the United States because his parents, being recent immigrants to the U.S., could not support him financially. To support himself, he had to hold a series of odd jobs at the university. His first job was to work as a janitor, later moved up to be a telephone operator, lab assistant, and library assistant, working roughly 25 h a week during the academic year to pay for his room and food. He received the legal minimum wage for his work at the university. After his third year at the college, he was most fortunate to get a job in a small industrial firm near his university that manufactured disposal plastic products such as cups and dishes. The best part of the job was the pay! The hourly wage at the company was 120% more than the compensation for student assistants at the university. He felt rich!

Moreover, he was in charge of his project with flexible working hours so that he could attend his classes at school on Mondays, Wednesdays, and Fridays, while working at the company the rest of the week, including Saturdays. He was the only "engineer" in the small company, although he had not yet completed his undergraduate studies. He worked with a dozen or so skilled machinists and technicians, who taught him a lot of practical skills and know-how.

One day, the president of the company asked him to design a new product that could replace a competitor's product that had been used in vending machines for dispensing hot coffee. The young engineer then learned, for the first time, about the problem his boss identified, that had to be solved. The problem was the following: The company decided to replace paper cups used in vending machines with a plastic cup. However, the cup made of thin polystyrene sheet by vacuum-forming could not replace the paper cup, because the cup made of the plastic sheet was too hot to hold with a bare hand when hot coffee is poured into it. Furthermore, the cup did not have enough rigidity to be held by a hand when it contained hot coffee. The alternative was to use a thick foamed plastic sheet (sometimes called Styrofoam that had high thermal insulation) to make the cup, but it was not acceptable, because the wall thickness of the cup made of foamed polystyrene was too thick, limiting the number of cups that can be stacked in the vending machine. The president of the company assigned him to develop a new solution. It was an exciting challenge for the young engineer, who had not yet graduated from college.

The young engineer's solution was to satisfy two FRs, i.e., stiffness and thermal insulation, by laminating foamed plastic sheet with un-foamed straight polystyrene sheet to provide both the required thermal insulation and rigidity. In addition to creating the product, he also designed and built a continuous manufacturing system for mass production of the laminated plastic products. It took about 2 years to finish the project and go into mass production. The product was a major commercial success. The company did very well with the new invention, making many products. The U.S. Patent Office granted a patent for the product and processes. He received a bonus that was equal to his weekly pay, which was appreciated but did not make him rich!

Many years later after he became a professor at the same university where he was a student, he and his family visited one of the manufacturing plants of the company and found that the same machine he designed and built as an undergraduate student, a la a development engineer, was still being used to make the product, except that there were many more of them humming at the same time! He was happy to show what he did many years ago to his wife and daughters.

Design Story 1.2:

As the above design story unfolded, across the town, a recent graduate of the same engineering school got a job at a major teaching hospital. While working there, he had this *inspiration* that the hospital could use a computerized information management system. He realized that the hospital, which was well known for its advanced medical care system throughout the world, was inefficient in its operation because the hospital lacked an integrated information system because all the information was written by hand and stored in file cabinets by people. Such information could not be shared among different departments of the hospital without human intervention.

He designed and implemented a central software system for electronic record keeping as well as providing diagnostic assistance to medical doctors based on the data collected from various tests done on a patient. He established a new company in 1968 to make a software system for automation and management of hospitals and healthcare. His company might have been one of oldest software systems company in the world. (Note: Bill Gates started Microsoft in 1975.)

Initially, the company struggled but eventually received funding from a local venture capitalist. Now the company is the leading software company in the healthcare industry in the United States. The company did superbly well, making him and his wife one of the wealthiest couples in the country. He and his wife have become generous philanthropists, supporting many worthwhile causes at universities; hospitals; and various educational, civic, and cultural organizations in the United States and other countries. Many of the recipients of their largess were glad that he had that inspiration and started a new industry.

Design Story 1.3:

Another young engineer established his company that tested imported merchandise for big department stores in the United States for quality assurance. He had learned from one of his classmates that large department stores had a problem controlling the quality of merchandise they were importing from overseas. They needed the confidence that the products they were about to buy in large quantities from a vendor in other countries were of good quality. His company tested various merchandise (ranging from clothing, furniture to even medicine) at the request of department stores.

The manufacturer of the merchandise wishing to sell its product to a department store in the United States paid this testing company to test and certify the quality of their products. When his company approved the quality of the product, the department store purchased the merchandise directly from the manufacturer. It was a perfect arrangement for this testing company, i.e., testing done at the request of large department stores but paid for by the manufacturers of various merchandise that is trying to sell their products to the department stores.

His company designed and invented many new testing methods and machines. They also established the standards for an acceptable quality of various products, creating an extensive database. The company became a reputable and highly successful merchandise testing company in the world. One of the reasons for success of this company was the reputation and personality of the founder. He always had impeccable reputation for hard work, honesty, and the highest ethical standards. Later, he and his wife sold the company to a large company at a high premium. With their immense wealth, they became philanthropists, supporting many worthwhile causes at universities, hospitals, and needy students in many countries.

Design Story 1.4:

There are other interesting stories related to design. Recently, students at a well-known university organized a team to create a solar-energy-powered electric car to solve the problem of global warming caused by CO_2 emission. They came up with their unique design for the solar-powered electric car, learning about many issues related to developing such new products. The students would have done a better job if they had known more about fundamental aspects of the design of such vehicles and solar power. If they had defined the FRs of such a car first (i.e., in a solution-neutral environment) without letting the pre-conceived notion of what such a vehicle should be like, they would have created a better vehicle. They could have learned the lesson from those who designed the "Sunraycer" that won the 1,867-mile Pentax World Solar Challenge (Wilson et al. 1989). The Sunraycer team defined FRs *first* without any specific design in mind, whereas other competitors had decided on the physical configuration first without clearly defining the FRs of such a vehicle and then tried to optimize the design afterward. Doing so, they encountered too many problems due to the coupling of FRs.

Design Story 1.5:

A young professor at a leading university presented a seminar on how to manufacture thin, single-crystal III–V semiconductors without defects. The idea he offered for making thin semiconductors was creative and smart. It had the potential of manufacturing thin-film semiconductors that can be used to make devices.

We have known for a long time that if we deposit a new layer of a known crystalline material (e.g., III–V semiconductor compound) on a crystalline substrate by vapor deposition, the newly deposited material assumes the crystal structure of the substrate. After the deposition of several layers of the crystalline material, if we could separate the newly deposited crystal from the substrate, it could be used to make a memory or logic device. The *problem* was that it was difficult to peel off the newly deposited semiconductor layer from the substrate.

The young professor's idea, which he developed while he was working at IBM, was to satisfy two FRs *independently from each other*, i.e., the FR of growing thin-film semiconductors and the FR of separating the thin-film semiconductor from the substrate. To satisfy the second FR of separating a newly deposited semiconductor layer, an intermediate atomic layer of graphene was deposited first on the solid semiconductor substrate. The thin graphene sheet is a two-dimensional material and does not bond to any material perpendicular to its surface because the interatomic force of graphene is planar. Then, if the semiconductor material is deposited on top of the graphene by vapor deposition, the newly deposited semiconductor would then assume the structure of the substrate crystal below the graphene sheet, but not bond to the graphene. Hence, when the semiconductor material is deposited on top of the graphene layer, the crystalline structure of the newly deposited semiconductor material on the top of the graphene would be the same as the original substrate below the graphene layer. Then, the freshly deposited crystal on top of the graphene sheet can be peeled off to make thin semiconductor devices. If the design can produce atomic scale-thin semiconductors on a mass production basis, it may open up a new chapter in mass production of semiconductor devices.

Design Story 1.6:

Famous researchers and professors got together at a research institute, which was established by a generous gift given by a leading industrialist and an alumnus of the university, to discuss the progress made in the field of brain science and technology related to autism. They were bright people with impressive credentials. Young researchers and their professors made presentations in front of these experts assembled from many different regions of the world. They presented the results of various measurements, correlations, hypothesis, and models. They got into heated discussions to clarify multiple concepts presented. What was clear from the presentations and subsequent discussions was that they could not define the cause or the *problem* that lead to autism. Until they can identify the problem, their research is likely to take longer to find a cure for autism. Their research, which is in their early stages, needs to be conducted to determine the problem. They should perhaps do more research based on hypothesis to narrow down the probable cause of autism. To do this type of hypothesis-based research, they will probably need to adopt "design thinking" to make more rapid progress.

Design Story 1.7:

In 2019, one of the most challenging issues in the world is the "cyberattack" by hostile governments to disable computer networks or steal the information stored in the computer systems of other nations. Many countries are engaged in such hostile attacks, hoping to tilt the public opinion. They either try to steal or compromise the information stored in the computer system of the targeted institutions. Certainly, the attempt to influence the U.S. election has dislocated the U.S. political system in 2016. Corporations and institutions are spending a vast sum of money to protect their information system from those who are attempting to steal the secret information and strategic plans stored in their computer systems. In some cases, the goal of the attacker is to destroy or disable specific computers to render the entire information system malfunction and thus destroy the infrastructure of their competitors.

This kind of cyberattack is of primary concern for governments, corporations, and even individuals. The problem is how to deal with cyberattacks and safeguard the information systems from these intruders. The attackers may use email systems and the Internet system to penetrate the information system of the organizations they wish to compromise. One of the major design issues in cybersecurity is the continuing escalation of attacking strategy to avoid newly installed defense systems, which require a response system that periodically updates and adjust the defensive strategy. One design approach might be to attack the source of the cyberintruders at their base.

This problem can be solved only through the superior design of the software system that can identify the attacking system, protect its information system, mislead the attacking system to self-destruct, and, at the same time, disable the attacking computer system.

Design Story 1.8:

One of the most critical issues of the twenty-first century is global warming. If it is unchecked, the temperature of the earth atmosphere will rise, creating many unacceptable calamities such as flooding, the rise of sea level, creation of desert, and many others. One of the major causes is the anthropogenic emission of carbon dioxide (CO_2) by automobiles and electric power plants. A widely accepted goal is to limit the temperature rise to below 2 degrees Celsius relative to the temperature of the atmosphere before industrialization. Professor William D. Nordhaus of Yale University received the Nobel prize in economics for his work on how to reduce carbon emission. His idea was to introduce a carbon tax to limit CO_2 emission. In 2016, 196 nations signed the United Nations Framework Convention on Climate Change (UNFCCC). Its implementation has not been easy, some countries refusing to join in, citing that its negative impact on the economy and the high cost of replacing fossil fuels with solar and wind energy.

It is a classic design problem. There are many FRs we have to satisfy to solve this global warming problem. We need to identify all the FRs we have to satisfy and the corresponding DPs. The carbon tax, although a creative idea, cannot solve the global warming problem by itself. As we will demonstrate in later chapters, when there are more FRs to be satisfied than the number of DPs (in this case, the carbon tax), the design is not acceptable, i.e., the problem cannot be solved. We will show that the number of DPs must be equal to the number of FRs that must be satisfied to solve the global warming problem. Thus, the carbon tax alone will not bring about an acceptable solution to global warming! We have to identify all the FRs that must be satisfied and then develop an equal number of DPs, which will satisfy the FRs without coupling them to each other.

Question 1.1:

"What is the common element in all these stories? How are they related to the main subject of this chapter, i.e., why design?".

1.3 Importance of Knowing How to Define the Problem Based on Design Goals

Every design task, regardless of the specific field of application, has a set of goals. In the case of the environment, the goal may be the reduction of greenhouse gases, whereas, for the head of a university, the goal may be making the university one of the best in the world. In the case of product development, the goal may be to make the most efficient electric vehicle. The goal of the government may be to provide universal healthcare to all citizens.

Once the goal is determined, the designer must ask, "What is the PROBLEM(s) that has to be solved to achieve the goal?" Once the problem is defined, we can proceed with the design task by going through the following four-step transformational processes:

(a) understanding the problem that needs to be solved in the customer domain;
(b) defining functional requirements {FRs} that must be satisfied to solve the problem identified;
(c) identifying design parameters {DPs} to satisfy the {FRs};
(d) selecting process variables {PVs} that can satisfy the {DPs}.

This transformational process occurs over the four domains of the design world: the customer domain, the functional domain, the physical domain, and the process domain. The relationship between the domain on the left and the domain on the right is "What" versus "How." In other words, {FRs} with respect to {DPs} represent "what we want to achieve," whereas {DPs} are "how we are going to satisfy {FRs}." Figure 1.1 illustrates this transformational process.

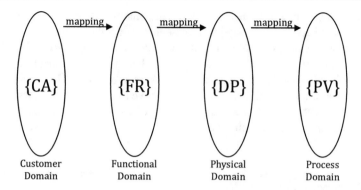

Fig. 1.1 Design is done to achieve the goals (i.e., the customer attributes, CA) stated in the customer domain. Typically, the PROBLEM that is preventing the achievement of the goal must be identified and solved. We state the goal in the form of functional requirements {FRs} in the functional domain that will solve the problem. Then we go through a series of transformational processes, i.e., from {FRs} to design parameters {DPs} in the physical domain, from the design parameters, {DPs}, in the physical domain to process variables {PVs} in the process domain. The terms DP and PV can be interpreted in different ways, depending on what we are designing, e.g., an organization rather than a machine

The importance of identification of the problem cannot be over-emphasized as the following story about the invention of the Watt steam engine illustrates: James Watt, who transformed the history of humankind, began his quest for mechanical power generation with the use of thermal energy by discovering the problem with then-existing Newcomen engine!

1.3.1 Invention of the Steam Engine by James Watt Changed the History of Humanity and Created the Science of Thermodynamics

From a historical point of view, the most critical invention made by human beings is the steam engine by James Watt. His invention was not only responsible for the Industrial Revolution in the eighteenth century but also chartered a new path for human history by awakening the human brainpower for scientific and technological thinking. The Watt engine freed humankind from hard physical labor and changed the trajectory of civilization through a series of scientific and technological advances that followed. Now 300 years after the invention of the Watt engine, science and technology are taking humanity to a hitherto unimaginable path that depends on science and technology, the outcome of which we cannot even fathom with any degree of certainty. The only thing we know for sure is that in the future, humankind will create new problems and new solutions that will accelerate the pace of change. The design will be central in this transformation of human history, as people will continue to use their creativity to design artifacts that will take humans to a new plateau of not only technological progress but also better understanding of humanity itself and societal fabric.

History attributed the beginning of the Industrial Revolution of the world to the invention of Steam Engine by James Watt in 1736. In some ways, James Watt was fortunate to be at the right place at the right time, in addition to being gifted with brainpower and persistence to solve a problem that led to his invention of the Watt steam engine. His genius was his ability to identify the problem (i.e., shortcomings) associated with the Newcomen engine (invented in 1712), which led to the invention of the Watt steam engine (1763–1775). At the time, the Newcomen engine was primarily used to pump water out of mine shafts.

History states that James Watt was asked to repair the Newcomen engine that belonged to the University of Glasgow. While repairing the machine, he found the major shortcoming with the Newcomen engine (see Fig. 1.2), i.e., its intermittent motion. As shown in Fig. 1.2, steam is injected into the cylinder of the Newcomen engine. Then, the valve from the boiler to the cylinder is closed, and cold water was injected into the cylinder to lower the temperature and condense the steam in the cylinder. The vacuum created in the cylinder due to condensation of the steam pulled the piston down. This downward motion of the piston, which was connected to the water pump of the mine, sucked the water from mine shafts. James Watt noticed that since one cylinder was used for both expansion and condensation of the steam, the Newcomen engine was slow and not efficient. This discovery of the problem by James Watt led to the invention of the Watt engine. His solution was to separate the two functions, i.e., expansion and condensation by adding a separate cylinder for condensation. This solution is consistent with the Independence Axiom of AD, which is a formalization and generalization of what James Watt did, although the origin of AD was not based on this observation of the Watt engine.

1.3.2 Design as a Common Human Activity in Many Fields

"Design is a universal human activity to satisfy human aspirations."

In 2006, researchers at KAIST (The Korea Advanced Institute of Science and Technology) identified the elimination of CO_2 emission from internal combustion (IC) engines as the central problem they must solve in order to alleviate the global warming problem. Electrification of ground transportation systems should eliminate about 30% of all anthropogenic CO_2 emission of the world by using electricity generated at more efficient electric power plants as well as using renewable energy sources such as wind, solar, and hydropower.

This goal of removing of anthropogenic emission of CO_2 has resulted in the invention of new kinds of electric buses, cars, and trains that receive electric power *wirelessly* from the underground power supply system to propel the vehicle. This technology is called the "On-line Electric Vehicle (OLEV)." The OLEV bus carries a small battery on board for operations of the vehicle on roads without the underground power supply system. The driver of the OLEV bus drives the vehicle

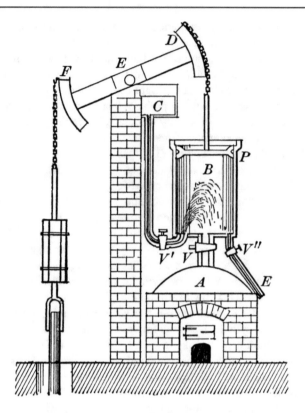

Fig. 1.2 Schematic drawing of the Newcomen engine. The sequence of operation: Hot steam is injected into the cylinder, followed by the closing of the valve. The piston of the cylinder then moves upward due to the internal pressure created by the steam. This piston is connected to the water pump of the mineshaft. When the steam in the cylinder condenses by the cold water injected into the cylinder, a vacuum was created in the cylinder, pulling down the piston. The downward motion of the piston pulled the piston of the water pump upward, pumping water out from the mineshaft. (Reproduced from Black and Davis 1913)

without ever worrying about recharging the battery because it is done automatically when the bus is on the top of the road with underground power supply system. Figure 1.3 shows a bus commercially operating in Gumi City in Korea.

In addition to the design issues related to technology, similar design needs exist in other fields such as organizations, economics, finance, public policy, and literature. For instance, a senior professor at a leading university got a telephone call from overseas, asking him to lead a university to the next level of academic excellence. He accepted the presidency of the university and redesigned the university through strategic planning with the support of some of the faculty members, eventually making it one of the best universities in the world. What the new president did first was to identify the problems the university had to solve through institutional transformation. After reaffirming the new goal of the university, he and

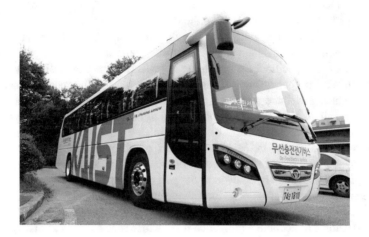

Fig. 1.3 OLEV bus in Gumi City in Korea

his team redesigned the university, including organizational structure, operational policies, financial structure, and personnel policies. They used the principles of AD. The university has indeed emerged one of the best innovative universities of the world.

The design is performed in many fields, although in some fields they may not call it "design" and use other synonymous phrases. It is interesting to note that recently, graduates of liberal arts colleges in many countries are eager to become writers of fictions, inspired by the work of Kazuo Ishiguro, the 2017 Nobel laureate who is the author of "The Remains of the Day." To write such a novel, the author had to design the book first before actually commencing the writing of the book.

Although the specific nature of their tasks appears to be vastly different, all of the people mentioned in this chapter have performed similar tasks! The first thing all of them had to do to achieve their goal was to identify the problem to be solved and then develop design solutions for the problem identified through a transformational process illustrated in Fig. 1.1. The engineers and scientists design their products, processes, and systems. The writers of fictions also design their book, i.e., identify the "problem (i.e., the theme of their story)," design the structure of the story to be written, and then write the narratives of the book. University administrators must also do similar things: design the goals, strategy, and policies, and organize the university for the execution of the plan.

Question 1.2:

Through DESIGN, humans have created modern society; fulfilled their aspirations, curiosity, technological and cultural advances; and extended human life. Unfortunately, people have also conceived the means of harming nature and human civilization through design. How do we design all of these different things? Are there common elements in all these designs?

In this introductory section of this chapter, we emphasized, repeatedly, the need to discover or identify the "problem," either before or after the goal of the design is established. Then the designer translates or transforms the problem into a set of specific objectives or goals the design must satisfy (or achieve). The goals are then transformed into specific FRs that must be satisfied through design in order to achieve the stated goals. Then, we have to search for specific means of satisfying the FRs, which is defined as DPs in AD. All designs must go through these steps. Fortunately, all designs, regardless of the field or the subject matter, involve similar thought processes and the same basic principles a good design must satisfy. In summary, to be useful in design, we must go through the actual process of designing and understanding the design process, similar to learning how to ride a bicycle, i.e., one has to try it, even at the risk of falling!

The process of the design described above applies in all fields that require design solutions. It is not a difficult task. Everyone can do it! In design, the experience can either be helpful or become a hindrance if the experience consists of purely random trial-and-error processes.

1.3.3   Two Different Solutions for the Same Problem

Space travel fascinates many people of all ages, both young and old. The idea of people going to the Moon was a big challenge in the 1960s. When Apollo 11 of the United States landed on the Moon for the first time, on July 20, 1969, it was a momentous and aspiring moment for all humankind. It gave confidence that human beings can claim space as part of the human habitat. It has undoubtedly inspired many young people all over the world to be interested in space travel and science.

In the early 1980s, the U.S. National Aeronautics and Space Administration (NASA) established the Space Shuttle Program in order to build a space transportation system primarily between Earth and the International Space Station. Figure 1.4 shows a space shuttle taking off the launch pad. It shows the orbiter vehicle (OV) that looks like an airplane attached to the external tank (ET), which carries oxygen and hydrogen in two spherical tanks inside the external tank. Two solid-fuel booster rockets are attached to the external tank on its two sides, which assist during the liftoff. The external tank, which is made of aluminum, has about half-inch thick polyurethane foam layer on its surface as thermal insulation in order to prevent the formation of ice on the cold surface of the external tank while waiting for launch. If ice forms, it can fracture during the ascent, which may hit the OV, damaging the ceramic tile on the OV that protects the vehicle from burning up during its re-entry into the earth's atmosphere. The surface area of the external tank is about the same as two football fields. The students, who visited the

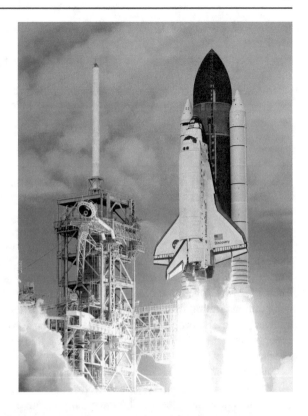

Fig. 1.4 The space shuttle discovery and its seven-member STS-120 crew head toward earth's orbit and a scheduled linkup with the International Space Station. (Reproduced with permission from Petrushenka 2019)

manufacturing facility in Louisiana, U.S.A., where the external tank was being built, were duly impressed by the size of the external tank.[1]

The problem with the Space Shuttle Program was its enormous cost. In comparison to the cost of launching communication satellites using a rocket, the cost of launching it using the space shuttle was much more expensive. NASA justified the cost because the space shuttle was needed to service the International Space Station. In order to reduce the cost, it was decided to reuse the solid booster rockets. They jettisoned the rockets mounted on the external tank fall into the ocean upon completion of their mission during ascent. Then they have recovered the jettisoned rocket for future use.

Another solution to the reuse of the solid rocket is to let it descent along a pre-programmed trajectory back to the launch pad, which has been demonstrated in 2017 by Space X, a company founded by Elon Mask. Conceptually, this technology appears to be more elegant because it eliminates the need to search the ocean for the

---

[1]As part of the contract between a NASA contractor and MIT, one of the students under the supervision of a faculty member developed a method of putting on thermal insulation on the external tank, which significantly reduced the cost of manufacturing.

recovery of used rockets. We have two different designs to solve similar highest level FRs.

The FRs of the Space Shuttle Program involved many additional functions than the Space X because it had to serve the International Space Station and launching of satellites. However, the problem of recovering used rockets is similar at the highest level of the design hierarchy. The lower level of FRs and DPs was different, yielding two different solutions.

1.4 Designing Without Explicit Goals and Problem Identification is Analogous to Sailing a Sailboat Without a Rudder

In a major global company that makes steering systems for automobiles, the management assembled their technical and marketing leaders to review their strategic direction for the development of their next generation of new products. Their goal was to be more competitive in the market place, especially in light of the competition coming from Chinese companies that were offering similar products at a lower price. The people gathered in the conference room of the company were all experienced and bright people. Various ideas and solutions were proposed and discussed.

Their products may be classified into the following four different kinds of systems: purely mechanical systems, electro-mechanical systems, all electrical systems, and hydraulic systems. The price ranges from a few hundred dollars per unit to a few thousand dollars. After 3 h of intense discussion, the meeting was concluded without developing any new major ideas and decisions. They decided to have another meeting in about a month. Unfortunately, these unsuccessful meetings are often a common occurrence in many companies. It is highly probable that the meeting failed to produce any concrete ideas because they concentrated on lowering the manufacturing cost of their products rather than reviewing their design after clearly defining the PROBLEM.

The situation discussed above is similar to trying to steer a sailboat without a rudder. The sailor will not go very far, or even worse, may not turn to the home base!

1.5 A Summary of the Creative Process

The first step in developing innovative design typically requires the establishment of the need (or the goal) and the identification of the problem that must be overcome to achieve the goal.

Based on the identification of the goal and the problem, we establish specific FRs that our design must satisfy to meet the goal. The next step in design is to come up with DPs that will enable us to satisfy the FRs. Then, we configure the designed system through the integration of various DPs as an integrated system. The integrated system may consist of hardware, software, information systems, natural elements, and others such as sensors. In some ways, it is an obvious way of coming up with good designs.

Most people confront many problems, large or small throughout their life. They have to solve them through design and perhaps by other means as well. The difficulty is that often they are trying to find solutions without first defining the problem. They may come up with various and contradictory claims and counter-claims, aggravating each other. If we can define "what the problem is," it may be easier to develop solutions to the problem identified. The ability to define the problem can be acquired by accumulating broad knowledge base, experience, and design thinking. One of the goals of this design book is to teach those who are not yet initiated into the field of design the ability to identify and define the problem and FRs.

Once the FRs are defined, most people can synthesize their unique solutions, unless they can find a quick solution from their "library" of past solutions that are similar to the current problem. When there are no obvious past examples that can be adapted, people should seek a new solution through "design" with confidence without being intimidated. The decision to either adopt an old existing solution or create a new "solution" depends on one's knowledge base or experience or the confidence that one can create something new from scratch that will be superior to the existing system. Many people instinctively want to create their unique solution. That may be a good aspect of human nature.

1.6 Importance of Design and Design Thinking

Design and design thinking are essential in dealing with all aspects of any system. Design thinking implies that a system must be designed first before analyzed. Sometimes based on the analysis, we may have to go back to the original design of the system to improve the design. Unfortunately, sometimes, engineers are mired in an analysis of wrong designs rather than changing the design. Engineering education sometimes biases students' thinking by giving well-defined problems at the end of each chapter, without explaining the design that led to the problem. To repeat, design thinking emphasizes the need to design first, followed by analysis. This chapter outlined how one should begin the design process.

We design two kinds of systems: technical and non-technical. Much of this book deals with technical and scientific design. However, the design of non-technical systems such as government and universities has equally significant consequences on society and humanity as much as technical systems. Institutions and governments must be designed well for them to serve their constituents as well as intended. Unfortunately, this is not always the case. In short, "Design Thinking" is equally applicable to all designs.

When we deal with systems, technical as well as non-technical, we must deal with synthesis and analysis. In designing new systems or modifying old systems, it is often instructive to consider the synthesis (or design) issues first before delving into an analysis of a subset of the overall system. One can spend a lifetime analyzing a poorly designed system, because coupled systems, i.e., poorly designed systems, are often mathematically intractable. Unfortunately, more people in all intellectual persuasions tend to delve into an analysis of lower level issues and then become bewildered by conflicting details of a poorly defined or designed system. To reiterate the significant point of this chapter: identify the PROBLEM(s) of a system that must be improved (in the case of an existing system) and then establish goals in the form of FRs that must be satisfied. Then find DPs that can satisfy the FRs, before undertaking a detailed analysis of lousy design, thinking that optimization will improve the system. An optimized, poorly designed system is still a bad design!

In many professions, the precedents provide guiding lights, and therefore they look for similarities of a case with an old example for decision-making. For instance, not too many political leaders in many countries have a technical or scientific background. In the United States, many of them have legal or business backgrounds. Occasionally, there were exceptions. Two of the past presidents of the United States, Herbert Hoover (1929–1933) and Jimmy Carter (1977–1981), had technical backgrounds. Hoover was a mining engineer and Carter was a nuclear engineer who served on nuclear submarines in the United States Navy. Even today, they are regarded as honest and ethical people with deep convictions. However, historians might not see their presidencies as successful ones. During their presidencies, the United States encountered economic difficulties. The Hoover administration had to deal with the world's worst depression of 1929. During the Carter period, inflation was out of control. Either they were unlucky or mismanaged the economy. Did they concentrate too much on individual detailed issues rather than the systems issues to develop suitable designs for economic policy? The simple conclusion may be that they focused too much on details before they really identified and understood the problems and then design their policies accordingly. We must identify the overall problem first and then design sound policies. Analysis of poorly designed systems typically is not enlightening. Accurate analysis of a poorly designed system cannot improve the poorly defined system. If the system is coupled, i.e., FRs are not independent, improving one FR may result in deterioration of other FRs, negating the intended effect.

It should be emphasized again here: The first step in developing innovative design typically requires the identification of the problem.

Once we know the problem, we establish the goals that our design must satisfy to solve it and other associated issues. (Sometimes, we set the goal first based on the "customer need" and then identify the problems that must be solved to achieve the goal.) These goals must then be stated as specific FRs that our design must satisfy. The final step in design is to come up with DPs that will enable us to fulfill the FRs.

The last step is to configure DPs through the integration of various DPs as an integrated system that may consist of hardware, software, information systems, natural elements, and others, such as sensors. In some ways, it is an obvious way of coming up with good designs. However, many companies have repeated the error made by some manufacturers, i.e., trying to be more competitive, without first discovering the specific problem faced by their company other than lowering the cost of manufacturing. This situation may not be only confined to manufacturing companies but also individuals as well.

Most people confront many problems, large or small, throughout their lives. They have to solve them through design and perhaps by other means as well. The difficulty is that often they are trying to find solutions without first defining the specific problem. They may come with various and contradictory claims and counterclaims, aggravating each other. If we can determine "what the problem is," it may be easier to develop solutions. The ability to define the problem can be acquired by accumulating broad knowledge base, experience, and design thinking. One of the goals of this design book is to teach the ability to identify and define the problem.

Once the problem is recognized and defined, most people can synthesize their unique solutions, unless they can find an immediate solution from their "library" of experience that is similar to the current problem. When there are no prominent past examples that can be adapted, people should seek a new solution through "design" with confidence without being intimidated. The decision to either adopt an old existing solution or create a new "solution" depends on one's knowledge base or experience or the confidence that one can create something new from scratch that will be superior to the existing system. Many people instinctively want to create unique solutions. That may be the meritorious aspect of human nature.

1.7 What is the Most Difficult Aspect of Learning Axiomatic Design?

Every era has certain businesses that dominate the economy. In the first half of the twentieth century, it was the automotive companies (such as Ford, General Motors, Toyota, and Daimler Benz). In the late twentieth century, manufacturers of computers (such as IBM and Microsoft) and semiconductor chips and integrated circuit devices (such as Intel) have dominated the economy and technology. In the first half of the twenty-first century, it was the era of high-speed Internet and social networking and telecommunication businesses (dominated by companies such as Amazon, Facebook, Google, Uber, and others) that have built their business using digital technologies and the Internet. In all cases, they were successful in creating new industries, because they could identify problems that need to be solved and came up with FRs and DPs for their businesses, using newly emerging technologies.

One of the most stumbling mental blocks in learning AD could be the lack of experience in defining the FRs for the problem identified in the customer domain. To some, defining FR is a trivial task, and to some others, it is a difficult task. To many, it is a new experience to think of design as the transformational process of going from problem definition to FR, going from FR to DPs, and from DPs to PVs. There could be many reasons for this difficulty—different depending on one's experience and educational background. Some people might have worked on problems someone else defined for them throughout their life. Students are often taught to solve the problem defined by others, especially in textbooks. In some countries, the college entrance examinations ask only analysis-oriented questions. Not surprisingly, students prepare for the exam accordingly. Also, in some cases, one might have spent most of their career, modifying, through trial-and-error processes, designs someone else has made. In many companies, high-level executives define the problem, and engineers/designers execute them. In universities, professors assign problems to be solved, and students are taught to solve them following well-established methods and processes. Also, throughout their education, students are taught that there is ONE correct solution, which is true in most cases of analysis-oriented subjects. However, in design, there can be many equally good solutions!

The best way of learning how to define the problem to be solved and establish a specific set of FRs is to go through the experience doing them a few times to internalize the process in one's brain. Pretty soon, it can become second nature to young students.

Design is ecumenical in the sense that the design methodology is not a field-specific subject. The same method and approach can be used in all fields that require synthesis and design, although the specific design task will depend on the nature of the problem and the FRs that we must satisfy. Some students claim that the most challenging part of learning and using AD is the process of coming up with FRs, which are derived from the problems that were identified in the customer domain. Some claim that they could delve into the design without specifying FRs, which may indicate that the person either modified or copied an existing design. When someone designs without specifying FRs, one may come up with a coupled design that does not withstand the test of times or fails to perform. One must invest time and effort to state FRs correctly and creatively. It is not difficult to learn how to state FRs, but it may take longer to state FRs than the designer has been accustomed to.

The basic rule in defining FRs is the following: Define FRs in a solution-neutral environment! That is, "DO NOT THINK OF THE SOLUTION FIRST BEFORE DEFINING THE PROBLEM AND THE FRs." When this simple rule is violated, the proposed design is simply an old reconstituted design.

Some designers and organizations spend "five minutes" in defining the design task and spend months or years to make the designed system work by correcting all the problems that continue to pop up because of the poor and unsystematic design practice. This practice leads to long development times and high costs. There are many well-publicized failures where a critical project failed to work, airplanes plunge into ground, cars stop all of a sudden leading to fatal accidents, and R&D projects had to be redone, all because the designers used their gut feelings to design some new products, purely based on their years of experience in designing systems and what they have seen before somewhere rather than defining FRs a priori.

Designing Orbital Space Plane (OSP)

A principal defense contractor in the United States received a government contract to design and manufacture the orbital space plane (OSP), which can replace the space shuttle that transported people and goods to the International Space Station. One of the primary goals of OSP is to reduce the cost and improve the versatility of space transportation. The manager in charge of the project decided to produce a better product at a lower cost. To achieve this goal, the visionary the leader of the OSP program chose to replace the past practice of repeating the "design-build-test" cycle of system development and production, because the company leadership found that such a practice is costly and invite major failures after they deploy the system. They hired a consultant to teach AD to their "lead engineers," about 250 engineers and scientists.

These highly experienced and skilled engineers and scientists learned AD rather quickly. However, it was much more challenging to teach experienced engineers and designers than undergraduate students because they tended to jump right into the physical domain, i.e., DPs and PVs, without ever defining what they want to achieve, i.e., FRs, explicitly. In many cases, many experienced designers and engineers often jumped right into solutions, i.e., DPs and PVs, without first establishing FRs and constraints, even when FRs are simple to state and in some cases, almost trivial. Sometimes, people try to state FRs after they come up with DPs, which is counterproductive in practicing AD. When FRs are not defined in a solution-neutral environment, the design may turn out to be a replication of a product that already exists. For innovation, it is of utmost importance to define FRs in a solution-neutral environment.

The experience of teaching AD has been that it is easier to teach undergraduate students than graduate students or experienced industrial engineers. The underlying reason might be that experienced people do not define FRs in a solution-neutral environment. They may instead think of a solution first based on their experience and justify their decision afterward.

In the corporate world, people who become top executives need the ability to define the problem and FRs from a systems point of view. They often have many competent people working for them who are well trained to solve specific problems if they are presented with well-defined problems. It is harder to find people who can define the problem the company needs to address. Even in academia, people who can lead an organization need the ability to identify the problem and create specific goals in the form of FRs. Sometimes, universities select students based on their ability to solve problems someone else defined for them, and then teach more of the same skill for another 3 or 4 years. Sometimes, the student rarely has the opportunity to identify the problem themselves and establish goals in the form of FRs.

1.8 List of Example Problems

Consider the following problems and think about how one might approach them to develop a design solution for each example. Some of these examples will require much thinking and work to develop the desired design solutions. In some cases, one may have to acquire some fundamental knowledge of the field by reading reference books or by getting information from the Internet. Most of all, one may have to THINK with an open mind in a *solution-neutral environment*! We should not forget is that all these design tasks can be achieved, given enough time and resources.

Example 1.1 Improvement of the Protocol System for Social Networks

Social networks (SN) such as Facebook and Twitter facilitate interaction between and among people as well as between people and business for fast social information distribution or disinformation. In the 2016 presidential election in the United States, certain groups or nations used these SN services to tilt the election by spreading distorted or fabricated information to American electorates. One of the issues we have to deal with is the privacy issue, because Facebook, for example, has accumulated so much data on individuals that some may use them for illegal purposes. How would we improve the protocol of SN to prevent such misuse of the SN systems?

Example 1.2 Water Faucet to Control Water Temperature and Flow Rate

We want to have a water faucet that will enable a person to control the water flow rate and the water temperature independently. How should we achieve these goals through the design of a new faucet?

Example 1.3 Operation of Emergency Room

In a typical emergency room (ER) of a hospital, as many patients as possible must be treated as quickly as possible. One problem faced by the hospital is that patients with many different kinds of illnesses come into ER without any prior notice, e.g., some because of the injury sustained in a car accident, another due to a flare-up of the chronic disease. Often, the doctors are so busy that patients must wait after checking in with the admitting nurse before the patient can see the doctor, especially if the illness appears to be chronic. Many hospitals use the FIFO (first in–first out) system to control patient flow in the ER unless someone is about to die, who should be given the highest priority. If one is to design a better triage system for the ER operation, what should the new system? Would an AD designer be able to create a better triage system to maximize the throughput rate of the ER?

Example 1.4 Global Warming

One of the societal goals is to solve the global warming problem by reducing anthropogenic CO_2 emission. Roughly 27% of CO_2 is generated by ground transportation systems and about 33% from electric power generating plants that burn coal. Suppose that our goal is the reduction of CO_2 as the primary design goal to deal with global warming. To achieve the goal, what specific actions would we undertake?

Example 1.5 Ski Bindings

Ski bindings enable a skier to transmit control loads from the boot to the ski to maneuver the ski while sliding on snow at varying speeds. One of the main problems is to avoid transferring loads from the ski to the boot that leads to injuries. They need to transmit control loads from the skier to the ski reliably and not transmit injurious loads from the ski to the skier. The solution is to have the binding release the ski from the boot under certain situations that lead to injury. Because the ski bindings do not perform these functions well, many skiers end in hospitals especially with knee injuries most to the ACL and from collisions after an inadvertent release of the ski by the binding. How would we solve this problem?

Example 1.6 3D Printing

One of the final outputs of design could be the manufacture of reliable goods. Some of these products have complicated three-dimensional shapes such as inside holes not connected to the outside surface. We have used, and often still use, various casting and machining processes to make these parts. The disadvantage of these traditional processes is the need to prepare expensive tooling, which necessitates that we make a large number of the same pieces to distribute the fixed manufacturing cost over a large number of parts to lower the unit manufacturing cost. How can we make these 3D parts using a general-purpose machine that can produce several products with minimal tooling and in small volumes on short notice?

Example 1.7 Money Circulation and Economy

To an engineer, it appears that one way of strengthening the economy is to increase the velocity of money circulation because the faster the money circulates, the higher will be the economic activity and increased economic growth. Thus, everyone within the economic system benefits as the velocity of money circulation increases. However, real rich people will only spend a small fraction of their wealth, whereas poor people do not have the money to spend. This situation limits the velocity of money circulation. Assuming that the wealth distribution is Gaussian, determine the ideal wealth distribution that will maximize the money circulation. As a designer, our task is to design several policies for increasing money circulation. State your FRs.

Example 1.8 Healthcare Delivery

A medical doctor has spent many years to deliver healthcare services to developing countries. One of the problems he has encountered is not the medical problem, but the logistics of delivery of medical care and medicine to remote areas. He is looking for "system engineers" who can solve the logistics problem working with MDs. What FRs should we try to satisfy in our design? How should we create a solution to this problem through the design of a system for delivery of medical care to remote regions?

Example 1.9 Global Warming

Many people in many countries are concerned about global warming. The Intergovernmental Panel on Climate Change (IPCC) of the United Nations determined that unless we can keep the temperature rise of Earth to within 2 °C relative to the temperature at the time of Industrial Revolution, many calamities will make the Earth much less habitable with more floods, hurricanes, forest fires, drought, and rising ocean submerging low lying lands. The consensus developed based on scientific data is that one of the major causes of these problems is the anthropogenic generation of CO_2. As a designer, what would you do to deal with this problem? What should be our goals to deal with the challenge created by global warming?

Example 1.10 Reduction of Plastic Consumption

A high-level executive of a major industrial firm that manufactures many products out of polymers (i.e., plastics) is searching for means of reducing the consumption of plastics to lower the cost of the company's products. Since the materials cost constitutes about 50% of the manufacturing cost, the executive reasoned that the company could lower the cost of their products by 5% if they can reduce the materials consumption by about 10%. Their products must look and perform the same as their current products. As a designer of manufacturing processes, develop a design for achieving the above-stated goal—first state the FRs you have selected.

Example 1.11 Mobile Harbor

Containerships carry as many as 16,000 containers (TEUs[2]) and cross the Pacific Ocean to deliver goods in containers to the United States and elsewhere. Many of these ships unload their containers in Long Beach, or Los Angeles harbors in California, which is then transported to the rest of the United States by freight trains because the Panama Canal was too narrow to accommodate these giant containerships. Now the Panama Canal has been widened, but the problem is not entirely solved, because the harbors in the eastern seaboard of the United States are not broad enough and deep enough to accommodate these large containerships. As a solution to this problem, mobile harbor (MH) was invented while visiting Singapore and developed at KAIST. The central idea for the MH is as follows: "Why should ships come into the harbor? Why not have the harbor go out to the ship?" Under this scheme, big container ships moor in deep waters rather than come into a harbor. The MH (see Fig. 1.5) that can handle 600 containers goes out to the containership to unload the containers and deliver them to their final destinations. MH has a relatively flat bottom rather than streamlined V-shape, which enables it to turn quickly in harbors, maneuver easily in shallow waters, and go to any place to unload the containers.

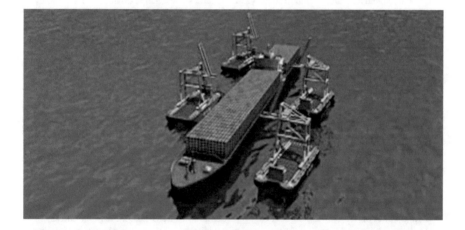

Fig. 1.5 Mobile harbor concept invented at KAIST (four mobile harbors are unloading containers from a large ocean-going containership in open sea to transport the containers from the ship to the shore)

To develop MH, we had to deal with two problems. The MH had to be firmly tied to the big containership during the loading and unloading of containers, so they move in unison in the rough and windy sea. A new design issue was how to tie the MH to the containership. Another problem is related to unloading the containers from the big ship to MH. The

---

[2]A **TEU** (20-foot equivalent unit) is a measure of volume in units of 20-foot long containers. For example, large container ships are able to transport more than 18,000 **TEU** (a few can even carry more than 21,000 **TEU**). One 20-foot container equals one **TEU**.

containers on the big containerships are lifted using a crane and steel rope. During the transfer of the container from the ship to MH, the container may oscillate due to the motion of the ship and MH. How should the containers be unloaded from the containership to MH on a windy day in a rough sea? What FRs should we satisfy?

In all of the above examples, better solutions may involve "design" of a new solution rather than adapting the past or existing designs. Some of these examples are not simple tasks and may require in-depth thinking and extensive work to provide the answer. They are given here to let the reader think about various issues involved in design. Many of the solutions will be systems that consist of many subsystems.

The purpose of this book is to teach the fundamentals of design to those interested in "developing superior design solutions." To achieve this goal, in the subsequent chapters, the design principles based on AD will be introduced with many examples and case studies. Many case studies show that projects executed based on the teachings of AD cost less and deliver a superior design.

1.9   Definition of Systems

The final output of design is a "system" that solves the problem and satisfies the perceived original need. A system is defined as an entity that generates a set of pre-determined outputs when a set of pre-defined inputs is supplied.

The operation of all systems consumes energy, i.e., the energy input to the system is higher than the energy output of the system. Some also are net consumers of materials and human resources. Some systems require financial resources to operate, and some are net generators of financial returns. The performance of a system is measured in terms of economic measures, or efficacy and fidelity in satisfying FRs, or social and human benefits.

Some systems are massive both in terms of the number of FRs they satisfy and their physical size. However, there is no relationship between physical size and the number of FRs they must fulfill. Some systems, such as semiconductor devices, are tiny physically, but they fulfill a large number of FRs. Some systems are measured in terms of people involved in operating the system.

Some systems are relatively simple, whereas some systems are complicated partly because of the number of FRs involved in a system and the nature of DPs chosen. Some systems are complex because they may not satisfy the FRs at all times. Sometimes a complicated system is also complex, but not always. For instance, the design of Boeing 787 is complicated because of the number of functions it must perform is very large as well as the number of parts that make up the airplane. However, they are not complex, because they satisfy their FRs with 100% certainty. On the other hand, the ignition key of a car manufactured by one of the largest automobile companies in the world could be extremely complex, if the probability of the key performing its functions is much less than 100%. Complexity increases when the system cannot satisfy FRs with 100% certainty.

The constituents of systems vary depending on FRs, DPs, and PVs. Exemplary system elements are physical elements, natural elements, software programs, biological units, humans, ideas (e.g., books), and some combinations of all of the above. Many systems operate within a set of constraints. There are two kinds of constraints: pre-existing external constraints and some constraints created during the design process or operation of the system.

1.10   Fundamental Principles of Design

The following two axioms constitute the basis of AD. All designs must satisfy them. We can separate good designs from unacceptable designs by checking whether or not they are consistent with these two axioms.

The Independence Axiom

Maintain the independence of FRs.

The Information Axiom

Minimize the information content.

Subsequent chapters explain and apply these axioms to various systems and problems.

1.11   Principle of Similitude of Systems

This book deals with many different systems, including mechanical, electrical, chemical, software, organizational, healthcare, and others. Once we understand the basic design principles and methodologies in one field, we should be able to deal with other design problems in many different fields. The reason we can treat many design problems in many diverse fields is that they are all systems with similar structures and characteristics. That is, the concept of design domain, the design axioms, and the design process apply to all design problems regardless of the specific field of application.

The Principle of Similitude of Systems may be stated as follows:

All systems follow the same design principles and processes, and therefore the same concept of design applies to all systems, although their specific functions, components, and usage may be domain-specific.

After students learn the materials presented in this book, they should be able to solve the 18 examples given in this chapter and be able to solve many other original design problems.

1.12 Importance of Knowing the Basic Laws and Principles of Science and Engineering

To be a creative designer of engineering artifacts, it helps if the designer has a strong background in basic disciplines of relevant engineering fields. Similar comments are equally valid for other disciplines. Without a strong knowledge of the related subjects, it is difficult to identify the problems that need to be solved and follow through the steps involved in the transformative process for the design of creative solutions outlined in this book.

The output of design is the functional requirements, {FRs}, which is what the designer wishes to satisfy through design. The inputs are the design parameters, {DPs}. If the design is related to physical things, the designer should have a fundamental understanding of natural laws and principles, constitutive relationships, and conservation principles. If the design involves information technology, the outputs are codes and background in algorithms should be invaluable. If the system is biological or medical, the designer should have background life science subjects such as biology. If the design is related to organizations, {DPs} may be organizational entities. After the design is completed, a more detailed mathematical modeling may be necessary to choose the correct values for DPs and PVs.

The results of the design we see are the assemblage of DPs. How DPs should be physically arranged is an issue that needs to be addressed, sometimes by examining the physical proximity in the case of mechanical design.

1.13 The Inverse Problem in Design: Extraction of Functional Requirements from Many Design Parameters

In the preceding sections of this chapter, the emphasis was on identifying the problem to be solved through design. In subsequent chapters, we will go through how the design can be done to solve the problem identified through the transformation of the problem to FRs, which are then transformed to DPs. Similarly, DPs will be transformed into PVs. We will show how FRs can be stated to represent the design task. We transform FRs to select appropriate DPs. This approach may be called the "direct" approach to design.

There is another approach to design, an "inverse" approach, i.e., going from existing designs to uncover the DP that can satisfy the desired FR. Usually, it is a difficult task to go from DP to FR, because a DP may satisfy many FRs. For example, the FR of a "coffee mug" can be many. It could be "hold hot coffee," "act as a paperweight," "commemorate a special event," and others. The fact that a DP can be related to many different FRs is one of the difficulties of "reverse engineering" because determining the FR from geometric shapes is challenging. However, with the enormous computational power of modern computers, we can manipulate a vast database and try many different combinations of existing DPs to satisfy FRs. In other words, the inverse method consists of going through a vast database of DPs to identify the design of a system that is close to the problem identified. This "inverse method" is possible because of the extensive data that can be processed by supercomputers and cloud computing. This approach is, in essence, the use of artificial intelligence (AI) to synthesize design solutions. With the increasing use of AI techniques, the inverse approach to design may be employed more in the future.

IBM has developed a machine named "Watson." Watson is an intelligent question answering (QA) computing system. IBM built it to apply natural language processing, information retrieval, knowledge representation, automated reasoning, and machine learning technologies to answers questions posed by people using natural language. It has access to 200 million pages of structured and unstructured content consuming four terabytes of disk storage. These machines can store an immense amount of data, which are used to answer questions posed by the user. IBM has been attempting to make Watson be the next generation of products that can generate new revenues for the company. It won chess games over the best human master chess player. Watson has been used in medical applications to guide medical practitioners as well. Google has its version similar to Watson that can provide answers to queries made by people. These technologies are possible because of large computers and easy access to the database produced by large networks and cloud computing. The difficulty lies in satisfying many FRs at the same time, which many design tasks require.

1.14 Optimization of an Existing System Versus Design of a New System

"Optimization of a poorly designed system yields yet another poorly designed system."

Many engineers, economists, and others in many different fields are engaged in the analysis and optimization of an existing system. They devoted significant effort to get the most out of existing systems, which were designed and have been used, sometimes, for decades.

There are many optimization techniques, mostly, mathematical, that have been developed. Typically, the mathematical approach is to express the problem in terms of an objective function with constraints. Even when there are many objectives, the problem is formulated for one objective function with many constraints for mathematical convenience and treatment. Such a brute force approach would not be applicable when an entirely new system must be designed to satisfy many FRs. James Watt would not have invented his steam engine if he tried to optimize the Newcomen engine.

1.15 Scope of the Book

The purpose of this book is to enable the reader to "design" on her/his own, with imagination and creativity, to satisfy human needs and societal aspirations. Human intellect is a powerful tool that enables human beings to achieve many things through design—it only requires the imagination and willingness to learn how the design should be done. This book outlines the steps involved in design based on AD to develop a rational design solution. The basic idea is to approach design systematically so as not to make wrong designs. There are well-known design mistakes that cost a great deal to re-do them to correct the errors, a la the design problem associated with control of Boeing 737 MAX. Many of these mistakes are often due to the coupling of FRs during the decomposition process. These coupled designs lead to accidents of nuclear power plants, crashing of aircraft, delayed construction of airports, and unreliable products.

This book presents the basic concepts involved in AD: the idea of four domains in the design world, the mapping between the domains, and the transformations involved during the design process. After the problem that needs to be solved is identified, the designer sets the ultimate goals of the design task in terms of functional requirements {FRs} and constraints (Cs). Then perform specific design tasks of identifying design parameters {DPs}. The idea of the design matrix is also introduced in this chapter. The design process, including the decomposition through zigzagging, is illustrated in this chapter. Many examples are given to clarify the new concepts presented.

The subject of "DESIGN" treated in this book is not limited to engineering, although many examples are derived from engineering and technology. Design is equally important in many other fields that involve synthesis to achieve a set of goals, such as in the design of software, organizations, and even in cooking gourmet foods. The same thinking and methodologies apply to all these subjects. That is, although the specific topics and subject matters are field-specific, all fields share the standard design process and the same design axioms.

1.16 Conclusions

The design is one of the most critical subjects in engineering. Synthesis of innovative products and solutions is the essential foundation for solving societal problems and advancing commerce, engineering, science, and social science fields. The ability to design well determines the quality of most things: products, processes, manufacturing, organizations, governments, technologies, the quality of life, and others.

Good designs depend, the foremost, on the quality of problem identification and definition. Once the problem is defined, the designer can proceed to the subsequent steps of design. The steps consist of the transformation of customer needs of the customer domain into functional requirements {FRs} of the functional domain, followed by transformation of {FRs} to design parameters {DPs} of the physical domain, and finally the transformation of {DPs} to process variables {PVs} of the process domain. The relationship between the domains is "What" and "How." The {FRs} in the functional domain is "what we want to achieve," whereas the {DPs} in the physical domain represent "how we are going to satisfy the FRs."

Similar design processes govern the design of diverse systems. A person who can design technical systems well can also apply the same skill to other design problems such as organizations, although specific issues are domain-specific.

Problems

1. In the twenty-first century, telecommunications and social network systems (SNS) have become the dominating information dissemination mechanism, displacing the printed media. As a result, the information distributed in SNS throughout the world can be corrupted by those with ill-intentions and nations as a warfare tool. Our job is to solve this problem to safeguard the system and make the information in the digital communication system from being corrupted. What FRs, would you satisfy this problem?
2. Faulty designs or poor designs cause many failures in various systems. The recent crash of Boeing 737 airplanes, the delayed opening of the new Berlin airport, and the Fukushima Daiichi nuclear power plant disasters are some of the well-publicized failures. These accidents occur despite numerous tests. What is the best way of preventing these failures?
3. If you are the president of your university, how would you improve the admissions process? What is the problem you are trying to solve? What functional requirements {FRs} should your university try to satisfy through their admission process?
4. Many companies are working on driverless automobiles. What functional requirements {FRs} should the designer of the automobile satisfy?
5. What do you think makes Starbucks so successful in selling coffee even though so many other companies had already been selling coffee before their emergence?
6. Define the FRs we must satisfy to teach AD well.

References

Black NH, Davis HN (1913) Practical physics for secondary schools. Fundamental principles and applications to daily life. Macmillan and Company, public domain

Petrushenka A (2019) The launch of the space shuttle. With fire and smoke. Against the background of the starry sky. Elements of this image were furnished by NASA. Photo licensed from Shutterstock, ID: 1480426817

Further Reading

Hatamura Y (2008) Learning from design failures. Springer

Senor D, Singer S (2009) Start-up nation: the story of Israel's economic miracle. Twelve Hachette Book Group

Suh NP (2001) Axiomatic design—advances and applications. Oxford University Press

Suh NP (2010a) On innovation strategies: an Asian perspective. The Glion Colloquium. https://glion.org/on-innovation-strategies-an-asian-perspective/

Suh NP (2010b) Theory of innovation. Int J Innov Manag (IJIM) 14:893–913. https://doi.org/10.1142/S1363919610002921

Suh NP, Cho DH (eds) (2017) The on-line electric vehicle: wireless electric ground transportation systems. Springer International Publishing

Wilson HG, McCready PB, Kyle CR (1989) Lessons of Sunraycer. Sci Am 260(3):90–97

What Is Design?

2

Nam Pyo Suh

Abstract

The design is a commonly used English word that describes a variety of different human activities, depending on the context and the field of interest. In this book, the word "design" refers to a series of creative activities that are related to solving a problem identified in the customer domain to achieve a goal through synthesis. The identified problem is solved through synthesis. A set of functional requirements (FRs) is established in the functional domain through the mapping between the customer domain and the functional domain. The FRs are then satisfied by selecting design parameters (DPs) in the physical domain through the mapping between the functional and the physical domains. The selected DPs must satisfy the Independence Axiom, i.e., FRs at a given level of decomposition must not affect other FRs by the selected DP or be affected by other FRs. DPs are, in turn, satisfied by selecting process variables (PVs) in the process domain through the mapping between the physical domain and the process domain. Thus, the design consists of a series of transformation processes, beginning from the goal and the problems identified in the customer domain to FRs of the functional domain, FRs to DPs in the physical domain, and DPs to PVs in the process domain. In this design process, analysis often follows synthesis for the quantification of design decisions made.

N. P. Suh (✉)
M.I.T., Cambridge, MA, USA
e-mail: npsuh@mit.edu

© Springer Nature Switzerland AG 2021
N. P. Suh et al. (eds.), *Design Engineering and Science*,
https://doi.org/10.1007/978-3-030-49232-8_2

2.1   Introduction

2.1.1   Why Design Theory (DT)?

Many engineers and scientists often wonder why we need design theory. Many of them are proud of their past accomplishments because they have designed many things based on their intuition and experience. However, consider the following simple example:

Disaster Faced by a Major Airplane Manufacturer in 2019

The CEO of an airplane manufacturer was a man of full confidence for having come up through the ranks of the company to become the leader of one of the largest airplane manufacturers in the world. More importantly, he was confident of his engineers, who have racked up years of experience. Overall their airplanes performed well in the field. Their new airplane, which was an extended version of their best-selling aircraft but with larger more fuel-efficient engines, was selling well.

Then, a disaster struck the company, bringing down their stock price and losing potential new customers to their rival company. Two of their planes fell from the sky, killing all the passengers and the flight crews! The pilots of the airplane could not control the aircraft during its ascent right after takeoff and thus plunging into the ground. Many organizations, in addition to the manufacturer of the airplane, began investigations. They will eventually come up with explanations and solutions after much testing and information gathering.

We cannot draw any firm conclusions without knowing the actual design of the control system developed by the airplane company and the data in the black box of the airplane. In the following example, we will illustrate how Axiomatic Design (AD) might be used to provide answers to the failure of an aircraft as a means of explaining the use of AD. To determine the real cause of failure, the airplane manufacturer usually works with authorities, analyzing all available data, and simulating with the real similar airplanes. They will also test the actual system operation using simulators. Based on these results, the airplane manufacturer will make appropriate changes in software and hardware to prevent future failures. However, all the persons perished in those accidents would never know what happened to them.

In this simulation of what might have happened, we will make up a fictitious case study to show the power of AD in the proper designing of complicated systems. The irony is that it is not difficult to develop the right system, but if one makes design decisions based on "gut feeling," one can make serious mistakes that are very costly both financially and also in terms of human lives.

Design of the airplane control system:

Assume that the pilots must control four functions of the airplane for its safe operation, which we will designate as FRs, i.e., FR1, FR2, FR3, and FR4. We will assume that the outputs are controlled using four input control variables, which we will designate as DP1, DP2, DP3, and DP4, respectively. Furthermore, we will assume that DP3 is automatically controlled by the system installed as part of the airplane control system, and thus the pilot cannot manually control DP3. However, the pilot can control DP1, DP2, and DP4. The relationship between FRs and DPs may be represented as

$$FR1 = a\,DP1 + b\,DP2 + c\,DP3 + d\,DP4$$
$$FR2 = e\,DP1 + f\,DP2 + g\,DP3 + h\,DP4$$
$$FR3 = i\,DP1 + j\,DP2 + k\,DP3 + m\,DP4 \qquad (2.1)$$
$$FR4 = n\,DP1 + q\,DP2 + s\,DP3 + w\,DP4$$

The above relationship may be rewritten in a matrix format as follows:

	DP1	DP2	DP3	DP4
FR1	a	b	c	d
FR2	e	f	g	h
FR3	i	j	k	m
FR4	n	q	s	w

(2.2)

Design matrix: Four FRs and Four DPs (a Full matrix)

*Suppose that they designed their control system such that the coefficients **a, b, c, ... w** are fixed and may not be varied during the flight. Furthermore, the airplane company sold these features (i.e., **a, b, c, ... w**) for an extra price as options. Therefore, some of the airplanes did not have all the features provided by a, b, c, ... w.*

Questions the reader should try to answer:

Case #1: *Suppose the design is such that all coefficients are zeroes except a, f, k, and w. The desired values of FR1, FR2, FR3, and FR4 are given as 5, 9, 3, and 8. The control task is to set the values of DPs (i.e., DP1, ... DP4) to satisfy FRs. What should be the values of DPs?*

The design matrix for this case is a diagonal matrix as shown below:

	DP1	DP2	DP3	DP4
FR1	a	0	0	0
FR2	0	f	0	0
FR3	0	0	k	0
FR4	0	0	0	w

(2.3)

A Diagonal Design Matrix for an Uncoupled Design

This diagonal matrix represents an ideal design, where one DP affects only one FR. The control of this kind of systems is the simplest. We should attempt to develop systems that are of this kind.

Case #2: *Suppose the design is such that all coefficients are non-zeroes (i.e., a full matrix). The desired values of FR1, FR2, FR3, and FR4 are still 5, 9, 3, and 8. The control task is to change one of the FRs without affecting any other FRs by varying appropriate DPs. What should be the values of DPs? What should we do if the coefficients vary from time to time? If we want to change only FR1 without changing other FRs, which DPs should we change to vary the FR1?*

Case 2 represents a coupled design. When one of the FRs is to be changed, it will be necessary to vary all the DPs simultaneously. Such an airplane will be hard to control in actual flight. The control of the aircraft by the pilot will be extremely challenging if the pilot does not know which DPs are changing because the computer onboard directly controls the DPs, i.e., if the pilot is out of the control loop. Even if he knows that the computer is in the loop, the pilot would not know how to control the airplane because the computer will change DPs.

Was this coupled design the reason the two Boeing airplanes plunged into the ground?

Case #3: Anything in human-made systems can malfunction. That is, one of the elements of the design matrix can malfunction, i.e., change arbitrarily on its own without any input from the pilot. In that case, an unexpected coupling may occur, or the plane may lose some of its functional capabilities. In that case, the pilot must be able to override the automated systems and operate the airplane manually before they lose control over the airplane.

For simplicity, we discussed three extreme cases in this example. Other cases will be covered in later chapters.

Think of the panic faced by the pilot! The pilot cannot see the design matrix and has to try to control the plane with his feeling, control lever, and engine speed. In this case, the situation was even worse. The automated control system also tried to control the plane, probably over-riding the inputs of the pilot—a classic example of a coupled design!

This example shows that the design with a diagonal matrix is the best design in terms of satisfying FRs by varying the input variables, i.e., DPs. When the matrix is a full matrix, it is complicated to vary only one FR with one DP, i.e., all DPs may have to be changed simultaneously, which increases the complexity of the design and operation of the system. Typically, it cannot be done. This kind of design is a coupled design. When many groups of engineers start changing the design without informing the "design architect"—by changing one or two elements of the design matrix—and without the group consensus, it will be extremely difficult to make the airplane controllable and safe when unexpected events occur. This coupling of FRs adds to the complexity of the airplane operation.

Without knowing the details of what happened to those two airplanes, one can only speculate that the failure of the aircraft might have been due to the coupling of FRs. This failure may be due to the wrong design of the control-system software. Pilots cannot avert disasters in such a case.

The vice president in charge of engineering or the president of the company should have asked a simple question: "Does the aircraft control system, which includes both hardware and software, satisfy the Independence Axiom? That question could have saved hundreds of lives!"

We devoted most of Chap. 1 to one issue: the importance of identifying the goal to be achieved and defining the PROBLEM in the customer domain to accomplish the goal. To repeat: identify and define the problem well, before embarking on the design activity! That is, the ability to identify the most critical problem that needs to be solved is the first and the most defining step for successful design and innovation. The preceding statement is true, regardless of the specific nature of the problem. Even if it takes several trials, it is less expensive and fruitful to spend time identifying the right problem at the early stages of design. Without James Watt's identification of the shortcomings of the Newcomen engine, the Industrial Revolution might not have begun in the latter part of the eighteenth century! Although many other people had used the Newcomen engine before James Watt did, they merely used it without recognizing and questioning its shortcomings. The power of observation, intelligent questioning of well-accepted wisdom, and penetrating logical reasoning are some of the essential requisites in defining the problem (or shortcomings) and creating innovative designs to achieve the goal identified in the customer domain.

In this book, we present a specific theoretical and practical approach to design based on AD theory. According to the theory, one should not jump into analysis or experimentation right away before a design solution is conceived or completed. When the problem is identified in the customer domain, the designer should think about the overall design issues, i.e., goals of the design and desired final output. The first step in AD should be the identification of THE PROBLEM, as discussed in Chap. 1. The subsequent steps of AD involve the transformation of the problem identified in the customer domain into FRs in the functional domain, followed by two additional transformations to generate DPs and PVs.

To be proficient in design, the designer should initially think broadly about many related issues to the design task, before settling on a design solution. It is highly advisable to consider all the peripheral matters before defining the problem to solve. It is also good to think deeply about the implications of the problem to be chosen. Any changes made to the problem definition or FRs and DPs have consequences, and therefore one should consider all alternate possibilities before making the final decision on design goals and problems. It is much cheaper and better to make changes in the early stages of design activity as soon as one realizes that there is a flaw or shortcomings in decisions made in the early design cycle rather than persist with a flawed design. This initial thinking process does not take much time.

2.1.2 Think in Solution-Neutral Environment!

Designers should select the problem in the customer domain and the FRs in the functional domain in a "solution-neutral environment," i.e., do not think about a solution before defining the problem! Many people come up with "a solution" first before determining the problem. In other words, one should not come up with a solution and then think about the problem that fits the solution. Similarly, one should not start to develop their design by copying their competitor's product or thinking about a solution first even before they commence the task of defining the problem. Many industrial firms have difficulties in making their people think in a solution-neutral environment. The "marketing groups," which are charged to develop broad guidelines for their desired new products, often "cheat" by studying their competitors' products and develop "specifications" for their new proposed products based on what they have already seen in their competitors' products. In many cases, such an approach yields systems or solutions that are nearly identical to its competitors' or their old product. It is hard to be competitive or creative this way!

A Story of Design Failure: The RIM Machine designed by an outstanding graduate student and his professor

Identifying the real problem and creating a new design that addresses the identified problem is not a trivial exercise, as one young professor learned the hard way! The following story is a real story that happened at a well-known technological university.

Many professors enjoy working with bright students in research because students often contribute to their research projects while also furthering their knowledge as well as learning through their participation in research. In an ideal arrangement, professors and students should become "partners-in-learning," which implies that both the professor and the student must be willing to learn new things while working on research. The professor teaches the student how to define the problem and how to think about it. When teaching is done through research, both the student and the professor learn. The professor has more experience, and thus can teach the student how to think and how to approach the unknown question. It also strengthens the university, since the involvement of students in research makes in the university a live theater for education and research. Through research, students learn to exercise independent thinking. Therefore, the young professor was delighted when a new graduate student signed up to work with him! The student was not only bright but also mature, having served for 5 years as an officer in the U.S. Army, after graduating from West Point, the military academy of the United States. For his doctoral research, the professor and the student jointly decided to develop a new machine for producing polyurethane parts. A large industrial firm sponsored the project. Polyurethane is one of the favorite materials in the automotive industry since it is easy to make complicated parts such as bumpers and fenders with polyurethane as well as reducing the weight of the vehicle—this reduction in weight results in the improved fleet gas mileage of automobiles.

To make polyurethane parts, two liquids, i.e., diisocyanate and polyol, a viscous resin, are mixed in a precise ratio to make solid polyurethane parts when these two components react in a mold. Turbulent mixing of two liquid components occurs when two liquid streams collide with each other at high speeds in a small chamber. The higher the impingement speed, the smaller is the turbulent eddy size, thus better mixing. Commercial machines used two precision gear pumps to deliver polyol and diisocyanate in a pre-set ratio at high flow rates for impingement mixing in the mixing chamber. The mixture then flows into a mold where the reaction is completed, forming a solid part. The fast-reacting mixture is then injected quickly into a large mold to produce polyurethane parts when the chemical reaction is completed. For his doctoral research, the student and the professor jointly decided to develop a new machine for producing polyurethane parts, because the industrial machines used precision gear pumps, which had to be replaced frequently due to wear.

The student worked very hard and was productive, thanks to his intelligence, personality, and the experience he gained in the U.S. Army. He quickly designed and built the machine and demonstrated its capability. The central idea behind the new design was to replace the high-speed precision gear pumps with accumulators and inexpensive gear pumps. In this newly designed machine, the resin and diisocyanate were pumped into two separate accumulators with a rubber pouch (shown in Fig. 2.1). The resin was injected into the accumulator slowly, using an inexpensive gear pump. A similar arrangement was also made for diisocyanate. As the pouch expanded with the injection of resin taking up the free

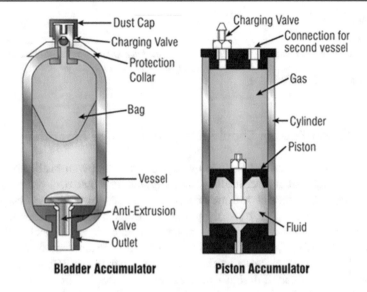

Fig. 2.1 Bag-type and piston-type accumulator. (Reproduced with permission from Casey (2009))

space of the accumulator, the gas pressure in the accumulator increased. When the gas in the accumulator was compressed to a pre-set high pressure, the valve was opened to discharge the resin at high speeds. A similar arrangement was made for diisocyanate. They mixed in the impingement mix chamber and then discharged into the mold. These accumulators eliminated the need for large, expensive gear pumps. The newly designed machine seemed to work as intended. After a couple of years of research, the student, a technician, and the professor jointly applied for a patent. The student received his Ph.D. after adding a detailed analysis of his machine. All the inventors were very proud and hopeful about the potential of their RIM machine. However, the industrial firm that sponsored the research never adopted the device for their production! After all that hard work and confidence in their design, it was very disappointing that the industrial people did not share their enthusiasm!

The industrial sponsor found that the new machine did not perform as well as the old industrial machine. It could not deliver the liquids in the set ratio, precisely and consistently. The student and the professor tried to figure out why the device they designed with such confidence did not perform as well as the commercial machine! It turns out that their new design was a wrong design! The original problem was well defined, but a wrong solution was proposed. All the hard work of the student and all the money the sponsor spent did not yield the desired result. Now we know the shortcoming of this newly developed machine: it violated the Independence Axiom. If they had known the design theory covered in this book, they might not have made the mistake of proceeding with the wrong design! Unfortunately, when this project was undertaken, the AD theory had not been developed. Unfortunate timing?

Question 2.1:

Based on the preceding saga of the RIM machine development, what do you think were the fundamental shortcomings of the design? Could you have known a priori *that the design had flaws? Would you have designed a better machine? Did the design violate any fundamental principles?*

2.1.3   Design Theory: Should It Be Axiomatic or Algorithmic?

A few years after the retired U.S. Army captain graduated with his doctorate and became a professor at another leading university, his former advisor began to think about a more fundamental and systematic way of dealing with the design and synthesis of systems. The basic theory-based design would be better than the intuition- and experienced-based design practice. He concluded that experienced-based design is a highly limited form of education and that university may not be the best place to teach experience-based design. Better places for learning experience-based design would be leading industrial firms with years of design experience. However, there is a role for university-based design education if universities can teach design based on fundamental design principles that can generalize the characteristics of excellent designs.

He reasoned that there are two different ways of teaching design: axiomatic and algorithmic.

In the algorithmic approach, we provide step-by-step instructions, which, if the student follows it, the student will arrive at an answer, a la software algorithm. Under an algorithmic design approach, one would design a system following a step-by-step algorithm. An example of the algorithmic approach to teaching can be found, for instance, in training "electricians." In this case, a young person (who might have graduated from a technical high school) works for a "licensed master electrician" for a few years to learn the "trade" by following the footsteps of the master electrician for a few years as an assistant. A similar approach is also used in large companies to train their technicians, draftsmen/designers, and machinists through apprenticeships. In these companies that have made similar machines for many years, there is a system of designing a specific class of machines (that might be called the algorithm), which was based on the knowledge gained while making similar machines, with minor variations, for many years. The shortcoming of an algorithmic approach is that it is challenging to develop so many algorithms for so many different cases and products, especially in rapidly changing industries that must introduce new systems to satisfy many different sets of FRs.

In the axiomatic approach, general design principles for design are created for all designs that satisfy different sets of needs and requirements. The axiomatic approach to design should apply to all designs regardless of the specific nature of the system to be designed. Such general principles should be valid in all fields and for all applications. The shortcoming of the axiomatic approach is that there are no algorithms that would yield the right answer if one were to follow it. In the axiomatic approach, broad general principles are given without a product-specific algorithm. If we had the design algorithms for the RIM machine, we might have produced a machine similar to the then-existing commercial RIM machine. However, that algorithm would not have created a better RIM machine than the then-existing industrial machines.

On the other hand, had we had the design axioms when we worked on the RIM machine, we would have been cautious not to create the accumulator-based RIM machine because it would have violated the design axioms! The RIM machine developed without the benefit of design axioms "coupled" FRs. The three FRs—function of maintaining a fixed ratio of two fluids, the function of providing high-quality mixing, and the function of controlling flow rates—all depended on pressure in the accumulators (which decayed as the fluid is being discharged) and material-specific properties such as viscosity and temperature of each liquid.

Had the AD theory existed at the time the Ph.D. student worked on the RIM project, they would not have developed the RIM machine that is based on the use of accumulators. Design axioms eliminate the need for expensive and extensive testing to find out the fundamental shortcomings of a system because the flawed design can be identified at the conceptual stage based on generalizable axioms! Unfortunately, even today, many companies make mistakes in system development by depending on their experience and intuition! There are some well-known examples of failure that have cost millions of dollars. These costly mistakes are a result of experientially based or intuitive designs. Students who learn and practice rational design presented in this book should not make these expensive mistakes!

AD is created based on the realization that all good designs always satisfy two fundamental axioms regardless of the specific nature of the design or the field of application. One has to do with the independence of FRs, and the other has to do with simplicity (or minimum) of information contained in the design. AD is based on the identification of common features that all good designs possess. The axioms are stated as follows:

The Independence Axiom:
Maintains the independence of FRs.

The Information Axiom:
Minimizes the information content.

The meaning of these two axioms will be made more apparent throughout this book. Many examples will be given to clarify the statements of these two axioms. These two axioms were extracted by identifying the common elements that exist in all good designs. It should be noted here that "cost" is not a FRs in nearly all designs, but the design that violates the Independence Axiom can become extremely costly, and many times, the system must be abandoned or redesigned and built.

2.2 Design: Transformational Process to Create Human-Inspired Systems

2.2.1 Definition of Key Words: Design, Goals, and Domains

The design consists of a series of the following actions and processes:

(a) *identifying a problem that needs new or improved solutions to achieve a set of goals;*
(b) *transforming the problem into a set of goals in the form of FRs to be achieved;*
(c) *fulfilling the goals with specific DPs within a given set of constraints;*
(d) *synthesizing the final embodiment in the form of hardware, software, systems, organizations, and policies through the integration of DPs, preserving the simplicity of the ultimate system; and*
(e) *maintaining the independence of FRs throughout the transformation process.*

The above definition of "design" is comprehensive and applicable to many different kinds of designs, ranging from systems, hardware, software, and organizations. Many examples given in this book should clarify the significance of these statements.

2.2.2 The Concept of Four Domains

The description of design given in Sect. 2.2.1 may be represented graphically as shown in Fig. 2.2.

Figure 2.2 shows the four domains of the design world, i.e., the customer domain, the functional domain, the physical domain, and the process domain[1]. We define the "PROBLEM" in the customer domain (e.g., James Watt's recognition of the shortcomings of the Newcomen engine).

---

[1]These four domains are applicable to all kinds of designs, including hardware, software, and manufacturing processes. The particular names assigned to the domains are due to the fact that when AD was first developed, most examples came from hardware- and manufacturing-related activities. We are using the same names, although this general concept is applicable to many other design tasks.

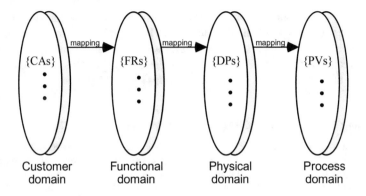

Fig. 2.2 Four domains of the design world

2.2.3   Goals

One of the prominent words used in the definition of design is the word "goal or goals." We establish the goals in the customer domain after we identify the perceived customer needs. After establishing the goals, we can identify the problem we must solve to achieve the goals. Based on the problem identified, we can create FRs in the functional domain that are consistent with the specific design goals. One of the tasks of a designer is to come up with "means" of satisfying the FRs, which will be called DPs in the physical domain.

2.2.4   Mapping from Domain to Domain: Functional Requirements, Design Parameters, and Process Variables

The problem defined in the customer domain is transformed into a set of FRs in the functional domain, which represent the "GOALS" of the design (e.g., in both the Watt engine and the Newcomen engine, one FR was for expansion of steam and another FR was for condensation of steam). Once FRs are identified in the functional domain, we identify and conceptualize DPs in the physical domain that can satisfy the FRs of the functional domain. Then, in the process domain, we choose PVs that can satisfy DPs or make DPs possible. We call this process of transforming the problem into FRs, FRs into DPs, and DPs into PVs the "MAPPING" between domains.

{FRs} in the functional domain may be considered as a vector with n components that defines the problem. Similarly, {DPs} in the physical domain constitute a vector, whereas {PVs} is a vector that defines the process domain[2]. Transforming the FR vector to the DP vector represents the design process. Similarly, we are designing the process when we transform {DPs} to {PVs}[3].

Example 2.1 Illustration of the Mapping Concept (Shoe Soles for Children's Shoes)

Background story: A recent immigrant to the United States just graduated from an engineering school with a bachelor's and master's degree. He joined the largest shoe-machinery company in the world, a successful and great company to work for, which was founded by two families many decades ago in Massachusetts, U.S.A. One of the good things about this company was that they did not do much defense-related work, and therefore even a recent immigrant could get a job there since they did not require its employees to have a defense-security clearance. They made nearly all the machines that are used in making shoes worldwide.

Until a few years before this young engineer joining the company, they had a monopoly in the shoe-machinery business by only leasing their machines rather than selling them. They even built factories for shoe companies with their machines in them and collected a royalty each time their machine was used to make shoes. They were active in research and obtained many patents to protect their business. Other companies could not break into this shoe-machinery business because of their business model. However, sometimes, good things do not last forever! The United States government sued the company for practicing monopoly and won. The company had to sell all their leased machines at a discount, which gave the company lots of cash. This loss of monopoly ultimately resulted in the company exploring ways of expanding its business under the new rules.

The problem (or the need) in the customer domain: The first assignment given to the young engineer was to develop the process for manufacturing children's shoe soles at a low cost. The shoe soles had to meet several requirements. They had to be flexible, lightweight, and wear-resistant. In the functional domain, the FR was to manufacture inexpensive shoe soles for children's shoes. In the process domain, he decided to use a variation of the commonly used injection molding process. The idea was to directly injection mold the foamed PVC (polyvinyl chloride) shoe soles to the upper (i.e., a stitched leather, which is stretched and mounted on a last to create the three-dimensional shoe shape) to satisfy the FRs of the shoe soles. In the process domain, he designed the manufacturing process that can yield the product with specific DPs.

The goal in the functional domain was quite clear:

FR = manufacture foamed PVC soles for children's shoes.

Mapping this FR in the physical domain (i.e., DP domain), DP may be stated as

---

[2]The bracket {x} is used to denote a vector in this book.
[3]Note that FR, DP, and PV are also written as *FR, DP,* and *PV* interchangeably throughout this book.

DP = Injection molded shoe soles.

We map this DP in the physical domain into a PV, which may be stated as

PV = Injection molding process.

The above set of FR, DP, and PV represent design decisions made at the highest level. This young engineer's task was to decompose these highest level FR, DP, and PV to mass-produce the injection-molded shoes with PVC soles with desired properties at low cost. To implement this design, we need more detailed designs. To produce detailed designs, we will decompose them to generate lower level FRs, DPs, and PVs, which is discussed in Sect. 2.3.4.

2.2.5   Design Axioms

We presented design examples from different fields in the preceding sections to show how the design should be conceived and executed. In the examples presented, we judged design based on the independence of FRs without much elaboration. We will try to formalize what we have done in previous sections by presenting the design axioms more formally.

Axiom is defined as

"The truths for which there are no counter-examples or exceptions."

We use two design axioms to be sure that the design decisions we make are the right ones. These two axioms were created based on the observation of common features or elements that all good designs possess.[4] Axioms, by definition, cannot be derived. All students are familiar with some axioms; for example, in Euclid's geometry, they learned that the shortest distance between two points is the straight line that connects these two points, which is an axiom because we cannot derive it, but we cannot find counterexamples.

In the examples given in the preceding section, we defined FRs to solve the problem stated in the customer domain and then selected DPs to satisfy the FRs. How would we know whether or not we chose the most suitable set of DPs? In the case of the shoe sole manufacturing, the example discussed in the preceding section, we were fortunate that the process designed to make the composite shoe soles with a foamed core and a skin layer worked as intended, although we did not invoke design axioms. In this section, we present design axioms that we must satisfy in creating rational designs more formally.

There are many questions that we must answer to be sure that our thought processes on design are progressing correctly. We have to know if we selected the

---

[4]For historical details, see Nam P. Suh, *The Principles of Design*, Oxford University Press, 1991.

right set of DPs for the given set of FRs. To be sure that our design can indeed achieve the intended design goals, we must be able to answer the following questions:

- Have we selected the right problem?
- How do we know we selected the right FRs and DPs?
- What are the fundamental requirements we must satisfy to be sure that we have made the right design decisions?
- What constitutes a good design?
- How do we know that our design is excellent?

The design rationale presented in this book is based on two design axioms: the Independence Axiom and the Information Axiom. These axioms were postulated by asking the following question: *"What were the common elements (or features) that were present in all successful designs?"*

These two axioms have been applied to a variety of different problems, the design of hardware, software, organizations, manufacturing processes, complicated systems, and others. Historically, axioms have provided the basis for scientific and technological advances in many fields such as geometry and thermodynamics. Newton's laws at the time they were advanced might be considered to be also axioms in that they were not based on scientific measurements of force and acceleration, i.e., they were conceptual. Perhaps the following two questions will remind the reader what axiom is and how axioms have advanced many fields:

Question 2.2:

Why is the straight line that joins two points the shortest distance?

The answer to the question is: In Euclidean geometry, an axiom states that the straight line is the shortest distance between two points. We believe in the axiom because we cannot find exceptions or counterexamples.

Question 2.3:

List three axioms taught in other subjects such as geometry and thermodynamics.

A design task may involve both synthesis and analysis. To do analysis, we invoke certain natural principles such as Newton's laws and thermodynamic laws. *They may be regarded as axioms. Axioms are defined as the evident truth for which there are no counterexamples and exceptions.* Of course, we apply all known natural laws and principles to develop design solutions, in addition to the Independence Axiom and the Information Axiom.

In AD, it was stated that there are two axioms: the Independence Axiom and the Information Axiom. They are stated again here in declarative form as follows:

The Independence Axiom

Maintain the independence of FRs.

The information Axiom

Minimize the information content.

These axioms were extracted by identifying the common elements that were always present in good designs, but not present in bad designs. This entire book is devoted to the use and application of these two axioms. They are applied to a variety of different tasks in many different fields.

Example 2.2 Water Faucet Design

Given the two faucets shown below that control the flow rate of water and the temperature of water, which is a better design?

We cannot answer the question until we know what the FRs of the design are. If we define the FRs to be the following:

FR1 = Control temperature;

FR2 = Control flow rate.

The faucet shown in (a) has two valves, one for cold water, and one for hot water, i.e.,

DP1 = Hot water valve;

DP2 = Cold water valve.

In this design, when one of the valves is turned to change the temperature of water flowing out the faucet, the flow rate changes as well. Thus, it violates the Independence Axiom. In the faucet shown in (b), the up-and-down position of the lever only changes the flow rate and turning the lever left and right only changes the temperature. The design shown in (b) maintains the independence of FRs, and thus is a better design.

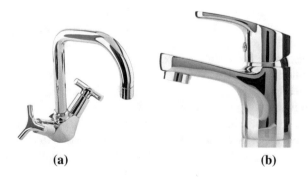

(a)   **(b)**

Fig. 2.3 Two water faucets: **a** two valves, one for cold water and the other for hot water, **b** One valve with two independent controls for flow rate and for water temperature. (Reproduced with permission from Kurguzova (2019a, b))

Example 2.3 Design of Cutting Tool

A variety of cutting tools are used for machine steel and other metals. Cutting speeds are affected by the quality of cutting tools. Industrial productivity is directly related to cutting speed, which is often limited by the wear of cutting tools. However, besides the wear of cutting tools, they must be able to withstand the cutting force without deflection and fracture. If the task is to improve the quality of cutting tools, what are the appropriate FRs that must be satisfied to improve the performance of the cutting tools? What are the DPs that can satisfy the FRs?

The FRs of a cutting tool may be stated as follows:

FR1 = Provide wear resistance;

FR2 = Prevent fracture;

FR3 = Have sufficient stiffness.

Many cutting tools were made of a single material such as high-speed steel, cemented carbides, and ceramics. Therefore, FR1, FR2, and FR3 could not be independently satisfied. These FRs must be then mapped in the physical domain by finding DPs, i.e., DP1, DP2, and DP3, which may be stated as

DP1 = Tool material;

DP2 = Tool material;

DP3 = Thickness of the cutting tool.

Since the same DP controls FR1 and FR3 because DP1 = DP2, we cannot satisfy the FRs independently, thus violating the Independence Axiom. As a consequence, a material that has an excellent wear resistance may lack toughness. Conversely, if we select a material with toughness, it may wear too fast. This is not an ideal tool design.

How should we improve the performance of cutting tools by satisfying the three FRs independently?

Examples 2.1 through 2.3 are given earlier to illustrate the concept of mapping from the functional domain to the physical domain. The question now is: are those designs good as per the Independence Axiom? A convenient way of deciding whether or not the proposed design solution is consistent with the independence Axiom is to examine the design matrix.

Note that design involves both synthesis and analysis, which reinforce each other. In the early stages of design, the detailed analysis may not be feasible or necessary until the design details emerge from conceptual design. The analysis becomes more critical after the overall initial conceptual design has been completed, although analytical thinking is always essential throughout the design process. However, a coupled design cannot be improved through analysis!

2.2.6 Design Matrix [DM]

The relationship between FR1 and FR2 of the water faucet may be written as

$$FR1 = A_{11} DP1 + A_{12} DP2$$
$$FR2 = A_{21} DP1 + A_{22} DP2$$
(2.4)

One way of representing the relationship between FRs and DPs is to construct a matrix between FRs and DPs. The water faucet shown in Fig. 2.3a is a coupled design, which has the following design matrix:

	Valve 1	Valve 2
FR1 (control the temperature of water)	X	X
FR2 (control the flow rate of water)	X	X

Since valve 1 and 2 affect both FR1 and FR2, it is a coupled design, violating the Independence Axiom.

We can represent Eq. (2.4) and the above table as follows:

$$\{FRs\} = [DM]\{DPs\}$$
(2.5)

{FRs} is a vector, consisting of two components: FR1 and FR2. Similarly {DPs} is a vector, consisting of two components: DP1 and DP2. [DM] is called the "Design Matrix."

To satisfy the Independence Axiom, the design matrix [DM] of a system must be a diagonal or a triangular matrix. From a mathematical point of view, when the matrix is diagonal, the governing equation is a set of the one-input one-output problem regardless of the number of FRs and DPs involved, which can be solved without much difficulty either analytically or numerically. When [DM] is a triangular matrix, we can get solutions to the design problem, if we vary DP in the sequence given by the triangular matrix. When [DM] is a full matrix, we have to find a unique (or compromised) solution, which is difficult to solve mathematically or evaluate and calibrate. As a result, even when a unique sweet spot for the design is found, the design requires tight tolerances to work correctly. Furthermore, as the system wears out, it can fail more readily than an uncoupled system.

2.2.7 Design Equation

Equation (2.5) relates the output, i.e., {FRs}, to input, i.e., {DPs}. A similar equation that relates vector {DP} to input vector {PVs} can be written. These will be called the design equations. The solution to these design equations is simple to solve if the design is uncoupled since there is only one output and one input variable. When the design is coupled, we have to solve many equations simultaneously, which may not be solvable. If the design equation is non-linear but uncoupled or decoupled, it can be solved either analytically or numerically. When the design is coupled, an analytical solution would be difficult to obtain since many equations must be solved simultaneously.

In practical terms, the following should be noted as a reminder to all designers. When there are n FRs to be satisfied, one may have n equations with n DPs. When the design is coupled, the design matrix is going to be a full matrix, and one may have to solve n simultaneous equations for a unique solution, which is a difficult task, especially when the equations are non-linear. Even if one can solve it, a slight change in one of the DPs will throw the entire system into chaos. On the other hand, if the design is uncoupled, each FR can be solved by itself, regardless of whether the equation is linear or non-linear.

Many systems we design have many FRs. If the design is coupled, the implementation of the system is likely to bog down, leading to system failures. The reason an international airport cannot be made to operate even after spending billions of more dollars and years of delay is a symptom of this problem, i.e., a coupled design.

2.2.8 Decomposition of Functional Requirements, Design Parameters, and Process Variables Through Zigzagging Between the Domains

In Sect. 2.2.1, we discussed the idea that in the design world, we have four domains: customer, functional, physical, and process domains. For the shoe sole example given in Example 2.1, we defined the FR in the functional domain, DP in the physical domain, and PV in the process domain. These were the highest level characteristic vectors that define each respective domain. When further details are needed for implementation, we must decompose FRs, DPs, and PVs further to generate detailed designs that can be implemented.

To decompose, we have to zigzag between the domains. For instance, after we define FR1 in the functional domain, we move to the physical domain to select the corresponding DP1. If the selected DP1 does not have sufficient details that can be implemented, we must return to the functional domain, and select children-level FRs, i.e., FR1.1, FR1.2, etc., by decomposing the highest level FR1. These children-level FRs may be thought of as the FRs of DP1. Figure 2.5 illustrates the zigzagging between the domains (Fig. 2.4).

After FR1.1 and FR1.2 are chosen, we need to go back to the physical domain and select corresponding DPs, i.e., DP1.1 and DP1.2, which are the children of the highest level DP. This zigzagging process must continue until sufficient details of the design that can be implemented are generated. This process is illustrated in Example 2.5.

Fig. 2.4 Zigzagging between domains to decompose FRs and DPs

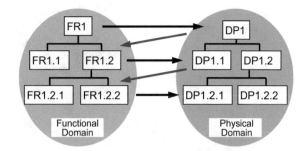

Example 2.1 (cont'd)

Continuation of the Decomposition of the Children's Shoe Sole Design

(To illustrate decomposition of FRs, DPs, and PVs through zigzagging.)

Going back to the example related to children's shoes, we completed the design at the highest level as follows:

FR = Manufacture foamed PVC soles for children's shoes;
DP = Injection molded shoe soles;
PV = Injection molding process.

These highest level FR, DP, and PV are rather conceptual without details, and therefore cannot be implemented without further details. In order to generate the details, we have to decompose FR, DP, and PV. The decomposition of FR, DP, and PV creates in each domain a tree-like structure with lower level FRs, DPs, and PVs.

The highest level FR may be decomposed as follows:

FR1 = Mold the entire shoe sole onto the upper;
FR2 = Make the sole flexible, i.e., pliable;
FR3 = Make the sole wear-resistant;
FR4 = Control the weight (i.e., density) of the sole.

Every designer might have decomposed the FR differently, resulting in different products that may perform the same highest level FRs.

The corresponding DP in the physical domain may be chosen to be the following:

DP1 = Injection molding against the upper mounted on last;
DP2 = Density of foamed PVC;
DP3 = Solid skin layer for wear resistance;
DP4 = Total weight of the PVC injected into the mold.

In Fig. 2.5, the cross section of shoe soles is shown. DP1, the injection molding, controls the shape of the molded shoe soles. To make the sole flexible (FR2), foamed PVC (DP2) is used by mixing PVC with a chemical blowing agent (which decomposes in the plasticating extruder section of the injection molding machine) to generate gas when it reaches the decomposition temperature of the blowing agent. To make the shoe sole wear-resistant, PVC in contact with the movable mold surface was prevented foaming by keeping the mold

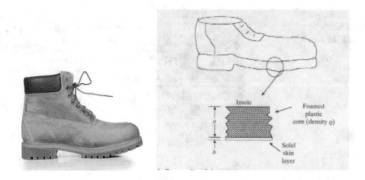

Fig. 2.5 A shoe sole (Boot reproduced with permission from Alexlukin (2019))

surface in contact with PVC cold. The flow front of PVC tends to foam and expand because of the low pressure at the flow front. Therefore, to prevent the expansion of the molten PVC while the molten plastic flows into the mold, the cross-sectional area of the mold was made very narrow by making the bottom of the mold (which is in contact with the bottom of the shoe sole) moveable. To increase the pressure on the plastic during injection and thus prevent it from expanding when the blowing agent decomposes, the cross-sectional area of the flow channel was narrowed by moving in the movable part of the mold. After the mold cavity is filled, the movable part of mold (which is in contact with the bottom of shoe soles) was moved out to expand the mold volume, and thus allowing the plastic to expand forming tiny bubbles everywhere, except the bottom of the shoe sole. During this expansion process, the bottom of the PVC sole in contact with the cold mold surface cannot expand because of the low temperature of PVC, thus forming a solid skin layer. To bond the molded shoe sole directly to the shoe upper mounted on the last, an adhesive is applied to the shoe upper mounted on the last, before the injection of PVC (Fig. 2.5).

Now that DPs are selected to satisfy FRs, we can check the relationship between FRs and DPs. One way of checking it would be to use a matrix relationship. A means of representing the relationship is to ask: "Does DP1 affect FR1? FR2? And FR3?" If it does, we put down X, and if not, 0.

	DP1	DP2	DP3	DP4
FR1	X	0	0	0
FR2	0	X	0	X
FR3	0	x	X	0
FR4	0	0	0	X

By rearranging the above sequence of FRs and DPs, we obtain

	DP4	DP2	DP3	DP1
FR4	X	0	0	0
FR2	X	X	0	0
FR3	0	x	X	0
FR1	0	0	0	X

It is a triangular matrix. According to the Independence Axiom, we need to maintain the FRs independent from each other, but since it is a triangular matrix, FR3 is affected by DP2. It states that the density of the foam core can affect the wear rate after the skin layer wears off. Therefore, we need to change the DPs in the right order to maintain the independence of FRs. In this case, we first control the foam core thickness for flexibility and then determine the skin layer thickness for wear resistance. We call such a design that requires a sequential change of DPs a "decoupled design." In this design, the sequence of change of DPs should be in the order of DP4, DP2, DP1, and DP3. Then the design matrix becomes triangular.

Note that we purposely chose the same number of DPs and the number of FRs for a good reason. It can be shown that in an "ideal design," *the number of FRs and DPs must be the same (Theorem 4)*.

As the foregoing paragraph stated, the PVs were as follows[5]:

PV1 = Injection of PVC with chemical blowing agent;
PV2 = Expansion of the mold volume by moving the bottom plate;
PV3 = Temperature of the mold that comes into contact with the bottom of the shoe sole;
PV4 = Expansion of the mold volume by moving the bottom mold plate.

In Fig. 2.5, the cross section of shoe soles is shown. DP1, the injection mold, controls the shape of the molded shoe soles. To make the sole flexible (FR2), foamed PVC (DP2) is used by mixing PVC with a chemical blowing agent (which decomposes in the plasticating extruder section of the injection molding machine) to generate gas when it reaches the decomposition temperature of the blowing agent. To make the shoe sole wear-resistant, a solid layer of PVC skin at the bottom of the shoe sole is created by making the mold surface that is in contact with PVC cold to prevent the expansion of PVC by the blowing agent. To prevent the expansion of the PVC during the injection of plastic into the mold, the cross section of the mold was made very narrow to build up the pressure on the plastic with blowing. After the mold is filled, the bottom part of the mold that is in contact with the bottom of shoe soles was moved to expand the mold volume, thus allowing the expansion of the plastic with the decomposed blowing agent. This process creates a foamed shoe sole with a solid skin layer. The adhesive is applied to the shoe upper mounted on the last, which bonds the molded shoe sole directly to the shoe upper mounted on the last. It should be noted that this project was finished in 3 months with field tests after the young engineer took over the project that had been going on for a couple of years, all thanks to the rational design of the process.

---

[5]The PVs can be selected if one has some knowledge on injection molding of foamed PVC. This is a rather specialized knowledge that must be acquired either by reading reference books or through actual practice. A special molding technique was invented to achieve PV1, PV2, and PV3, which was named the "high-pressure injection molding." It will be described in Chap. 7

Example 2.4 Illustration of the Mapping Concept (Global Warming)

In this example, the goal is to keep the temperature rise of Earth to within 2°C above its temperature at the time of the Industrial Revolution[6]. The problem we identified to solve in the customer domain is global warming to slow down the temperature rise of Earth. Global warming is primarily due to the anthropogenic emission of CO_2. Now we need to "map" this need to reduce CO_2 into the functional domain and we need to define a set of FRs in the functional domain to reduce CO_2 emission.

In the functional domain, we may establish the following FRs as a means of solving the problem identified in the customer domain:

FR1 = Replace internal combustion (IC) engines with electric drives;
FR2 = Generate electricity with solar energy;
FR3 = Generate electricity from wind power;
FR4 = Plant trees.

Note that the designer chooses the FRs. Other designers may choose a different set, which may be larger or small than the four FRs listed above. The quality of the ultimate design will depend on the choice of FRs. Each designer will attempt to solve the problem identified in the customer domain in different ways. Therefore, in design, there is no unique solution, i.e., uniqueness theorem does not hold. There may be many equally acceptable solutions as long as they satisfy the same set of FRs. We will later cover the Information Axiom, which may be used to evaluate two equally good designs from the viewpoint of the Independence Axiom, but one particular design may be superior to the other from the simplicity point of view, which is what is measured by the Information Axiom.

To satisfy the four FRs identified above, we have to come up with DPs in the physical domain (i.e., transform FRs into DPs). How many DPs should we select to satisfy the four FRs chosen? What would you pick as DP1, DP2, DP3, and DP4? Should we have more (or less) than four DPs? What should be the relationship between the FRs and DPs? How should we represent the relationship between FRs and DPs? These questions may be difficult to answer at this stage of learning AD, but we will answer all these questions later in this book.

Different designers may select a different set of DPs to satisfy the FRs. Suppose that a designer selected the following set of DPs to satisfy the FRs chosen:

DP1 = Electrical ground transportation system;
DP2 = Solar cell "farm" for the generation of electricity;
DP3 = Windmills along the shore to generate electricity;
DP4 = Designated national tree planting day.

Sometimes it is hard to distinguish FRs and DPs. It is suggested that always state FRs starting with a verb and DPs with a noun.

Once we select DPs, FRs and DPs are related as

$$\{FR1, FR2, FR3, FR4\} = DM\{DP1, DP2, DP3, DP4\} \tag{2.6}$$

The FR vector, i.e., {FRi} is related to the DP vector, i.e., {DPi} by the design matrix DM.

---

[6]On December 12, 2015, 195 nations at the United Nations Conference on Climate Change in Paris (Conference of Parties COP21) agreed to reduce their CO_2 emission to limit the rise of the earth's temperature to below 2 C above the pre-industrial level.

Equation (2.6) may also be expressed as

$$FR1 = A_{11} DP1 + A_{12} DP2 + A_{13} DP3 + A_{14} DP4$$
$$FR2 = A_{21} DP1 + A_{22} DP2 + A_{23} DP3 + A_{24} DP4$$
$$FR3 = A_{31} DP1 + A_{32} DP2 + A_{33} DP3 + A_{34} DP4 \quad (2.7)$$
$$FR4 = A_{41} DP1 + A_{42} DP2 + A_{43} DP3 + A_{44} DP4$$

In indices notation, Eq. (2.7), may be written as

$$FR_i = \sum_j A_{ij}DP_j, \quad where\ i\ and\ j\ are\ 1, 2, 3, 4 \quad (2.8)$$

{FRs} and {DPs} are vectors, and DM is a matrix that relates these two vectors. The nature of DM determines whether or not the proposed design at this highest level is acceptable or not. If the design violates the Independence Axiom, it is not acceptable. The Independence Axiom states that the FRs must be independent of each other.

A straightforward way of checking the independence is to construct the design matrix and check if a DP affects FRs. For example, does DP1 affect FR4? If the answer is affirmative, we put down X and if not, 0.

	DP1	DP2	DP3	DP4
FR1	X	0	0	0
FR2	0	X	0	0
FR3	0	0	X	0
FR4	0	0	0	X

(2.9)

The designer decides whether there is a relationship between a DP and an FR, making certain assumptions. In the above example, it was decided that DP2 (solar power) does not affect FR1, because, in the early days of installing the electric car system, they will rely on the power sources currently used. Eventually, if the entire electrical power generation is done using solar, the power generation may affect the transportation system.

The above design represented by Eq. (2.9) has a diagonal matrix, and therefore each FR can be changed by varying one DP without affecting any other FRs. Such a design is much easier to manage and optimize than when some of the off-diagonal elements are non-zero. This kind of design is called "uncoupled design," which is the most desirable design. Although there are many FRs, each one of them can be treated as a one-input/one-output problem, which makes it much easier to optimize, control, and operate.

Once we define DPs, we have to map them in the process domain and identify means of satisfying the DPs. We call them PVs. For instance, PV1 should provide a means of enabling DP1. Possible PV1 could be "rechargeable batteries" or "wireless electric power transmission."

Assembly of DPs into a physical system

DPs must be assembled into a whole system. In the case of solid components, this process may be aided by determining the interaction between DPs to put them into geometric proximity during assembly of the parts, if the design involves hardware. For this, we can determine the interaction between DPs, creating a matrix similar to that given by Eq. (2.10). Such a matrix is called the geometric proximity matrix (GPM) or design structure matrix

(DSM). The table states that there are physical interactions when the element of the matrix is non-zero. For example, DP2 and DP4 may be close together physically. It does not imply that there is a functional relationship between FR2 and FR4. Sometimes, it takes a great deal of effort to package all the components that go into the automobile engine compartment, which is limited in space.

	DP1	DP2	DP3	DP4
DP1	a	c	e	g
DP2	c	d	0	h
DP3	e	0	n	f
DP4	g	h	f	m

$$(2.10)$$

Given the GPM, DP1 should be surrounded by DP2, DP3, and DP4, if there is appropriate space. Similarly, DP4 can be placed in close proximity of other DPs. DP2 and DP3 do not need to be placed in close proximity.

Example 2.5 Illustration of the Mapping Concept (Mass production of glass bottles)

Suppose you are in charge of developing a mass manufacturing system for the production of glass bottles by blow molding molten glass gobs. Molten glass runner at about 1100 C (note: runner is sometimes called parison in plastics blow molding industry) is extruded as the round rod, which must be cut to gobs using a special cutting tool which shears the glass runner (the shearing tool is similar to scissors with two blades). The gobs are then inserted into a mold where it is molded into a bottle by blowing air into the gob, i.e., similar to blow molding of plastic bottles. After the glass bottle solidifies in the mold, it is transported away from the machine. The desired production rate is 100 bottles per hour. The cutter must cut the glass parison within a tight tolerance without leaving any residues of glass particles on the parison surface, which, if left on the surface, would then show up as defects on the bottle surface. The problem we are concerned with is that the shearing tool must be replaced frequently due to the wear of the cutting tool, which slows down the production rate and create defective parts. Our job is to design the entire system for shearing off the glass runner.

Determining the highest level FRs:

Our job is to improve the glass/gob cutting operation to minimize the wear of the shearing tool to cut the parison. We begin by asking: "What are the FRs of the cutting operation?" Each designer may come up with a different set of FRs based on the designer's understanding of the problem in the customer domain.

Suppose that we chose the following FRs:

FR1 = Control the diameter of the runner;
FR2 = Measure the length of the runner where it must be cut;
FR3 = Shear off the runner when the runner reaches the pre-set position;
FR4 = Lubricate the cutting operation;
FR5 = Control the temperatures of the glass, lubricant, and the cutting tool.

We will know whether or not this set of FRs is complete after we complete the design by choosing the right set of DPs. In some cases, the final verdict will come when the actual shearing operation is done to test the design. Even if the above five FRs are not complete, this systematic approach will enable us to spot any mistakes made. Our experience shows that in most cases, design done this way is complete and performs the intended functions well.

Mapping of FRs into DPs at the Highest Level:

Having defined the FRs of our design, we need to map the FRs into the physical domain by identifying the corresponding set of DPs. As we try to select the corresponding DPs, we should note that the control of temperature is critical, because the glass has a narrow glass transition temperature where the glass behavior changes drastically from a viscous–elastic state into a glassy state. As an initial attempt to designing a right shearing tool for the molten glass, we may select the following DPs to satisfy the FRs chosen:

DP1 = Diameter of the extrusion die opening;
DP2 = Optical gage;
DP3 = Mechanical shear with sharp blades;
DP4 = Water-based lubricant with surfactants, corrosion inhibitors, and water-soluble oil;
DP5 = Temperature controllers for glass, machines, and shearing blades.

Note that each one of these FRs and DPs must be further decomposed to develop further details since DPs cannot be implemented for lack of detailed designs.

Also, note again that FRs are stated starting with verbs and DPs begin with a noun in order to easily identify FRs and DPs.

Design Matrix

For the chosen FRs and DPs, we must construct the design matrix and investigate if the proposed design at this highest level satisfies the Independence Axiom, i.e., is it an uncoupled or decoupled design. Design matrix links the {FR} vector to the {DP} vector. The design matrix is shown below, which indicates that the design at this level is an uncoupled design:

	DP1	DP2	DP3	DP4	DP5
FR1	X	0	0	0	0
FR2	0	X	0	0	0
FR3	0	0	X	0	0
FR4	0	0	0	X	0
FR5	0	0	0	0	X

Decomposition

This design at this level does not have sufficient details, except DP1 and DP4. Therefore, other FRs and DPs need to be further decomposed. Ultimately, it should show all the detailed designs through continuous decomposition until the implementable details are designed. This subject is discussed further in a later chapter.

Example 2.6 Money Circulation for Economic Growth

In the customer domain, the problem we identified is the slow economic growth of a small country in Asia. Our goal is to solve the problem through a new design of its taxation and economic policies.

Some economists seem to believe that one way of promoting the economic growth of a nation is to increase the circulation of money (sometimes called the velocity of money circulation). The rationale seems to be the following: When the money circulates, people with money either buy or sell goods and services. Thus, the faster the circulation money, the greater is the economic activity, and hence faster economic growth. The question is how a taxation system should be designed to increase the speed of money circulation. We will assume this assumption to be accurate and determine how we may develop economic policy based on AD.

Poor people spend all their income but still cannot buy all the things required for a decent living because they make less than what is needed to maintain "middle-class life." People in the top 1% spend as much money as they please, but they cannot use all of their income, because their income is far higher than the amount of the money they need to maintain their luxurious lifestyle, and therefore they circulate only a small fraction of their annual income. Rich people may directly deposit their money to collect interest on the money, which may not affect money circulation in a significant way. Your task is to transform the economy of this nation. We need to transform the problem identified in the customer domain into a set of FRs in the functional domain and a set of DPs in the physical domain in order to design an economic system that will maximize the economic growth rate of the country by increasing the velocity of money circulation, assuming that this is sound economic policy.

Your task as a renowned economist is to transform the problem we identified in the customer domain into a set of FRs in the functional domain and a set of DPs in the physical domain. The goal is to transform the economic system and accelerate the economic growth rate of this country by increasing the velocity of money circulation.

The following facts about this country are known: There are five income groups: A, B, C, D, and E. Group A is the lowest income Group; B the second lowest income group, which makes twice as much as those in Group A; Group C makes three times that of B; Group D makes five times that of Group C; and Group E makes 100 times that of Group D. Income of Group C is just enough to support a typical family. The population distribution in each one of the economic income groups is as follows: A = 100,000; B = 5,000,000; C = 1,000,000; D = 50,000; and E = 300. People in Group C spend all the money they make to take care of their minimum expenses. Groups A and B need more money to achieve middle-class living quality but do not have the necessary income. The goal is to design fiscal and monetary policies through design to maximize the velocity of money circulation.

The new tax system will be designed to achieve the following three FRs:

FR1 = Maximize the velocity of money circulation;
FR2 = Invest in public infrastructure, including national defense;
FR3 = Provide incentives to all groups to work efficiently and effectively.

The DPs may be stated as follows:

DP1 = Monetary policies;
DP2 = Investment policies for a public good;
DP3 = Fiscal policies.

These highest level FRs and DPs must be decomposed to develop detailed designs that can be implemented, because FR1, FR2, FR3 and DP1, DP2, DP3 are still conceptual and do not provide sufficient details for us to implement.

To achieve the goal of having a strong economy, we need more details than the design done so far. We will decompose FR1, FR2, and FR3 as well as DP1, DP2, and DP3. Different designers may come up with different sets of lower level FRs, depending on how they decompose them based on their understanding of the problem and issues involved.

We decided to choose the following children-level FRs to address the problem of maximizing money circulation, i.e., FR1 (maximize the velocity of money circulation):

FR11 = Give subsidies and tax credits to Groups A and B;
FR12 = Establish a progressive income tax rate for Groups C, D, and E;
FR13 = Reduce the tax rate on the net income that exceeds the preceding year's income;
FR14 = Levy fixed % tax on all income groups for healthcare;
FR15 = Levy fixed % tax on all income for social security.

For FR2 (invest in public infrastructure, including national defense), we selected the following as the next-level FRs:

FR21 = Invest in infrastructure building;
FR22 = Fund national defense;
FR23 = Provide free education from primary to tertiary education;
FR24 = Invest in 5% of GDP in extensive R&D;
FR25 = Strengthen patent policies;
FR26 = Provide free public transportation.

For FR3 (provide incentives to all groups to work efficiently and effectively), we decided to choose the following as the next-level FRs:

FR31 = Provide free education for primary, secondary, and tertiary education;
FR32 = Legislate a minimum pay policy that is tied to the inflation rate;
FR33 = Promote merit-based reward system;
FR34 = Implement a generous overtime pay policy.

To satisfy these FRs, we need to select the means of satisfying them by choosing the right set of DPs in the physical domain. Again note that DP1 is chosen to satisfy FR1, and so on.

One possible set of DPs that are chosen to satisfy the children-*level FRs listed above are as follows:*

DP11 = Special tax incentives for Groups A and B;
DP12 = Progressive tax rate for Groups C, D, and E;
DP13 = Tax incentive system for exceptional achievers;
DP14 = Healthcare tax;
DP15 = Social security tax;
DP21 = *Infrastructure fund*;

DP22 = Defense budget;
DP23 = Strong public educational institutions;
DP24 = Competitive R&D funding;
DP25 = Patent policy for public good;
DP26 = Public infrastructure;
DP31 = Public education system;
DP32 = Mandatory minimum pay system;
DP33 = Civil servant examination systems;
DP34 = Overtime pay legislation.

Questions 2.4:

How do we know that we have selected good DPs? Do the selected DPs constitute an acceptable set of DPs? What is the role of the Information Axiom in designing these systems?

2.3   Design Process in Creating Various Systems

To summarize the design process:

The first step is to have a clear understanding of the problem that requires a design solution (in the customer domain). From this problem statement, we establish design goals in the form of FRs. After the designer chooses FRs, the DPs must be selected that can satisfy the FRs. Then, to be sure that the DPs are correctly chosen, we create the design matrix (DM) to check for the independence of FRs. Then, we assemble DPs into a system for ease of use, physical compatibility, physical contiguity, geometric compatibility, transfer of forces, electrical compatibility, etc. In other words, in the case of physical products, DPs must be "packaged" into a physical assembly, e.g., the engine compartment of cars is packaged to house most mechanical components such as engine, electricity generator, air-conditioning compressor, etc., to fit under the hood.

2.3.1   Revisiting the Water Faucet Design

Example 2.2, two water faucet designs were shown to ask which design is superior in satisfying two FRs, one controlling the water flow rate and the other for controlling temperature. We stated that the design that satisfies the temperature and the flow rate independently is a superior design as per the Independence Axiom. We will now go back to the water faucet design and discuss the actual design process.

The FRs for the water faucet may be stated as follows:

FR1 = Control water flow rate = Q;
FR2 = Control temperature = T.

The desired design is an uncoupled design that will enable us to write the design equation as

$$\left\{ \begin{array}{c} FR1 \\ FR2 \end{array} \right\} = \left\{ \begin{array}{c} Q \\ T \end{array} \right\} = \left[\begin{array}{cc} A11 & 0 \\ 0 & A22 \end{array} \right] \left\{ \begin{array}{c} DP1 \\ DP2 \end{array} \right\} \tag{2.11}$$

We should try to choose DP1 and DP2 that will give us a diagonal design matrix. Then, we can proceed to determine what the coefficients A11 and A22 should be in order to satisfy FR1 and FR2.

One way of achieving the independence of these two FRs might be to control the cross-sectional areas of the valve through which hot water and cold water flow. If Ah is the cross-sectional area of the valve through which hot water flows through and Ac is that for cold water, then Q and T are functions of Ac and Ah as

$$Q = f(Ac + Ah)$$
$$T = g(Ac/Ah)$$

Thus, Eq. (2.11) may be written as

$$\left\{ \begin{array}{c} FR1 \\ FR2 \end{array} \right\} = \left\{ \begin{array}{c} Q \\ T \end{array} \right\} = \left[\begin{array}{cc} X & 0 \\ 0 & X \end{array} \right] \left\{ \begin{array}{c} DP1 \\ DP2 \end{array} \right\} = \left[\begin{array}{cc} X & 0 \\ 0 & X \end{array} \right] \left\{ \begin{array}{c} f(Ac + Ah) \\ g\left(\frac{Ac}{Ah}\right) \end{array} \right\} \tag{2.12}$$

Equation (2.12) states that if FR is to control water flow rate, we vary f(Ac + Ah), and if we want to vary the water temperature we vary g(Ac/Ah). A valve design must be such that it will control the total flow rate of water without affecting the temperature of the water and vice versa. To achieve the design goal, we need to develop a mechanism that will let the flow rate change without affecting temperature by keeping the ratio of cross-sectional areas remain the same, while the sum of the cross-sectional areas changes. Conversely, it must be able to change the ratio of the cross-sectional areas without affecting the total flow rate.

Now we must develop the design that will define DP1 and DP2 more explicitly. The design question now becomes what kind of mechanism will provide us DP1 that will let us vary the (Ac + Ah) without affecting (Ac/Ah) and DP2 that will affect (AC/Ah) without affecting (Ac + Ah).

One of the mechanisms that will let us achieve these design goals is shown in Fig. 2.6

Then, the design equation, Eq. (2.11), may be written as

$$\left\{ \begin{array}{c} FR1 \\ FR2 \end{array} \right\} = \left\{ \begin{array}{c} Q \\ T \end{array} \right\} = \left[\begin{array}{cc} X & 0 \\ 0 & X \end{array} \right] \left\{ \begin{array}{c} DP1 \\ DP2 \end{array} \right\} = \left[\begin{array}{cc} X & 0 \\ 0 & X \end{array} \right] \left\{ \begin{array}{c} \phi1 \\ \phi2 \end{array} \right\} \tag{2.13}$$

Equation (2.13) verifies that the water faucet is an acceptable design because the DM is a diagonal matrix.

Fig. 2.6 Uncoupled water faucet design (©Oxford Publishing Limited. Reproduced with permission of the Licensor through PLSclear (Suh 2001))

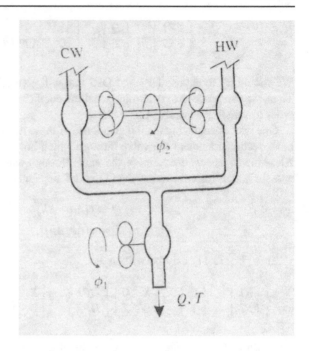

2.3.2 Design of a System for Salary Raise

Many organizations, including universities, give annual salary raise to their employees. It is in recognition of the contributions they have made to the organization during the previous 12 months and also to adjust for the inflation of living costs. The central administration typically allocates a lump sum for each unit of the organization with the approval of the board of directors (or trustees). Each group then distributes to its employees by the head of the unit based on an established rationale. The salary administration must be fair to the employees as well as for the organization to achieve the goal of improving performance and rewarding expected contributions. Our job is to design a salary raise system that performs these tasks.

Design Task:

PROBLEM to be solved through design (in the customer domain)
Usually, the available pool of funds for the salary raise is not sufficient to give a significant increase to everyone. Furthermore, the organization must recognize those who have made significant contributions to achieving the goals of the organization. Therefore, those who have made more significant contributions to the organization should receive a higher raise. Such a system may be called a merit-based system. However, those who think they received smaller raises than they deserve can criticize the system. One temptation for the administrator to avoid

criticism is to give a uniform raise based on their current salary, which violates the goal of advancing the organizational goals through a merit-based reward system.

GOALS of the salary distribution (in the functional domain)

Having defined the *problem*, we need to define the goals we have to achieve through design.

FR1 = Assess the contributions made by each employee;
FR2 = Reward based on specific contributions.

Implementation of the goals (DPs of the salary system)

DP1 = Merit-based salary system consisting of six groups of merit;
DP2 = A Gaussian distribution, giving the two times the average raise to the best performing and 20% of the average raise to the least effective employees.

Constraint: To determine the average raise, the total sum of the raises to be given must be the same as the available fund to be distributed.

2.4   Role of System Architect in Managing Large System Development

When the system to be designed is vast and complicated (for example, the on-line electric vehicle), many people participate in the execution of the project. To manage such a large system development with many FRs, it is necessary that a system architect is appointed. The primary job of the system architect is to make sure that any member of the design and management team introduces no coupled design.

Since there may be a large number of FRs and DPs with many layers of decomposition, different groups of people are in charge of different subsets of the project. When they make design decisions, they tend to make them by considering their tasks alone. However, their judgment may affect the design decisions made in some other branches of the design team. These mistakes usually increase the cost of the project substantially and lengthen the development period. Therefore, someone has to monitor whether or not the decisions made by everyone working on the project are proper from the systems point of view, i.e., prevent the inadvertent introduction of DPs that couple FRs of the system. Such a person is the system architect.

The role of the system architect is to construct the master design matrix for the entire project and check if any design decisions have inadvertently introduced the coupling of FRs by any participant in the design project. To achieve this goal, the design architect must construct a master design matrix for the entire system and must follow all the branches of design and the rationality of the design decisions made by checking for the inadvertent coupling of FRs. When KAIST[7] developed the on-line electric vehicle (OLEV) and mobile harbor, system architect teams monitored the decisions made by various team members, thus preventing the introduction of coupled designs.

2.5 Uncertainty and the Information Axiom

In this chapter, we discussed the implication of the Independence Axiom in designing various systems, including mechanical, electrical, economic, and organizational systems. No in-depth discussion was presented on the Information Axiom. Information Axiom states that a better design is the one with less information content. According to the second axiom of AD, a robust system that satisfies the Independence Axiom has required less information than coupled systems that violate the Independence Axiom. When two designs that satisfy the Independence Axiom are compared, the design with less information content is the best one.

The Information Axiom deals with the "robustness" of a design, reliability of designed systems, optimization of the system, and complexity of a system. Robustness implies that the system is easy to make and operate and reliable. We will show that a system that satisfies the Independence Axiom inherently requires less information to construct and to operate. Therefore, when we design a new system, we must make sure that the Independence Axiom is not violated before we concern ourselves with the Information Axiom. In Chap. 8, we will discuss the Information Axiom and its implications in great depths. We will show how the Information Axiom can be used to choose the design range and the system range to develop an optimum design for faster economic growth.

In Example 2.6 (money circulation for economic growth), we designed a fictitious taxation system as a way of illustrating how AD may be used in non-technical fields. We considered the effect of increasing the velocity of money circulation as a way of increasing the economic growth of a nation, assuming that indeed the velocity of money circulations will affect economic activity. (In economics, there seems to be a diversity of opinions among economists on many economic matters.) The simple example illustrated how the taxation system could be designed to increase the circulation rate by changing the tax rates, tax credit, and tax brackets. In Chap. 11, we will show how the Information Axiom can be used to choose the design range and the system range to develop an optimum design for faster economic growth.

---

[7]KAIST is an acronym for the Korea Advanced Institute of Science and Technology.

2.6   On Design of Machines that Can Design

In recent years, many companies have introduced AI-based technologies and products (e.g., IBM's Watson, self-driving cars, machines that employ facial recognition, and many others), but so far most design decisions are made by people other than routine graphics that use robust modeling tools.

Question 2.5:

Do you think someday intelligent machines can develop complicated systems, taking over the functions human beings are performing today? Following the sequence of the design described in Chaps. 1 and 2, (i.e., identification of the problem, distillation of FRs, selection of DPs without violating the Independence Axiom, and choosing PVs to satisfy DPs), which part or parts are likely taken over by an intelligent design machine?

Already routine design functions (e.g., graphics that are part of known products such as airplanes and automobiles) are performed by computer-assisted machines. However, the original highly creative problem identification is still in the realm of human ingenuity. No one can predict the future of technological and scientific innovations when we realize how much human ingenuity has advanced these fields during the past 350 years.

One thing is clear! As we systematize the logic and procedure of design through the development of theories such as AD, it can be the basis for creating a "Thinking Design Machine" that performs many routine functions of design such as playing the role of system architect. It may create a design matrix (DM), suggesting better FRs and DPs, identifying coupled designs and decoupled designs, coming up with a proper sequence of operations when decoupled designs are involved, and assembling DPs into a unified physical system. Computers are powerful tools, especially when we have to deal with massive data that can facilitate the design process.

Human creativity has done amazing things. It is difficult to imagine the day when machines can replicate (or replace) the incredible intellectual advances people like Einstein, Watts and Crick, Shannon, and others made during the past century. If one may be permitted to speculate on what the future holds, human ingenuity will continue to lead high-level thought processes that are essential in genuinely creative designs.

2.7   Conclusions

Synthesis builds on the human ability to quantify and understand broader social and natural issues. In this chapter, we strived to show the role of design, not only in engineering but also in many other fields. Leaders in all fields must possess the ability to design since their responsibility often requires the ability to integrate and synthesize based on the analytical database provided by various groups within the organization. Head of industrial firms, university presidents, and national political leaders must understand the complementary role of synthesis and analysis in creating systems. Some leaders possess both synthetic and analytic capabilities. However, if one can have only one, i.e., either analytic or synthetic capability, it may be better to choose a leader with a strong ability to synthesize available information to generate a new design or solutions.

Educational goals of a university must be diverse, educating people who are analytic thinkers, also people who are more talented in synthesis, and even people who are comfortable in both analysis and synthesis. Creativity is needed both in analysis and synthesis. The ability to design well must be nurtured through education, practice, and deep thinking.

It is much harder to teach synthesis for many different reasons. Therefore, even in engineering schools, design or synthesis education has received marginal emphasis. Many students are expected to learn design and synthesis in the industry. However, the industry cannot provide a formal pedagogy in design. As a result, many engineers learn design through experience. More formal teaching of design is needed in many countries.

There are a few important messages that we hope to convey in the first three chapters of this book. First, the design is a process of creating solutions. Second, we show how the design should proceed. In Chap. 7, the Independence Axiom is discussed in depth to explore the significance of the independence of FRs. In Chap. 8, the Information Axiom is examined to show how design can be made more robust. In later chapters, these two design axioms are applied to a variety of engineering problems to illustrate the AD process of creating solutions.

Problems

1. The 2014 report of the Intergovernmental Panel on Climate Change (IPCC) of the United Nations stated that the emission of anthropogenic greenhouse gases must be reduced by 40–70% in 2050 in comparison to the emission level of 2010 to limit the earth's temperature rise below 2 °C relative to the pre-industrial level. Define FRs that your country must satisfy to reduce CO_2 emission by 50%.

2. Identify potential problems of driverless cars and then define the FRs and constraints of such a system for an ideal driverless car.

3. In many countries, unemployment or under-employment of young people is a significant social issue. The goal established by the government is a 50% reduction in the unemployment rate of college graduates. Define FRs and DPs to alleviate the problem.

4. The supply of clean potable water is a significant issue in many parts of the world. Traditional desalination processes such as evaporation technology and reverse osmosis (RO) processes are too energy-intensive. For the country, you are a resident of, develop FRs and DPs to deal with the portable water problem.

5. University education is important. There are many problems associated with providing higher education: cost, inadequate preparation of incoming students, and lack of jobs for college graduates. You just became the Minister of Education of your country. Define the problems faced by your country in improving

university education. Develop a set of FRs that can solve this problem. Identify corresponding DPs.

6. Social networks (SN) play a vital role in forming public opinions. Unfortunately, some manipulate the public opinion for personal gains using SN. Design an SN system that can filter out erroneous information.

7. When you drive a car and try to steer it to either right or left, the car tilts, indicating that the steering function is coupled to the tilting of the vehicle. Stiffer suspensions are used in sporty cars for tight steering, while the softer suspension is in limousines for comfort. The suspension and steering systems are coupled with designs. Can we develop a design that uncouples steering and tilting?

8. Construct the design matrix for the problem discussed in Example 2.6: money circulation for economic growth.

Bibliography

Alexlukin (2019) Yellow leather stylish shoes isolated on white background. Photo licensed from Shutterstock, ID: 96707662

Casey B (2009) Advice for maintaining hydraulic accumulators. Machinery Lubrication. https://www.machinerylubrication.com/Read/2305/hydraulic-accumulators

Kurguzova O (2019a) Mixer cold hot water. Modern faucet bathroom. Kitchen tap. Isolated white background. Chrome-plated metal. Photo licensed from Shutterstock, ID: 529620055

Kurguzova O (2019b) The water tap, faucet for the bathroom and kitchen mixer, isolated on a white background. Chrome-plated metal. Side view. Photo licensed from Shutterstock, ID: 524192626

Further Reading

Farid A, Suh NP (eds) (2016) Axiomatic design in large systems. Springer, Cham, Switzerland

Fiege R (2009) Axiomatic design: Eine Methode zur serviceorientierten Modellierung. Gabler Verlag

Park GJ (2007) Analytic methods for design practice. Springer

Suh NP (2001) Axiomatic design—advances and applications. Oxford University Press

How Do We Design?

3

Nam Pyo Suh

Abstract

The design of systems foreshadows the outcome of human efforts in many fields. Many successful designs (e.g., the U.S. Constitution, automobile, airplane, telephone, Internet, electric power, electric grid system, a banking system, university, refrigeration, atomic bomb, computer, microelectronics, new materials) have altered the course of human history. This chapter describes how a system can be designed, following the design process outlined in Chaps. 1 and 2.

The designer envisioned in this book is a person with a large, clean canvas on which to design a system freely and creatively, unhindered, and unencumbered by any prior bias and preconceptions. The role of the designer is analogous to that of a composer of a symphony, who uses creativity, inspiration, and knowledge to orchestrate the entire process of creation and performance of music. When they achieve their goals successfully, their work can mesmerize thousands of music lovers for centuries. The result of the designer's work must be a complete, practical, and realistic system that embodies the most rational, creative, and imaginative thoughts. The design should yield the solution(s) for the problem identified within a set of bounds (i.e., constraints such as cost, safety, reliability, rules, and regulations). History shows that the work of great designers has changed the course of nations, technology, and humanity, perhaps as much as the composer and the scientist who are still affecting humanity decades after they had done their work.

This chapter shows how Axiomatic Design (AD) has been used to create solutions to various problems in diverse fields, technical and non-technical. Some are simple examples, such as the design of ashtrays to complicated subjects such as the design of wireless electric power transfer for on-line electric vehicle (OLEV). Regardless of the problem, the same thought process is used in designing these items. The use of AD theory has shortened the time and cost of

N. P. Suh (✉)
M.I.T., Cambridge, MA, USA
e-mail: npsuh@mit.edu

© Springer Nature Switzerland AG 2021
N. P. Suh et al. (eds.), *Design Engineering and Science*,
https://doi.org/10.1007/978-3-030-49232-8_3

developing new products, systems, processes, and organizations. A series of different examples of designs illustrate the design process. They demonstrate how the designer begins the design process with a clear goal in mind and solves the problem through the use of ingenuity, creativity, and practicality within a given set of constraints. Perhaps most importantly, the AD shows the designer how to avoid making wrong decisions.

After studying this chapter, the reader should know the following:
(1) What we must do to achieve the design goal(s). (2) The first step in design is defining the problem we must solve to accomplish the design goal. (3) A clear understanding of the characteristics that distinguish each domain, i.e., FR, DP, PV. (4) The transformational process of mapping between the domains. (5) Design matrix. (6) Importance of satisfying the Independence Axiom. (7) The similitude of all design tasks, i.e., the same processes used for both the design of technologies and organizations. Perhaps equally important: how to imagine and even dream of what appears to impossible things!

One of the Most Important Questions to Think About throughout This Chapter:
This chapter presents some of the essential theorems, including the one on an ideal design. These theorems state that in an ideal design, the number of FRs and the number of DPs must be equal to each other with a diagonal matrix between the FR vector and DP vector. Then, mathematically, the optimization of design should be simple and straight forward, i.e., transform any matrix into a diagonal matrix, which is possible mathematically. However, in design, such mathematical operations cannot and should not be done. Why?

3.1 Universal Nature of Design Tasks

Chapter 2 presented the four domains of the design world. All designs can be regarded as a cascade of activities starting from the customer domain, where the goal of design is established. Also, in the customer domain, the problems that must be overcome to achieve the goal are explicitly stated. The identified problem is then mapped into the functional domain, which is characterized by the functional requirements (FRs). The set of FRs constitutes the characteristic vector {FRs}, which represents the design goals. Design is the activity of choosing FRs and satisfying the chosen FRs.

After the FRs are chosen, then they are transformed into a set of design parameters (DPs). Each DP is chosen to satisfy a given FR. A set of DPs, represented as {DPs}, constitutes the characteristic vector {x} that satisfies the FR vector, {FRs}, in the physical domain. Finally, DPs are mapped into the process domain by choosing process variables (PVs). {PVs} is also the characteristic vector in the process domain that satisfies {DPs}. This transformation process from the problem identification to the establishment of FRs, similarly from FRs to DPs, and

DPs to PVs embodies the design process discussed in this book. This process of design, which may be called the GPFDP (Goal-Problem-FR-DP-PV) transformation process, is universally applicable in all design activities. Therefore, as stated in Chap. 1, the Principle of Similitude of Systems applies to all systems. This chapter illustrates how these ideas for design have created new systems such as:

- new products;
- new technologies;
- new systems;
- ultra-precision machines such as a lithography machine;
- new organizations, including a government agency and venture firms, and
- strategies.

Design Story 3.1: Battleship Design and the Design of a Winning Battle Strategy

Throughout history, there were many wars between and among nations. Preparing for battles or trying to defend oneself from invaders, many countries invested enormous financial resources and devoted precious human capital to the military and armaments. As a by-product of the R&D investment in developing new weapons, many innovative technologies have been created throughout human history, especially since the 1940s.

The story described in this sub-section is based on a real story that happened in the sixteenth century. The goal of this storytelling is to illustrate rational thinking that led to innovative ship design, albeit for military purposes, as well as a winning military strategy.

Historically, neighboring nations often fought wars or had various conflicts. This story is about two neighboring nations geographically close to each other but separated by sea. One of these nations that had a more extensive population base invaded the other country several times during the past 500 years. One of these occurred in the mid-sixteenth century. The invading nation assembled a large fleet of naval ships and invaded its neighboring country. Notwithstanding a large fleet they deployed for the battle, they lost the war. Why?

The credit must be given to the commanding admiral of the smaller country, who led their smaller navy to victory, defeating a much more powerful navy with many more ships. The admiral had done two things right to win the battle: innovative ship design and the design of winning war strategy. Surprisingly, what he did was consistent with AD.

The commanding admiral of the smaller nation might have known several important things: (1) the invading navy would have a larger number of warships than he had; (2) the ships of the opposing navy would have a conventional streamlined hull shape designed for faster speed with the least amount of resistance; (3) these ships could not make sharp turns quickly because of the hull shape, and (4) it would take a long time to reload their guns after each shot.

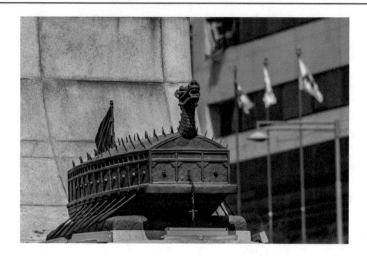

Fig. 3.1 Model ship with a flat bottom for ease of maneuver (i.e., turnaround) known as the turtle ship, the design of which is credited to Admiral Yi Sun-Sin. It was built around 1590. (Reproduced with permission from Papilionem 2019)

Based on these observations, the admiral designed a warship that had a flat bottom and iron deck, as shown in Fig. 3.1. These ships with a flat bottom, rather than a streamlined ship hull, could turn around quickly.

The admiral engaged his enemy's naval armada in the open sea. He then pretended as if his ships were retreating from the fight. He led his ships into a narrow strait where the water flowed fast due to the retreating tide. The invading navy chasing after these flat-bottomed ships had to line up in the strait because the channel width was too narrow to accommodate many ships.

When the ships reached a narrow section of the strait, the admiral engaged the invading navy in a fight by firing guns broadside of the invading ships, hitting vessels one at a time. As soon as the flat-bottomed ship fired its weapon, the ship was able to quickly turn around and then fire again, using the guns that had been pre-loaded. By keep rotating his naval ship and reloading the guns, they could sink the enemy vessels one by one. The ships of the opposing navy did not have quick maneuverability and the capability to rapidly fire.

Since the ships with flat bottom could turn around quickly and fire almost continuously, which the invading ships could not, they could demolish the other side. Thus, the invading naval ships suffered a major defeat.

The FRs for the admiral's fighting strategy might have been the following:

FR1 = Engage in fight with one enemy ship at a time;
FR2 = Quickly rotate the ship;
FR3 = Uninterrupted firing of guns (from both sides of the ship).

The DPs were:

DP1 = Narrow sections of the strait (where the current flow of water is fast due to large difference in high and low tides);
DP2 = Flat bottom ship (rather than the streamlined ship);
DP3 = Fast rotation of the ship.

The design of the ship is illustrated in Fig. 3.1.

It should be noted that the relationship between FRs and DPs can be represented by the following matrix (note: X indicates that there is a relationship between the FR and the DP):

	DP1	DP2	DP3
FR1	X	0	0
FR2	0	X	0
FR3	0	0	X

The design of the war strategy, including the ship design, was uncoupled. The warships with the flat bottom and the war strategy were the creation of the admiral.

The admiral defeated the invading navy and won the war, becoming a national hero to this day. However, soon after his triumph, his government put him in jail because some politicians spread unfavorable innuendos and rumors to protect their political positions and interest in the kingdom. Unfortunately, such injustice has occurred in too many countries.

Design Story 3.2: Student Enrollment in an Academic Department of a Well-Known University

Many land-grant colleges in engineering and technology were established at the end of the American Civil War around 1865. One of these universities became a leading university in the world. Initially, it had two engineering departments: civil engineering and mechanical engineering. Both departments became one of the highest ranked engineering departments in the world. In the late twentieth century, the mechanical engineering department had about 65 professors. Many of these professors were the leaders of their respective fields. However, many undergraduate students would not choose this department as their major field of study. They would go into other engineering fields such as electrical engineering and computer science. This low enrollment created a massive headache for the department chair. The professors' opinions had three different kinds of views, each with a different diagnosis of the problem. The faculty members of the department argued over this issue and tried many different things for three decades without a solution.

Then a new department head was appointed to lead the department. One of the first things he did was to identify the problems that were the barriers to attracting undergraduate students to the department. One of the issues identified was that the curriculum was not suited to deal with contemporary issues of the engineering field. It was the curriculum the professors went through when they were students 20 to 30 years ago. Students wanted to study the topics related to their era, but the curriculum was not flexible enough to accommodate their interest because there were too many required subjects that the professors thought were important based on their experience.

A new curriculum had to be developed to enable students to construct their personalized curriculum with a minimum set of required common subjects by identifying the FRs of the curriculum. One of the FRs was: "Allow flexibility in establishing students' academic programs." Having identified this FR, a new DP was introduced. The new DP was: allow students to construct an individualized curriculum, selecting 50% of their academic courses from any one of the six academic fields outside of their department, substantially reducing the number of required subjects of the old curriculum. To administer this new curriculum, a professor who had a multidisciplinary academic background became the professor in charge of this unique undergraduate educational program, i.e., (PVs). This change of the educational program increased the number of undergraduate students enrolled in the department by a factor three. The department became one of the most popular academic departments in the university.

3.2 Some Useful and Simple Corollaries and Theorems

As a result of the Independence Axiom and the Information Axiom,[1] we can state corollaries, and derive theorems, some of which are simple and yet useful to remember. Corollaries and theorems can be derived from the axioms. We will state them here. The readers of this chapter should strive to derive them based on the axioms. The definitions of corollary and theorems are as follows[2]:

Corollary:

1. a proposition inferred immediately from a proved proposition with little or no additional proof;
2. something that naturally follows from axioms or other propositions that have been proven;
3. something that incidentally or naturally accompanies or parallels;
4. some corollaries and axioms may be interchangeable.

---

[1]For those interested in knowing how the design axioms were created in 1976, see (Suh 1990, pp 17–22).
[2]"… it is useful to distinguish between theorems and corollaries in mathematics vs in design science. Mathematics, as natural science, states axioms, theorems, and corollaries in a descriptive manner. This is because the underlying field itself simply seeks to true statements on the natural world and its underlying world. In contrast, design science has a prescriptive nature. Its goal is to guide the designer with the guidance of what good design is. For that reason, in AD the axioms, theorems, and corollaries are stated in a prescriptive manner rather than a descriptive manner." (Farid and Suh 2016).

Theorem:

1. a formula, proposition, or statement in mathematics or logic deduced or to be deduced from other formulas or proposition;
2. an idea accepted or proposed a demonstrable truth often as a part of a general theory;
3. a theorem is valid if its referent axioms are valid.

Some corollaries of the Independence Axiom (i.e., maintain the independence of FRs) and the Information Axiom (i.e., minimize the information content) of AD are the following:

Corollary 1: (Decoupling of Coupled Design)

Decouple or separate parts or aspects of a design solution if FRs are coupled or become interdependent in the design proposed.

Corollary 2: (Minimization of FRs)

Minimize the number of FRs and constraints.

Corollary 3: (Integration of Physical Parts)

Integrate design features in a single physical part if FRs can be independently satisfied in a proposed solution to reduce the information content.

Corollary 4: (Use of Standardization)

Use standardized or interchangeable parts if the use of these parts is consistent with FRs and constraints.

Corollary 5: (Use of symmetry)

Use symmetrical shapes and/or components if they are consistent with the FRs and constraints.

Corollary 6: (Largest Tolerances)

Specify the largest allowable design range in stating FRs.

Corollary 7: (Uncoupled Design with Less Information)

Seek an uncoupled design that requires less information than coupled designs in satisfying a set of FRs.

There are many theorems, but only a limited number will be listed here.

Theorem 1: (Coupling Due to Insufficient Number of DPs)

When the number of DPs is less than the number of FR, either a coupled design results, or the FRs cannot be satisfied.

Theorem 2: (Decoupling of Coupled Design)

When a design is coupled due to the greater number of FRs than DPs, it may be decoupled by the addition of new DPs to make the number of FRs and DPs equal to each other, if a subset of the design matrix containing n x n elements constitutes a triangular matrix.

Theorem 3: (Redundant Design)

When there are more DPs than FRs, the design is either a redundant design or a coupled design.

Theorem 4: (Ideal Design)

In an Ideal Design, the number of DPs is equal to the number of FRs.

Theorem 5: (Need for New Design)

When a given set of FRs is changed by the addition of a new FR, or sub-
stitution of one of the FRs with a new one, or by selection of an entirely
different set of FRs, the design solution given by the original DPs cannot
satisfy the new set of FRs. Consequently, a new design solution must be
sought.

Theorem 6: (Path Independence of Uncoupled Design)

The information content of an uncoupled design is independent of the
sequence by which the DPs are changed to satisfy the given set of FRs.

Theorem 7: (Path Dependence of Coupled and Uncoupled Designs)

The information contents of coupled and decoupled designs depend on the
sequence by which the DPs are changed and on the specific paths of the
changes of these DPs.

There are many additional theorems, some of which are presented in the appendix
of this chapter.

These theorems and corollaries are important, because they guide the designer's
thoughts as they search for best or acceptable design. For instance, Theorem 4 states
that in an ideal design the number of FRs and DPs must be the same. This theorem
is simple and important to remember.

3.3   Lesson on "Design It Right, i.e., No Coupled Design!"

More frequently than we realize, many designers create coupled designs, thinking
that they can optimize it through modeling and optimization. Then, they try to make
the flawed design work through extensive analysis, modeling, "optimization,"
testing, and other means—wasting time, effort, and resources as well as damaging
their professional reputation. Their coupled design may even end up leading to
fatalities (e.g., airplanes plunging into the ground!). Those who do not understand
the design axioms may work hard, spend lots of money (often someone else's), and
end up creating a poorly functioning and unreliable product. Then, they produce a
lengthy and complicated instructional manual, hoping to minimize complaints from
those who end up buying the "broken" system. Advice: create an uncoupled design
from the beginning. If a coupled design is introduced inadvertently, identify the
coupling early and change the design to an uncoupled design! The following
example illustrates the importance of creating uncoupled or decoupled design:

Engineers and scientists at the Diamond Light Source of the United Kingdom
published an excellent paper on the importance of the Independence Axiom. They
decoupled a coupled design. In short, they first came out with a coupled design, and
then they analyzed it to optimize the system. However, the system optimized based
on their analysis failed! Later, they learned about AD, redesigned it to eliminate the
coupling of their FRs. It solved their problem! Their paper describes what they have

gone through for the benefit of others who make a system complicated by creating a coupled system, wasting time, money, and resources!

It should be noted that their problem is similar to designing a water faucet that will control temperature and the flow rate of water independently from each other! Often when a coupled design feature is found, the best thing to do is to develop a new design that is uncoupled rather than tweaking the system to make the flawed design work, which will not work well as long as the design is coupled. Their abstract reads as follows (Reproduced from Drakopoulos et al. (2015), originally published open access under a CC BY license: https://journals.iucr.org/s/issues/2015/03/00/ie5138/):

"I12 Joint Engineering, Environmental, and Processing (JEEP) is a high-energy imaging, diffraction and scattering beamline at Diamond. Its source is a superconducting wiggler with a power of approximately 9 kW at 500 mA after the fixed front-end aperture; two permanent filters aim at reducing the power in photons below the operating range of the beamline of 50–150 keV, which accounts for about two-thirds of the total. This paper focuses on the design and simulation process of the permanent secondary filter, a 4 mm thick SiC disk. The first version of the filter was vulnerable to cracking due to thermally induced stress. Therefore, a new filter based on an innovative concept was proposed: a water-cooled shaft rotates, via a ceramic interface, the SiC disk; the disk operates up to 900 $^\circ$C, and a copper absorber surrounding the filter dissipates the heat through radiation. We utilized analysis data following the failure of an initial prototype to model the heat flow using FEA successfully. This model informed different iterations of the re-design of the assembly, addressing the issues identified. The operational temperature of the final product matches within a few degrees Celsius the one predicted by the simulation."

The schematic of their optical and functional layout of the I12 JEEP beamline is shown in Fig. 3.2.

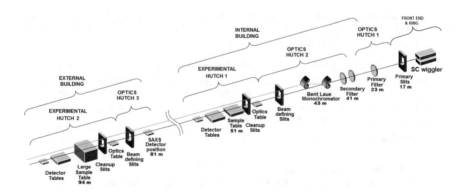

Fig. 3.2 Schematic optical and functional layout of the I12 JEEP beam line. (Reproduced from Drakopoulos et al. 2015, originally published open access under a CC BY license: https://journals.iucr.org/s/issues/2015/03/00/ie5138/)

Fig. 3.3 A round SiC disk is attached to a disk holder made of copper with circulating water. The round disk is positioned and attached to the copper holder with molybdenum interface material. Three FRs and two DPs is a coupled design since there are more FRs and DPs (a theorem). (Reproduced with permission from Tizzano et al. 2018)

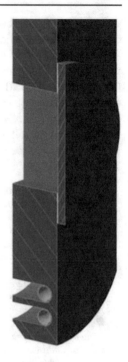

Design Issue: The purpose of the second filter is to reduce the power coming in from the primary filter from 6.2 to 2.6 kW. The filter made of a 4-mm-thick SiC disk (shown in Fig. 3.3) is attached to the Cu carrier with a molybdenum interface binder. There are three FRs for the secondary filter:

FR1 = Lower the power level from 62 to 2.6 kW;
FR2 = Transmit heat to cool the filter;
FR3 = Hold the SiC disk in place.

The original design made by engineers and scientists at the Diamond Light Source of the United Kingdom is shown in Fig. 3.3. The SiC disk is bonded with a molybdenum binder to the copper fixture, which is cooled by circulating water. The energy absorbed by the SiC disk (to reduce the power transmitted by 3.8 kW) is transmitted to a copper fixture by conduction to maintain its operating temperature low.

The DPs are as follows:

DP1 = Thickness of SiC disk;
DP2 = Heat conduction from SiC to the copper fixture through the molybdenum binder;
DP3 = Molybdenum Binder = DP2.

Since there are three FRs and only two DPs, we know that it is a coupled design, because the number of DP is less than the number of FRs (A theorem). The design matrix may be represented as:

	DP1	DP2
FR1	X	0
FR2	0	X
FR3	0	X

It is a coupled design because there is only one DP, i.e., the molybdenum binder, for two FRs, i.e., FR2 and FR3. As a result, both FR2 and FR3 were not satisfied, and the SiC disk cracked due to the temperature rise and thermal stress induced due to the differential expansion of the SiC disk and the copper holder. Before constructing the design shown in Fig. 3.2, the scientists and engineers performed extensive analysis and optimization to be sure that the design was going to work as intended. However, after the construction, they found that the designed system failed to satisfy FR2 and FR3.

Because they had cracking and other problems with the coupled design, they applied AD and came up with a new uncoupled design, which is shown in Fig. 3.4.

In this uncoupled design, SiC disk (shown in blue) is sandwiched between two copper disks (shown in brown, with copper tubing circulating water) to remove heat. Heat transfer occurs through the large surface area in contact between the SiC sandwiched between the two copper plates. The DPs are

DP1 = Thickness of SiC disk;
DP2 = Heat conduction from the SiC surface to copper plates on both surfaces of the SiC;
DP3 = Two copper plates bolted together.

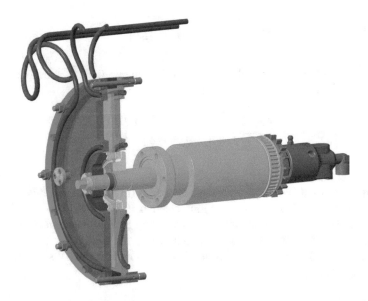

Fig. 3.4 New uncoupled design. SiC disk (shown in blue) is held in place by sandwiching the SiC disk between two copper plates (shown in brown), which are cooled by circulating water. (Reproduced with permission from Tizzano et al. 2018)

This is an uncoupled design, i.e., the design matrix is a diagonal matrix.

This design performed well. The lesson of this example is: if the design violates the Independence Axiom, the design is a flawed design that cannot be solved through optimization.

This design was later modified for ease of mounting the disk assembly and also to promote additional heat transfer through the rotating shaft (Papilionem 2019).

3.4 Mathematical Optimization and Design

It was stated that FRs is a vector, {FR}, and DPs is a vector, {DP}. What relates these two vectors is the design matrix [DM], which may be expressed as

$${FR} = [DM] {DP} \tag{3.1}$$

When there are two FRs, there should be two DPs, as per Theorem 4. The best design, i.e., an ideal design, then is the one where the FRs are independent from each other, i.e., the design with a diagonal matrix, i.e.,

$$FR1 = (A11)DP1$$
$$FR2 = (A22)DP2$$

$$\text{or} \quad {FR} = \begin{bmatrix} A11 & 0 \\ 0 & A22 \end{bmatrix} {DP} \tag{3.2}$$

If we design without the Independence Axiom in mind, the relationship between {FR} and {DP} may be stated as follows:

$$\begin{Bmatrix} FR1 \\ FR2 \end{Bmatrix} = \begin{bmatrix} A11 & A12 \\ A21 & A22 \end{bmatrix} \begin{Bmatrix} DP1 \\ DP2 \end{Bmatrix} \tag{3.3}$$

Equation (3.3) can be mathematically manipulated to make it a diagonal matrix, like Eq. (3.2), by determining characteristic values (in mathematics, it is referred to as "eigenvalues"). However, the resulting changes in DPs would be such that they could not be implemented physically. What a pity that the mathematical transformation cannot be applied in design! Otherwise, the designer's task would be straightforward. In design, we have to choose the right set of DPs to prevent the coupling of FRs.

Example 3.1

Suppose that FR1 and FR2 in Eq. (3.3) are given as 5 and 10, respectively. Furthermore, the proposed design yielded the following *diagonal* design matrix:

$$\begin{Bmatrix} FR1 \\ FR2 \end{Bmatrix} = \begin{bmatrix} 1 & 0 \\ 0 & 5 \end{bmatrix} \begin{Bmatrix} DP1 \\ DP2 \end{Bmatrix} \quad \text{(Note : This is an } uncoupled \ design.)$$

What should DP1 and DP2 be? The correct answers are DP1 = 5 and DP2 = 2. In this case, if FR1 is to be changed, the only thing we have to do is change DP1. FR1 and FR2 are independent from each other.

Now the design matrix for another design is a *triangular matrix* given as follows:

$$\begin{Bmatrix} FR1 \\ FR2 \end{Bmatrix} = \begin{bmatrix} 1 & 4 \\ 0 & 5 \end{bmatrix} \begin{Bmatrix} DP1 \\ DP2 \end{Bmatrix}$$

(Note: This design is called the *decoupled design, because the design matrix is a triangular matrix.*)

What should DP1 and DP2 be?

In this case of "decoupled design,"

$$FR1 = 5 = 1 \times DP1 + 4 \times DP2$$
$$FR2 = 10 = 5 \times DP2$$

DP2 must be determined first, which should be 2. And then we can determine DP1 as

$$DP1 = 5 - 8 = -3$$

Therefore, in this case of a *decoupled design*, we have to vary DPs in a proper sequence, i.e., we have to vary DP2 first and then determine DP1. As long as we follow this sequence, FR1 and FR2 are independent from each other.

Suppose now, the design matrix is a full matrix as given below:

$$\begin{Bmatrix} FR1 \\ FR2 \end{Bmatrix} = \begin{bmatrix} 1 & 4 \\ 3 & 5 \end{bmatrix} \begin{Bmatrix} DP1 \\ DP2 \end{Bmatrix}$$

In the above design, FR1 and FR2 are coupled to each other. If we change one of the DPs, it will affect both FRs, i.e., a coupled design. In this coupled design, there is only one set of DP1 and DP2 that will uniquely satisfy FR1 and FR2. Similarly, if one of the FRs is changed, both DPs must find a new design spot, i.e., change their values, to satisfy the new value of the FR. When DPs represent physical things, it becomes an enormous task to change them.

Example 3.2

The design that is easiest to implement is the one where all elements of the design matrix are zero, except A1, B2, C3, and D4, as shown below. In this case, we change D11 and

DP12 to satisfy FR11 and FR22, which are the children FRs of FR1, which enable us to satisfy FR1. This is an uncoupled design, which satisfies the Independence Axiom.

		DP1		DP2	
		DP11	DP12	DP21	DP22
FR1	FR11	*A1*	0	0	0
	FR12	0	*B2*	0	0
FR2	FR21	0	0	*C3*	0
	FR22	0	0	0	*D4*

Now, suppose that the design has two additional design elements, A4 and D1, as shown below. In this case, if we vary DP22 to satisfy FR2, FR1 also changes. Similarly, if DP11 is changed to satisfy FR1, FR2 also changes. This is a coupled design. This design should not be implemented.

		DP1		DP2	
		DP11	DP12	DP21	DP22
FR1	FR11	*A1*	0	0	*A4*
	FR12	0	*B2*	0	0
FR2	FR21	0	0	*C3*	0
	FR22	*D1*	0	0	*D4*

The above example is a straightforward design in that we had to decompose FRs and DPs only once. However, if Boeing 737 Max had many layers of decomposition and many of the off-diagonal design elements were non-zero elements. The pilot would have had difficult times to control the airplane if the pilot was not aware of the fact that a computer was controlling one of these elements independently of the pilot's command! That is why satisfying the Independence Axiom is essential. Unless we construct a master matrix of the entire design to trace all the design decisions made, it will be impossible to determine if the design is satisfactory. Many companies, instead of constructing the design matrix for the entire system, resort to the practice of developing products following the repetitious cycle of "design-build-test-redesign to correct mistakes-test" to develop their products. Such an approach to design and development is costly and unreliable.

In executing a sizeable complicated system design with many FRs, it will be necessary to appoint a "system architect," whose team constructs the entire design matrix and checks all the design decisions made by any member of the project team. When the system architect determines that a particular design decision made by one of the project teams has introduced the coupling of FRs, the architect should instruct the team that introduced coupling to develop another design that does not create such a coupled design.

Example 3.3

In the mathematical world, we can take any square matrix and determine its eigenvalues (i.e., characteristic values). However, in design, we cannot make a coupled design and manipulate it mathematically to find "characteristic values (i.e., eigenvalues)" to uncouple a coupled design. If we could discover eigenvalues in design through mathematical manipulation, any bad design can be made into a good design that satisfies the Independence Axiom, but unfortunately, in the design world, that cannot be done.

Suppose we have two FRs for a water faucet design: FR1 = control temperature, FR2 = control flow rate. If the design of the water faucet has a cold water valve and a hot water valve, we cannot independently satisfy FR1 and FR2 without changing two valves continuously to get the right temperature and the flow rate. This design is a coupled design with a full design matrix, i.e., DP1 affects both FR1 and FR2. Likewise, DP2 also affects both FR1 and FR2. Then, the design equation may be written as

$$\begin{Bmatrix} FR1 \\ FR2 \end{Bmatrix} = \begin{bmatrix} A11 & A12 \\ A21 & A22 \end{bmatrix} \begin{Bmatrix} DP1 \\ DP2 \end{Bmatrix}$$

The elements of the design matrix are non-zero elements.

In a pure mathematical world, the above equation may be transformed into

$$\begin{Bmatrix} FR1 \\ FR2 \end{Bmatrix} = \begin{bmatrix} A11 & A12 \\ A21 & A22 \end{bmatrix} \begin{Bmatrix} DP1 \\ DP2 \end{Bmatrix} = \begin{bmatrix} 1 & 0 \\ 0 & 1 \end{bmatrix} \begin{Bmatrix} DP1* \\ DP2* \end{Bmatrix}$$

where DP1* and DP2*, which are sometimes called the "characteristic values" or "eigenvalues."

For instance, we encounter this kind of transformation in applied mechanics. Stress σ_{ij} and strain ε_{ij} are second-order tensors. In the two-dimensional case where i and j vary from 1 to 2, σ_{ij} represents an ellipse with a major axis and a minor axis. Along with these principle directions, only the normal stress and strain are present with no shear components. However, a mathematical transformation cannot be done in the case of design to determine the characteristic values, because DP1* and DP2* represent something that does not have any physical significance. This difficulty of finding DPs that is physically meaningful is the reason why design is challenging, i.e., we have to choose the right DPs a priori based on our understanding of the "physical or the real" world to satisfy the Independence Axiom.

Similarly, the same comments apply to the software world. Many software companies have had problems that stem from their misunderstanding of this issue. Software developers know that coupling FRs create a spaghetti code, but they find that it is complicated to uncouple legacy codes because it is difficult to determine the logic behind the existing legacy codes.

The lesson of this example is simple and straightforward but important: satisfy the Independence Axiom by selecting a correct set of DPs to satisfy FRs from the beginning. In most cases, uncoupled design cannot be created through mathematical manipulations.

3.5   Design of Technological Products

"The purpose of this section is to illustrate that even a system that appears to be complicated or complex can be designed by following the process used to design a simple system such as the water faucet. We have to use a systematic process to check for the coupling of FRs because as the number of FRs and the number of the layer of decomposition increase, the probability of creating coupled design increases."

Many companies, university researchers, individual inventors, and government laboratories design and develop new technologies. Anyone with some science and engineering background can create new technologies. The person(s) should identify the problem(s) in the customer domain, be able to transform the problem into a set of FRs, and then select appropriate DPs to create a system that fulfills the FRs. Then, they have to deal with PVs such as investment and personnel. In this section, two examples will be presented to show how new technologies can be designed and created.

3.5.1   Design of Easy Open Beverage Can

Bauxite is the raw material that is used to produce aluminum through an electrolytic process of separating aluminum atoms from oxygen atoms, which is an energy-intensive process. The cost of electricity is the most significant contributor to the manufacturing cost of aluminum. The largest fraction of aluminum produced worldwide, i.e., about 60% of the aluminum produced worldwide, is used to make beverage cans. The rest is used to manufacture airplanes, buildings, and the like. Although they tried, it has not yet penetrated the automobile market. 70% of an aluminum can is recycled.

A manufacturer of aluminum beverage can has continued to reduce the amount of aluminum used to make a can to be able to compete with cheaper materials such as steel and plastics. Aluminum is the most expensive material among the three. The ability to make a thin-walled can cheaply enable the aluminum industry to dominate the beverage can business. The aluminum ingot is made to a thin sheet, from which a disk is punched out, which is then deep drawn into a thin-walled cylindrical tube with a bottom. Then, the top of the cylinder is rolled to reduce its diameter. The top of the can is made separately, which is then attached to the main body.

An aluminum beverage can with an easy-open tab is shown in Fig. 3.5. What are the FRs of this can? What are the constraints? Why is the top of the can narrower than the rest of the body? Why is the bottom of most aluminum cans not flat but rather concaved-in?

The major constraints are relatively easy to identify:

Constraint 1 = Minimize the overall cost of manufacturing;
Constraint 2 = Use a minimum amount of aluminum;
Constraint 3 = Allow recycling of used aluminum.

The FRs of an aluminum beverage can are more challenging to identify because the geometry does not reveal all the FRs. The FRs for the easy opening can appear to be the following:

Fig. 3.5 Aluminum beverage
can. (Reproduced with
permission from Gossip 2019)

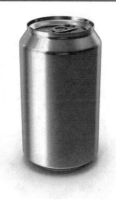

FR1 = Contain the radial internal pressure of 30psi;

FR2 = Allow easy opening of the can;

FR3 = Allow easy stacking of the can;

FR4 = Coat the inside of the can to prevent the beverage
    acquire the taste of aluminum;

FR5 = Allow printing on the outside of the can;

FR6 = Make the diameter of the top of the can as small
    as practical to minimize the consumption of aluminum;   (3.4)

FR7 = Make the bottom of the can to be concave in to contain the pressure;

FR8 = Enable stacking of cans on top of each other;

FR9 = Contain the pressure at the bottom of the can;

FR10 = Contain the pressure acting on the lid;

FR11 = Attach the tab for ease of opening the can;

FR12 = Join the lid to the body of the can.

Exercise 3.1:

An engineer of a major aluminum producer attended a special program for engineers in the industry on AD at a university. During one of the discussions, he stated that the beverage can satisfies 12 FRs. However, he realized that the company was struggling with its product because he could only identify 11 DPs. While attending the class, he figured out what the missing DP was and thus was able to develop an uncoupled design. Assuming that the above 12 FRs are what he had identified as FRs, what are the 12 DPs? Does the can satisfy the Independence Axiom?

3.5.2   Removal of Kidney Stone with a Robot

Some people suffer severe flank and lower back pain because of kidney stones, which are hard deposits of minerals and salt that stick together in the kidney, or the urinary tract. Some stones are small being in the order of 5 mm or less, which

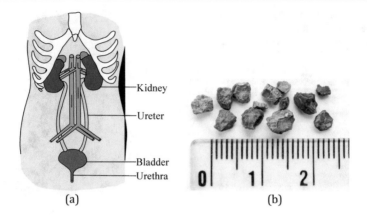

Fig. 3.6 a A schematic drawing of kidneys, bladder, and ureter in the human body. (Reproduced from NIH: National Cancer Institute 2009.) **b** Kidney stones (Reproduced with permission from Lorne 2019)

generally pass through the urinary system by themselves, but they can be much larger, several stones filling the entire kidney (see Fig. 3.6). The common symptoms are severe back and flank pain, stomachache, blood in the urine, and nausea or vomiting. A well-known technique of removing the stone is to use the ultrasound to crush the stone and then let the urine to carry the stone out of the kidney or the urinary tract.

A well-known professor in the field of robotics at a leading science and technology university in the world decided to develop a robotics technology to solve the kidney stone problem. His technique worked so well that he decided to establish a new venture firm with his former students to commercialize his technology. He raised the initial capital in his country to start the business. He and his team visited major hospitals, venture capitalists, and major universities in many countries to show-tell his technology. His patented technology combines vision to identify the stone in the kidney or the urinary tract with a mechanical means of transporting the stone out of the patient. It also can crush the stone in the kidney. In some cases, the robot can grab the stone in the kidney and transport it out of the patient. Before inserting the robot through the ureter (the duct that connects the kidney to the bladder and finally urethra, a soft lining tube may be inserted through the ureter.

Without knowing how the professor initially designed his surgical robot for kidney stone removal, we may attempt to create it based on the teachings of AD and using the information he verbally explained what his robot does over a lunch in Boston, Massachusetts, U.S.A., during his visit to the Massachusetts General Hospital (MGH) and a high-tech company. The benefit we have is that we know what he designed and made, although we have not seen the actual robot and do not know the detailed design of the robot.

The goal of the design is clear: remove kidney stones from human beings. The overall constraint is that it has to be safe, i.e., extremely safe. The FRs, for this robot may be stated as follows:

FR1 = Flexible robot that can be inserted into the kidney through ureter and urethra;
FR2 = Protect the lining of ureter and urethra;
FR3 = Provide camera at the end of the robot;
FR4 = Attach a clamp mechanism at the end of the robot to grab the stones;
FR5 = Transmit mechanical means of manipulating the clamp mechanism;
FR6 = Provide light to capture the image.

Now we have to come up with DPs to satisfy the above FRs. Conceptually, we can visualize many different physical configurations. For example, a robot made of a soft-flexible and corrugated "long tube," in which electric wiring is placed for LED lighting in the kidney and to control the end effector (e.g., a mechanical suction device that sucks in the stone into the tube and transport to outside), the illuminating light at the head of the robot, a camera that can see the inside of kidney, the mechanism that sucks the stones into the tube, and the means of pressurizing/de-pressurizing the corrugated tube to insert the tube into kidney. The robot can "crawl" toward the kidney through cyclic pressurization of the soft, flexible, corrugated tube. The tube can stretch and move forward slowly when pressurized. When the tube is de-pressurized, the tube will stay stationary. By repeating the pressurization cycle, it may reach the kidney. Another possible insertion method may be to put a flexible but stiff wire in the tube and push the front end of the tube.

Exercise 3.2:

Based on the above description of the robot, define DPs that can satisfy the six FRs stated above.

3.5.3   Ash Tray in Automobiles

About four or five decades ago, smoking of cigarettes was prevalent among people, especially young people. Therefore, passenger cars had to have an ashtray in the dashboard of a vehicle. What would be a useful design feature? What FRs should the ashtray satisfy?

Suppose that we want to make it convenient for the driver to use the ashtray by letting it pop out of its stored position when the front of the ashtray is pushed in slightly to unlock it. To lock it in, the driver pushes it about a halfway then the ashtray is pulled into the locked position. Then, when the driver wants to use it again, the driver pushes it in slightly to have the ashtray pop out of the closed position to its open position. For an ashtray that can perform these two functions, what should be the FRs? We may state them as follows:

FR1 = Push in the front of the ashtray (that is in a locked position) to have it unlocked and pop out to the fully open position;

FR2 = Push in the front of the ashtray in its open position about halfway to move it into move into its closed and locked position.

The corresponding DPs are

DP1 = Unlocking mechanisms;
DP2 = Locking-in mechanisms.

The design matrix is diagonal, indicating that it is an uncoupled design. FR1 and FR2 should be decomposed since we need to have more detailed designs for DP1 and DP2 to be able to implement it.

FR1 and FR2 may be decomposed as

FR11 = Unlock the ashtray from its locked position;
FR12 = Push the ashtray out when activated;
FR21 = Pull the ashtray in and lock it when it is pushed in toward the closed position;
FR22 = Lock the ashtray in the closed position.

The decomposed DPs, the corresponding FR11 and FR11, FR21, and FR22, may be chosen as follows:

DP11 = Unlocking mechanism (release cam);
DP12 = Stiff spring (which releases the stored energy);
DP21 = Locking mechanism (locking cam);
DP22 = Compression of a soft spring.

The actual mechanism is sketched in Fig. 3.7.

The design matrix for this design is given below. It has a diagonal matrix, indicating that the design is an uncoupled design. In this design, one DP satisfies a specific FR and no other FRs, thus satisfying the Independence Axiom. In an uncoupled design, each FR is independent of other FRs. This is an essential characteristic of the uncoupled design.

		DP1		DP2	
		DP11	DP12	DP21	DP22
FR1	FR11	X	0	0	0
	FR12	0	X	0	0
FR2	FR21	0	0	X	0
	FR22	0	0	0	X

$$(3.5)$$

In the above design matrix, X indicates that there is a relationship between FR and DP. For instance, DP11 affects FR11 only. This design matrix demonstrates that we have an uncoupled design, which is acceptable as per the Independence Axiom.

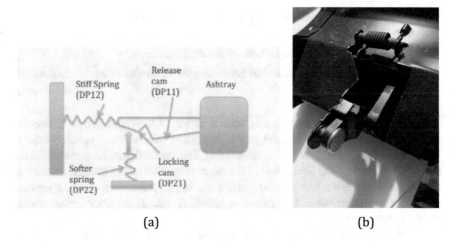

Fig. 3.7 **a** Sketch of an ashtray design; **b** Photograph of an automobile ashtray with coil spring rather than a linear spring sketched in (**a**). In this commercial product, the linear spring is replaced by coil springs to make the product more compact

3.5.4 Design of a Collapsible Steering Column for Automobiles

Automobiles use steering systems that turn the front wheels to change the direction of the vehicle motion. There are many commercial steering systems with different designs, ranging from simple mechanical systems to power-assisted steering systems. Power-assisted systems use either electric or hydraulic power. The price of steering systems varies over a wide range, as much as by order of magnitude. We will illustrate the design process by considering the design of a simple steering column of an automobile.

The steering column must transmit the rotational motion of the steering wheel at the command of the driver. It must also protect the driver in the event of a frontal collision of the vehicle. When the car comes to a sudden stop due to the frontal impact, the driver's chest may hit the steering wheel of the vehicle due to the forward inertia of the body. The goal of the design is to protect the driver by making the steering column collapse when the impact occurs. At the same time, the column must be strong and stiff enough to allow the regular operation of the vehicle.

The {FRs} of a simple steering column are

FR1 = Transmit steering motion by the driver to the front wheel;

FR2 = Collapse the steering column to protect the driver in a frontal collision;

FR3 = Absorb energy during the collapse of the steering column;

FR4 = Allow the telescoping motion of the steering column adjust to the drivers position.

$$(3.6)$$

A rough sketch of the design is shown in Fig. 3.8, which shows a steering column that consists of two steel tubes. A portion of a smaller metallic tube is inserted tightly inside a larger metallic tube. The serrated interface transmits the rotational motion of the inner tube to the outer tube. The larger tube is attached to the car body through a bracket that holds a bearing in place to allow the rotational motion of the outer tube. The two-tube assembly rotates together under normal steering operations. When a major frontal collision occurs, the smaller tube inside the larger tube slides down inside the large tube, plastically deforming the narrowed down section of the larger tube, and thus dissipating energy to protect the driver as the chest of the driver slams down the steering wheel. The steering wheel position is fixed by attaching the inner tube to the inside hole of a bearing. A steel bracket that holds the inner tube is attached to the car body. To telescope the steering wheel, the bolt that holds the steel bracket to the car body is loosened to allow the inner tube to move in and out of the larger tube.

The DPs corresponding to FRs are as follows:

DP1 = Serrated interface between the inner tube and outer tube (to transmit the rotational motion of the inner tube to the outer tube, allowing relative axial movement);

DP2 = Pin attached to the outer tube that breaks when the inner tube is pushed down under high force (when the drivers body hits the steering wheel and pushing the inner tube downward);

DP3 = The narrow section of the outer tube (which absorbs energy as the inner tube attached to the steering wheel is pushed down during frontal impact, which deforms the outer tube plastically deforming it and dissipating energy);

DP4 = A journal bearing (the inner hole of which is attached to the inner tube of the steering column) and the outside is attached to another tube that is attached to the car body through a bolt and an elongated hole, which allows telescoping of the steering wheel to adjust its position to match the drivers height.

$$(3.7)$$

The design matrix for the design is as follows:

	DP1	DP2	DP3	DP4
FR1	X	0	0	0
FR2	0	X	0	0
FR3	0	x	X	0
FR4	0	0	0	X

$$(3.8)$$

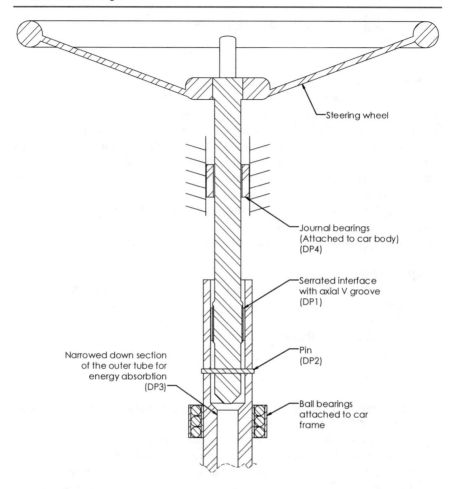

Fig. 3.8 A schematic drawing of the collapsible steering column. It consists of two tubes: the inner tube is connected to the steering wheel at one end and the other end of the inner tube is inside an outer tube. A shearable pin connects the inner tube and the outer tube. The inner tube and the inside surface of the outer tube are serrated, which prevents the slippage while transmitting the rotational motion. The other end of the outer tube is connected to the front wheels through a steering mechanism (not shown). The inside diameter of the outer tube narrows down. During the collision, the smaller tube is pushed down, breaking the pin, and, as it is pushed down inside the outer tube, the plastic deformation of the outer tube absorbs the impact energy

The design matrix is triangular, indicating that it is a decoupled design. The pin that holds the outer tube to the inner tube absorbs a small amount of energy when it breaks due when the chest of the driver hits the steering wheel upon impact. It is an uncoupled design.

3.5.5 Design of a Technology that Reduces Material Consumption

Problem

One of the well-known manufacturers in the United States uses several freight-car loads of plastics to make a variety of their products every day. They surmised that if they can reduce their plastic consumption by 10% in making their products, it would have a significant impact on the profitability of their products. Many of their products are injection-molded or extruded thermoplastics. The constraints are the following: the product shape cannot change from those currently manufactured, the toughness of their product must remain the same to prevent cracking of the parts when they are dropped, and the production rate must be competitive. In other words, the product shape cannot change, and yet it must use less material with similar mechanical properties. How should we proceed?

Design Solution:

Based on the description of the problem given above, we have to be able to define FRs. They may be stated as follows:

FR1 = Reduce material consumption;

FR2 = Maintain mechanical properties within an acceptable range; (3.9)

FR3 = Keep the geometric shape the same as the currently produced parts.

Now we have to come up with DPs that can satisfy the FRs. What DPs would you choose to satisfy the above three FRs?

To select good DPs that will create innovative products, it is useful to know about other related disciplines. Sometimes, the designer may read reference books; go into Google for information; ask friends, co-workers, and colleagues for suggestions; and most important of all, "think" of fundamental principles, one has learned in science and engineering.

One possible set of DPs may be selected as shown below:

DP1 = Plastic parts with a plethora of tiny bubbles;

DP2 = Bubble size; (3.10)

DP3 = Injection molding process.

The rationale for choosing the above set of DPs is as follows: (1) By introducing a large number of tiny bubbles, voids take up space, thus using less material. (2) When the bubble diameter is less than a critical size, its toughness is not negatively affected, because they may arrest cracks, and therefore the material may even be tougher than the solid plastic parts. (3) By using a conventional injection molding process, we can keep the geometric shape the same. This kind of material has been invented at a university and currently used in industry worldwide to make automotive parts. The tiny bubbles of about 20 microns in diameter are introduced dissolving CO_2 in molten polymer and suddenly releasing the pressure to nucleate tiny bubbles.[3]

The design matrix for this material that is commercially known as microcellular plastics is shown in the following:

	DP1	DP2	DP3
FR1	X	X	X
FR2	0	X	x
FR3	0	0	X

$$(3.11)$$

The above matrix given by Eq. (3.11) indicates that it is a decoupled design, and thus this design does not violate the Independence Axiom if we follow the sequence given above to FRs, i.e., change DP1 first; then DP2; and finally DP3 to change FR1, FR2, and FR3 independently from each other.

Figure 3.9 shows the cross section of a microcellular plastic. It has about 10^9 bubbles per cubic centimeter. The bubble size is about 10 to 30 microns. It is currently produced by extrusion of plastics or by injection molding.

Exercise 3.3:

Develop ideas as to how we can put in about one billion bubbles of 10 microns per cc of plastics on a mass production basis using either by extrusion or by injection molding processes.

3.5.6 Wireless Electric Power Transmission System to a Bus in Motion

Problem

Suppose that your university has decided to replace the diesel buses from your campus with electric buses to reduce CO_2 emission and help in solving the global warming problem.[4]

---

[3]See the review article: "Microcelluar Plastics" at Wong et al. (2016).

[4]One of the significant issues of the twenty-first century is global warming. According to IPCC, we must keep the temperature rise of the earth to below 2C relative to its temperature at the time of the Industrial Revolution. One of the major causes of weather change is the accumulation of anthropogenic generation of CO_2. We must reduce the CO_2 emission to prevent the weather change, which is the primary cause for the rise of sea level, forest fire, preservation of agriculture, and many other calamities. Roughly, 27% of CO_2 is generated by internal combustion (IC) engines, and about 33% by coal-burning electric power plants. To reduce the CO_2 emission by automobiles that are powered by IC engines, we need to replace it with electric vehicles, which will reduce anthropogenic emission of CO_2 by nearly a half. After considering the vast consumption of lithium needed if lithium batteries power all the cars, we decided to employ electric vehicles that receive electrical power wirelessly from external electrical power sources embedded under the ground.

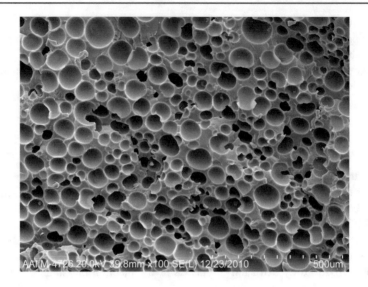

Fig. 3.9 Cross section of microcellular plastics. (Reproduced with permission from the Trexel Corporation)

Design Solution:

After considering all the factors involved in the electrification of the transportation system, it was decided that the best option is to use the wireless transmission of electric power from an underground power supply system to the bus either in motion or stationary. A proposed design idea was to install the power supply system underground just below the road pavement and transmit the electric power to moving buses while the vehicle is on the top of the power supply system beneath the road. We need to transmit about 100 kW of power to the bus over a distance of over 20 cm. Since such a wireless electric bus system is not commercially available, it was decided to design the system as a university research and development (R&D) project. The bus will have a small lithium–ion rechargeable battery onboard for limited mobility even when the bus is on the road without the underground power supply system. Our job is to design such a system that is robust, reliable, and low cost.

There are many FRs that such a transportation system must satisfy to work well as shown in Eq. 3.9.

FR1 = Propel the vehicle with electric power;

FR2 = Transfer electricity from an underground electric cable to the vehicle;

FR3 = Steer the vehicle;

FR4 = Brake the vehicle;

FR5 = Reverse the direction of motion;

FR6 = Change the vehicle speed;

FR7 = Provide electric power when there is no external electric power supply;

FR8 = Supply electric power to the underground cable.

$$(3.12)$$

The constraints the final design should not violate are

C1 = Safety regulations governing electric systems;

C2 = Price of OLEV (should be competitive with cars with IC engines);

C3 = No emission of greenhouse gases;

C4 = Long–term durability and reliability of the system;

C5 = Vehicle regulations for space clearance between the road and the vehicle.

$$(3.13)$$

The DPs chosen to satisfy the highest level FRs given by Eq. (3.12) are as follows:

DP1 = Electric motor;

DP2 = Wireless power transfer system;

DP3 = Mechanical steering system;

DP4 = Hydraulic braking system;

DP5 = Electric polarity;

DP6 = Motor drive;

DP7 = Rechargeable battery;

DP8 = Electric power supply system.

$$(3.14)$$

The relationship between {FRs} and {DPs} is given by

$$\{FRs\} = [DM]\,\{DPs\} \qquad (3.15)$$

For the eight FRs and DPs chosen for OLEV, the design matrix [DM] is given in Eq. (3.16) by checking whether or not a given DP affects the specific FR:

	DP1	DP2	DP3	DP4	DP5	DP6	DP7	DP8
FR1	X	X	0	0	0	X	X	X
FR2	0	X	0	0	0	0	0	X
FR3	0	0	X	0	0	0	0	0
FR4	0	0	0	X	0	0	0	0
FR5	0	0	0	0	X	0	0	0
FR6	0	0	0	0	0	X	X	0
FR7	0	0	0	0	0	0	X	0
FR8	0	0	0	0	0	0	0	X

$$(3.16)$$

Design Matrix [DM] for the OLEV.

As mentioned before, X indicates that an FR is affected by a DP. For example, DP2 affects FR1 in the design represented by Eq. (3.16).

Our part of the project is to design the wireless power transmission system from an underground power supply system to moving or stationary buses, i.e., FR2. Other FRs for moving buses can be satisfied using existing technologies.

Decomposition of FR2 and DP2:

At the time this project was undertaken, there was no existing technology for FR2 (transfer electricity from an underground electric cable to the vehicle) and DP2 (wireless power transfer system). Therefore, we have to design a new system that can transmit heavy electric power (>100 kW) over a considerable distance (~25 cm) by identifying children of FR2 and DP2 through the decomposition of FR2 and DP2.

In physics, we learned that when electric current flows through conducting wire, a magnetic field is created around the wire. Conversely, if we wrap copper wire around a rod made of ferromagnetic material (e.g., a ferrite) with high permeability and send an electric current through the electric coil surrounding the ferrite core, a magnetic field is created in the rod. One end of the rod becomes the "north (N) pole" and the other end becomes the "south (S) pole" just like the North pole and South pole of the earth's magnetic field. Between the N pole and the S pole, we create a magnetic field, emanating from one pole and terminating at the other pole as shown below for a U-shaped ferrite core as shown in Fig. 3.10. By using alternating current in the coil, we generate an oscillating magnetic field above the ground. If we then catch the alternating magnetic field at the bottom of the bus, we can transfer the power wirelessly if we capture the magnetic field energy and can generate electric power on the bus.

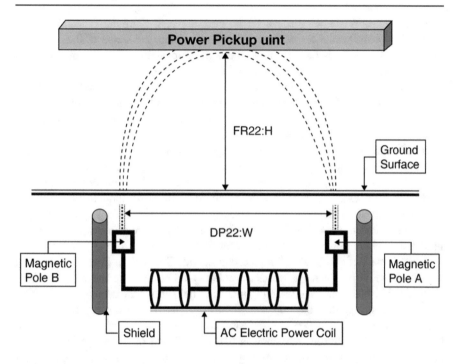

Fig. 3.10 Design of the wireless electric power transfer system based on "Shaped Magnetic Field in Resonance" (SMFIR) principle

We may decompose FR2 into second-level FR2s as follows:

FR21 = Create an alternating magnetic field above the ground;

FR22 = Control the shape of the magnetic field;

FR23 = Control the power level of the magnetic field;

FR24 = Pick up the energy of the magnetic field by the vehicle;   (3.17)

FR25 = Confine the electromagnetic waves between the vehicle and the
        underground power supply system (shielding of EMF);

FR26 = Deliver the electricpower to the vehicle while it is in motion.

Figure 3.10 shows the magnetic field outside of the electromagnet with a ferrite core with high permeability. It illustrates the concept of sending power over a distance H wirelessly. First, a two-dimensional oscillating magnetic field is created above ground by sending oscillating electric current around a ferrite core of the underground power supply system. The distance between the magnetic poles W determines the magnetic field shape above the ground. The greater the distance, the higher is the reach of the magnetic field. Once the field shape is determined, the field strength can be adjusted by controlling the electric power that generates the magnetic field. When we place a ferrite core above the ground (attached to the vehicle) opposite to the ferrite core below the surface, the shape of the magnetic field above the ground changes due to the high permeability of the ferrite core, i.e., more magnetic field permeates through the ferrite core above the ground. The oscillating magnetic field energy in the ferrite core is then captured by a set of electric conductors "wrapped around" the ferrite core of the power pickup system attached to the vehicle. Because the power pickup system is tuned to have the same natural frequency as the power supply system below the ground, the magnetic field forms a continuous loop from the power supply system to the power pickup system because they are in resonance. Note that the power transfer efficiency is maximum only when the power pickup system is in resonance with the underground power supply system. Only at resonance, a continuous magnetic loop is created from Magnetic Pole A to Magnetic Pole B through the top power pickup system without interference and a phase lag. We tune the system by varying the capacitance and inductance of the power pickup unit on the bus.

For the magnetic field to reach a certain height, H (FR22 in Fig. 3.10), we can adjust the width between the magnetic poles W (DP22). If we use an alternating electric field to generate an alternating magnetic field above the ground, we can pick it up by using a conducting coil attached to the bus. The frequency is chosen to maximize the electric power transmission at a minimum energy loss during the transmission. The chosen frequency is between 20 and 60 kHertz, because, at a higher frequency, the loss of power may be too significant. This technology, which was developed at KAIST, is named SMFIR (shaped magnetic field in resonance).

DP2 was decomposed into second-level DPs as follows:

> DP21 = Electromagnet design—ferrite core inside electric field;
> DP22 = Distance between magnetic poles (W);
> DP23 = Amplitude of the electric current that generates the magnetic field around the underground ferrite core;
> DP24 = Resonating magnetic energy pickup unit on the vehicle;
> DP25 = (Passive or active) shield for stray electromagnetic field;
> DP26 = Two-dimensional magnetic field that does not vary along the direction of vehicle motion.

DP2 was decomposed into second-level DPs as follows:

DP21 = Electromagnet design − ferrite core inside electric field;

DP22 = Distance between magnetic poles(W);

DP23 = Amplitude of the electric current that generates the magnetic field
around the underground ferrite core;

DP24 = Resonating magnetic energy pickup unit on the vehicle;

DP25 = (Passive or active)shield for stray electromagnetic field;

DP26 = Two-dimensional magnetic field that does not vary along
the direction of vehicle motion.

$$(3.18)$$

The constraints that the design could not violate were

C1 = Maximum allowable EMF level : 62.5 mGauss;

C2 = Maximum weight of the pickup unit;

C3 = Electric shock resistance of the system;

C4 = Temperature rise should not exceed 20 degrees Celsius;

C5 = High magnetic permeability of the core material m;

C6 = Minimize power loss.

$$(3.19)$$

The design matrix for FR2s and DP2s is given in Eq. (3.20).

	DP23	DP21	DP26	DP24	DP25	DP22
FR23	X	0	0	0	0	0
FR21	X	X	0	0	0	0
FR26	0	X	X	0	0	0
FR24	0	0	0	X	0	0
FR25	0	0	0	0	X	0
FR22	0	0	0	0	0	X

Second-level Design Matrix for OLEV

$$(3.20)$$

The design at the second level of FR2 and DP2 is a decoupled design. Therefore, DPs must be varied in the specific sequence specified in Eq. (3.20), i.e., DP23 should be set first to satisfy FR23 before setting the value of DP21 to satisfy FR21. Figure 3.11 shows the schematic arrangement of the SMFIR design that is given by the design matrix.

To satisfy FR21 (create an alternating magnetic field above the ground), DP21 (electromagnet design—ferrite core inside the electric field) is the ratio W/H, which must be much larger than 1, i.e., W/H > > 1. FR25, the shielding of EMF, can be satisfied by either reactive or passive shielding. Passive shielding would consist of placing a barrier in the ground and grounding the EMF picked up around the receiving unit; reactive shielding would include generating a signal that is opposite to the EMF emanating from the receiver unit.

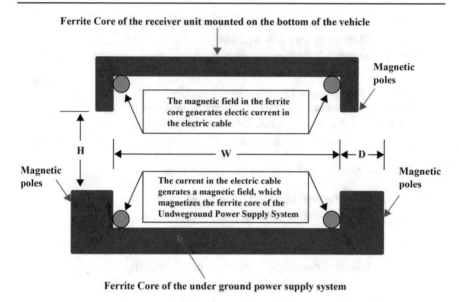

Fig. 3.11 Schematic design of SMFIR. To have the strongest field extend from the underground magnetic pole to the pole of the pickup unit on the vehicle (FR21), L should be much larger than H. Having the electric current flow perpendicularly to the ferrite cores (parallel to the direction of motion of the vehicle) satisfies FR26

The actual physical arrangement of the electric coil is shown through which the current flows to generate the magnetic field in the ferrite core by aligning magnetic domains. Because the ferrite core has low magnetic permeability, the magnetic field is concentrated in the core. One end of the core becomes the S pole and the other becomes the N pole. Since the electric current that flows in the cable is alternating current (AC), the magnetic field above the ground also oscillates. The magnetic poles alternate between N and S. To create a magnetic field that is strongest above the ground, pointing toward the vehicle rather than directed toward the magnetic poles, the distance H from the magnetic pole in the ground to the poles of the pickup unit on the vehicle should be smaller than the distance W between the magnetic poles of the underground power supply system (see Figs. 3.10 and 3.11).

The frequency of the field must be carefully chosen. It should be high enough to reach the necessary height and low enough to minimize loss of energy in the conductors and ferrite core. The initial frequency chosen was 20 kHz. The wire for electric current in the underground cable has to be Litz wire, which is a type of cable used in electronics to carry alternating current at frequencies up to about 1 MHz, to reduce the skin effect and proximity effect losses in conductors. For high-speed trains, the chosen frequency was 60 kHz. The advantages of using 60 kHz are as follows: if the current of the embedded power line is maintained the same as for the 20 kHz case, the cost and weight of the power pickup system can be reduced by about 1/2 of the 20 kHz design, because the induced voltage will increase by three times. On the other hand, if the induced voltage of the power pickup system is the same as the 20 kHz case, the cost and weight of inverter and embedded power cable can be decreased by about 1/2 because the current of the inverter and embedded power cable decreases by 1/3.

SMFIR is unique in its transmission of electric power to moving vehicles, i.e., FR26. This feature is achieved by creating a two-dimensional magnetic field (DP26) that is not a function of the direction of vehicle motion, i.e., the magnetic field generated is a two-dimensional planar field perpendicular to the vehicle's direction. Therefore, the pickup unit mounted on the vehicle sees the same magnetic field while the vehicle is moving, independent of the vehicle's position along the direction of motion, and the vehicle's motion does not affect power transfer and its efficiency. Thus, OLEV receives electric power while in motion or stationary. Furthermore, the height of the magnetic field is controlled by placing magnetic poles at a pre-determined distance apart.

The power transfer efficiency of SMFIR decreases when the magnetic poles of the receiver unit mounted on the bottom of the vehicle are not aligned with the poles of the underground power supply system. However, because these poles are far apart (~ 25 cm), the transmission efficiency is not too sensitive to slight misalignment, unlike the magnetic induction between two circular rings.

Many wireless power transfer systems use circular coils for both the transmitter and the receiver, which requires that the centers of two coils are well aligned, and the coils close together for maximum power transfer. Such a device can be used only when a vehicle is stationary. FR24 (pick up the energy of the magnetic field by the vehicle) and DP24 (resonating magnetic energy pickup unit on the vehicle) must be decomposed to the next level to define the lower level FR24s and DP24s. One way to decompose the FR24s is

> FR241 = Control the impedance of the pickup coil to that of the incoming magnetic field;
> FR242 = Control the natural frequency of the pickup coil to match that of the magnetic field;
> FR243 = Control the temperature of the pickup coil within an acceptable range;
> FR244 = Control the flow path of the magnetic field.

DPs must be selected to satisfy these FRs. Since the pickup unit must be designed using a coil and ferrite core, it can be characterized as an RLC circuit built inside a ferrite core. We can choose capacitance to satisfy FR241, inductance to satisfy FR242, a convective air channel for FR243, and a shaped ferrite core for FR244. Many physical configurations are possible, all variations on this basic idea. There are also many constraints at this level of design that cannot be violated. The details of these design issues are discussed in detail in subsequent chapters.

3.5.7 Design of Ultra-Precision Lithography Machine

One of the most advanced technologiesis the lithography machine that prints electric circuits (e.g., transistors) on semiconductor chips, either silicon-based or gallium arsenide III–V semiconductors. Commercially, many of the current lithography equipment use a 193 nm UV light source. Lithography machines that use UV lights can print billions of transistors on postage-stamp-size silicon. The density of these transistors is so high that the storage density of memory space and the speed of computation are no longer the limiting factor in many applications. Also, transistors with dimensions as small as 5 to 7 nm can be printed on semiconductors, using EUV (extreme ultraviolet) light source with a wavelength of 13.5 nm. A commercial machine is shown in Fig. 3.12. These machines are so precise that everything used in these lithography machines must be extremely accurate. It is difficult to measure the curvature of lenses and alignment of all components, etc., used in lithography because of the ultra-precision required. The light source must have a short wavelength to be able to make the critical dimensions of the line width of the circuit as narrow as possible. Now the preferred technique is to use EUV (extreme ultraviolet) as the light source, which eliminates the need for multiple deposition/etch processes and multiple masks.[5] The ambient air in these fabrication facilities in which these lithography machines are operated must be almost particle-free. Also, to increase productivity, the power of light source matters. The industry has been trying to increase the brightness of EUV to 250 watts.

To increase productivity, the components in these lithography machines must move at very high speeds. For instance, the silicon wafer must be loaded on a platen by a robot, and then the platen moves the wafer at high speeds to the location where the wafer will be subjected to UV light to make the circuit. The platen must attain a top speed from a stationary position. As given by Newton's second law, when the platen and associated components are accelerated very fast, it involves large forces. These forces make the machine vibrate, which may affect these precision lithography machines.

Exercise 3.4:

Consider a platen attached to a linear electric motor, on which a silicon wafer is mounted. Suppose that the platen moves with an acceleration of 30 g. We cannot allow any vibration of the machine, because we are printing electric circuit patterns of 10 nm in width. Design a mechanism that eliminates the mechanical vibration of the device under these operating conditions.

---

[5]There used to be several companies that used to make these lithography machines. A couple of Japanese companies (Canon and Nikon), ASM Lithography (ASML) of the Netherlands, and a few others were significant suppliers of lithography machines. Now ASML dominates the lithography business globally because of its advanced technologies. In 2016, ASML sold about 140 lithography machines, making its market share to be around 60%. Each lithography machine can cost approximately $110 million. It takes an entire Boeing 747 cargo plane to transport the machine.

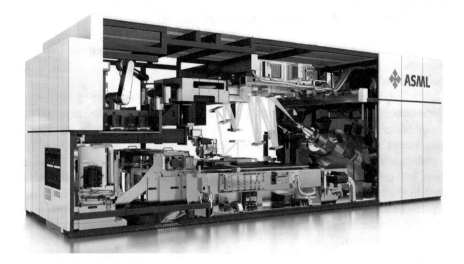

Fig. 3.12   A lithography machine for semiconductor wafer manufacturing (Permission granted by ASML)

3.6   Design of Organizations

Public and private organizations perform diverse functions in society and a nation. They constitute systems that deal with a variety of different problems and issues they confront during their operation. The design of their organization determines its effectiveness. Some of these organizations are government agencies and private entities, either for-profit (e.g., industrial companies) or non-profit organizations (e.g., universities). These organizations function within the laws governing organizational entities of a country, which are different from country to country and from region to region. In the United States of America, the constitution, which is the ultimate guarantor of the rights, goals, and limits of these organizations, is an amazing design of governing principles.

In this section, the design of two different kinds of organizations will be illustrated. In Chap. 21, the design of other organizations will be more thoroughly examined, including the design of universities. One of the significant differences in designing organizations is the primary role of people in an organization. In many cases of organizational design, often the DPs and PVs involve people with free will. Therefore, sometimes, organizations do not perform as designed initially because people in the organization may not function or behave as assumed initially.

3.6.1 Design of a Government Organization

Suppose someone is suddenly appointed to head up a government agency that supports engineering research at universities throughout the country, although she has not served in the government before. What should she do?

The simple answer is that she must go through the four domains of the design world, which were presented in Chap. 2 and design the policies, procedures, and the organization within the broad bounds and constraints that exist within the overall government policy and within the bounds established by the law. Once she establishes the policies and programs for her organization, she must administer them well to serve the public to the best of her ability. One significant constraint, at least in the case of the United States government, is that she does not have much time to do all these things unless she works hard and prepares her actions even before she assumes the job. As the common saying goes, "you have to run as soon as you hit the ground."

Before she assumes the job, she may have time to prepare her plan of action while waiting for her nomination by the president of the country after the background check, which may take about 6 months (in the case of the presidential appointment in the United States, clearance by security agencies and presidential personnel office is needed), and confirmation by the U.S. Senate. During this time, it will be highly desirable to acquire the current and historical information about the agency she is about to join and think about what she wishes to achieve in the job. If she has no idea as to what she wants to do to contribute to the nation, it will be wise not to take on such an assignment. Then she must plan! She may wish to identify the problem(s) the agency must address in the customer domain, and then formulate specific goals by establishing the FRs of the organization. Talking to important constituents of her agency may be a good idea to get a sense of how they would react to her designs as well as learn about their thoughts and concerns. This process is needed to find out the problem she must deal with in the customer domain.

After FRs are established in the functional domain, she must create an organizational structure (i.e., DPs) in the physical domain that will enable the execution of the chosen FRs. Then, in the process domain, she has to establish PVs (resources, budget, and personnel), which will be needed to support the DPs. This way we are mapping from the customer domain to the functional domain, from functional domain to physical domain, and finally from the physical domain to process domain (where resource issues such as funding and personnel are addressed). As she transforms from domain to domain, she must check to be sure that there are no coupled designs (i.e., the coupling of FRs as per the Independence Axiom). Since she will need financial and personnel resources, she should secure the necessary resources and support of other government agencies of the U.S. government and the U.S. Congress. She then should execute the policies and programs logically, fairly, and legally for the public good, as she swore to do at the time of her appointment.

Case Study 3.1: The Story about the Design of the NSF Engineering Directorate:

The purpose of this case study on organizational design is to illustrate the following:

1. importance of knowing the PROBLEM(s) as discussed in Chaps. 1 and 2;
2. importance of defining FRs to address the problem;
3. developing an organizational structure in terms of DPs to fulfill FRs;
4. importance of addressing resource issues: personnel and budget;
5. importance of addressing potential criticisms that usually follow when decisions are made that change the direction of an organization.

These five issues should be addressed in the design of organizations, because in many situations of organizational design, most attention is given to DPs, i.e., the creation of organizational structure, without articulating the goals of the organization in the form of FRs. Once FRs and DPs of the organization are appropriately addressed, one of the most critical tasks of the person heading up the organization is related to resource issues, i.e., budget, staffing, and facilities.

Item 5 is unavoidable when changes are introduced to any organization. Since some have benefited by the existing organization, any change made may affect them negatively or in some cases, adversely. Sometimes, some of those affected negatively by the changes introduced may even take personal attacks. It can consume a great deal of mental and physical energy to deal with negative attacks, either overtly or behind the scene. One way of avoiding Item 5 is to maintain the status quo and maintain existing organizations and try to make the influential stakeholders "happy" until the end of the tenure. Perhaps such a person should not take on the job since organizations must move forward to serve the people for whom the organization exists.

A Real Story:

The National Science Foundation (NSF) is a United States (U.S.) government agency that provides research funding primarily to universities in the United States. It was established in 1950 to enable universities to continue to make the critical scientific and technological contributions to the country as they had done during the Second World War. NSF supports research in science, engineering, and education. Its budget is relatively modest in comparison to other R&D agencies such as the National Institute of Health (NIH), Defense Advanced Projects Agency, and U.S. National Aeronautics and Space Agency (NASA). However, it is the largest agency that supports only extramural research at universities, whereas NIH and NASA have important intramural programs. It promotes research in physics, mathematics, chemistry, biology, materials, engineering, and education. The Engineering Directorate was established in the late 1970s. Before that, it was part of the Mathematics, Physics, and Engineering Directorate.

In the early days of its establishment, basic scientists dominated NSF, perhaps because, during the Second World War, scientists played critical roles in developing new weapons. Beginning in the 1970s, NSF attempted to strengthen the support for engineering research. However, NSF had difficulties in defining its role in engineering. By 1984, the United States had formidable competition from abroad, especially in manufacturing-related industries and NSF was under pressure to strengthen its engineering programs. To chart a new course for engineering, President Ronald Reagan appointed an engineering professor as the first presidential appointee in charge of the Engineering Directorate of NSF as Assistant Director (AD) of NSF for Engineering. What should he do to strengthen the engineering community of the United States?

Introduction to the NSF Engineering Directorate:

NSF was established to achieve the following three primary missions: (1) to promote progress in science and engineering; (2) to provide health, welfare, and prosperity to the people; and (3) to secure the national defense.

In the early days of NSF, engineering was part of the Directorate for Mathematics, Physics, and Biology. Then, it became a separate directorate in the late 1970s. Even then, engineers at NSF defined its role as "applied science," and thus fields such as design and manufacturing were not supported. Furthermore, it dwelled on engineering issues of the first half of the twentieth century, even though microelectronics, semiconductors, and biology were revolutionizing the world of science and technology. The then-existing policies were in part established because well-known engineering professors had undue influence on the NSF Engineering Directorate, emphasizing those topics that were important in the first half of the twentieth century. This practice forced young professors to work on old engineering problems to get funding. The people in the White House, who were responsible for science and engineering policies in President Reagan's administration, thought that the NSF should strengthen its support for engineering R&D to make the United States more competitive in the world.

Problems Identified in the Customer Domain:

The problems the new AD for Engineering identified through extensive consultation with professionals in industry, academia, and the government were the following:

1. The NSF mission was, as defined in the NSF Act of 1950, (1) to promote progress in science and engineering; (2) to provide health, welfare, and prosperity; and (3) to secure the national defense. The NSF Engineering Directorate was primarily serving the interest of existing engineering educational programs. It was organized like a mirror image of a typical engineering college and forgot about their primary mission related to the future well-being of the nation.
2. Funding was given primarily to well-known senior professors in engineering who were solving (or resolving slightly different approaches) the problems of the past to improve the accuracy rather than dealing with the future progress of engineering and technology in a rapidly changing world. Young professors who were yet to establish their reputation had difficulty in getting NSF grants. To write credible research proposals with many references, they tended to extend their doctoral thesis work rather than venturing into new challenging fields.

3. *Research in the design and innovation of technologies was neglected entirely.*
4. *Emerging and critical technologies were neglected, although these areas will become important in the future. Many grants supported engineering problems of the first half of the twentieth century.*
5. *The budget was allocated in proportion to the number of proposals received in a given area. Consequently, new fields and creative ideas did not get much funding, because the number of proposals in these emerging and critical areas was small, and therefore there was no budget allocated for newly emerging and innovative fields. For example, there was no funding for research in design or emerging technologies (e.g., biotechnology). As a result, many universities did not hire professors in these emerging engineering fields.*
6. *Cross-disciplinary research did not get any funding, including the fields in which the collaboration between academia and industry is of paramount importance.*
7. *Although NSF is a government agency to deal with national issues, NSF Engineering was not providing funding research areas that are important for the U. S. competitiveness in the twenty-first century. Funding went to those who submitted thick proposals that received high scores in peer review rather than proposals with creative and risky ideas.*
8. *The number of women in engineering was inadequate because they shied away from engineering because of its traditional image, i.e., engineers wearing hard hats.*

These were the problems that had to be dealt with to be sure that NSF fulfills its mission, as outlined in the NSF Act of 1950.

Design Solution:

Defining FRs in the Functional Domain:
Based on the problems identified, the FRs for the NSF Engineering Directorate were defined as follows:

FR1 = Advance engineering science base;
FR2 = Support engineering fields where the science base needs to be developed;
FR3 = Support emerging technologies;
FR4 = Advance critical technology areas for U.S.competitiveness;
FR5 = Promote collaboration between universities and industry;
FR6 = Strengthen the support for young researchers,
minority researchers, and women researchers.

$$(3.21)$$

Constraints: There are many constraints when one attempts to reorganize any organization, especially government agencies. It is especially difficult when the FRs deal with newly emerging subjects for which there are no large groups of researchers and professional societies (e.g., at the time of reorganization, nanotechnology). Furthermore, if the budget has to be changed by more than a fixed amount, it has to be approved by the director of NSF, the Office of Management and

Budget of the White House, and the Congressional Committee that oversees NSF, which may take a long time for approval. An equally important constraint was personal. He promised his family that he would work at NSF for only 1 year and return home, mostly for financial reasons. Therefore, the reorganization had to be done during the first 3 months of his tenure at NSF. No one believed that such an ambitious redirection of a government agency could be achieved in less than 2 or 3 years. It was reorganized, received the approval of OMB and Congress for budgetary changes, and implemented in 3 months, a record that defied the prevailing culture of Washington! The new structure and policies of the NSF Engineering fundamentally changed the NSF engineering support structure.

When a new direction for an organization is implemented, what people often search for are the DPs and PVs rather than FRs. DPs, which are created to achieve FRs, are represented by an organizational chart. PVs are resources such as personnel and budget that are needed to support DPs. However, to design an effective and efficient organization, we must establish FRs first and then develop DPs. That is, in the design of organizations, DPs are the organizational entities that exist to achieve (or satisfy) a given set of FRs. For example, DP3 that must satisfy FR3 (i.e., "support emerging technologies") could be called the "Division for Emerging Technologies."

Exercise 3.5:

(a) Define DPs for the above set of six FRs chosen for the new NSF Engineering Directorate. DPs will be entities called "divisions" within which we will have "programs" for various sub-topics of engineering. For example, DP1 could be "Division for Engineering Sciences." Remember that the DPs must satisfy the Independence Axiom, i.e., FRs must remain independent from each other by creating proper DPs that do not couple FRs. (b) Construct the design matrix. Is the design coupled?

Exercise 3.6:

Based on the DPs chosen, design an organizational structure. Remember that the Division Directors must report to AD for Engineering. In each division, there may be many "Programs," each with a Program Director. The total budget for the Engineering Directorate is $800 million a year. How and on what basis should the budget be allocated to various FRs?

Essence of the Design Process for Organizational Design

We demonstrated through this organizational design was to show the process of applying the design methodology using the design of the organization as an example. The steps involved were in the GPFDP sequence: (1) establish the goal, (2) define the problem, (3) establish FRs to solve the problem identified, (4) develop DPs to satisfy the FRs, and (5) identify PVs (i.e., resources in the form of personnel and financial resources). We have to make sure that the FRs are not coupled to each other during this design process. We will now repeat this process over and over again for all sorts of different designs involving machines, processes, and systems, in addition to other organizations.

It is good to remember that unlike the design of machines and manufacturing processes, the design of organizations that affects people can become controversial, especially if the budget has to be cut in some favored traditional areas. Money matters even in academia, often over-ruling their rational judgment! Often these well-established fields have champions—often better known scholars, who believe that their field is the most important among all academic disciplines. Such a conviction is often necessary, but we need a balanced perspective in all matters we deal with, but usually, our behavior follows instincts rather than a fair rationale. This NSF AD, who did not fully appreciate the sensitivity and politics of the academic community, was severely criticized for his actions by some professors. Sometimes, this is the price one has to pay to achieve what appears to be the right thing to do to achieve the institutional goals.

Micro-Management of an Organization

If by mistake, one creates an organization that is a coupled design (i.e., an organizational structure that couples FRs to each other), the person who is in charge of any one of the FRs cannot decide without affecting other FRs that are coupled to it. In this case, the decisions made by one of the division heads may affect those made by others, creating conflicts and tensions among them. Then the person who is in charge of all FRs ends up managing all the details of the entire organization. Such an organization cannot function effectively. Such a manager is sometimes called a "micro-manager," which should not be taken as a compliment! An organization that must be micromanaged tends to be inefficient as well as ineffective, often with unhappy and frustrated staffers.

Exercise 3.7:

Suppose that you have been asked to be the president of your university to make it to make it one of the best research universities in the world. What are the problems the university has you must deal with to achieve the goal of making it one of the leading universities in the world? What are the FRs you will try to satisfy? What DPs would you choose to satisfy the FRs? Where would you get the necessary resources (PVs) you will need to achieve your goals? Show how you would perform the PFDP transformation to make your university a great university.

3.6.2 Design of High-Technology Industrial Firms

Most people would agree that during the past 40 years, there have been explosive growths of new high-technology industries, especially in the United States. Many well-known companies, such as Microsoft, Google, Intel, Apple, Broadcom, Samsung, Boeing, and Amazon, have changed the world. The combined revenue of these companies is far larger than the total income of more traditional companies such as General Motors, General Electric, IBM, Hitachi, Ford, and BMW. Some of the new companies have demonstrated that new industrial firms based on technology innovation can make significant contributions to society and make their investors wealthy. Therefore, many young students hope to start their own companies during their careers.

Only a few new venture firms, out of thousands, become successful. Many factors determine the outcome of new ventures. However, the most successful companies are those that have designed their business goals and strategy well. They were also "lucky" in terms of timing, financing, and market receptivity for their products. The most important elements behind the successful companies are the correct identification of the "problem," selection of a right set of FRs, selection of appropriate DPs in the physical domain, and securing (or generation) of financial resources (PVs) for proper execution.

Case Study 3.2: Creation of Successful High-Technology Company

Problems identified in the Customer Domain:

A well-known high-technology firm grew rapidly because of its superior proprietary products, dominating some of the high-technology product areas. They made
computers, semiconductors, digital printers, measurement devices, and others. They
competed with other high-technology firms, which had also diversified into many
product areas. Then, new firms that only specialized in a limited number of product
areas entered the market place, competing with this large company with many
different products in highly competitive markets. To be more competitive, this old
firm with an extensive portfolio had to invest more and more in research and
development (R&D) to stay competitive. Eventually, this large firm realized that it
must divest some of its divisions that were no longer competitive because of the
severe competition. They sold their semiconductor device division to a private
equity firm, which generates funds from institutions such as universities to invest in
profitable areas and return handsome profits to the investors.

A private equity firm, which bought a division of this large company, launched a
new semiconductor manufacturing company. They hired a brilliant and capable
CEO for this new company. The new CEO organized the new company and made it
profitable in a couple of years. Then, he took the company public selling its shares
to the public. The private equity firm sold its shares at a considerable profit and left
the company.

The CEO of this new company developed a set of FRs and corresponding DPs to
make the new company successful. If you were the CEO, what would you choose
as your FRs and DPs?

Design Solution:

The CEO of this newly formed company developed a new set of FRs for the
company. The highest level FR was the following:

FR = Become a dominant manufacturing company in semiconductor chip
     products for the telecommunications and enterprise systems (i.e., storage
     equipment).

The corresponding DP was

DP = High-technology semiconductor chip manufacturing company in
     telecommunications and storage.

The following were the next-level FRs:

FR1 = Dominate a few selected product areas in the market place;
FR2 = Consolidate R&D and other activities to increase efficiency and reduce
      cost;
FR3 = Show a substantial profit and raise the stock price;
FR4 = Acquire other semiconductor companies that are in a related business;
FR6 = Increase profit margin by offering high-performance products.

He then selected the DPs to satisfy the above set of FRs.

Concluding Note:

This new company became hugely successful. The stock market rewarded this company by increasing its stock price. It soon acquired a larger semiconductor company that had been around for about three decades and became one of the dominant semiconductor device companies. This newly merged company became one of the dominant semiconductor companies in the world. The company CEO donated large gifts to his alma mater.

3.7   Conclusions

In this introductory chapter, many examples of design—both technical and non-technical—are used to illustrate the design process involved in creating various systems. It is shown that the design of systems, regardless of the specificity of the field, is a transformational process of going from problem identification to FRs, FRs to DPs, and DPs to PVs, in short, the "PFDP transformation." We have illustrated this typical transformational process for various designs such as organizations, transportation systems, and others. During this transformational process, we must maintain the independence of FRs as per the Independence Axiom to create designs that are robust and easily implementable. Construction of design matrix can help in identifying coupled designs, especially when the design involves many FRs and many layers of decomposition. It was emphasized that the design process is common to all designs, regardless of the field of application.

Problems

1. Design an alternate steering column that may be better than the one shown in Sect. 3.5.4.
2. In design, it was stated that we cannot make a non-diagonal design matrix into a diagonal matrix through mathematical manipulation in most cases. Is this statement valid?
3. In many countries, political problems arise because educational opportunities for children depend on family income levels. Usually, better educational opportunities are available to children from financially better-off families than those from financially struggling families. Better educated people end up getting better paying jobs and get more opportunities to advance in society. Design a system where all children will get equal opportunities in education. State your FRs and DPs clearly. Construct the design matrix for your design. Is your design a good one that provides equal opportunities?
4. If you were the CEO of the above semiconductor company, what would you pick as your DPs to satisfy the FRs? For the DPs chosen construct the design matrix. Is your design uncoupled? Decoupled design? Coupled design?

5. Design a new venture firm that specializes in artificial intelligence (AI) in the field of financial auditing of industrial firms. Identify the problem (in the customer domain). List the FRs of your new venture firm in the functional domain that can solve the problem. Then, list DPs in the physical domain that will satisfy the FRs. Finally, list the investment you will need to finance your new venture firm (PVs in the process domain). Construct the design matrix for your design. Is your design acceptable?

6. At the Diamond Light Source of the United Kingdom, they have been developing high-energy imaging, diffraction, and scattering beamline. Its source is a superconducting wiggler with a power of approximately 9 kW at 500 mA after the fixed front-end aperture; two permanent filters aim at reducing the energy in photons below the operating range of the beamline of 50–150 keV, which accounts for about two-thirds of the total. How would you remove the heat generated in the permanent filters? Propose a design solution.

7. One of the modern technologies that have changed the world is the airplane with jet engines. Now we can reach almost anywhere within 24 h because these planes fly at nearly the speed of sound, i.e., sub-sonic. They are quite efficient. However, they produce more CO_2 than other transports per passenger per mile flown than any other transports. Therefore, we need to reduce fuel consumption and thus CO_2 emission.

The jet engines mounted typically on the aircraft wings are quite big and heavy. The engine size is determined by the power the airplane needs to reach the liftoff speed within a fixed length of the runway. However, once it reaches the cruising altitude, it uses only a tiny fraction of its power, since the pressure drop across the plane and air drag on the aircraft body is rather small. The massive engine needed for takeoff increases the drag on the airplane. Propose designs that can reduce the drag or the engine size.

8. The engineers at the Diamond Light Source published a paper on the design and simulation process of the permanent secondary filter, a 4-mm-thick SiC disk used in the system. The first version of the filter was vulnerable to cracking due to thermally induced stress, so a new filter was designed based on an AD. The new design solved their problem. Review the following paper and comment on their design. Propose another design that can accomplish the same goal.

Reference: W. Tizzano∗, T. Connolley, S. Davies, M. Drakopoulos, Design and FEA of an innovative rotating SiC filter for high-energy X-ray beam,, Mechanical Eng. Design of Synchrotron Radiation Equipment and Instrumentation MEDSI2018, Paris, France JACoW Publishing ISBN: 978-3-95,450-207-3. https://doi.org/10.18429/JACoW-MEDSI2018-THOAMA04 [G. E. Howell Diamond Light Source, OX11 0DE Didcot, United Kingdom].

Appendix

Additional Theorems (Note: some of the theorems are related to information, which is presented in Chaps. 8 and 11).

Theorem 8 (Independence and Tolerance)

Design is an uncoupled design when the design range is greater than $\sum_{i=1, i \neq j}^{n} \left(\frac{\partial FRi}{\partial DPj} \right) \Delta DPj$, *in which case, the non-diagonal elements of the design matrix can be neglected from design consideration.*

Theorem 12 (Sum of Information)

The sum of information for a set of events is also information, provided that proper conditional probabilities are used when the events are not statistically independent.

Theorem 13 (Information Content of the Total System)

If each DP is probabilistically independent of other DPs and affects only its corresponding FR, the information content of the total system is the sum of the information of all individual events associated with the set of FRs that must be satisfied.

Theorem 14 (Information Content of Coupled versus Uncoupled Design)

When the state of FRs is changed from one state to another in the functional domain, the information required for the change is greater for a coupled process than for an uncoupled process.

Theorem 16 (Equality of Information Content)

All information content that are relevant to the design task are equally important regardless of their physical origin and no weighting factor should be applied to them.

Theorem 17 (Design in the Absence of Complete Information)

Design can proceed even in the absence of complete information only in the case of decoupled design if the missing information is related to the off-diagonal elements.

Theorem 18 (Existence of an Uncoupled Design)

There always exists an uncoupled design that has less information than a coupled design.

Theorem 19 (Robustness of Design)

An uncoupled design and a decoupled design are more robust than a coupled design in the sense that it is easier to reduce the information content of designs that satisfy the Independence Axiom.

Theorem 20 (Design Range and Coupling)

If the design ranges of uncoupled or decoupled designs are tightened, the designs may become coupled designs. Conversely, if the design range of some coupled design are relaxed, the designs may become either uncoupled or decoupled designs.

Theorem 22 (Comparative Robustness of a Decoupled Design)

Given the maximum design ranges for a given set of FRs, decoupled designs cannot be as robust as uncoupled designs in that the allowable tolerances for DPs of decoupled design are less than those of uncoupled design.

Bibliography

Drakopoulos M, Connolley T, Reinhard C, Atwood R, Magdysyuk O, Vo N, Hart M, Connor L, Humphreys B, Howell G, Davies S, Tim Hill and GW, Pedersen U, Foster A, Maio ND, Basham M, Yuan F, Wanelik K (2015) I12: the Joint Engineering, Environment and Processing (JEEP) beamline at Diamond Light Source. J Synchrotron Radiat 22:828–838
Farid A, Suh NP (eds) (2016) Axiomatic Design in large systems. Springer, Cham, Switzerland
Gossip (2019) Template aluminum soda can isolated on white background, mockup, can for beer and carbonated drinks. 3D rendering. Photo licensed from Shutterstock, ID: 1300349536
Lorne E (2019) Kidney stones after ESWL intervention. Lithotripsy. Scale in centimeters. Photo licensed from Shutterstock, ID: 179862602
NIH: National Cancer Institute (2009) SEER training modules: Anatomy & physiology. https://training.seer.cancer.gov/anatomy/urinary/components/,publicdomain
Papilionem K (2019) Geobukseon (Korean Turtle Ship) replica sculpture in Gwanghwamun agora. Photo licensed from Shutterstock, ID: 1425185789
Suh NP (1990) The Principles of Design. Oxford University Press
Tizzano W, Connolley T, Davies S, Drakopoulos M (2018) Design and FEA of an innovative rotating SiC filter for high-energy X-ray beam. In: Proceedings of Mechanical Engineering Design of Synchrotron Radiation Equipment and Instrumentation (MEDSI2018) in Paris, France, JACoW Publishing, pp 306–312
Wong A, Guo H, Kumar V, Park CB, Suh NP (2016) Microcellular Plastics. Wiley. pp 1–57. https://onlinelibrary.wiley.com/doi/pdf/, https://doi.org/10.1002/0471440264.pst468.pub2

Further Reading

Suh NP (2001) Axiomatic design—advances and applications. Oxford University Press
Suh NP (2005) Complexity. Oxford University Press
Suh NP, Cho DH (eds) (2017) The on-line electric vehicle: wireless electric ground transportation systems. Springer International Publishing

Design Representations

4

Paolo Citti, Alessandro Giorgetti, Filippo Ceccanti, Fernando Rolli, Petra Foith-Förster, and Christopher A. Brown

Abstract

The results of design activities must be transmitted to people who need them for their tasks, e.g., manufacturing, construction, software development, etc. The objectives of this chapter are to understand how design information should be represented and conveyed using standards, geometric drawings, design matrices for the complete system, DP_i/DP_j matrices, and industry-specific functional diagrams. The goal of this chapter is to introduce how the design information is typically conveyed to its ultimate user.

Proper descriptions of design must address the needs of the users of the design results. For example, the manufacturing group may need the information on the geometry of each part, acceptable tolerances for each dimension, materials, the hardness of each piece, the complete assembly of the system, etc. On the other hand, those charged with the task of evaluating and implementing the design may need information on the entire assembly of parts, operating procedure, power requirements, etc. To facilitate these processes, different professional groups have established commonly used methods, conventions, and practices.

The "design information" is typically represented using representation methods that are used in a given profession, sometimes adapted by each company to deal with their specific needs. This chapter reviews some of the

P. Citti · A. Giorgetti (✉) · F. Ceccanti · F. Rolli
Department of Engineering Science, Guglielmo Marconi University, Rome, Italy
e-mail: a.giorgetti@unimarconi.it

P. Foith-Förster
Fraunhofer Institute for Manufacturing Engineering and Automation IPA, Stuttgart, Germany

C. A. Brown
Department of Mechanical Engineering, Worcester Polytechnic Institute, Worcester, MA, USA

© Springer Nature Switzerland AG 2021
N. P. Suh et al. (eds.), *Design Engineering and Science*,
https://doi.org/10.1007/978-3-030-49232-8_4

fundamental representation methods of design that have been developed by various professional groups, typically non-government entities. For instance, there are national professional organizations such as the American Society of Mechanical Engineers (ASME) that have established the standards for certain products such as pressure vessels and boilers to assure the safety of certain products. Globally, there is the International Organizations for Standardization (ISO), an international non-governmental organization that has established voluntary international standards, which facilitates world trade by providing common standards worldwide.

In this book that emphasizes Axiomatic Design (AD), the relationship between functional requirements (FRs) and design parameters (DPs) is the basis for product design. In AD, the design process begins with the identification of FRs first, followed by the development of DPs, which are specifically chosen to satisfy the FRs. Therefore, in AD, the relationship between FRs and DPs forms the core of design representation, in addition to the representation of geometric shapes in the case of the design that involves solid objects. A design matrix is a form of design representation that describes the relationship between the functions and physical entities. The design matrix between FRs and DPs is the most effective means of identifying the coupled designs that are to be avoided in AD.

To highlight the powerfulness of the design matrix representation and the wide applicability of AD, several families of representations, as stated above, have been considered. In particular, the chapter is structured in such a way to explain, in a first instance, what should be the connections between designing with AD and representing the results. The concept of module and tolerance will be introduced. Therefore, representation families will be presented: standard mechanical drawing, piping and instrumentation diagram (P&ID), and software. A case study is presented as well, to bring a real example of a complete application of AD. The choice to illustrate both mechanical drawing and software representation comes to the authors' will to emphasize that the design process should follow a structured approach, in particular, the AD one, regardless the nature of what is designed.

Proper descriptions of a design must address the needs of a variety of users of the design information. Some may only be interested in knowing the functional and physical relationships in terms of FR and DP hierarchy. Some may need to exact geometric details of the designed parts in terms of DPs, their tolerances, the geometric shape, and their relationships. Some may need the information on the assembly of DPs, i.e., information on DP_i/DP_j relationships. The objectives of this chapter are to describe how design information is typically represented and conveyed using standards, geometric drawings, design matrices, DP_i/DP_j matrices, and industry-specific functional diagrams.

4.1 Introduction: Design Representations and Their Purposes

A Real Story

In the late 1950s, a financially struggling engineering student got a job in a small local machine shop near his university. It was a god-sent job because he was struggling financially to pay for his dormitory room and meals. The job paid much better than what he was getting from other odd jobs. It was also unusual. His job was to draw up the machines the head machinist built without any drawings. He would look at a machine or a photograph of a machine, and proceed to make a similar machine by machining the parts with steel or aluminum without any drawings. This practice was contrary to what his school taught him. He was taught to draw the assembly drawing as well as part drawings for someone to make the part based on the drawings that had nominal dimensions and tolerances. However, his boss at this company proceeded to produce parts without drawings. He took a photograph of a machine that was similar to what he had in mind. Then, without any drawings, he would proceed to make various machines such as vacuum-forming machines, punching press, molds, and so on. For a few years, the company liked him, because without hiring any designer or engineer, he produced to manufacturing equipment for vacuum-formed plastic parts and punching press quickly. The company wanted to have a record of what he had made. The company decided to hire someone to draw up what he just made without any drawings! That is the reason the company hired this young aspiring engineer.

This young "engineer" went around the machines, examining the parts the "chief engineer" had already made to produce paper documents for what he had already made. It was a very difficult job! Measuring parts that had been already machined and assembled, and then drawing them on a piece of paper was not only dull but could easily be misleading, because the geometric information did not reveal functions of the part, i.e., FRs. He could only measure nominal dimensions and had no information on the tolerances . He just assumed that the tolerance was around ±0.005 inches in the case of linear dimensions. As the company's business grew, the management realized that they could no longer depend on this archaic method of making machines and machined parts without designing the machine or the part first on paper. The management changed their policy: design machine parts first on paper and then make the machine based on the drawing that had all the information on materials, dimensions, and tolerances. This new approach was much more reliable and less expensive than the previous method, i.e., start cutting a piece of metal without the benefit of having drawings that specified tolerances and nominal dimensions.

In some ways, history repeats itself. It turns out that a similar situation existed in the late eighteenth century. Then, muskets were made without standardization and interchangeable parts. Artisans uniquely created each gun, and none of the parts could be exchanged with similar parts in other guns made by the same manufacturer. Every musket was "custom made." Therefore, they could not supply the number of muskets needed for wars. Then, the idea of interchangeable parts was finally introduced, which required drawings of the parts with nominal dimensions, tolerances, and material specifications, which were needed to standardize the components and increase manufacturing productivity. Each piece was made separately within a tight tolerance and assembled with other mass-produced parts because they were interchangeable.

Mechanical technologies have come a long way since then. Now in semiconductor manufacturing, we are dealing with nanometer-scale dimensions with fractions of nanometer accuracy for mass production of integrated circuits (IC) with a very high yield of acceptable products. The required accuracy of these chips is a fraction of nanometers. Indeed, these amazing technologies would not be possible without the capability to represent the design graphically for a single part as well as a system of parts. The drawings must carry all the information needed to manufacture the part. Sometimes, extensive documentation is required to specify all the conditions that must be satisfied in manufacturing these parts that produce integrated semiconductor parts.

Almost everything humans do or produce is *designed first*, either formally or informally. Representations of design embodiments are required elements of design. Final design representations communicate design solutions to others. They represent the outcome of syntheses processes. When the design is done for a client, the design representation is an integral part of the contract. When the design of a product is done for manufacturing within a company, it becomes the basis for designing and planning the production system or the factory.

Sometimes, especially during the early phase of design, the design is sketched as an abstract and idealized model of the design concept for future implementation. They describe reality in a simplified and pragmatic way to allow for scientific or technical analysis or description or exploration. Final design representations should communicate the details of the design intent, results of analyses, calculations, alternatives, and decisions carried out during the design phase. There are three main uses of representations during the life cycle of a product:

1. support for design processes and documenting progress;
2. final documentation of completed design solutions;
3. inputs for manufacturing process design and quality assurance.

First, design solutions are not created for the first time after design problems are completely solved. Representations evolve with developments of solutions during zigzagging decomposition processes between FRs and DPs, as described in the previous chapters. *Second*, representations guide design processes. They represent progress in solution developments. Also, they can provide a record of how solutions were reached. Usually, more than one candidate for a design solution should be considered. Reasons for selections and rejections of candidate solutions should be recorded. Good representations of evolving designs help designers follow effective, structured design processes that can build on experience. *Third*, representations of designed products are instruments for transferring manufacturing-relevant information from designers to manufacturing and industrial engineers, who are responsible for designing production systems and processes, including quality assurance.

Good design representations do not, per se, mean that design solutions are good. Design representations merely document the design embodiment. They do not alter it. A poor design could be well documented and still be insufficient to accomplish the CNs. Good design solutions start with good problem statements, followed by appropriately structured, functionally oriented design processes. Based on the CNs, different FRs and, consequently, different DPs, might be considered for good design solutions.

Design representations use special semantics for explaining things that have been designed, like process, objects, and functions. These special semantics can be combined in different ways for different purposes. Different semantic systems are used, based on what is designed. Typically, representation systems are chosen for their effectiveness in communicating the features of each design process step. Conventional graphical representations of product design solutions, such as 2D and 3D drawings, e.g., as produced by CAD software, are well-established notation systems used to represent an object's physical dimensions, i.e., DPs. Note that while CAD often refers to "computer-aided design," this is not "design" in the sense used here. CAD is rather computer-aided drafting or drawing.

Drawings fail to record design intents, i.e., FRs. Drawings show only physical aspects of components and assemblies. Drawings also fail to explain how DPs influence FRs and which ones they influence. These deficiencies in graphical-only design representations make it impossible to modify DPs without risking unintended consequences, a result of violating axiom one, albeit inadvertently because the FR-DP relation modules are not communicated. It is essential to make extra efforts, integrating design intent, FRs, and FR-DP modules into design representations, to represent solutions more fully.

Axiomatic Design (AD) offers more complete and useful representations of design solutions, through FR-DP modules and hierarchies. These are the semantics for functional–physical representations of design solutions. AD's module-junction diagram and flow diagram further deliver object and process representations of design solutions.

The following section elaborates on AD semantics for representations that facilitate robust, adjustable, controllable design solutions that avoid unintended consequences and have the highest probabilities of success.

4.2 Design Representations for Applying the Axioms

4.2.1 Axiom 1, Maintaining Independence, Function– Physical Representations, and Module Junction Diagram and Flow Diagram

Complete design solutions need to indicate the design intent for each physical feature, and they need to show the interactions between physical solutions and design intents. In AD processes, this starts by writing text to record FR–DP pairs. Relations between FRs and DPs are then described mathematically in the design equation within a design matrix.

Design matrices progress with design processes. Design matrices encapsulate design decisions, and the progress made toward complete design solutions. Full design matrices contain all the individual design equations between each FR and all the DPs that influence it.

Design matrices can be used to check quickly for the satisfaction of the Independence Axiom. FR–DP interactions can be summarized together in design matrices with Xs and 0s, representing significant interactions or lack of them, as described in the previous chapters. If a particular DP is influencing a certain FR, it is indicated by an X in the appropriate position in the matrix or, not, shown by an 0.

An uncoupled design has a matrix with Xs only on the diagonal. DPs can be adjusted in any order to fulfill FRs without iterating to correct unwanted influences of DPs on FRs. Off-diagonal Xs indicate unwanted influences of DPs on FRs. Triangular matrices show decoupled designs, which must be adjusted in a specific order to avoid iterating. If a matrix indicating unwanted influences cannot be arranged by linear algebra to be triangular, then the design is coupled.

Knowing, quantitatively, how each FR is influenced by each of the DPs independence can be maintained as prescribed by axiom one, adjustability and controllability are provided and unintended consequences can be avoided.

AD provides a unified representation, including the various levels of decomposition of FRs, based on modules. *Modules are defined in terms of FR–DP or DP–PV relationships. A module is the row of the design matrix that calculates the value of an FR when it is provided with inputs of corresponding DPs.* Hence, the design modules show how each FR is satisfied by its corresponding DP and may be affected by the other DPs.

An FR is satisfied if there is a function M such that FR = M(DP). Therefore, interactions among use cases, DPs, can be interpreted as system inputs. For simplicity in notation, the operator * can be introduced. This operator represents, in equivalent modular form, mapping relationships (FR–DP or DP–PV), even for non-linear systems at high abstraction levels. Then the following simplification can be used: FR = M(DP) = M * DP.

In complex systems, consisting of many modules, this simplification is useful for identifying the types of relationships existing between the various modules. Three types of relationships can be considered. The relations between the modules of a system are defined as uncoupled (S—summation junction) when FRs are mutually exclusive, i.e., independent. This situation is equivalent to having a diagonal matrix design (Eq. 4.1):

$$\begin{Bmatrix} FR_1 \\ FR_2 \end{Bmatrix} = \begin{bmatrix} a & \\ & b \end{bmatrix} \begin{bmatrix} DP_1 \\ DP_2 \end{bmatrix} \rightarrow \begin{cases} FR_1 = M_1 * DP_1 \\ FR_2 = M_2 * DP_2 \end{cases} \tag{4.1}$$

Figure 4.1 illustrates the graphical representation in terms of the flowchart diagram for the system of Eq. (4.1).

In practice, relations between modules of systems correspond to connections parallel to these modules.

Similarly, relationships among system modules are defined as decoupled (C—control junction), if the system of equations corresponds to a triangular design matrix. In this case, connections between modules of a system are a bit more complex.

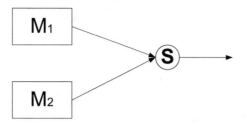

Fig. 4.1 Flowchart diagram for an uncoupled system where M_1 and M_2 modify DP_1 and DP_2 to satisfy FRs 1 and 2, respectively, and S is a summation junction

$$\begin{Bmatrix} FR_1 \\ FR_2 \end{Bmatrix} = \begin{bmatrix} a & \\ b & c \end{bmatrix} \begin{bmatrix} DP_1 \\ DP_2 \end{bmatrix}$$
$$\rightarrow \begin{cases} FR_1 = aDP_1 = M_1 * DP_1 = f(DP_1) \\ FR_2 = bDP_1 + cDP_2 = M_2 * DP_2 = f(DP_1, DP_2) \end{cases} \quad (4.2)$$

where

$$M_2 = b\left(\frac{DP_1}{DP_2}\right) + c \quad (4.3)$$

This path starts from module M_1 and develops to module M_2.

The modules corresponding to the same DPs can be connected in series. They are sub-assemblies of modules arranged with respect to the execution of main information paths of systems. Therefore, overall graphical representations of systems are equivalent to flowcharts, constituted by subsets of modules in series, connected in parallel. Modules M_1 and M_2 are connected in series. This means that the output of M_1 constitutes the input for M_2. Figure 4.2 shows the graphical representation as a flowchart diagram of the system in Eqs. 4.2 and 4.3.

Connections among system modules are coupled (F—feedback junction) when FRs are not independent. In this case, system behavior can no longer be represented by simple connections of modules in series or in parallel. In order to define the system status, some modules need to have a return. In these situations, there is a feedback relationship between the various modules. In terms of matrices, connections of this type can be represented by scattered matrices.

$$\begin{Bmatrix} FR_1 \\ FR_2 \end{Bmatrix} = \begin{bmatrix} a & d \\ b & c \end{bmatrix} \begin{bmatrix} DP_1 \\ DP_2 \end{bmatrix} \rightarrow \begin{cases} FR_1 = aDP_1 + dDP_2 = M_1 * DP_1 \\ FR_2 = bDP_1 + dDP_2 = M_2 * DP_2 \end{cases} \quad (4.4)$$

where

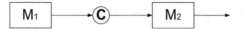

Fig. 4.2 Flowchart diagram for a decoupled system

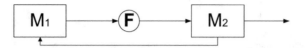

Fig. 4.3 Flowchart diagram for a coupled system where F is a feedback junction

$$\begin{cases} M_1 = a + d\left(\frac{DP_1}{DP_2}\right) = f(DP_1, DP_2) \\ M_2 = b\left(\frac{DP_1}{DP_2}\right) + c = f(DP_1, DP_2) \end{cases} \tag{4.5}$$

In graphical form, Eq. 4.4 is represented by the flowchart in Fig. 4.3.

This module representation with AD is particularly interesting. It can be represented graphically as a module-junction structure diagram or as a flowchart. In this treatment, there is recourse to representations of system modules, like flowcharts. This typology of representation has extensive use. It can also be used in industrial and mechanical systems design. It is a representational equivalent of a design matrix. Moreover, modular representations can be particularly effective in describing complex systems, consisting of components of different natures.

Flowcharts of system modules facilitate integrated designs of non-homogeneous parts. Each module constitutes an abstract entity. However, these diagrams give considerable relevance to connections among various components of systems, regardless of their nature. In this way, it is possible to pursue integrated designs, which allow the contextual and coordinated development of mechanical, electronic, and software components. In fact, the decomposition of FRs can be carried out to define designs of individual components and interfaces between components.

Design matrices and modules for each FR that compose them need to connect with other representations can be applied in each engineering field. Mechanical drawings, process maps, etc. are included with design matrices for more complete representations of design solutions.

4.2.2 Axiom 2, Minimizing Information Content and the Concept of Tolerances

DPs are physical solutions to design problems. They can be almost any sort of thing because the science of design is applicable in practically all fields. DPs can include physical and electrical components, industrial processes, healthcare delivery, and monitoring of operations. Regardless of the application, in almost all designs, there will be parameters more critical than others for success. There can be uncertainties in determining independence and in estimating the probability of success for calculating information contents for the candidate solutions. These uncertainties can be enough, such that, even starting from common CNs, it is possible to get different design solutions of indistinguishable quality.

The success of a complete design is measured by its ability to satisfy the original CNs. Success is measured in decompositions by abilities of DPs to fulfill FRs and of PVs to produce DPs. In most cases, CNs are represented by things like satisfying needs, component life, sustainability, and interfaces with other components. Based on these, and considering potential constraints, such as cost, maximum weight and maximum dimensions, many different design solutions that satisfy all points and axiom one might be developed within specified tolerances. Probabilities of achieving these tolerances can be used for calculating information contents and ranking solutions to determine the best design through Axiom 2. Metrics are essential for this.

Good metrics reduce uncertainties in determining information content. With metrics, all potential design solutions can be ranked by their information contents, i.e., probability of success. Uncertainty in knowing probabilities of success limits the ability to distinguish information contents for candidate solutions, which limits the application of information content, i.e., Axiom 2 for ranking candidate solutions.

Short Metrics Examples

To understand how metrics can work in design, imagine designing an electrified transport system to replace traditional internal combustion buses and taxis in a downtown environment. Regardless of other DPs to be chosen, the power line voltage delivered to the transport unit must match the electric motor specifications. Power drops or spikes that could damage the motors need to be addressed. The power supply should be as constant as possible, within limits that the motors can withstand. The tolerance for the power supply variance depends on what the motors can tolerate while maintaining functionality. These considerations establish tolerances on DPs.

Consider, as another example, mechanical components subjected to cyclic bending loads that can cause fatigue failures, like a shaft. Fatigue cracks generally initiate on the surface and cycle by cycle; they grow until the component fails. Maximum stress on shafts subjected to bending loads is initially on the surface, until a crack starts, then they are at the crack tip. Surface integrity is critical because surfaces are where cracks initiate. Tolerances on surface topographies should be specified by designers to ensure the required component life. Typically, this is done by specifying maximum values for roughness parameters. Because surface characterizations are vital for design success, the roughness characterization parameters to be used in each situation should be specified by designers. The selection of topographic characterization parameters to be specified for a given situation is based on several considerations, including materials, processes used to create the surface, and surface accessibility, which should all be specified in representations of design solutions.

An approach to reducing uncertainty is stress estimation. The best solution can be selected by evaluating the performance of each candidate design with finite element method (FEM) analyses. In which case, metrics, such as maximum stress, maximum strain, and maximum displacement, can be used to determine information contents of each design solution.

Another approach could be to build prototypes to test design solutions physically in real working conditions, i.e., pilot tests. Different kinds of metrics, such as the number of cycles to the break, maximum load withstood, and hours to failure, can be adopted to score candidate design solutions.

Note that different detailed metrics, such as maximum stress and the number of cycles to failure, address standard high-level performance metrics, such as component life. From this perspective, simulations and tests can be used either to enrich designers' knowledge for improving design solutions or to confirm and freeze a design solution concluding the design phase and starting the production phase. Iterative steps can be design phases, where the axioms are applied to design representations consistently through all attempts, which is why design representations are essential during design development phases.

A brief history of the concept of tolerance

The concept of tolerance was born during the first industrial revolution to supply guns for the military more efficiently. Before that moment, "quality control" was carried out directly by artisans during fabrication. Therefore, there was no need to check dimensions and shapes, because, in the case of incongruencies, artisans would correct them immediately, to get the desired components and systems functioning properly.

When demands for products increased, production paradigms evolved. From a one-person artisanal work, goods started to be produced in sub-assemblies. The creators of this production method are usually identified in Honoré Blanc and Eli Whitney. Sub-assemblies were pre-assembled modules of components designed to be put together when the final product was needed. Also, modules could be mixed to make different kinds of guns. This production paradigm modification, even though it seems natural, introduced several aspects completely ignored until then. One of them was tolerancing. Because modules were supposed to be assembled, their dimensions and all their interfaces needed to satisfy interface and clearance requirements.

This need was satisfied by thinking of dimensions of modules such that, with all the stack-ups of dimensional variations, the resulting modules could be assembled into a properly functioning gun. This apparent smart dimensioning is the first massive application of the modern tolerance concept.

The concept of tolerance is fundamental in design because it connects the design world, which is always an abstraction with semantics modeling reality, and the real world, with uncertainties and constraints. Tolerancing is fundamental to design because calculations, considerations, and selections are usually carried out only in ideal and simplified environments. The real world is, on the contrary, an imperfect and complex environment in which designed products will live their entire lives. Therefore, design solutions should consider intrinsic, real-world imperfections, and provide robust choices for robust design solutions. Like design performance, there are metrics for design robustness. Axiom two is all about probabilities of success in achieving tolerances and robustness to the selection of design solutions.

Whenever there are critical DPs, regardless of what is designed, their values require tolerance intervals. Tolerance intervals are the ranges in which values can vary, while satisfying the CNs. Tolerance interval definitions comprise manufacturability, performance, safety, and lifetime.

Regardless of why tolerance is used, designers should identify DPs, i.e., features, that need special tolerances, which require special PVs, because these features can increase information content. Specification of tolerances that challenge capabilities of conventional PVs can introduce additional costs in prototyping and manufacturing. Therefore, the number of tolerances specified should always be defined considering the criticalities of specific applications. They should be defined according to the target performance. Target performance defines tolerances, and tolerances define cost. Therefore, if tolerances are defined, based on CNs and FRs, to be as large as possible and still supply required values, the costs of products come down.

4.2.3 V-Model, Design Process Representation to Guide a Structured Design Process

In conventional industrial practice, designs often evolve iteratively from a first prototype without a dedicated analysis of FRs and feasibility testing of design solutions, as can be achieved by applying the axioms. The success of such a design process relies purely on the designers, who might find satisfactory solutions by chance or experience. Systems-engineering methods promote representations of actual design processes to support designers with a structured approach. Instead of luck or designers' experience, design processes should be driven by decomposition of design process functions and concerted design process steps.

A popular design process representation in industry is the V-model. Originally defined for software development, it breaks the design process into three phases (Fig. 4.4). The alignment of the phases in the form of a V gives the procedure its name.

During the first phase, a specification and decomposition of FRs lead down to the level of a detailed design of system modules. This becomes the basis of the implementation phase, located in the tip of the V, where design representations (i.e., system models) are created and realization takes place. Different product domains may be realized independently (e.g., mechanical, electronical, and software realization). The third phase is dedicated to integration and testing. It is located on the right flank of the V-model. Consequently, each of the first phase's specifications and decomposition steps on the left flank of V has a testing and integration counterpart.

The V-model can be run through several times during a design project. Depending on the design progresses, outputs of the V-model could be laboratory prototypes, functional prototypes, pilot-run products, and so on, until the final design stage is reached.

The benefit of the V-model is its representation of a structured, requirements-oriented, design process. Product architectures are defined as realization begins to integrate components from functional decompositions into

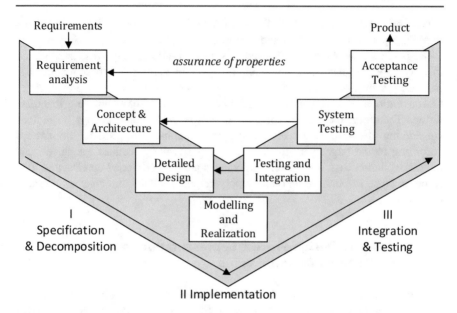

Fig. 4.4 V-model design process representation (as introduced by Gausemeier and Moehringer (2002))

physically realizable units. Another benefit of the V-model is that it promotes testing for multiple levels of integration of physical subsystems. However, the V-model misses iterations between phases. However, in AD, needs for iterations are largely eliminated by application of the axioms during functional decompositions and physical integrations. Its underlying concept is that of a sequential design process. As a rule of thumb, early testing and user involvement in the evaluation of the design are discouraged until the late design phase of the right flank of V.

AD also promotes a structured design process, focusing on customer needs, functional–physical decompositions, and physical integrations. The design process is represented by customer, functional–physical, and process domains, populated by zigzagging between them (Fig. 4.5). Through application of the information axiom, every single mapping of an FR to a DP solution into the physical domain is associated with verification of its probability of success in satisfying its respective FR. To find out about system ranges, testing of design solutions can be indispensable. Consequently, testing can be included in design steps in AD, and zigzagging between domains allows for iterations when necessary.

AD processes continue through the domains as required, to reach a final design stage via prototypes of increasing maturity and detail, until the solution is obvious.

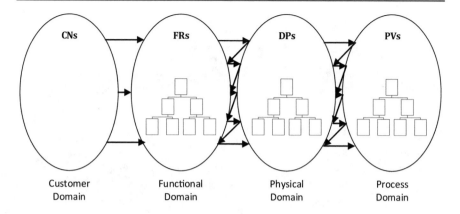

Fig. 4.5 Axiomatic Design domains

4.3 Examples of Design Representations in Industrial Environment

This section introduces example design representations: The first example shows how a technical drawing is created from a design decomposition and matrix. The second explores piping and instrumentation diagrams.

4.3.1 Mechanical Product Design: From the Design Matrix to the Mechanical Drawing

Consider a vehicle braking disk design solution starting from an FR "brake the vehicle." The example shows how, starting from a high-level FR "Brake the Vehicle," it is possible to complete the detailed design of the component brake disk. A brake disk (Fig. 4.6) is part of a sub-system, the braking systems, that allows vehicles to stop. Braking is an FR to be developed for vehicles. A portion of the design matrix is shown in Table 4.1.

This high-level representation is not detailed enough for drafting a technical drawing, or for generating a solid model. Therefore, only by considering lower level FRs and DPs it is possible to draft a technical drawing. The line related to FR_n is expanded in more detail in Table 4.2.

This example shows how technical drawing drafting processes should proceed. The design brake disk sub-assembly is represented by its technical drawing (Fig. 4.7), annotated with numbers corresponding to FR–DP pairs. Ideally, decompositions are taken far enough so that specific dimensions and tolerances can be calculated, before completing component drawings.

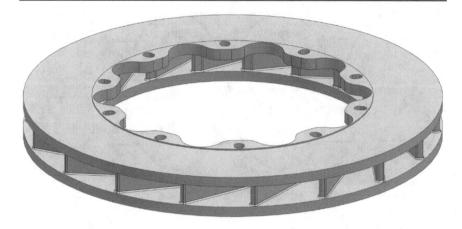

Fig. 4.6 Brake disk

Table 4.1 A section of the design matrix for braking

		DP$_{n-1}$	DP$_n$	DP$_{n+1}$
		...	Brake the system	...
FR$_{n-1}$	...			
FR$_n$	Brake the vehicle		X	
FR$_{n+1}$	...			

Table 4.2 A portion of the decomposition of the brake system

		...	DP$_n$	DP$_{n.1}$	DP$_{n.1.1}$	DP$_{n.1.1.1}$	...
		...	Brake system	Disk brake system	Self-cooling disks	Determine roughness level	...
...	...	...	...	...	...	...	...
FR$_n$	Brake the vehicle	...	X				...
FR$_{n.1}$	Provide adequate breaking power density	...		X			...
FR$_{n.1.1}$	Dissipate friction heat	...			X		...
FR$_{n.1.1.1}$	Maintain stable contact between sliding surfaces	...				X	...
...	...	...	...	...	...	...	...

In Fig. 4.7 DPs are highlighted in red with arrows to the features. Physical integrated in of DPs are depicted. DP numbers link to the FRs, which indicate design intents. Knowing design intents, features on designed artifacts can be changed, without risking unintended consequences. Definitions of actual

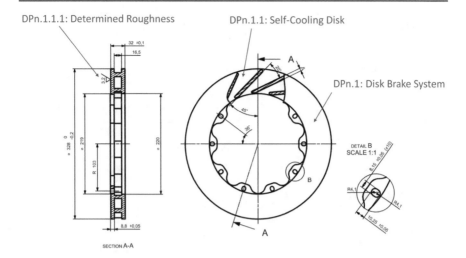

Fig. 4.7 Technical drawing of the brake disk and identification of DPs (in red)

dimensions, such as the disk thickness, disk diameters, and the number of holes for connecting disks to vehicles, are defined with consideration of other FRs and their modules, showing how they are influenced by the DPs.

4.3.1.1   Mechanical Drawing General Rules

Semantics for representations of design solutions, i.e., rules for interpreting symbols, are discussed here for mechanical drawings. There are many rules to be followed, including standardized communication methods, for drawings. These rules make the many kinds of technical representations of design solution languages, like musical scores. These representations transcend ordinary human languages. Just as it is not necessary to speak Italian to play music written by Vivaldi, it is not necessary to speak Italian to understand technical drawings and manufacture components for Fiat. Technical drawings are special methods of communicating, and similar rules are followed, regardless of what is designed.

Consider mechanical drawings, like the braking disk example. In the following example, we examine the most important aspects of this kind of design representation. The first consideration about mechanical drawing is how 3D components are represented on paper in 2D. The answer is with multiple views.

Consider parallel projections. These look at a component from an exact point and remove perspective effects, i.e., vanishing points, which consider perceived diminishing of sizes with distance from the observer. Components are represented by looking at them from as many views as needed to understand its entire shape.

The next question is about how views are arranged on drawings. There are two standardized conventions shown in Figs. 4.8 and 4.9, the first angle projection according to ISO, the International Standards Organization, and the third angle projection according to ASME, and the American Society of Mechanical Engineers.

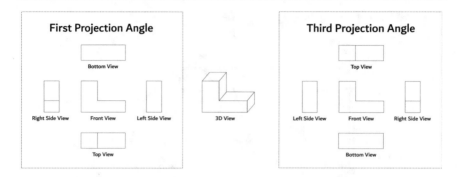

Fig. 4.8 Projection angles

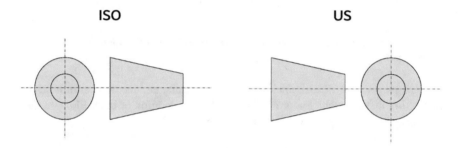

Fig. 4.9 ISO and ASME representations

Knowing which convention, ASME or ISO, is used in the drawing is fundamental to understanding it properly.

Usually, notes are inserted in title blocks as shown in Fig. 4.10. These notes are a crucial part of any mechanical drawing. Title blocks are usually placed on the bottom right side of a drawing. They contain all the notes necessary for understanding the drawing content, such as the projection angle, component name, and scale.

Component dimension can be either explicit or implicit, determined by adding or subtracting explicit dimensions. There are only two rules to follow when dealing

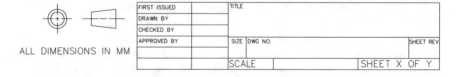

Fig. 4.10 Title block

with component dimensioning: include all dimensions, and only define dimensions once, either explicitly or implicitly, never both.

Consider details of all the different dimensions reported in the brake disk in Fig. 4.7, particularly:

- Numbers express linear dimensions. The measurement unit can be either millimeters or inches. Inches all have the symbol, ", after the number, e.g., 3".
- Indications, such as 36°, express an angular dimension, as in the disk example, this is the angular difference between two adjacent holes connecting the disk to the boss.
- Numbers proceeded by the symbol, ø, e.g., ø219, indicate a diameter. Diameters can also be represented with a number without the ø symbol, but in that case the measures should be referred to a diameter of a drawn circumference, e.g., 206 in the brake disk example, which means that all the hole centers are placed on a circumference of 206 mm in diameter.
- When dimensions are followed by smaller number values with a sign or signs, such as $8.15^{\pm0.05}$, it means that a dimensional tolerance has been specified, on that specific measure, which must be satisfied when making that component. This means that the nominal dimension 8.15 mm can vary within the range specified by the tolerance, in the example ±0.05 mm. The specification of dimensional tolerances usually indicates that those dimensions are important for the function of that component. Dimensional tolerances are given only where they are important for fulfilling FRs.
- When a dimension is followed by a multiplication symbol and a number, such as $8.15^{\pm0.05}(\times10)$, it means that the dimension is valid for all the ten similar features in the view. In the brake disk example, the holes that fix the disk to the boss are specified on only one feature and apply to the rest of them, although written only once.
- Surface topographies are defined through specific symbols indicating surface roughness at fine scales, waviness at larger scales and lay, or directionality, according to ASME standard B46.1 on surface texture. There are many topographic characterization parameters that represent different geometric components of roughness, waviness, and lay (see also ISO 25178, ISO 21920, ASME B46.1, and Y14.36M).
- Usually, surface properties, mainly textures, are indicated by placing symbols on drawings of surfaces that are specified. The number above the triangle traditionally is the arithmetic average roughness, Ra, the most used topographic characterization parameter. In Fig. 4.11, the symbol means Ra should not exceed 12.5 μm.

Another fundamental attribute found on mechanical drawings is geometric tolerances on form. Unlike dimensional tolerances, these are applied on surfaces, and not on dimensions, like lengths, widths, and heights. Geometric tolerance on form, as the name suggests, specify how much the actual shape of a surface can differ from nominal. As with dimensional tolerances, surface tolerances are only specified

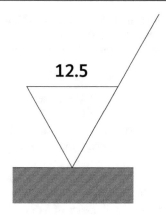

Fig. 4.11 Traditional indication of surface roughness

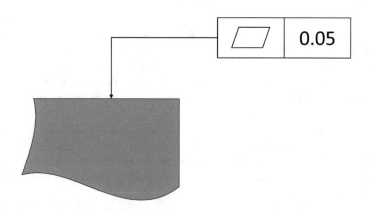

Fig. 4.12 Example of a geometric tolerance on component form for a surface

when shapes are critical for function. An example of a geometric tolerance is shown in Fig. 4.12. The face indicated by an arrow should have a flatness of 0.05 mm. This means that all points on that surface should be between two ideal planes 0.05 mm apart.

Geometrical tolerances are divided into two groups: self-referenced and cross-referenced. Flatness is a self-referenced tolerance. An example of a cross-referenced tolerance is parallelism, shown in Fig. 4.13.

In cross-referenced tolerances, there is always a reference surface, called the datum, which is labeled A in Fig. 4.13. Tolerances are specified with respect to the datum. In Fig. 4.13, the face indicated by the arrow should be parallel with respect to datum A with a tolerance of 0.1 mm. This means that all the points on the surface subjected to the tolerance should be between ideal planes 0.1 mm apart, parallel to the datum A.

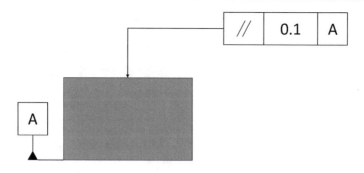

Fig. 4.13 Cross-referenced geometric tolerancing

Artifacts may have more than a datum, like a plane, a face, and a center. If possible, the datum is independently defined. On other applications, each datum needs a certain sequence of definitions. Therefore, the design will be decoupled and a sequence on drawing and manufacturing needs to be followed. For example, a datum center may depend on a face datum. If specifications do not follow the correct sequence for the datum, then dimensions and tolerances will form coupled designs. Coupling of dimensions and tolerances incur extra manufacturing costs. Costs can arise because drawings define lower values for tolerances than necessary, and because specified designs are impossible to manufacture. Impossible designs cause parts to be rejected without the manufacturing enterprise understanding why. It is because a design problem caused a manufacturing problem.

Moreover, in assemblies without movements between components, geometric tolerances should be defined for worst-case scenarios, which allow tolerance bonuses. The worst-case scenario in GD&T is the maximum material condition (MMC), which is identified in the tolerance by a circle with an M inside. For example, a hole could be as short as allowed and a stud that should fit in it is as large as allowed. Maximum material conditions, in many cases, provide the worst case. This condition allows manufacturing to save non-conforming parts that can be reworked, to ensure that when tolerances are at their worst condition, the component still functions properly. These are just two examples of the most common geometrical tolerance that could be necessary for design solution representations. Note that not all the kinds of dimensioning listed above have the same importance.

Figure 4.14 shows some symbols commonly found in technical drawings. They are potentially required to successfully represent design solutions, i.e., DPs. For a detailed description of each symbol refer to mechanical drawing books and manuals.

Tolerance independence is another fundamental principle to be considered. Dimensional tolerances and geometric tolerances should be considered separately. This influences design processes. When dealing with real components, both dimensional and geometric tolerance specifications might be required at the same location. In this case, careful definitions of tolerance intervals can avoid conflicts

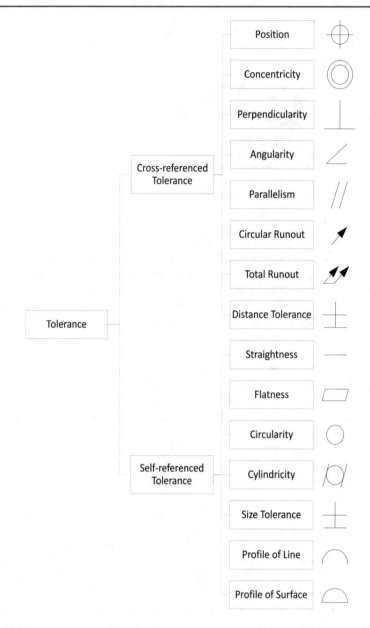

Fig. 4.14 List of geometric tolerances

with axiom one. Complete dimensional information is vital for representing DPs. Surface properties and tolerances are specified only when they are required to assure function, because they incur manufacturing costs.

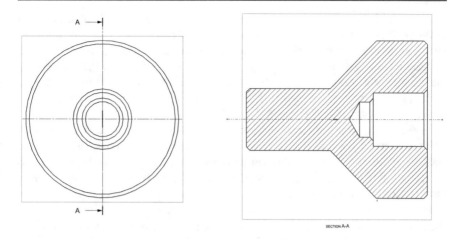

Fig. 4.15 Example of a section representation along A-A left

In principle, physical tolerances on DPs should be derivable from functional tolerances on the FRs, and traceable through design equations. These equations are design modules that show how an FR is influenced by DPs. FRs should have functional tolerances that indicate the acceptable range for satisfying the CNs. Tolerances can be mapped to DPs using the appropriate module.

When an FR is influenced by more than one DP, and DPs influence more than one FR, then tolerances on the DPs might need to be considered with two or more FRs. The partitioning of the tolerances should follow axiom two so that they provide the least information content for the system.

In practice, tolerances are often based on experience with similar designs. Guidance can also be found in the literature. For example, ANSI/ASME B4.1 is a standard guide for tolerancing cylindrical features. It gives textual descriptions corresponding to functions, FRs, and then it gives physical tolerances for DPs, so that components function as intended.

Representations of designed components have been considered, i.e., how to describe sizes and shapes of DPs with dimensions and tolerances. These concepts are valid for any possible view used in a drawing. Components with internal features are considered below.

Internal features are not visible from outside. To view inside a component section is used. A section is a view, or portion of a view, in which a component is opened virtually to see inside. All the above concepts can be applied to exposed interiors. There are two ways to show interiors: traditional section views and break-out section views.

Traditional section views consist of virtual cutting of whole components following the plane specified through a section line. Section lines can be either simple or dashed. Section lines are defined on a view, and section drawings consist of additional views of cut components.

The left side of Fig. 4.15 has a section line. Section lines are typically long dash-dot lines extending beyond components where two arrows, one per extension, indicate the section orientation. Arrows at section line extremities in Fig. 4.15 indicate that the section shows the right side of the component. On the right side of the drawing, the section itself is shown. Usually section views are indicated by a name like "Section X-X," where X is the letter near the arrows indicating the section orientation, e.g., Section A-A.

In section drawings, all intersections between cutting planes and solid material are represented by filling with a crosshatch pattern. Different types of crosshatch patterns are used to indicate different parts and materials, and therefore a discontinuity in filling indicates an interface between two parts. In this way, section views are characterized by section lines in one view, and actual sections in separate views.

Break-out section views help to reduce the number of views required for a complete representation. Break-out sections are defined directly on views on which sections are made. Therefore, there is no need for an additional view in which the section line is defined. Figure 4.16 illustrates the advantages of break-out sections in drawing simplification.

The choice of one or the other kind of representation is completely up to designers.

The most important aspects are drawing readability and understandability. Drawings represent design solutions, which are products of design phases, they should be clear and free from misunderstanding. Representations complying with

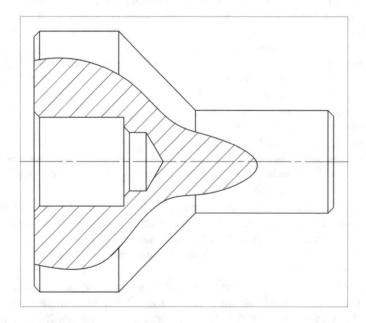

Fig. 4.16 Break-out view

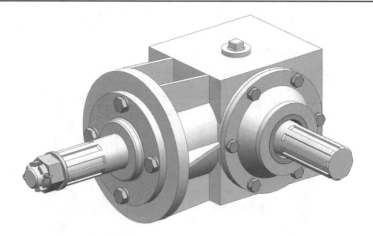

Fig. 4.17 Example of a system made with multiple components: Gearbox

axiom two should minimize the information content and in so doing, maximize the probability of success in correctly communicating intentions of design solutions. Intentions are clearer when corresponding decompositions are supplied with the drawings. This is an essential requirement for any good AD solution representation.

The last topic regarding the design representation of mechanical components is assembly drawings. These show how elements of decompositions are physically integrated, with relationships between multiple components, in one drawing. An example of a gearbox is shown in Fig. 4.17.

Assembly drawings follow the same rules already discussed for component drawings, such as view orientations and section views. Assembly drawings, however, have different scopes than component drawings. They satisfy different CNs for the representation of design solutions. Component drawings are intended to completely represent single components, with all the details of its dimensions and shapes.

Typically, components are physically integrated, i.e., assembled, into systems that fulfill FRs at a higher level. Satisfying CNs and fulfilling FRs typically require an assembly of components, and design representations should include assembly drawings.

As mentioned above, assembly drawings and component drawings have different purposes. Therefore, they contain different kinds of information. Assembly drawings should identify components that comprise a system, and show how these components are arranged in a complete assembly. An example of an assembly drawing is shown in Fig. 4.18.

Individual components are identified with numbers, in balloons. Code numbers in the balloons should indicate numbers of individual DPs as they appear in the decomposition.

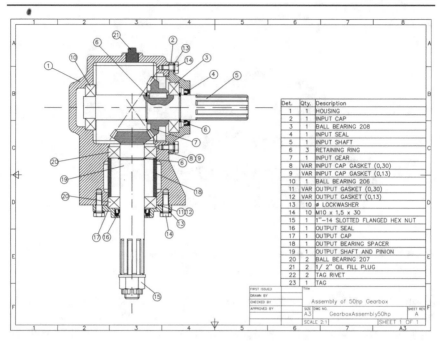

Fig. 4.18 Example of an assembly drawing of a gearbox

Lists of components, also called a bill of materials (BOM), are important because they reference what is needed to deliver functioning products.

4.3.2 Industrial Environment: Piping and Instrumentation Diagram (P&ID)

Piping and Instrumentation Diagrams (P&ID) come with well-defined semantics in the language of process industries. They represent details of piping, process equipment, instrumentation, control devices, and all their interconnections. P&IDs are chosen as an example here because their applicability is wide in industry, and because they represent connections between design processes and representations.

P&IDs show how a designer wants to arrange equipment, instruments, control devices, etc., and how to connect them to get a system to provide its FRs. Many systems are represented through P&IDs, e.g., water cycles inside a power plant that uses steam turbines, oil inside hydraulic/oleodynamic actuators, and an automatic fire-extinguishing system.

Every P&ID representation is detailed and characterized by specific symbology. Because of their high level of precision in representation, P&IDs are suitable and effective in many applications, such as

- planning and construction of power and manufacturing plants;
- operations processes;
- maintenance and modification of processes;
- reference documentation for mechanical technicians and safety personnel;
- reference documentation for HAZOP (hazard and operability study) studies; and
- control of documentation formally issued at various stages of the project.

It is interesting to note that this kind of design representation has been thought to be exhaustive from many perspectives at the same time. Looking at P&IDs, it is possible to understand simultaneously how systems are arranged and controlled, how to plan maintenance, and what the critical parts are.

P&ID representation of an air supply system is shown, as an example, in Fig. 4.19.

Air supply systems are used in industries to obtain a clean air supply for the operations, e.g., pneumatic circuit and conditioning systems. An array of instruments is used to condition air supply, and each component has a specific task. The system functions as follows:

- air passes through a filter (used to clean the air) and arrives to a compressor;
- a compressor (actuated with a motor) takes filtered air and compresses it;
- compression makes the air hot, so a cooling system is needed (aftercooler);
- a cooling process condensates moisture from the air. So, moisture needs to be removed with a separator;
- then the air is sent to a receiver, which removes the dirt and oil from it;
- the air is sent to the dryers to remove the remaining moisture.

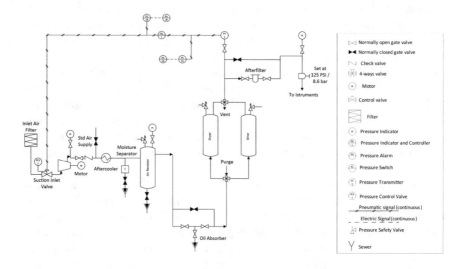

Fig. 4.19 Example of a P&ID representation of an air supply system

- Finally, the air pressure is regulated to target values for operational needs.

Each component is represented in a specific way usually referred to normative (pneumatic system, hydraulic/oleodynamic, electric, instrumentation devices, etc.).

As briefly observed in the example, reading a P&ID diagram can be complicated when readers are not so confident with this kind of representation. However, symbols are standardized, and their meaning is listed in ANSI/ISA S5.1 and ISO 14617-6. Furthermore, each component symbol can be enriched with detailed information, such as dimensions, lengths, and temperatures.

4.4 Case Study: Design and Manufacture of Mechanical and Chemical Polishing Machine (CMP) by Four Graduate Students

Background Story: A major industrial firm in the semiconductor manufacturing equipment industry was interested in getting into a related but new business in the semiconductor processing equipment industry. After considering several possibilities, they decided to buy a small company that manufactured equipment that polished semiconductor surfaces between deposition processes to make the surface "atomically" smooth for the next manufacturing step. This process is called CMP (chemical–mechanical polishing), which polishes the semiconductor surface after each deposition of a new layer of materials to make a semiconductor device. After each round of deposition of materials on the semiconductor surface, it was polished flat before the next deposition can commence.

This business was thought to be growing. In order to increase the density of devices and shorten computational times, deposition layers were increasing, and dimensions of devices were getting smaller. They wanted to buy a small company in Southern California, but they were asking for an unreasonable price. Therefore, a decision was made to let MIT design and build a prototype machine to learn the intricacies of CMP processes and consider the possibility of going into the business with a better tool. For MIT, it was an opportunity to teach students how to design such a complicated large commercial scale machine based on the AD theory. It was determined that such a machine could be built in about 2 years while teaching graduate students how to design and manufacture such a precision machine. CNs were to demonstrate the CMP process using a machine that is better than existing commercial machines.

Five graduate students were assigned to the project. The students had finished undergraduate studies at several different universities and had just entered graduate school at MIT. None of them had any prior industrial experience. To provide proper faculty supervision, an adjunct professor with years of industrial experience was invited to supervise the students. The professor in charge of the project believed that the students could do a successful job and learn what they need to know by executing the project, because he had developed complicated industrial processes and mass production systems when he was a senior at an engineering school. He believed in his students.

One student was assigned the development of the control system for the complete system, including building circuits and devices, although he majored in mechanical engineering. Another student was in charge of designing the entire mechanical system in cooperation with two other graduate students. One of the students, Jason Melvin, did such a great and extensive work that his doctoral thesis committee accepted his thesis as a doctoral thesis rather than letting him go through the typical routine of getting a master's degree first and then writing another thesis to receive a Ph.D. degree. Some of his PowerPoint slides are added below for illustrative purposes.

The students started by defining the highest level FRs based on what they learned by studying industrial machines on the market. They decomposed to the lowest level FRs and DPs, developing the design matrix during the decomposition process. In Fig. 4.20, the design of one of these components and the FRs and the DPs are shown. The according flow diagram for the spindle design is shown in Fig. 4.20.

The finished disk had to be perfectly flat without dished-in parts for subsequent manufacturing operations, using optical imaging to create transistors and other devices. One critical variable in getting an optically flat surface is controlling the pressure exerted on the disk. The decomposition of $FR_{3.2.1.2}$ is done to control the pressure distribution, as shown in Fig. 4.21.

Figure 4.22 shows the detailed assembly design for wafer career. It enables the transport of the wafer and applies the right pressure distribution during the polishing operation.

Note that only a few parts are shown to illustrate the design process based on AD.

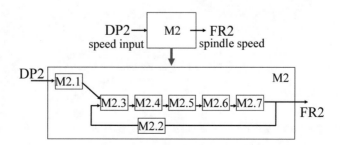

Fig. 4.20 Spindle flow diagram. (Reproduced with permission from Melvin (2003))

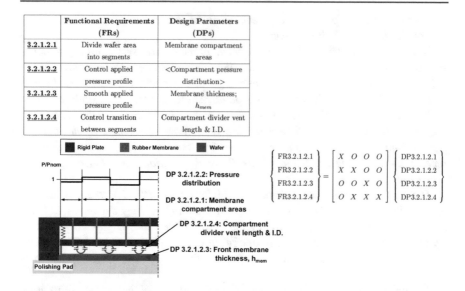

	Functional Requirements (FRs)	Design Parameters (DPs)
3.2.1.2.1	Divide wafer area into segments	Membrane compartment areas
3.2.1.2.2	Control applied pressure profile	<Compartment pressure distribution>
3.2.1.2.3	Smooth applied pressure profile	Membrane thickness; h_{mem}
3.2.1.2.4	Control transition between segments	Compartment divider vent length & I.D.

$$\begin{Bmatrix} FR3.2.1.2.1 \\ FR3.2.1.2.2 \\ FR3.2.1.2.3 \\ FR3.2.1.2.4 \end{Bmatrix} = \begin{bmatrix} X & O & O & O \\ X & X & O & O \\ O & O & X & O \\ O & X & X & X \end{bmatrix} \begin{Bmatrix} DP3.2.1.2.1 \\ DP3.2.1.2.2 \\ DP3.2.1.2.3 \\ DP3.2.1.2.4 \end{Bmatrix}$$

Fig. 4.21 Design of the system that controlled the radial polish rate. (Reproduced with permission from Melvin (2003))

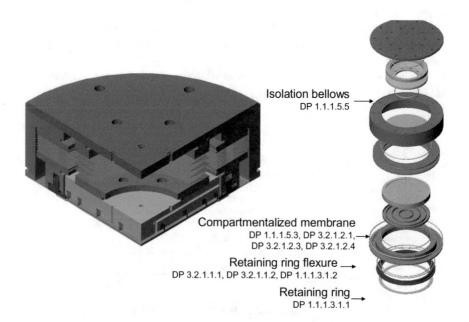

Fig. 4.22 Design of wafer carrier components. (Reproduced with permission from Melvin (2003))

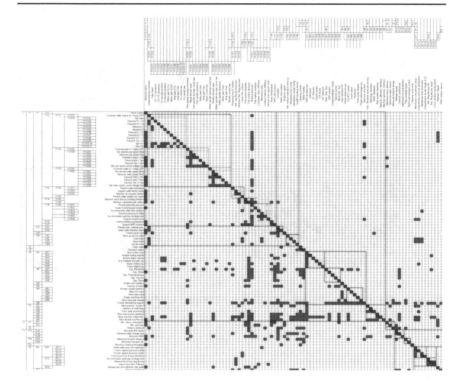

Fig. 4.23 The design matrix for the CMP machine. (Reproduced with permission from Melvin (2003))

The design matrix is shown in Fig. 4.23, indicating if there is any coupling, which requires re-design. Based on the design matrix, Melvin made the necessary and appropriate changes to be sure that the machine would function as intended. In many firms, they make the part and try it out to see if it works appropriately, which is a costly and time-consuming process, rather than checking it during the design stage to find any design flaws done by checking the design matrix.

The final assembled machine (right) and solid modeling (left) are shown in Fig. 4.24. The control system was designed and built by Douglas Lee as part of his thesis for his Science of Master's degree in mechanical engineering at MIT. The machine was designed, built, and tested in 2 years. CNs to develop a better-than-market CMP process machine could be met. Industry sponsors were surprised that students with no prior industrial experience could achieve such a feat in 2 years. **The secret is:**

THROUGHOUT THE DESIGN PROCESS, DO NOT CREATE A COUPLED DESIGN! CONSTRUCT DESIGN MATRICES TO BE CERTAIN THAT THERE IS NO COUPLING IN THE DESIGN DECISIONS MADE!

Solidworks model   Fabricated machine

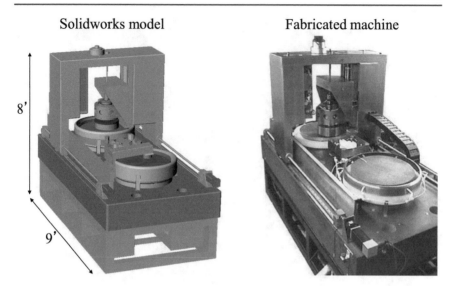

8'

9'

Fig. 4.24 The completed machine. The CAD model on the left and the final fabricated machine on the right. (Reproduced with permission from Melvin (2003))

4.5 Software Design

In previous sections, traditional design representation techniques have been introduced and analyzed. Traditional, in that they are referred to representations of classic components and processes. Because these have been studied for a long time, the basic ways in which they are represented are largely frozen.

In the last decades, however, less traditional products have experienced exponential growth in terms of numbers, relevance, and fields of application, ranging from industry to everyday use. In fact, one of the most important products, maybe *the* most important product, developed, produced, and sold in the last 50 years, is software. Today, almost everything is managed by, or must interact with, software. There is software for every application, and, more recently, with the growth of artificial intelligence applications, software for software management has been released as well.

Software is so important that it is impossible to overlook how software designs can be represented. Explanations follow on how software is usually represented, relationships of design structure matrices (DSM), and applications of modulus concepts in design processes. Reference is made to direct correspondence between unified modeling language (UML) diagrams and design matrixes resulting from decompositions of FRs. Relations between FRs and DPs or DPs and PVs decompositions are shown graphically in module-junction structure diagrams. Through these, a class diagram of systems can be built, on the basis of the existing correspondences between module concepts in AD and concepts of class in object-oriented programming. These make the axiomatic approach compatible with object-oriented programming techniques so that design solutions can be optimized in all phases of software life cycles.

4.5.1 Operational Context

Software is a result of human creativity, which is made up of intangible procedures, and yet pervasive across many human activities. The development of software systems is a complex process involving several actors, according to production cycles, that can follow different models, with multiple intermediate phases. Each development phase is characterized by interactions of skilled professionals who often have completely different roles, experiences, and cultural backgrounds.

The success of development projects depends on stakeholders engaging in dialog. Thus, just the availability of skilled developers does not guarantee success, if contractors fail in communicating clients' needs (CNs) to project analysts. Analysts must formalize CNs into FRs for their developers, who, in turn, must correctly translate FRs into DPs and PVs.

Software engineering emphasizes modeling languages and semantics that facilitate design processes. Representative forms of output design defined by the unified modeling language (UML) are particularly noteworthy. This modeling language was introduced in the late 1990s by the Object Management Group (OMG), in order to unify and standardize various software modeling techniques in use at that time. Object-oriented programming defines abstract software objects, which interact by exchanging messages. Systems can be designed with modular architectures. At each level of abstraction, these systems can be defined by simple diagrams. In this context, UML allows designers to analyze, describe, specify, and document software systems, even complex ones, using visual models, called diagrams. UML is in continuous evolution, and has different forms of graphical representation, depending on the intent. It simplifies dialog among stakeholders involved in software development processes. Project customers and contractors can understand one another through well-defined, clear rules. However, simple representations of cognitive artifacts do not provide all the tools needed to improve projects. In some cases, excessively specific representations of projects could also inhibit creative charges of stakeholders, who might not have an incentive to consider alternative solutions.

AD goes beyond simple, formal representations of projects. AD allows the selection of representations of products that are not simply resulting from the author's creativity or experience. Axiom one guarantees logical coherence of representations themselves, while axiom two selects the solution with the least complexity. However, not all types of UML diagrams are compatible with AD. After all, AD requires representations that are not simply descriptive of the project. For AD representations, unequivocal relationships can be inferred among various components. Therefore, on a case-by-case basis, it is necessary to adapt UML modeling to AD. Not to distort representative techniques, only to redefine them within the scope of design intents to be pursued. Each form of design output representation is specific to adopted software development processes and phases being represented. In this regard, an examination of axiomatic forms of representation of software design cannot ignore contextualization of adopted production processes.

4.5.2 Software Representation—UML

AD is well suited to optimize the software system designs based on object-oriented programming techniques. This is because the AD approach is based on decomposing FRs. For simplification, we can identify at least three levels of FR decomposition for software development. These levels can correspond to three specific classes of representations of software systems (Fig. 4.25).

The first class of representations should describe the conceptual designs of systems. It can be formalized in several ways. It starts by introducing system use cases, i.e., formalizations of specific operation modes to be designed. Each case represents a high-level FR, also from an AD perspective. This definition introduces two types of UML diagrams, use case diagrams and collaboration diagrams. In UML language, it is a matter of two distinct forms of formal representations of the same system. Diagrams of use cases represent general operations of systems and users. This type of representation of a software system has prevailing descriptive nature.

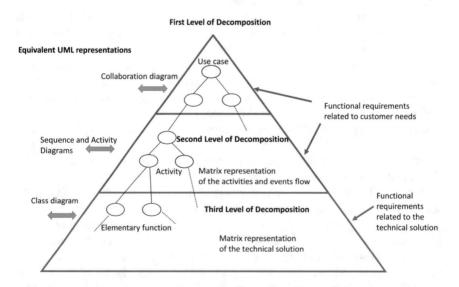

Fig. 4.25 Axiomatic decomposition levels and related software representations

A collaboration diagram has more quantitative elements than a matrix. It constitutes a graphical representation of collaborative interactions among various use cases. Every collaboration between use cases is activated by sending a message, which allows the execution of elaborations. Both types of diagrams provide high-level general representations of systems to be designed. They are used to make structures of systems understandable to non-technical users, such as project clients. They represent standards in the UML 2.0 modeling language, approved by the international OMG committee. The second class of representations defines logical system designs. It corresponds well to the second level of axiomatic decompositions of FRs. In this case, the second-level design matrix can be represented graphically by a sequence diagram. This diagram describes sequential flows of activities inherent to the system to be implemented. This type of representation of a software system constitutes a standard in the modeling language UML 2.0, approved by the international committee OMG. It is always a high-level description intended for analysts, particularly. These professionals act as a bridge between the customer and the developers who are responsible for implementing the procedure. The third class of representations starts to describe, instead, physical designs of systems. In this case, the third-level decomposition matrix of FRs begins detailed representations of objects of the system, consisting of methods, elementary functions, and datasets applied to them. This representation is addressed to the developers of the system, which already describes a design solution. In this case, the third-level design matrix can be graphically represented by a class diagram in UML. The class diagrams allow for formulating descriptions of operations of software systems based on abstract entities called classes.

A class can be constituted by two or more objects. Each object is defined by data structures, called attributes, and by active procedures on such data, called methods, according to what is defined or declared by the respective classes. However, as a simplification in the course of the discussion, we consider the terms "classes" and "objects" as synonyms, even if an object is an instantiation of a class. Also, class diagrams constitute standards in UML 2.0, approved by the international committee, OMG. The entire functional decomposition process is top-down. It starts with high-level requirements and goes on to define detailed technical specifications.

The writing phase of the source code is bottom-up. In this case, from the implementation of the elementary object, processes move on to developing interfaces, and up to overall system implementation. The whole process is iterative. The redefinition of an FR, here a use case, or its incorrect interpretation, involves the overall recycling of the process. The redefinition of use cases corresponds to changing the behavior of a system. This means reviewing the entire system.

4.5.3 Equivalence Between Forms of Representation

Software systems designed with object-oriented programming techniques can also have modular representations compatible with AD. To put this into practice, it is necessary to introduce a useful simplification to UML.

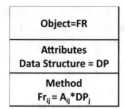

Fig. 4.26 Module M representation

One key phrase "Objects with indices" is used to represent all levels of FRs, i.e., class, object, and behavior. For example, classes or objects may be called Object i, which is equivalent to FR_i. The behavior will be denoted as Object ij to represent a second-level FR_{ij}. Therefore, each module (M) is an object that holds data structures (DPs) and functions that refer to that structure (A_{ij}), as seen in Sect. 4.2.3. Therefore, a generic module (M) is defined as the row of the design matrix (Eq. 4.1), which yields the FR of the row when it is multiplied by the corresponding DP, i.e., data. In practice, a module is an object, which contains the data and the methods that implement FRs (Fig. 4.26). Data structures correspond to data files, while (A_{ij}) are transactional functions, i.e., methods.

Starting from these definitions a series of graphical correspondences can be introduced between modular representations through flowchart diagrams and class diagrams in UM. These correspondences can translate representations of projects in terms of AD, both in the matrix and modular form, in an equivalent form of class diagrams. Regarding Eqs. 4.1 and 4.2, we can consider, respectively, Figs. 4.27 and 4.28 to analyze correspondences with class diagrams.

4.5.4 Example of a Software Representation

Consider the implementation of web services that allow family doctors to monitor the progress of therapies of patients at home with chronic hypertension. Considering clinical cases of hypertension control, in the first phase, consider only two people: a patient and a general practitioner. The stories of both people can be collected in semi-structured interviews. By putting these two interviews together, processes that involve them both can be schematized. The general scenario of the system (Fig. 4.29) can be defined. Each case of identified use must have at least one activation element, i.e., participant. Symbols for participants are little person icons. The two people of the system are also participants in the general scenario because, with their actions, they activate home management processes for blood pressure control. For the example shown, five main use cases are identified, which describe the main functioning of the system. They are represented in Fig. 4.29 by ovals.

In summary, the process is activated by periodic measurements of blood pressure by the patient at home. Every 10 days, a report is sent to a platform, which is

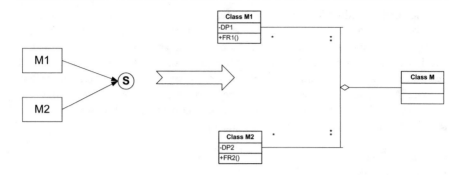

Fig. 4.27 An uncoupled software system like flowchart diagram and class diagram

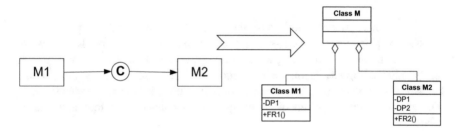

Fig. 4.28 A decoupled software system like flowchart diagram and class diagram

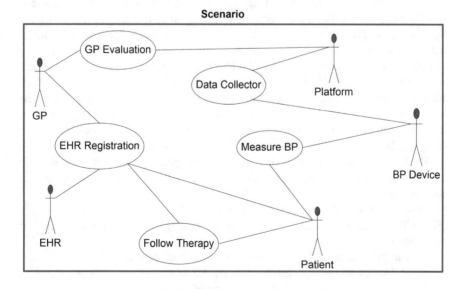

Fig. 4.29 Use case diagram describing the general treatment of hypertension

responsible for sending it to the general practitioner, GP, i.e., family doctor. The GP analyzes the report. If the pressures are considered abnormal then medication dosage can be changed, another medication can be prescribed, or a visit with a specialist can be scheduled. These are recorded in the patient's health record (EHR) and a message is sent via email and text message to the patient. Patient signs in to their EHR accounts and picks up the prescriptions. This identifies primary and recurrent activities. These activities can be summarized in the following synthetic semiformal description (high-level case story):

- measure BP;
- data collector;
- GP evaluation;
- EHR registration; and
- follow therapy.

This general system scenario describes relationships between two people using the system. This representation is simplified and easy to understand. Relationships between components on the diagram are descriptive. However, they are not suitable for directly feeding AD decomposition processes. Therefore, UML diagrams should be identified that can have graphic representations directly referable to matrices. At this level of detail, representations of systems as collaboration diagrams can be adequate.

Collaboration diagrams are graphical representations in UML of software systems. They are used to represent interactions, or collaborations, between various use cases of systems in main modes of operation. Such modality is shown in the diagram of the general scenario of the system of Fig. 4.29. However, to make it entirely compatible with AD, conditions, consisting of considering only interactions that produce elaborations in interaction use cases, must be imposed. Collaborations between use cases X and Y can be defined as the use case X enabling processing in use case Y. In other words, use case X interacts or cooperates with use case Y only when it activates a method causing use case Y to change its state. This forcing allows design processes to focus on events that involve processing. From the general scenario of Fig. 4.29, consider relative use cases of systems and place them in square matrices. In the same way, collaborations can be placed in columns of the same matrix. Then the design matrix of Table 4.3 can be obtained.

Black Xs in Table 4.3 are internal elaborations specific to the use case. Red Xs represent methods that, starting from a specific use case, activate a process in another use case.

From Table 4.3, the equivalent collaboration diagram can be obtained easily (Fig. 4.30). Here, use cases are indicated by rectangles, while arrows represent collaborations.

AD can provide modular representations of use cases related to general treatments of hypertension. As shown in Sect. 4.2.1, the matrix design related to Table 4.3 can also be represented as a system of equations.

Table 4.3 First-level design matrix describing the general treatment of hypertension

	DP$_1$ collaboration measure BP	DP$_2$ collaboration data collector	DP$_3$ collaboration GP evaluation	DP$_4$ collaboration HER registration	DP$_5$ collaboration follow therapy
FR$_1$ measure BP	X				
FR$_2$ data collector	**X**	X			
FR$_3$ GP evaluation		**X**	X		
FR$_4$ HER registration			**X**	X	
FR$_5$ follow therapy				**X**	X

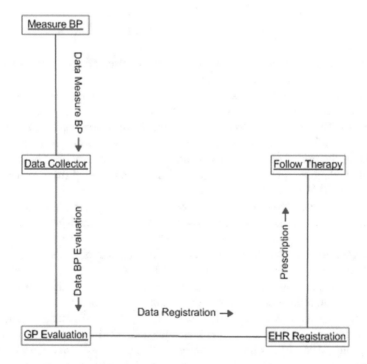

Fig. 4.30 Collaboration diagram describing the general treatment of hypertension

Fig. 4.31 Flowchart diagram
of Eq. 4.6. system

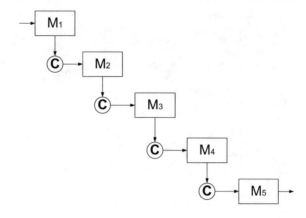

$$\begin{Bmatrix} FR_1 \\ FR_2 \\ FR_3 \\ FR_4 \\ FR_5 \end{Bmatrix} = \begin{bmatrix} X & & & & \\ X & X & & & \\ & X & X & X & \\ & & X & X & \\ & & X & X & X \end{bmatrix} \begin{Bmatrix} DP_1 \\ DP_2 \\ DP_3 \\ DP_4 \\ DP_5 \end{Bmatrix} \qquad (4.6)$$

Starting from previous equations, a modular representation in terms of a flow-chart diagram can be provided as shown in Fig. 4.31.

A new decomposition of FRs can be carried out from the use cases in Table 4.3. Use cases are broken down into actions. A higher level of detail is added (Table 4.4). The proposed decomposition is not the only one possible. Professional experience guides designers through analyses and decompositions of FRs. Thus, AD allows the use of quantitative comparison tools of alternative solutions, based on matrix algebra, such as reangularity and semiangularity from Principles of Design (Suh 1990).

In this case, the second-level design matrix is equivalent to the UML sequence diagram in Fig. 4.32. Its construction is simple. The sequence diagram describes the exchange of actions and messages related to the use case diagram of Fig. 4.29. In this diagram, actions are distributed between participants of the system, patients, medical devices, platforms, EHRs, and GPs. In practice, actions are attributed to specific participants in the process that activates them. Going through Fig. 4.32, each participant refers both to a main action and other actions, which are initialized following interactions with other participants in the system. Actions referring to the same participant are the same color. Messages addressed to other participants are straight lines, dashed lines instead represent those that constitute a return.

Representations of output design can be re-elaborated in terms of flowchart diagrams (Fig. 4.33). This form of representation holds different conceptual levels together. Taking the functional decomposition of Table 4.4 as a reference, the following systems of equations relative to the blocks M_1, M_2, M_3, M_4, and M_5 can be written as follows:

Table 4.4 Second-level design matrix describing the general treatment of hypertension

| | | DP₁ collaboration measure BP | | | DP₂ collaboration data collector | | DP₃ collaboration GP evaluation | | | DP₄ collaboration EHR registration | | DP₅ collaboration follow therapy |
		$DP_{1,1}$ daily BP	$DP_{1,2}$ periodic data pressure report	$DP_{1,3}$ ES BP report to platform	$DP_{2,1}$ collaboration registor BP report	$DP_{2,2}$ collaboration send message to GP	$DP_{3,1}$ collaboration get report	$DP_{3,2}$ collaboration analyse report	$DP_{3,3}$ collaboration prescription	$DP_{4,1}$ collaboration register prescription	$DP_{4,2}$ collaboration send message (prescription)	$DP_{5,1}$ collaboration get prescription
FR_1 measure BP	$FR_{1,1}$ read BP	X										
	$FR_{1,2}$ periodic data pressure report	X	X									
	$FR_{1,3}$ send BP report to platform		X	X								
FR_2 data collector	$FR_{2,1}$ registor BP report			X	X							
	$FR_{2,2}$ send message to GP				X	X						
FR_3 GP evaluation	$FR_{3,1}$ get report					X	X					
	$FR_{3,2}$ analyse report						X	X				
	$FR_{3,3}$ prescription							X	X			
FR_4 EHR registration	$FR_{4,1}$ register prescription								X	X		
	$FR_{4,2}$ send message (prescription)									X	X	
FR_5 follow therapy	$FR_{5,1}$ get prescription										X	X

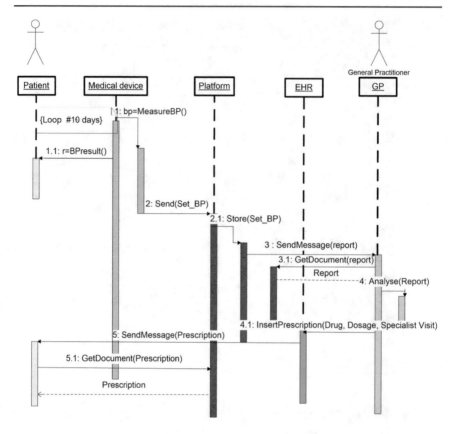

Fig. 4.32 Sequence diagram describing the general treatment of hypertension

$$\left\{ \begin{array}{c} FR_{1.1} \\ FR_{1.2} \\ FR_{1.3} \end{array} \right\} = \begin{bmatrix} X & & \\ X & X & \\ X & X & X \end{bmatrix} \left\{ \begin{array}{c} DP_{1.1} \\ DP_{1.2} \\ DP_{1.3} \end{array} \right\} \tag{4.7}$$

$$\left\{ \begin{array}{c} FR_{2.1} \\ FR_{2.2} \end{array} \right\} = \begin{bmatrix} X & \\ X & X \end{bmatrix} \left\{ \begin{array}{c} DP_{2.1} \\ DP_{2.2} \end{array} \right\} \tag{4.8}$$

$$\left\{ \begin{array}{c} FR_{3.1} \\ FR_{3.2} \\ FR_{3.3} \end{array} \right\} = \begin{bmatrix} X & & \\ X & X & \\ X & X & X \end{bmatrix} \left\{ \begin{array}{c} DP_{3.1} \\ DP_{3.2} \\ DP_{3.3} \end{array} \right\} \tag{4.9}$$

$$\left\{ \begin{array}{c} FR_{4.1} \\ FR_{4.2} \end{array} \right\} = \begin{bmatrix} X & \\ X & X \end{bmatrix} \left\{ \begin{array}{c} DP_{4.1} \\ DP_{4.2} \end{array} \right\} \tag{4.10}$$

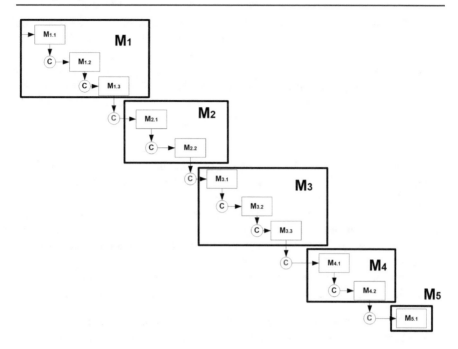

Fig. 4.33 Flowchart diagram describing the general treatment of hypertension

$$FR_{5.1} = XDP_{5.1} \qquad\qquad (4.11)$$

The flowchart in Fig. 4.33 can be represented in terms of class diagram. In this case, the modules M_i are replaced by classes (Fig. 4.34).

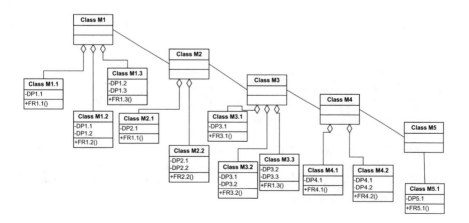

Fig. 4.34 Class diagram describing the general treatment of hypertension

In summary, software system representations in terms of UML diagrams are equivalent to AD forms of design representations. This is possible because object-oriented programming techniques allow systems with modular architectures to be implemented. Throughout software life cycles, representations of design solutions in terms of project matrices or flowcharts of modules can easily be translated into an equivalent UML diagram. These equivalences allow software design activities to be framed within broader scope of engineering studies.

Problems

1. Nowadays, tablets have become one of the most important devices for entertainment, since they allow us to watch films and series, as well as net surfing and social media. The most important problem with tablets is that they need, usually, to be held in place. Thus, how should we design a tablet holder? On the market there are lots of solutions, some of them patented and some others not. However, are they good designs? What about to try to design a tablet holder using AD?

   Consider a customer as a person who uses the tablet mainly to watch movies or other media while lying down. Consider the following customer needs:

   - CN1: Fits on as many different beds and couches as possible;
   - CN2: Holds tablets/other smart devices of various sizes and weights;
   - CN3: Pushes easily out of the way when the user is in need of getting up;
   - CN4: Adjusts easily while remaining stable.

   To facilitate the work, we also propose some FRs defined basing on the CNs:

   - FR1: Attaches securely between any hard surface and a cushion;
   - FR2: Holds tablets/smart devices up to 14 inches and 1 kg. One of the largest and heaviest tablets on the market today is the Toshiba Excite 13;
   - FR3: Pushes out of the way with minimal force, when the users are in need of getting up;
   - FR4: Adjusts with minimal force while remaining stable.

   A student can also try to figure out different FRs.

   Try to represent a design solution basing on this information.

   For further detail, you can find an example in: Helgason H, Þórarinsson T, Ingvason S, Foley JT (2018) "Design of a tablet holder with the help of Axiomatic Design" International Conference of Axiomatic Design 2017, MATEC Web of Conferences.

2. Adjustable desks are a valid solution to reduce prolongated sitting time. This fact, basing on recent studies, has been demonstrated to be helpful for people's health. As well as in the previous exercises, we would like to try to design an adjustable height desk using AD.

Even in this case, the market offers lots of solutions, but in this exercise, we would like to compare, at the end of the exercise, commercial solutions with the obtained design representation.

Even in this case, CNs, as well as FRs, will be provided.

- CN1: Adjustable desk that suits people in common sizes;
- CN2: The desk has to be steady so you can lean on it while working;
- CN3: It should be affordable;
- CN4: It should have electrical sockets;
- CN5: The top panel should endure hammer beatings and fluids without deteriorating.

In this exercise, we shall also consider some constraints as follows:

- C1: Total cost cannot exceed 400 USD;
- C2: It can be manufactured in a workshop.

FRs proposed are the following:

- FR1: Positions a work surface vertically;
- FR2: Stays stable when worked on;
- FR3: Locks in position;
- FR4: Powers appliances;
- FR5: Endures hammer strikes and fluid spills on the surface.

The student is supposed to define a design representation basing on these FRs (or on other FRs defined basing on the CNs).

For further detail, you can find an example in: Foley, J.T., Símonarson, A.F., Símonarson, H.T., Ægisson, L.F., and Goethe, A.T. 2017, "Adjustadesk—An Adjustable Height Desk," MATEC Web of Conferences.

3. Consider the following representation of a simple plate with two holes (Figs. 4.35 and 4.36):

    What is the difference between the two design representations? What is supposed to specify dimensioning in the second design representation? What would this representation tell about the difference in FRs that these fulfill?

4. Consider the following representation of a cylinder (Fig. 4.37):

    Think about a reason why the internal part of the cylinder has more specification about tolerancing than external? State this in terms of the FRs that might need this tolerance to be fulfilled satisfactorily by this specification on a DP.

5. Imagine needing to realize the assembly represented in section in Fig. 4.38.

    The element 1 and element 2 are represented by the following drawings (Figs. 4.39 and 4.40):

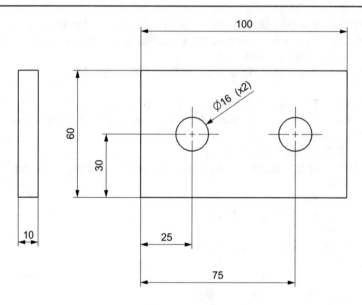

Fig. 4.35 Representation A of a plate with two holes

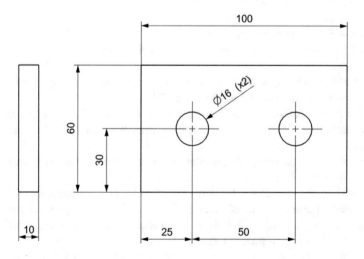

Fig. 4.36 Representation B of a plate with two holes

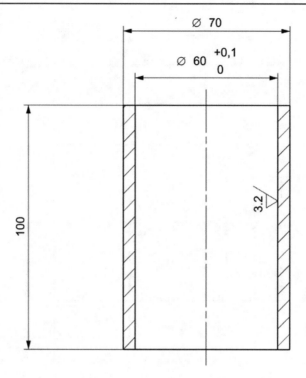

Fig. 4.37 Representation of a cylinder

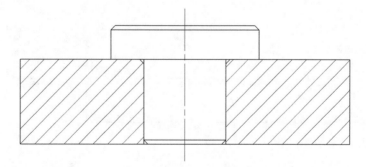

Fig. 4.38 Representation of a system composed of two elements (a single-hole plate—element 1 and a cylindrical pin—element 2)

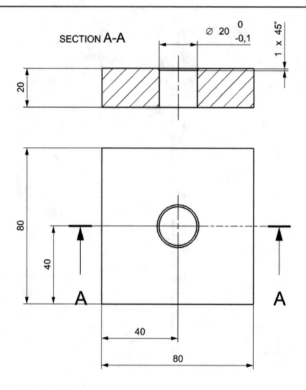

Fig. 4.39 Representation of element 1

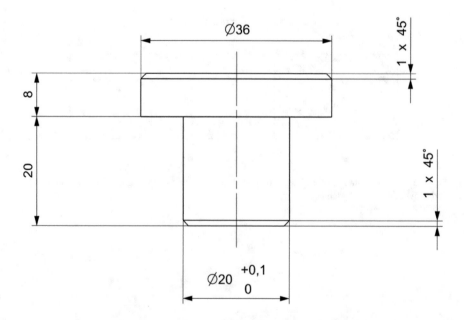

Fig. 4.40 Representation of element 2

Is it possible to say something about the connection between 1 and 2? What could be the DP represented by the hole and pin tolerancing? Do you have any idea of how to assemble the two parts?

6. Explain why AD may be an optimization tool in software system design processes.

7. Construct the design matrix for an FR–DP relationship of a case study related to home administration of drug infusion in pediatric oncology which is described below.

Problem:

The interviews with the actors (healthcare workers, parents, young patients) of the process allowed to identify the primary and recurrent activities for this process. These activities can be summarized in the following use cases:

- checking for drug availability (locker state, non-automated);
- change of therapy;
- change of modality;
- change of drug;
- prescription of drug by the hospital doctor;
- withdrawal of drug at the hospital pharmacy; and
- administration of drug by parents or healthcare professional (nurse, doctor).

Practically, the administration of a drug is activated by the management device. At this point, the system detects that the drug is about to end and sends the alert to the control center. The control center contacts the hospital doctor who prescribes the medicine administered by the hospital pharmacy where the patient's parent goes to collect it. At the end of the process, the availability of the drug is updated.

8. Decompose the FRs related to the design matrix of the abovementioned problem, in order to construct a modular representation of the process in terms of flowchart.

9. Draw for the abovementioned problem the representations in terms of class, collaboration, and sequence diagrams, starting from the previously defined design matrices.

References

ANSI/ASMEB4.1-1967 (2009) ANSI/ASME B4.1-1967 (R2009) Preferred limits and fits for cylindrical parts
ASME Y14.36-2018 (2018) ASME Y14.36-2018 Surface texture symbols
Gausemeier J, Moehringer S (2002) Vdi 2206—a new guideline for the design of mechatronic systems. IFAC Proc 35(2):785–790. https://doi.org/10.1016/S1474-6670(17)34035-1
ISO1302 (2002) ISO 1302:2002 Geometrical product specifications (GPS)—indication of surface texture in technical product documentation

ISO21920 (2020) ISO/DIS 21920 Geometrical product specifications (GPS)—Surface texture: profile
ISO25178-2 (2012) ISO 25178-2:2012 Geometrical product specifications (GPS)—Surface tex-ture: areal
Melvin JW (2003) Axiomatic system design: chemical mechanical polishing machine case study. PhD Defense Presentation Slides
Suh NP (1990) The principles of design. Oxford University Press

Further Reading

Bell E, Davison J (2012) Visual management studies: Empirical and theoretical approaches. Int J Manag Rev 15:167–184. https://doi.org/10.1111/j.1468-2370.2012.00342.x
Booch G, Rumbaugh J, Jacobson I (1999) The unified modeling language user guide. Addison-Wesley Professional
Brown C (2011) Axiomatic design applied to a practical example of the integrity of shaft surfaces for rotating lip seals. Procedia Eng 19:53–59. https://doi.org/10.1016/j.proeng.2011.11.079
Brown C, Hansen H, Jiang X, Blateyron F, Berglund J, Senin N, Bartkowiak T, Dixon B, Le Goïc G, Quinsat Y, Stemp W, Thompson M, Ungar P, Zahouani H (2018) Multiscale analyses and characterizations of surface topographies. CIRP Ann. https://doi.org/10.1016/j.cirp.2018.06.001
Do SH, Suh NP (2000) Object-oriented software design with axiomatic design. In: Thomp-son MK (ed) First international conference on axiomatic design, Institute for Axiomatic Design, Axiomatic Design Solutions, Inc., Cambridge, MA, pp 278–284. https://axiomaticdesign.com/technology/icad/icad2000/icad2000_027.pdf
Foley JT, Símonarson AF, Símonarson HT, Ægisson LF, Goethe AT (2017) ADjustadesk—an adjustable height desk. In: Slătineanu L (ed) 11th international conference on axiomatic design (ICAD), MATEC Web of Conferences, Iasi, Romania, 01002, p 7
Girgenti A, Pacifici B, Ciappi A, Giorgetti A (2016) An axiomatic design approach for customer satisfaction through a lean start-up framework. In: Liu A (ed) 10th international conference on axiomatic design (ICAD), Procedia CIRP, Elsevier ScienceDirect, Xi'an, Shaanxi, China, vol 53, pp 151–157. https://doi.org/10.1016/j.procir.2016.06.101
Helgason H, Þórarinsson T, Ingvason S, Foley JT (2018) Design of a tablet holder with the help of axiomatic design. In: Puik E, Foley JT, Cochran D, Betasolo M (eds) 12th international conference on axiomatic design (ICAD), MATEC web of conferences, Reykjavík, Iceland, p. 7
Melvin JW (2003) Axiomatic system design: chemical mechanical polishing machine case study. Doctor of Philosophy in Mechanical Engineering, Massachusetts Institute of Technology, 77 Massachusetts Ave., Cambridge MA 02139, USA
Oberg E, Jones FD (1916) Machinery's handbook volume 1916. Industrial Press
Object Management Group (2017) Unified modeling language specification (2.5.1). https://www.omg.org/spec/UML/About-UML/
Parretti C, Pourabbas E, Rolli F, Pecoraro F, Citti P, Giorgetti A (2019) Robust design of web services supporting the home administration of drug infusion in pediatric oncology. In: Liu A, Puik E, Foley JT (eds) 12th international conference on axiomatic design (ICAD), MATEC web of conferences, Sydney, Australia, vol 301, p 00013. https://doi.org/10.1051/matecconf/201930100013
Pecoraro F, Luzi D, Pourabbas E, Ricci FL (2017) A methodology to identify health and social care web services on the basis of case stories. In: Proceedings of IEEE E-health and bioengineering conference (EHB), Sinaia, Romania
Pimentel AR, Stadzisz PC (2006) A use case based object-oriented software design approach using the axiomatic design theory. In: Thompson MK (ed) 4th international conference on axiomatic

design, ICAD2006, Axiomatic Design Solutions, Inc., Firenze, Italy, p 8. https://axiomaticdesign.com/technology/icad/icad2006/icad2006_29.pdf

Reed D, Bohemia E (2012) Representations of design outputs in cross-functional teams. International conference on engineering and product design education. Artesis University College, Antwerp, Belgium, pp 425–430

Simmons C, Maguire D (2012) Manual of engineering drawing, 4th edn. Butterworth-Heinermann

Suh NP (1998) Axiomatic design theory for systems. Res Eng Design 10:189–209

Suh NP (2001) Axiomatic design—advances and applications. Oxford University Press

Vulliez M, Gleason M, Souto-Lebel A, Quinsat Y, Lartigue C, Kordell S, Lemoine A, Brown C (2014) Multi-scale curvature analysis and correlations with the fatigue limit on steel surfaces after milling. Procedia CIRP 13:308–313. https://doi.org/10.1016/j.procir.2014.04.052

Problem Definition

5

Ang Liu

Abstract

The first step in developing an innovative design is to know the problem we are trying to solve. Once we know the problem, we need to establish the goals our design must satisfy to solve the problem. Sometimes, we establish the goals first and then determine the problems we must solve to achieve the goals. These goals must then be stated as functional requirements (FRs) in the functional domain that our design must satisfy. In some ways, it is an obvious way of coming up with good designs. However, many companies have made errors by trying to be more competitive, without first discovering the real problem faced by their products. The information on their existing products may come with diverse and contradictory claims and counterclaims, aggravating each other. If we can define "what the problem is," the problem can often be solved through design. The ability to define the problem can be acquired by accumulating broad knowledge base, experience, and repeating the steps outlined in Axiomatic Design (AD). One of the goals of this chapter is to teach those who are not yet initiated into the field of design the ability to identify and define the problem.

5.1 Problem Definition in Engineering Design

5.1.1 Characteristics of Problem Definition

Problem definition is one of the most critical steps in design. It is an open-ended process. Given the same set of customer needs and design constraints, a variety of different problems can be formulated by different designers. It depends on their

A. Liu (✉)
Sydney, Australia
e-mail: ang.liu@unsw.edu.au

© Springer Nature Switzerland AG 2021
N. P. Suh et al. (eds.), *Design Engineering and Science*,
https://doi.org/10.1007/978-3-030-49232-8_5

experience, background, and knowledge. For example, in order to treat cancer, one person may define it as a biological problem that should be solved by "designing a biological experiment to understand the genesis and propagation of cancer." Alternatively, another person may define the problem as a pharmaceutical problem of "designing a new drug to retard cancer development." Another person may characterize it as a public healthcare problem and formulated it as "design a public campaign to discourage smoking." For engineers, multiple engineering problems can be formulated, such as "designing a scanning machine to identify and visualize stage-1 cancer," "designing a big-data platform to analyze a person's potential risk of developing cancer," "designing a medical device to remove cancer completely," and so forth. In another example, the same goal of "addressing climate change" can be converted into a scientific problem of "designing an assessment framework to evaluate the influence of global warming," a policy-making problem of "designing an environmental policy to reduce the greenhouse gas emissions," a political problem of "designing a political discussion to develop a consensus among global political leaders," or an engineering problem of "reversing the trend of global warming through climate engineering."

Problem definition is an iterative process. No problem definition will remain valid forever. As new data, information, and knowledge are acquired, people should be prepared to revisit and revise your problem definition. For example, the success of century-old IBM (International Business Machines) can be attributed to its strategic shift of core business by continuously focusing on the emerging, high-value, profitable new markets. In other words, IBM repeatedly redefined its essential problem from typewriter to personal computer, to IT service, to artificial intelligence (AI), and so on. The development of new problem definition can be triggered by new technological development. Every time a breakthrough technology is introduced, not only it solves existing problems, but also it introduces new problems. For instance, the advancement of additive manufacturing (3D printing) is promoting the development of material science.

Problem definition serves to bridge ideality and reality. The former refers to the ideal state you desire to achieve without any limitations in the distant future, whereas the later means the possible state you can afford to achieve against various constraints at present. A problem should be defined in light of the ideality, while the problem should be solved following the reality. Those successful company, organization, and person, with no exception, are all keenly driven by an ambitious vision of ideality. For example, the ideality of BMW is to produce the "ultimate driving machine," whereas the ideality of Toyota is to "lead the way to the future of mobility." The ideality of Elon Musk is "immigration in Mars," and his projects (e.g., Space X, electric vehicle, and Hyperloop) were all intended to serve such an ideality in the reality.

The design problem is a multi-faceted notion. Generally speaking, a complete problem definition involves customer need (CN), FRs, design constraint (DC), and problem context. Firstly, new artifacts are developed to satisfy unmet customer needs. In order to generate new values, impacts, and profits, it is imperative to fully understand your target customers and relevant stakeholders, concerning their voices of what is desirable and undesirable. Secondly, the unstructured customer voices should be translated into a set of well-defined FRs that can be assigned to engineered systems. This is where engineers come into play to leverage their engineering knowledge and design thinking to connect the customer domain and the physical domain. Thirdly, different from art design, engineering design is always performed against various limitations. Therefore, a variety of design constraints should be identified to limit the choice of FRs and design parameters (DPs). Lastly, a problem definition is unique in a particular context. The same problem should be defined differently in different contexts. When the context changes over time, the problem should be redefined correspondingly. Among the four critical components of problem definition (i.e., customer need, FRs, design constraint, and problem context), FR is arguably the most important but difficult decision to make in problem definition. Different from CNs and DCs that are mostly imposed by the third parties (e.g., client, management, supplier, government, and union), FRs are entirely decided on your own based on your engineering knowledge, experience, and creativity.

5.1.2 Good Problem Definition Leads to Design Innovation

Design Story 5.1:

As illustrated in Fig. 5.1, iPod was one of the most successful product offerings in the development history of Apple Inc. It is widely agreed that the subsequent successes of iPhone and iPad were more or less built upon the foundation of iPod. The original problem definition for iPod, proposed by Steve Jobs, was to design a portable device that could *"carry 1,000 songs in the pocket."* As a result of such a problem definition, the engineers at Apple were inspired to solve multiple "un-conventional" problems, such as *"where to download 1,000 songs in a legal way,"* *"how to pay for so many songs,"* *"how to deal with the copyright issue,"* *"how to index and search so many songs,"* etc. Through solving these problems, not only Apple engineers developed sophisticated hardware, but also it created the media library of "iTunes." Thereafter, the definition of iPod continuously evolved from a portable music player to a multimedia digital player, and eventually to today's multi-purpose pocket computer. It should be noted that, in the year of 2011, MP3 player was by no means an entirely new concept. Many competitors had their own product offerings of MP3 player. Assume the problem definition given to the engineers had been to *"develop an MP3 player with an Apple logo,"* it should not be too surprising that a set of very different problems would have been addressed, such as "storage capacity," "battery life," "sound quality," etc.

Design Story 5.2:

RSI (repeated stress injury) is a common problem caused by using the computer keyword. As the name suggests, RSI occurs when a routine motion that stresses the body is repeated. Over time, stress accumulation will lead to injury. Ergonomic

Fig. 5.1 Case study of iPod design. (Reproduced with permission from Delyk 2019)

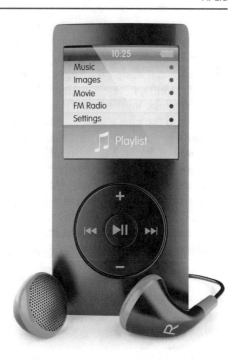

keyboard, as a traditional solution, was designed to address the problem of "how to provide users with the most comfortable (or least stressful) typing position." In other words, the focus of problem definition lies in the keyword of "stress." A few years ago, this design task was given to a group of KAIST students, and another innovative solution was created. By focusing on another keyword of "repetition," they redefined the problem as "*how to interrupt the repetition of the same gesture.*" As a result, they developed a "floating keyboard" that is characterized by a subtly moving plane to help unlock stressful muscles and engage other muscles. This concept has been applied to other industries. Take the office chair for example, by replacing the static piece of furniture with a yoga ball, the user subtly engages other muscles to keep an unstable balance, and hence reducing the RSI. This is called a yoga ball chair, as illustrated in Fig. 5.2. In addition, the footwear industry has seen this trend as well with "rocking shoes" that promote engaging ankle muscles in a way traditional shoe cannot.

A good problem definition enables you to discover those invisible innovation opportunities. As illustrated in Fig. 5.3, although the three products (i.e., smartwatch, jogging stroller, and yoga ball chair) belong to entirely different product categories (i.e., wearable device, children product, and office furniture), they can actually be recommended to the same target customer, because they are all intended to fulfill the same purpose (i.e., "perform exercise while multitasking") by solving a variety of different problems.

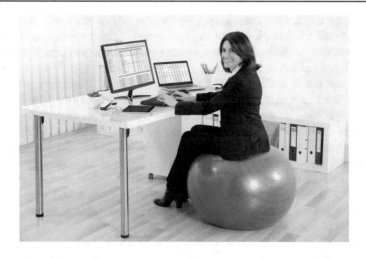

Fig. 5.2 Case study of yoga ball chair. (Reproduced with permission from Popov 2019a, b)

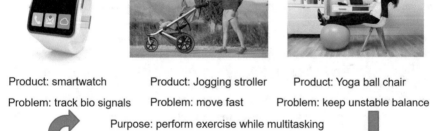

Product: smartwatch   Product: Jogging stroller   Product: Yoga ball chair

Problem: track bio signals   Problem: move fast   Problem: keep unstable balance

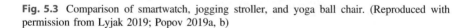

Purpose: perform exercise while multitasking

People: a young mother who has a full-time job

Fig. 5.3 Comparison of smartwatch, jogging stroller, and yoga ball chair. (Reproduced with permission from Lyjak 2019; Popov 2019a, b)

5.2 Definition of Customer Need

5.2.1 Who Are the Target Customers and Relevant Stakeholders?

Problem definition should be collaboratively developed between you with a group of target customers and relevant stakeholders. On the one hand, customer voices should be solicited, analyzed, and interpreted to consolidate the basis of problem definition, as Steve Jobs once proposed, *"you've got to start with the customer experience and work backward to the technology."* On the other hand, problem definition cannot be dictated only by customer voices, as Steve Jobs once proposed, *"you can't just ask customers what they want and then try to give that to them. By the time you get it built, they'll want something new."* Therefore, the rational attitude toward customer inputs should be "always listening to your customers, avoid being uttered by their voices, and make your own decisions."

Problem definition begins with involving target customers and relevant stakeholders. Generally speaking, there are three models of customer involvement (Kaulio 1998): design for customer (i.e., the process of creating new product based on customer's preferences), design with customer (i.e., the process of engaging customers in evaluating new products), and design by customer (i.e., the process of empowering customers to build individualized products by themselves).

Given an ill-defined problem statement, the first question to ask is *"who are the target customers."* Apparently, depending on your answer to this question, problem definition will be driven toward different pathways, because different customers more or less demand different things. In practice, brainstorming is a common method for identifying target customers. As illustrated in Fig. 5.4, a simple 4-P method can also be followed to search for target customers. Specifically, a set of four interrelated questions are asked in sequence: *"what is the name of a product," "what problem is the product designed to solve," "what purpose is the problem intended to serve,"* and *"who are the people behind the purpose."* By repeating this process, you will practice your divergent thinking to think outside the box. It should be noted that, in industry, Big Data analytics is growingly employed to recognize target customers, analyze customer preference, and build customer personas.

Take the toy design for example, who are the real target customers? Is it parent, children, toy store, or all of them? An obvious answer is children, who however has no money to pay for the toys he/she really prefers. An alternative answer is the parent, who has more purchase power than the child. In reality, nevertheless, most

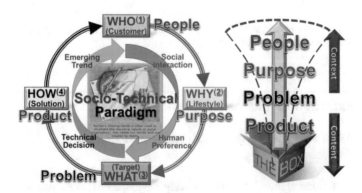

Fig. 5.4 4P Model to identify target customers and relevant stakeholders

of the children simply won't play the toys bought by the parent, which are primarily intended to "*stimulate intelligence and creativity*" (i.e., a typical customer need of most parents). Interestingly enough, in certain markets, grandparents are the most generous customers who are willing to pay for those very expensive toys. A smart designer like yourself should never underestimate the decision of target customers, because your choice will directly/indirectly affect the subsequent decisions of production, packaging, distribution, retailing, repairing, and recycling. For example, if you chose grandparent as your primary target customer, it may not be a good idea to sell the product online (e.g., Amazon), since most of the grandparents still prefer the conventional shell shopping experience.

In addition to target customers, it is equally important to involve the relevant stakeholders. Although the relevant stakeholders will not directly buy or use your product/service, their decisions will influence the design with respect to where, when, how, in what ways, and under what conditions the product can and cannot be sold, used, and maintained. For example, the relevant stakeholders of stroller design include government, supplier, car manufacturer, school, airline, grocery store, and so forth. A square design structure matrix, where the domain elements are the relevant stakeholders, can be created to indicate the conflicting or mutual interests between any two stakeholders. For example, passenger and airline share conflicting interests for the space airplane seat, while airline and airport share mutual interests for airplane safety.

Exercise 5.1:

If you were one of the chief designers of Boeing 787 Dreamliner, who are your real target customers? Is it passenger, pilot, airline, airport, Federal Aviation Administration (FAA), Transportation Security Administration (TSA), Department of Homeland Security, or simply all of them? Be careful, your answer to this question will drive the direction of a billion-dollar project.

Exercise 5.2:

If you were the dean of a leading engineering school, in the event of redesigning the existing curriculum for the accreditation purpose, who are your real target customers? Is it college student, faculty member, professional staff, industry partner, university president, government official, or simply all of them? If your answer is "all of them," is there a way to make everyone happy? What will you do in front of conflicting customer needs?

Exercise 5.3:

If you were the CEO of a global car ride-sharing service provider, can you name a list of key stakeholders who are relevant to the development, test, commercialization, and regulation of self-driving taxi technologies? Do they have any conflicting or mutual interests?

5.2.2 How to Solicit Customer Voices?

After you have involved a group of target customers and relevant stakeholders, some design methods can be followed to solicit their voices. Firstly, the lead user theory can be used to involve those lead users who possess in-depth knowledge of both "know-what" and "know-how" (Franke et al. 2006). Secondly, ethnographic studies can be conducted to observe and discover how and in what ways customers utilize, interact, and alter a product, being situated in a particular context. Ethnography is commonly used in social science to investigate how a particular culture is developed based on social interactions. It can also be employed in product design to understand user habits. Thirdly, you can interview customers to directly solicit their voices. In comparison with the traditional interview approach that occurs in a formal setting (e.g., conference room), contextual inquiry is a more user-centered method, which enables you to discover some contextual information. Focus group is a group interview approach, through which, dynamic interactions between peer users are leveraged to trigger common opinions and implicit findings that cannot be revealed by individual interviews. However, the success of a focus group session hinges on an experienced moderator. Lastly, surveys can be conducted to solicit customer opinions and aggregate their preferences. On the one hand, surveys are the most frequently used method in practice. On the other hand, surveys are by no means the most effective method. Not only you should have in-depth knowledge to design a set of meaningful survey questions, but also you should find a way to escape from the Arrow's Paradox when aggregating the survey responses.

The abovementioned methods all require direct interactions between you and the customer. Due to the rapid development of e-commerce and social networking, there emerged a huge volume of crowd-sourced online customer voices in the format of product reviews. Take a popular product "Kindle Paperwhite eReader" for example, over 58,000 product reviews are published on Amazon. Product reviews can be collected from a variety of online channels such as e-commerce platform, search engine, APP store, social media/networking, video sharing website, product forum, and so forth. Rich information can be abstracted from the product reviews. Take a typical review on Amazon for example, the data that is potentially useful for problem definition includes product rating, reviewer ranking, review content, photo and video, comment and Q&A, and peer evaluation of the review's helpfulness. Since the vast majority of product reviews are contributed by end users, the contents are oftentimes unstructured and inconsistent. Therefore, massively crowd-sourced reviews must be carefully analyzed through qualitative data analysis. A complete qualitative data analysis process consists of data collection, transcription, segmentation, categorization, and coding.

Customer voice includes customer need, want, expectation, complaint, reflection, emotion, etc. We are most interested in customer needs, especially the unmet customer needs that cannot be fulfilled well by any existing solution. Maslow's Hierarchy of Human Needs, which is one of the most fundamental theories in psychology, can be followed to classify CNs into different categories (i.e., "self-actualization," "esteem," "social needs," "safety and security," as well as "physiological needs"). Through the classification of CNs, you will be guided to filter those distracting noises that are unnecessarily customer needs (you are "forced" to double-check the vitality of those CNs that cannot be classified into any of the categories).

Exercise 5.4:
Given the task to design a coffee machine, how do you propose to solicit customer voices? Which method(s) will you select? How do you combine different methods?

5.2.3 Understand Customer Voices to Capture Innovation Opportunity

The above-solicited customer needs should be extrapolated in consideration of various macro-environmental factors based on the PEST framework (i.e., the political, economic, socio-cultural, and technological factors). By doing so, the purpose is to rank-order the CNs in terms of their probabilities of triggering breakthrough innovations. Since most of the political factors (e.g., government regulation, environmental law, tax policy, etc.) and economic factors (e.g., economic growth, interest rate, inflation, etc.) are not directly related to a typical engineering design project, as much as possible, you should focus on the socio-cultural and technological factors.

One of the most important socio-cultural factors is the lifestyle meaning behind a product. For example, the success of iPhone can be attributed to not only its functions but also the lifestyle meaning it represents in the customer's mind. Since the intangible lifestyle meaning is socially constructed via back-and-forth interactions, it must be examined in a particular context. For example, the coffee culture is notably different in different contexts (e.g., in the USA, UK, and Australia). Hence, a coffee machine should be designed differently to reflect such variations of lifestyle meaning. In addition, you should make sense the CNs in light of the ongoing social trends such as the sharing economy, human multitasking, product–service integration, etc.

With respect to the technological factors, in the interest of promoting innovations, the CNs should be unfolded in consideration of the ongoing technological trends. For example, multiple smart products can be interconnected, through the Internet of Things (IoT), to perform functions collectively and collaboratively that cannot be performed by any individual product. The Big Data analytics and machine learning algorithms can be leveraged to recognize, record, and analyze the complex human behaviors. A variety of sensors can be employed to make a product more aware of the surrounding contexts such as the physical context (e.g., time, location, weather, etc.), social context (e.g., peer product, complementary service, resource supply, etc.), and user context (e.g., user demographics, habit, mood, etc.). The additive manufacturing technologies make it possible to produce some complex structures that cannot be manufactured before. The digital twin enables the designer to compare a product's expected behaviors (i.e., that are derived from functions) and actual behaviors (i.e., that are derived from structures) in real time.

5.3 Definition of Functional Requirement

Problem definition is essentially a translation process from customer voices to engineer voices. The vast majority of customer voices are poorly defined, ill-structured, highly inconsistent, mostly biased, and full of noises. By contrast,

engineer voices should be clearly defined, well organized, and consistently phrased.
Engineers communicate through the language of FRs.

5.3.1 How to Represent Functional Requirements?

Function represents the purpose of design. By using FRs to describe an artifact, you are guided to diverge your thinking to explore a broader solution space for more possibilities. For example, if a watch is described as an artifact to "tell the time," then you are naturally inspired to think "are there any other means to tell the time"? As a result, more alternative solutions will automatically emerge, such as computer, smartphone, clock, etc. It should be noted that, in comparison with novice designers, expert designers are characterized by their awareness and ability to describe artifacts in terms of FRs in place of the physical name, appearance, material, and structure.

Functions are assigned to an artifact as its requirements, and hence, namely, FRs. Not only the same FR can be assigned to different products, but also the existing artifact can be assigned with new functions through iterative problem definition. Take the evolvement of mobile phone for example, initially, it was only assigned a few basic FRs, such as <make phone call>, <send message>, <manage contacts>, etc. Gradually, new and higher FRs were assigned, such as <take phone>, <respond email>, <manage calendar>, etc. Finally, mobile phone became smartphone that carries a variety of "smart" functions, such as <navigate direction>, <play game>, <browse Internet>, etc. As a matter of fact, it can be argued that today's popularity of smartphone is largely attributed to the great availability of smartphone apps, which enabled the users to customize the functions of their smartphones.

The formulation of FRs should follow some basic principles:

(a) FRs should be represented in the format of <verb + object>.
(b) FRs should be described in a solution-neutral fashion.
(c) FRs should be specified by a range of target value (i.e., design range).

Firstly, FRs should be represented in the format of <verb + object> or its variations as follows:

- Function = <Verb + Object>.
- Function = <Verb + Object1> to/from/with/through <Object2>.
- Function = <Verb + Object> in <context>.
- Function = <Verb + Object> against <constraint>.

Secondly, in order to inspire novel ideas, FRs should be formulated in solution-neutral fashion. By doing so, it enables you to explore a broader solution space in the concept generation phase. In practice, it is helpful to show your FRs to some fellow engineers and ask whether they can immediately associate the FRs with an existing product/service. If their answer is "yes," it is an indicator that you should step back and reformulate your FRs.

Thirdly, every FR should be associated with a quantifiable design range. In practice, specifying a design range requires a wealth of design knowledge, experience, and even in-depth research. It is important that the design range is carefully determined because it will be compared with the system range to compare multiple alternative DP options.

- FR_1 = Adjust the seat angle between $10°$ and $80°$;
- FR_2 = Support 15–20 kg (weight of a baby);
- FR_3 = Stop motion within 1–2 s;
- FR_4 = Convert human force (value range) to torque;
- FR_5 = Prevent direct sunshine by 50–70%;
- FR_6 = Carry 10–15 kg grocery;
- FR_7 = Hold a water bottle of 2–3 kg;
- FR_8 = Unfold the stroller (to what extent?);
- FR_9 = Make seat waterproof (volume of liquid);
- FR_{10} = Limit degree of freedom ($4°$–$5°$);
- FR_{11} = Dissemble seat within 15 s;
- FR_{12} = Install seat as car seat within 20–30 s;
- FR_{13} = Absorb shock impulses by 80%.

It should be noted that function formulation is an iterative process. It is common that you will need to revisit and revise your FRs once new market is cultivated, new knowledge is acquired, new constraints are imposed, and new decisions are made.

5.3.2 How to Extract Functional Requirements from Existing "Things"

FRs are intangible and solution-neutral. Therefore, it is cognitively difficult to formulate FRs without any tangible thing in mind. This is especially true for novice designers who have inadequate design knowledge and experience. In practice, it is common that young designers tend to extract FRs based on the observation, abstraction, and interpretation of existing things.

FRs can be extracted from not only engineered systems but also biological systems. Biologically inspired design is one of the most widely adopted design approaches. For example, "FR" can be extracted based on the human body to describe the roles played by different organs. It should be noted that the <verb + object> format is strictly followed to formulate the FRs of these organs.

- **Nose**: Breathes fresh air and senses smell;
- **Mouth**: Breathes fresh air, tastes food, speech, facial expression, etc.;

- **Larynx**: Generates sound, swallows food;
- **Heart**: Pumps blood;
- **Lungs**: Pull oxygen, push CO_2 gas out, add air to blood, etc.;
- **Stomach**: Digests food, absorbs small molecules, controls secretion, senses nutrition, etc.;
- **Liver**: Synthesizes protein, breaks down insulin, detoxifies chemicals, secretes bile, etc.;
- **Kidneys**: Clean blood, regulate blood pressure balance water, activate Vitamin D, filter water;
- **Small Intestine**: Digests food, absorbs nutrition.

It is interesting to point out that these internal organs are all functionally independent of each other, even though they are physically integrated, in a highly sophisticated manner, by the blood vessels. This can be considered as a vivid example of how the Independence Axiom applies for biological systems as well. From this perspective, cancer can be viewed as a redundant organ (or DP) that only consumes resources (or adding process variables (PVs)) without contributing to any useful function. As a matter of fact, one of the major challenges of treating cancer is how to identify cancer at a very early stage. This challenge is more or less attributed to cancer's functional invisibility.

The FRs extracted from an existing artifact (or biological system) can be reformulated, reorganized, and then recommended to the new artifact. For example, many functions of smartphone were extracted from its peer products such as computer, camera, PDA, etc. The FRs carried by the coffee grinder, milk frother, and mug warmer can be transferred to a coffee machine.

Exercise 5.5:
Can you specify a range of acceptable values for the above-listed FRs of different organs of human body?

Exercise 5.6:
Can you extract multiple candidate functions from other home appliances and recommend them to the robotic vacuum cleaner?

5.3.3 How to Classify Functional Requirements into Different Categories?

FRs should be classified into different categories. By doing so, it facilitates you to evaluate the weights and priorities of different FRs. According to the Kano customer satisfaction model, product features can be classified into three kinds: excitement function, performance function, and basic function. The Kano model is a qualitative measure of human psychological reactions (excitement) to a product based on Maslow's hierarchy of needs. Firstly, basic features are features that are required in a product or it won't sell. On the other hand, even the basic feature is available, customer reaction is neutral. For example, a customer will never purchase a car without any brakes. Basic features are often a result of government regulations. The second feature is the performance feature. The more performance features a product has, the more customer is willing to pay. Based on the car example, the performance features include gas mileage, air-conditioning, horsepower, airbags, etc. Thirdly, excitement features are a mirror image of basic features—if the product lacks them, the customer will not be disappointed because they didn't expect them in the first place. If a product has excitement features, the customer has to have it! An example would be a self-parking car. As time progresses, today's excitement feature will become tomorrows' performance feature, which eventually becomes basic features. With social media, this timeframe has accelerated tremendously! In certain cases, yesterday's basic feature may come back and become tomorrow's excitement feature. For example, consider a cigarette lighter in a car, while the technology hasn't changed, consumers can now use the cigarette lighter to charge electronic devices. In practice, the Kano model can be integrated with customer surveys to collect relevant information for accurate classification.

Secondly, according to the Long Tail model, FRs can be classified into two categories: popular functions and unpopular functions. Function popularity can be measured in terms of how many products are carrying the same function and how frequently the function is used by the customer. According to the traditional design thinking, the designers should focus on the 20% most popular functions, based on the principle of Pareto efficiency. The Long Tail model, however, suggests that you should focus on the 80% unpopular functions. It is increasingly difficult to maintain user excitement simply by providing popular functions because popular functions tend to be the focus of social media. As a result, most of the popular functions will soon lose their surprising effect, and therefore become performance features. Accordingly, customer excitement is increasingly stimulated by the "unpopular" functions that are tailored precisely to the unique demographic, need, and preference. Therefore, heavier weight should be assigned to the unpopular functions that are anticipated to trigger customer excitement.

During the classification process, the redundant FRs should be eliminated. In practice, redundant FRs refer to those functions that are undesirable to customers and the functions that can be better fulfilled by another artifact. It should be noted that redundant FR is not equivalent to unpopular FR. The former is measured by the customer desirability, whereas the latter is measured by the usage frequency. According to the previous studies of the Long Tail model, in many cases, customers tend to gain a much higher satisfaction when an unpopular function is met.

Exercise 5.7:
What are the 20% popular functions and 80% unpopular functions of a smartphone? What are the exciting function, performance function, and basic function of a smartphone?

5.3.4 How to Structure Functional Requirements?

The classified FRs should be organized into a design structure. Hierarchy is a commonly used structure to organize FRs. Hierarchy is a structured arrangement of entities based on their abstraction levels and dependency relationships. AD prescribed three basic principles for organizing FRs into a hierarchy, namely, "complete" (i.e., no necessary FRs are missing), "minimum" (i.e., no redundant FRs are included), and "independent" (i.e., no functional couplings exist). The functional hierarchy can be created by alternating the analysis and synthesis operations through a zigzagging process.

Generally speaking, FRs are organized according to their dependency relationships and abstraction levels. Specifically, the general FRs should be accommodated in the upper layers of the hierarchy, whereas the specific FRs should be placed in the lower layers of the hierarchy. The parent FRs should be placed above the children FRs. The relationships between FRs at adjacent layers of the hierarchy are the "part-of" relationship. By organizing FRs into different layers, the problem definition is decomposed into different levels, respectively. Figures 5.5 and 5.6 illustrate the functional hierarchies of stroller and baby incubator, respectively.

Exercise 5.8:
*Can you formulate a set of FRs for a **robotic vacuum cleaner**, organize the FRs into a functional hierarchy, and check to what extent these FRs are independent of each other?*

Exercise 5.9:
*Can you formulate a set of FRs for a **3D printer**, organize the FRs into a functional hierarchy, and check to what extent these FRs are independent of each other?*

Exercise 5.10:
*Can you formulate a set of FRs for a **self-driving car**, organize the FRs into a functional hierarchy, and check to what extent the FRs are independent of each other?*

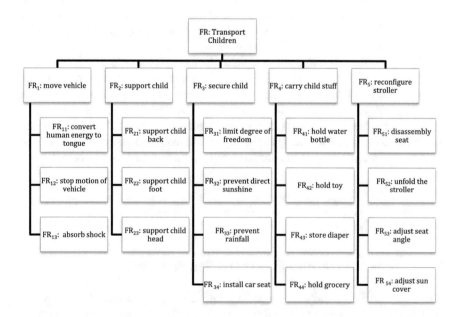

Fig. 5.5 Functional hierarchy of stroller design

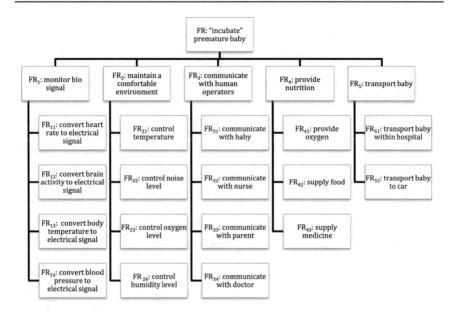

Fig. 5.6 Functional hierarchy of baby incubator

5.4 Definition of Design Constraint

Design constraint serves to define the boundary conditions of a design problem. Not only it limits the formulation of irrational FRs, but also it prevents infeasible solutions from being generated or selected. Design constraints should be clearly differentiated from FRs.

5.4.1 What Is Design Constraint?

Problem definition involves defining not only FRs but also design constraints. The former serves as objectives to illuminate the direction of ideation, whereas the latter serves to define the boundaries of solution space. Different design theories and methodologies model constraints in different ways. For example, AD treats "weight" as a constraint that limits the choice of DPs and PVs (Suh 2001), the function–behavior–structure ontology treats "weight" as a behavior derived from physical structures (Gero and Kannengiesser 2004), and the analytic hierarchy process treats "weight" as a criterion to select the best design alternative (Saaty 2008). It is most challenging to identify and manage constraints during the problem definition stage when everything remains intangible, subjective, and dynamic.

In problem definition, most of the design constraints are intangible and difficult to determine. Constraints are factors that would limit an artifact from achieving a more ideal state (i.e., performance, reliability, robustness, etc.). Accordingly, the instantiation, specification, and management of design constraints hinge on two necessary conditions: a specific goal and a tangible system. In the context of engineering design, the former means an initial intent or thought (i.e., customer need), whereas the latter means a completed artifact (i.e., DPs). In the problem definition phase, however, the intent is yet to be solicited, clarified, and analyzed, whereas the artifact is yet to be created, evaluated, and optimized. As a result, design constraints cannot be stated in an explicit, quantitative, and precise manner. For example, in the problem definition phase, it is difficult to accurately estimate the delivery time of a working prototype, though deadline is an important constraint for any product development.

In problem definition, design constraints could be easily confused with FRs. FRs are the real target of engineering design, whereas constraints are bounds to viable solutions, which are intended to fulfill the FRs. Different from FRs that should always be formulated and maintained independent of each other, it is difficult to make various design constraints entirely independent of each other. For example, the cost of an artifact is contributed by all the components, while it is mostly unnecessary to decompose cost into "sub-cost" and allocate them for different components. In terms of the relationship between FR and DC, according to AD, it becomes more efficient to select FRs when design ideation is appropriately constrained. Whatever the case may be, innovative design must be driven by FRs and limited by design constraints.

According to AD, design constraints are classified into "input constraints" and "system constraints." Input constraints are designer-independent and must be complied by all design solutions. On the other hand, system constraints are introduced by your own decisions, and therefore they are designer-dependent and context-dependent. The major distinction between input constraint and system constraint hinges on the original source. If a constraint comes from the explicit requirements imposed by relevant stakeholders other than yourself, it is classified as an input constraint. In contrast, if a constraint comes from your own decisions, it is classified as a system constraint. The difference between input constraint and system constraint can be illustrated by the comparison between "budget" and "cost." At first glance, "budget" and "cost" seem to mean the same thing. However, they belong to different categories of constraints. Budget means a financial plan of expenses for designing an artifact, whereas cost means the number of resources for producing the artifact. In practice, a budget is mostly decided by the management and imposed on you. Therefore, it should be attributed as an input constraint. In contrast, cost is primarily determined by your own decisions in terms of your unique choice and synthesis of components, structures, materials, manufacturing process, etc. As a result, cost should be attributed as system constraint.

Constraints can be either internal or external of an artifact. Design begins with an initial though that keeps growing toward a sophisticated artifact. The artifact's evolution is constrained by both internal and external forces. Internal constraint is a part of the artifact; hence, it limits the evolution of the artifact from the inside. For instance, the choice of combustion engine will limit a car's emission performance and fuel efficiency. This internal constraint can only be altered if the combustion engine is replaced by, for example, electric motor. In contrast, external constraint is not a part of the artifact, and as a result, it bounds the evolution of the artifact from the outside. For instance, if an artifact's structure cannot be manufactured by the readily available machine tools, then the machine tools will become an external constraint. In particular, government regulation is a typical external constraint, which can prevent illegal products from being developed.

Various design constraints are classified into four categories: internal input constraint, external input constraint, internal system constraint, and external system constraint (Liu et al. 2019).

- Internal input constraint: constraint that is a part of the artifact, though it is not chosen by you but imposed to you by the third-party stakeholders. For example, as per the government regulation, seat belt is a mandatory part of a car seat independent of the designer's decision.
- External input constraint: constraint that is not a part of the artifact, while it is included in the design task or problem statement. For example, if a product is developed for a particular country, the country's local culture and regulation will impose constraints to product design.
- Internal system constraint: constraint that is chosen by you to be a part of the artifact, which will intentionally or unintentionally limit behaviors of the artifact. For example, the seat belt alarm is purposefully added to constrain the driver–car interactions.
- External system constraint: constraint that is not a part of the artifact, which is introduced by your previous decisions. For example, the oil grade will limit a car's fuel efficiency, though oil is not a part of car. In other words, bad decisions will introduce unnecessary constraint.

5.4.2 Examples of Design Constraint

Uber is is a popular smartphone app that provides peer-to-peer ride-sharing services. As a smartphone app, the performance of Uber is inherently limited by the internal constraints of smartphone. For example, the GPS will limit Uber's ability to locate the user in areas where the GPS signal is weak, the battery life will limit the long-time usage of Uber, and the Big Data analytics will limit Uber from finding the best match between driver and rider among numerous possibilities and calculating the best route against the dynamically changing traffic. In the meantime, the development of Uber has been limited by some external constraints. An apparent external constraint is government regulation that varied in different contexts (i.e., different countries and cities). For example, some countries have explicit laws against any kind of phone usage during driving; some countries forbid UBER cars from picking up passengers in the international airport; and some counties require that the Uber drivers should be hired as employees in place of contractors. In the early days, the expansion of Uber was constrained by the resistance of taxi drivers.

Take the toy design for example, since the target customers are mostly children, toy design is bounded by a number of hard constraints that cannot be violated in any circumstance. Material is an external constraint imposed by government regulation. Most of the governments have mandatory standards in terms of which materials cannot be used in toy design. Size is a critical internal constraint. For example, a minimum size is imposed on the LEGO bricks to prevent child choking. The size constraint varies in accordance to the child age.

> **Exercise 5.11:**
> *Can you identify a list of design constraints for the child car seat, and specify a maximum or minimum value for each constraint?*

> **Exercise 5.12:**
> *Acceleration is an important measure of a car's performance. Can you identify a list of design constraints that will limit a car's acceleration performance?*

> **Exercise 5.13:**
> *Can you identify a list of design constraints that will limit the performance of a delivery drone to transport packages? For each constraint, can you specify a maximum or minimum value?*

5.5   Definition of Problem Context

Problem definition is situated in a particular context. A variety of contextual information should be collected, analyzed, and integrated in order to characterize the uniqueness of problem definition. A unique problem is only valid in a particular context. As the context changes over time, the problem should be redefined accordingly.

5.5.1   What Is Design Context?

The notion of "context" has been investigated from different disciplinary perspectives. By definition, context refers to the situation in which something occurs. For problem definition in engineering design, context can be regarded as a collection of information that characterizes a particular situation or scenario, within which a product/service interacts with the users in appropriate ways to satisfy their demands against certain constraints. Contextual information can be acquired in different ways such as the explicit way (e.g., direct communication among product, user, and environment), the implicit way (e.g., user survey, product review, and usage report), and the statistical means (e.g., data analytics to discover meaningful patterns shared by many products).

The commonly applicable design contexts include the following:

- **Physical context**: Information about the surrounding environment, in which the product is being used, such as temperature, humidity, weather, etc.;
- **Social context**: Information about how users interact with each other, such as with whom, when, where, in what occasion, and under what condition the product is being used;
- **User context**: Information about end users, such as user demographics, knowledge, mood, habit, preference, cognition, health, etc.;
- **Interaction context**: Information about the user–product interactions, such as browsing history, personalized setting, graphical user interface, etc.;
- **Operational context**: Information about a product's operational state, such as battery life, computing power, intelligence level, maintenance, etc.

Contextual information can affect problem definition in various ways. Firstly, user context can affect the selection of target customers, and social context can affect the solicitation of customer voices. For example, contextual inquiry is proven to be a more effective method than formal interview, because it occurs in the field when the product is being used by customers. Therefore, some invisible contextual information can be revealed. Secondly, the physical context can affect the formulation of FRs. Even the same FR should be defined differently against different contexts. For example, watch is generally used to fulfill the FR of "tracking time," while the accuracy requirement of tracking time varies significantly in different contexts, such as Olympic Games, stock trading, business meeting, lecture in the classroom, etc. Lastly, context can affect the definition of design constraints. The most apparent example is government regulation, which varied significantly in different countries.

Contextual information is especially useful for designing context-aware smart products. The advancement of information communication technology paves the way for the increasing popularity of smart products (e.g., smart car, smart home, smartphone, etc.). A critical facet of product intelligence is context-awareness. Context-awareness means a product's ability to accurately interpret a particular situation, in which, to intentionally perform appropriate actions and avoid inappropriate behaviors. So far, many context-aware information systems have already been developed to make personalized recommendations against different contexts. In the future, it is expectable that more and more context-aware smart product/service will be developed. For example, a user-context-aware robot vacuum should purposefully avoid interfering user activities within the home environment, and a social-context-aware robot vacuum should recognize nearby peer products and available resources.

New artifacts are created not only for the real contexts but also for the imaginary contexts, such as the movie themes and holiday themes. For example, from time to time, LEGO offers special sets designed for certain movie themes such as the Disney theme and the Star War theme. During the Christmas season, customers tend to purchase various holiday products such as Christmas tree. In most of the American universities, bookstore is one of the most profitable departments, where a

Fig. 5.7 Square watermelon.
(Reproduced with permission
from Volkov 2019)

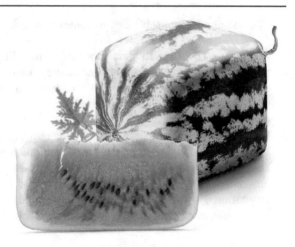

variety of souvenirs (e.g., T-shirt, coffee mug, etc.) with the university logo are sold at high prices. Such souvenirs are mostly designed according to the context of university culture.

5.5.2 Example of Design Context

As illustrated in Fig. 5.7, square watermelon is a popular product that was "invented" in Japan. It is produced by letting the baby watermelon grow inside a transparent square cube. The original intention of "designing" the square watermelon was to enhance space efficiency in small refrigerators and facilitate transportation. Compared to the regular watermelon, square watermelon occupies a much smaller space. However, because of the high cost of growing square watermelons, in practice, they can only be afforded by the rich families and hence go beyond the original design context of "small refrigerator."

> *Exercise 5.14:*
> *Can you create a list of contextual information that is relevant to the design of child car seat? In other words, under what contexts the child car seat will be used?*

> *Exercise 5.15:*
> *Can you reflect the history and define the design context of iPhone by Apple?*

> *Exercise 5.16:*
> *Can you define the design context of the kimchi refrigerator, which is a very popular product in South Korea?*

5.6 Examples of Problem Definition

Consider the following problems and think about how you might approach them to develop a design solution for each example. Some of these examples will require considerable thinking and work to develop the desired design solutions. In some cases, you may have to acquire some fundamental knowledge of the field by reading reference books or by getting information from the Internet. Most of all, you may have to think with an open mind!

Example 5.1 Mars Exploration Rover

In light of the successful launch of Falcon Heavy by Space X, NASA is interested in initiating another ambitious mission to explore Mars. Key equipment is an autonomous exploration rover. Assume you were the Director of NASA, can you prepare a one-page proposal to lobby the Congress for support of this project? What are the FRs and design constraints?

Example 5.2 Urban Farming System

Farming is one of the earliest human endeavors to alter the environment to satisfy basic human needs. Before the Industrial Revolution, farming plays a critical role in driving the historical development of human society. In modern society, however, farming is no longer accessible to ordinary people who live in the megacity. Against this background, can you develop a problem definition for designing a small-scale farming system that can be sustained in urban apartments? Who are the target customers? What are the design constraints? How is the new context different from traditional farming in the filed?

Example 5.3 Smart Factory

Making factories more intelligent is one of the key value propositions of Industry 4.0. The advancement of new technologies such as sensor, actuator, Big Data analytics, and artificial intelligence paves the way for the development of smart factory, which is characterized by information transparency, autonomous operation, decentralized decision-making, etc. Assume you were the CEO of a global auto manufacturer, can you frame a problem definition for designing a brand new smart factory?

Example 5.4 Mobile Learning Management System

Learning management system (LMS) is widely used in higher education for both teacher and student to manage learning activities in the cyberspace. Traditionally, the LMSs are mostly designed for the context of computer access. In light of the increasing popularity of smartphone and hence the transition of student attention from computer to smartphone, can you frame a problem definition for designing a mobile LMS? What is the new design context, and how is it different from the old context?

Example 5.5 Samsung Store

The Apple Store successfully revolutionized customer's impression of retailing. Assume you were the CEO of Samsung Electronics, in order to compete with Apple, can you frame a problem definition for designing a Samsung Store, which will be given to your senior managers and chief designers? Who are the target customers? Who are the relevant stakeholders? What are the customer needs? What are the design constraints? What are the FRs? What is the problem context?

Example 5.6 Access to Clean Water

Access to clean water is one of the 14 grand challenges for engineering in the twenty-first century, which were identified by the National Academy of Engineering in the USA. Every year, more deaths are caused by lack of clean water than wars. Assume you were the director of a global NGO foundation, can you design a 5-min presentation to highlight the significance of this grand challenge, and call for innovative, affordable, and reliable engineering solutions to address it?

Example 5.7 Kitchen Product

Of all the rooms in your home, kitchen is the center of energy, creativity, and comfort. In the coming decade as our habits change, the kitchen as we know it will evolve drastically. Today's youth, especially college students, tend to avoid cooking by themselves in the kitchen because it is time-consuming, inconvenient, and intuitive. This is evidenced by the fact that the food delivery service is becoming increasingly popular worldwide. Can you frame a problem definition for designing a new smart appliance that can facilitate cooking in the kitchen?

Example 5.8 Pet Entertainment System

Dog/cats have been a fundamental part of many households and are known to be quite active and responsive to their owners. However, oftentimes, owners must have periods of absences due to other commitments such as jobs and study, leaving their dog/cats at home alone. Can you develop a problem definition for designing a new system that can entertain or accompany dog/cat when their owners are away from home? Who are the target customers and relevant stakeholders? What are the FRs? What is the problem context?

Example 5.9 Bicycle Security on Campus

Bicycles are one of the most popular transportation means on the university campus. However, bicycle security has been a long-standing problem on the university campus. Can you create a problem definition for designing a new system that can prevent bicycles from being stolen or damaged on campus?

Example 5.10 Research Submarine

Some researchers need to carry out expeditions to explore the deep ocean. Can you develop a problem definition for designing a research submarine for scientific purposes?

Example 5.11 NGO for Climate Change

Climate change is one of the greatest challenges for humanity. Can you create a problem definition for developing a not-for-profit organization that is intended to promote social awareness in climate change? How do you propose to tailor the problem definition differently for different contexts (i.e., developing country and developed country)?

In the above examples, the success of design largely depends on how, in what ways, and to what extent a good problem definition is formulated. As much as possible, your problem definition should cover all aspects concerning customer need, FRs, design constraint, and problem context. For design instructors, these examples, as well as their variations, can be assigned as the topic of project-based learning.

5.7 Summary and Conclusion

Chapter 5 illustrates the critical role of problem definition in driving the design process toward more innovative solutions. It has been repeatedly proven by numerous product development successes as well as failures that a good problem definition is a necessary condition of design innovations. The quality of problem definition determines the direction of subsequence design activities such as concept generation, evaluation, and selection. Problem definition involves the iterative formulation, specification, reformulation, and mapping of customer needs, FRs, design constraints, and design contexts. It requires both divergent thinking and convergent thinking to develop a good and unique problem definition. Divergent thinking is needed to expand the searching for innovating opportunities, customer voices, boundary conditions, and contextual information. Convergent thinking is equally needed to convert the unstructured, separate, and inconsistent information into a set of well-defined FRs.

References

Delyk O (2019) MP3 player audio musical portable headphones Walkman iPod iPhone, Apple isolated 3D. Photo licensed from Shutterstock, ID: 272031950

Lyjak B (2019) Mother with child in baby stroller enjoying summer sunset and mountains landscape. Jogging or power walking woman with pram. Beautiful inspirational mountains landscape. Photo licensed from Shutterstock, ID: 1045287292

Popov A (2019a) Side view of a relaxed businesswoman stretching her arms. Photo licensed from Shutterstock, ID: 1083974525

Popov A (2019b) Young businesswoman sitting on Pilates ball working in office. Photo licensed from Shutterstock, ID: 396426541

Volkov V (2019) Cubic watermelon with slice on a white background. Photo licensed from Shutterstock, ID: 106115846

Further Reading

Franke N, Von Hippel E, Schreier M (2006) Finding commercially attractive user innovations: a test of lead-user theory. J Prod Innov Manag 23(4):301–315

Gero JS, Kannengiesser U (2004) The situated function-behaviour-structure framework. Des Stud 25(4):373–391

Goldratt E (1999) Theory of constraints. North River Press

Kaulio MA (1998) Customer, consumer and user involvement in product development: a framework and a review of selected methods. Total Qual Manag 9(1):141–149

Liu A, Wang Y, Teo I, Lu S (2019) Constraint management for concept ideation in conceptual design. CIRP J Manuf Sci Technol 24:35–48

Saaty TL (2008) Decision making with the analytic hierarchy process. Int J Serv Sci 1(1):83–98

Suh NP (2001) Axiomatic design—advances and applications. Oxford University Press

Suh NP (2010) Theory of innovation. Int J Innov Manag (IJIM) 14:893–913. https://doi.org/10.1142/S1363919610002921

How Should We Select Functional Requirements?

6

Nam Pyo Suh

Abstract

The preceding chapters provided broad outlines of the design of various systems based on Axiomatic Design (AD). Two axioms were the basis of making design decisions: the Independence Axiom and the Information Axiom. The process of AD consists of the transformation of the problem identified in the "customer domain" into a set of functional requirements (FRs) in the "functional domain," which was in turn transformed as design parameters (DPs) in the "physical domain" that are chosen to satisfy FRs. DPs were, in turn, transformed into process variables (PVs) in the "process domain" to fulfill DPs. The mapping process was illustrated.

Once the highest FRs and DPs are finalized at the highest level of the system design hierarchy, we may have to decompose FRs and DPs, if the selected FRs and DPs lack sufficient details to complete the design. This decomposition process must continue until the design has enough details that can be implemented. To decompose, we should zigzag between FR and DP domains. Similarly, DP versus PV can be decomposed through zigzagging.

The resulting designs were classified as uncoupled, decoupled, and coupled designs. Coupled designs violate the Independence Axiom and, thus, should not be implemented. They are unreliable and require monitoring, resulting in the waste of resources, cost overruns, and delays in implementation. When a system design is uncoupled, it can readily be satisfied because each FR is a function of only one DP, irrespective of the total number of FRs and DPs that the system has to satisfy. The design matrix is constructed to identify coupling. Throughout these chapters, "real-life" examples were presented.

The quality of the design is determined by how well the problem is identified and how FRs are selected. Although every step of the transformation is essential,

N. P. Suh (✉)
M.I.T., Cambridge, MA, USA
e-mail: npsuh@mit.edu

© Springer Nature Switzerland AG 2021
N. P. Suh et al. (eds.), *Design Engineering and Science*,
https://doi.org/10.1007/978-3-030-49232-8_6

the selection of FRs ultimately determines the functional quality of the design output. It is helpful to have an in-depth understanding of basic sciences, engineering, and other relevant fields to be proficient in system design. It may also take different kinds of information, depending on the field. In designing commercial products, market information on the current state and prospect is critical in selecting the right set of FRs. In other fields, such as the economy, the set of information required to choose the right set of FRs would be entirely different. However, the basic system structure is similar. The domain-specific knowledge is field-specific.

In this chapter, the process of selecting FRs is elaborated further. One of the essential concepts to remember in selecting FRs is the idea of choosing them in a "solution-neutral environment," that is, the designer should not think of a design solution first and then define FRs for the assumed solution. Given the critical importance of selecting the right set of FRs for the problem identified, the designer should have a broad knowledge base and also access to extensive "database for scientific facts and various technologies," including the commercial database for existing products.

6.1 Importance of "Solution-Neutral Environment" in Selecting Functional Requirements

The preceding chapters provided broad outlines of the design of various systems based on AD. Two axioms were the basis of making design decisions: the Independence Axiom and the Information Axiom. The process of AD consists of the transformation of the problem identified in the "customer domain" into a set of FRs in the "functional domain," which was in turn transformed as DPs in the "physical domain" that are chosen to satisfy FRs. DPs were, in turn, transformed into PVs in the "process domain" to satisfy DPs. The mapping process was illustrated.

Once the highest FRs and DPs are finalized at the highest level of the system design hierarchy, we may have to decompose FRs and DPs, if the selected FRs and DPs lack sufficient details to complete the design. This decomposition process must continue until the design has enough information for implementation. To decompose, we should zigzag between FR and DP domains. Similarly, DP versus PV can be decomposed through zigzagging.

The resulting designs were classified as uncoupled, decoupled, and coupled designs. Coupled designs violate the Independence Axiom and, thus, should not be implemented. They are unreliable and require monitoring, resulting in the waste of resources, cost overruns, and delays in implementation. When a system design is an uncoupled design, it can readily be satisfied because each FR is a function of only one DP, irrespective of the total number of FRs and DPs that the system has to satisfy. The design matrix is constructed to identify coupling. Throughout these chapters, "real-life" examples were presented.

The quality of the design is determined by how well the problem is identified and how FRs are selected. Although every step of the transformation is essential, the selection of FRs ultimately determines the functional quality of the design output. It is helpful to have an in-depth understanding of basic sciences, engineering, and other relevant fields to be proficient in system design. It may also take different kinds of information, depending on the field. In designing commercial products, market information on the current state and prospect is critical in selecting the right set of FRs. In other fields, such as the economy, the set of information required to choose the right set of FRs would be entirely different. However, the basic system structure is similar. The domain-specific knowledge is field-specific.

In this chapter, the process of selecting FRs is elaborated further. One of the essential concepts to remember in selecting FRs is the idea of choosing them in a "solution-neutral environment," that is, the designer should not think of a design solution first and then define FRs for the assumed solution. Given the critical importance of selecting the right set of FRs for the problem identified, the designer should have a broad knowledge base and also access to extensive "database for scientific facts and various technologies," including the commercial database for existing products.

Example 6.1 Lesson Learned: Role of *Solution-Neutral Environment* in Developing On-Line Electric Vehicle (OLEV)[1]

In Chap. 3, the basic design of OLEV (on-line electric vehicle) was presented by giving details of the design of the shaped magnetic field in resonance (SMFIR). In this chapter, the background story will be presented to illustrate the difficulties one may encounter in undertaking innovative R&D projects to show the importance of thinking in a "solution-neutral environment" in creating innovative products.

As mentioned in a previous chapter, in 2006, KAIST (Korea Advanced Institute of Science and Technology) designed a new plan to make it one of the best universities in the world in science and technology. To achieve this goal, one of the FRs chosen for the new KAIST strategic plan was to solve some of the most critical problems of the world in the twenty-first century. One of the issues identified was "global warming." To solve this problem, we decided to replace all internal combustion (IC) engines used in automobiles with electric drives (EV). Such a shift from IC to EV would reduce the anthropogenic emission of CO_2 by about 27%. Also, to avoid many problems associated with using a large number of batteries to propel all-electric vehicles, the decision was made to transmit electric power wirelessly to the vehicle from underground electrical power supply systems. We named it the on-line electric vehicle (OLEV). KAIST approached the government of the Republic of Korea for significant funding ($\sim$ about \$25 million during the first year, a large sum of money for research and development, by any measure).

---

[1]OLEV was partly introduced in Chap. 3 to illustrate the design process.

When the Korean government tentatively agreed to fund this OLEV project pending the congressional budget approval, two unexpected things happened. First, none of the KAIST professors who were specialists in electric power would be willing to lead this project, stating that the idea of transmitting 100 kW of electric power wirelessly over a distance of $20 \sim 25$ cm could not be done technologically. They claimed that the idea was meritless, although they were too polite to use these words! Therefore, the KAIST administration organized a project team led by professors who were not specialists in heavy electric power engineering. They did a great job because they were able to design a new system based on the first principles of electromagnetism and AD.

The second event was much more serious. Some of the professors at other universities, who were working on battery-powered electric automobiles, mounted a significant opposition to the KAIST project. They mobilized a member of the National Congress (equivalent to the U.S. Congress) with a Ph.D. in physics from a university in the U.S. and former professor of physics in Korea to mount a significant opposition campaign to the KAIST OLEV project. They argued that such massive electric power (~ 100 kW) could not be transmitted wirelessly over a distance of over 20 cm, similar to the argument presented by some specialists in KAIST. (For proprietary reasons, we could not reveal the basic idea behind OLEV.) They unduly interfered with the project proposal review process to stop the funding of the KAIST project. KAIST president was called in to answer questions at a special meeting of the National Assembly (i.e., counterpart the U.S. Congress) of Korea. The opposition to OLEV was based on their claim that the proposed idea was not technically feasible. This incident is similar to the opposition mounted in the United States against the NSF Engineering Research Centers (ERC) program when it was launched in 1985, albeit based on a different argument.

The professors who opposed the OLEV project were not thinking in a "solution-neutral environment." Instead of thinking about the goal of transmitting vast electric power over a considerable distance in a solution-neutral environment, they were thinking of the well-established designs that have been used in electric power transformers, where the primary coil is adjacent to the secondary coil. OLEV was based on the idea of creating an oscillating magnetic field of required shape and strength by controlling the distance between the two magnetic poles. The idea was generated based on the principles taught in undergraduate physics courses by people who were not specialists in heavy electric power transmission.

The KAIST project ultimately received its funding after a great deal of effort to overcome the opposition of influential professors at two leading universities and some members of the National Congress. It took 2 years—a short time after receiving the grant to develop OLEV and install it in Seoul Grand Park and entertain people around the park. Throughout the execution of the project, we made sure that there was no coupling of FRs by creating "system architects," who monitored design decisions made by various groups to be sure that no one in the design team introduced coupled designs. Now OLEV buses are running in five cities in Korea. AD played a significant role in achieving this feat.

Thinking in a solution-neutral environment is essential for creative design, which is a difficult thing to do for people with extensive design experience. The human instinct is to go directly to a solution without defining FRs.

Example 6.2 Space Life Support Systems[2]

The closed system human life support architecture now implemented in the International Space Station has been virtually unchanged for 50 years. In contrast, brief missions such as Apollo and Shuttle have used open-loop life support. As mission length increases, greater system closure and increased recycling become more cost-effective. Closure can be gradually increased, first recycling humidity condensate, then hygiene waste water, urine, carbon dioxide, and water recovery brine. A long-term space station or planetary base could implement nearly full closure, including food production. Dynamic systems theory supports the axioms by showing that fewer requirements, fewer subsystems, and fewer interconnections all increase system stability. If systems are too complex and interconnected, reliability is reduced, making operations and maintenance more difficult.

Using AD, we need to show how the mission duration and other requirements determine the best life support system design, including the degree of closure in a solution-neutral environment. The highest level FR and DP are as follows:

FR = Support human life in space;
DP = Life support system.

The next-level FRs and DPs may be stated in a solution-neutral environment by decomposing FR1 and DP1 as follows:

FR1 = Provide atmosphere (transmit oxygen to humans[3]);
FR2 = Provide water (maintain healthy level of water in humans);
FR3 = Handle waste (remove gas waste products);
FR4 = Suppress fire (restrict combustion to designated areas);
FR5 = Provide food (maintain healthy level of nutrition in humans).

DP1 = Atmosphere system;
DP2 = Water system;
DP3 = Waste system;
DP4 = Fire system;
DP5 = Food system.

H.W. Jones states the following:

"A key method of the AD approach is to match each requirement with its design implementation at each stage of the top-down elaboration of the requirements. The lower level requirements are more specific and detailed. This approach is a deliberate direct contrast to the usual method of creating a detailed multilevel requirements tree, freezing it, and then developing the hardware design to meet that set of detailed requirements. It is supposed, but rarely happens, that the requirements are developed without assuming some system design."

"While it helps in clarifying requirements, the main purpose of going back and forth between requirements and systems in the AD approach is to ensure maximum decoupling of each requirement from the systems implementing other requirements. The extent of decoupling obtainable can be limited by the environment and the available hardware systems."

---

[2]From Jones (2017).
[3]FRs in italics were suggested alternate statements by a reviewer of this chapter.

The design matrix [DM] for the above FRs and FPs is given as follows by Jones (2017):

	DP5: Food system	DP4: Fire system	DP3: Waste system	DP1: Atmosphere system	DP2: Water
FR5: Provide food	X				
FR4: Suppress fire		X			
FR3: Handle waste	X (food and packaging waste)		X		
FR1: Provide atmosphere		X (De- and re-pressurize)		X	
FR2: Provide water			X (extract water)		X

The above design given by H. W. Jones is a decoupled design given by the above design matrix. This design matrix satisfies the Independence Axiom.

Example 6.3 Consequences of Operating with Wrong FRs: Eastman Kodak Company

The importance of selecting the right set of FRs cannot be over-emphasized. Consider the case of Eastman Kodak. It was one of the most successful companies until about 1980. They dominated the camera and film business. They employed thousands of people and created the City of Rochester, New York. (The founder of the company, George Eastman, even gave a sizable gift to MIT to build the current campus on the bank of Charles River in Boston, changing the name from Boston Polytechnic Institute to the Massachusetts Institute of Technology. Without the money, MIT might have become a part of Harvard!) There were outstanding engineers, scientists, managers, and executives who made Eastman Kodak a leading industrial firm in the world. They pioneered silver-halide-based photography technologies well into the twentieth century.

Today, the company does not exist anymore. It is not appropriate to blame anyone or a group of people. However, the board of the company should bear the most blame because it is their function to be sure that the company is headed in the right direction by hiring an able leader as the Chief Executive Officer of the company. Apparently, "they dropped the ball." In many of these situations, however, it is the CEO who should bear the primary responsibility, because CEO's job is to steer that company toward success by taking appropriate actions to make the company successful. CEOs of companies are highly compensated because CEO's actions indeed determine the success of corporate goals. One of the last CEOs at Kodak, the board of directors hired, had made his reputation in semiconductor and electronics business, and yet he persisted, thinking that the silver-halide system could compete with the electronic photography business. He chose a wrong set of the highest level FRs!

When the electronic camera was being introduced, the upper management of Eastman Kodak continued to believe in the silver-halide system of making images on thin polymeric films and printing them on photographic paper. The irony is that Eastman Kodak was one of the first companies to develop electronic photography.[4] In hindsight, it is clear that the top management of Kodak chose a wrong set of FRs. They believed in the superiority of the silver-halide system because the company continued to improve the silver-halide system. Also financially, they had so much invested in old photography business based on the silver-halide system that they could not believe that digital technology could ever overtake their traditional business and obsolete their massive capital investment. When the digital camera was becoming popular, they even imported a top manager from electronics and semiconductor business, but he also became a convert to the old silver-halide system of photography. They did not fathom how fast semiconductor technology would miniaturize images (i.e., pixels per inch) and how digital technology would transform the communication technology involving images. Therefore, they did not fully support their digital technology group, although they got into digital photography first, because they could not foresee such rapid progress of electronic photography and demise of the old photography business in the marketplace. Because of the mindset of the top executives of Eastman Kodak, the lower level managers set the goal of saving cost and increasing productivity as their goals.[5] Many of them have done outstanding jobs, but they were not the captains of the ship.

The cited example above illustrates the importance of "knowledge" and the ability to make the right decisions in selecting the right set of FRs based on the available knowledge on a periodic basis. It also illustrates the conflict in decision-making between the short-term profits and creating new business by gutting an existing business that is bringing in cash, profits, and the current prosperity. The top management of Eastman Kodak failed to protect its employees and investors by having made a wrong decision and ultimately led to the demise of such a great technology firm. It is clear that when the CEO had a chance to choose a new set of FRs upon becoming a new CEO of Kodak, he stuck with the FRs his predecessors had chosen, which eventually bankrupted the company. The mystery is why a person who had a strong career in the semiconductor and electronics industry chose to stay with the silver-halide system. Is this because the system rewards the CEOs based on their short-term performance? This story highlights the importance of selecting the right person as the CEO of a company, who has the intellect, experience, and the ability to design a long-term strategy for the company.

Exercise 6.1: Design of Driverless Car

Many companies are developing driverless cars, such as the one shown below. Is the driverless car a good design? State FRs and constraints in a solution-neutral environment (Fig. 6.1).

---

[4]An engineer at Eastman Kodak, Steven Sasson, invented and built the first self-contained electronic camera. It used a charge-coupled device image sensor in 1975, which was initially used in mainly military and scientific application. Later, it was used in medical and news applications.
[5]This emphasis on cost-saving led to the creation of the microcellular plastics by MIT under the sponsorship of Eastman Kodak and other companies in the MIT-Industry Polymer Processing Program. Today, MuCell (tradename of Trexel, Inc., for microcellular plastics) is used in automotive industry to reduce the weight of cars so as to increase the fuel efficiency of automobiles. Reference: Wong et al. (2016).

Fig. 6.1 Driverless car.
Reproduced with permission
from Tim (2020)

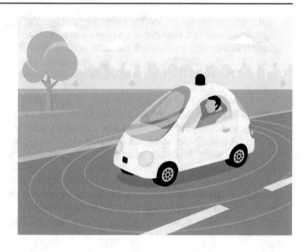

Exercise 6.2: Unbeatable Combination: Human and Machine Intelligence

Many things people do every day depend on a combination of human and machine intelligence. People decide what to do, and machines take over the task and deliver the results to the person. For instance, people order goods through the Internet, and automated systems take over the order and deliver the good to the door step of the person who ordered it.

One of the least developed areas in human society is "politics." Politicians often lie to people and argue with other politicians with lots of heat but with limited enlightenment to resolve issues and establish policies. We wish to develop an intelligent machine system that can settle political arguments and make decisions. Develop FRs and constraints that can improve the democratic decision-making process.

Exercise 6.3: Admission to Leading Colleges

Colleges and universities accept students for their freshman class each year. Many students apply for admission to the colleges they would like to attend. Colleges use several different criteria for admission. Along one axis, they measure the scholastic aptitude of the students by several different means such as entrance examination, high school grades, and letters of recommendation. Along the orthogonal axis, they attempt to measure personal characteristics for future success, such as student activities, letters of recommendation, particular unique talents, and extracurricular activities. The problem that colleges and universities are facing is that the number of qualified students exceeds the number of students they can accept. Design an admissions system for screening students by stating FRs and DPs in a solution-neutral environment.

Exercise 6.4: Mission to Moon

The space agency of the United Nations decided to colonize the Moon by establishing a base where people can stay for an extended period. To achieve this goal of colonization of the Moon, heavy equipment and supplies must be transported to the Moon from Earth. There are two options. The first option is to use a large enough booster rocket to carry the cargo from Earth to Moon in one shot by being able to escape the gravitational force of the

Earth. Then, once it reaches a point where the gravitational pool of the Moon is greater than that of the Earth, it will travel to and ultimately go into Moon's orbit for final landing on the Moon by slowly descending to the lunar surface. The second option is to use smaller rockets to take the payload to an orbit around Earth in several launches. Then, assemble the parts into a larger container in space while circling the Earth. When the entire space vehicle is assembled in the earth orbit, it can fire a rocket to propel it to Moon.

If you are the director of this Moon mission, which option would you choose? Why? List FRs in solution-neutral environment and develop DPs that can satisfy the FRs. Discuss the pros and cons of these two different approaches.

Exercise 6.5: Stabilizing the Weather

It is desirable to change the weather pattern of Earth to prevent global warming. Weather is controlled by a series of instabilities in the atmosphere. When instability is initiated in a local region (e.g., due to the abnormally hot zone in the equator), it will create fast circulating vortices. These become tornados that will gather more and more energy by entrapping vapor from the ocean surface and then unleash the condensate when it encounters a cold atmosphere, creating a large pressure gradient and additional instability in the atmosphere. If these unstable natural phenomena can be created by first initiating local instabilities at a preselected region (e.g., west coast of Northern Africa), we may be able to change the weather pattern of Earth. How would you change the desert in North Africa next to the Atlantic Ocean into a green forest with many trees, making use of human-made instabilities in the atmosphere? List FRs and DPs at the highest level.

Exercise 6.6: Energy Storage

One of the issues in using electric power generated by solar and wind is the storage of excess electrical energy when the electric power generated is higher than the demand. Ideally, we should be able to store excess energy and use it when the demand is greater than supply. How would you store electric energy that may exceed the demand by tens of million watt-hours? List your FRs and DPs.

6.2 Functional Requirements and Zigzagging between Domains to Generate Lower Level Functional Requirements through Decomposition

At the highest level of design, the FRs may be stated based on the problem identified in the customer domain. However, we cannot identify the lower level FRs, without first identifying the corresponding DPs that can satisfy the FRs identified at the highest level. The lower level FRs can be stated after we first select and define the DPs at a higher level. These FRs are children-level FRs that represent the functions of the DP at one higher level. Therefore, mapping and zigzagging are essential concepts that the designer should be familiar with since they are the fundamental tools of AD.

Example 6.4 Designing Chemical–Mechanical Polishing (CMP) Machine for Silicon Wafers[6]

In manufacturing semiconductors, there are many steps involved. One of the processes is the chemical-mechanical polishing (CMP) process. Flat silicon wafers (diameter of up to 12 inches) is first coated with a thin layer of photoresist by spinning the wafer at high speeds after the photoresist is put on the surface. Then, electric circuits are printed on the photoresist with a lithography machine, using a short wavelength light (e.g., typically ultraviolet light (UV)) that goes through a mask with open slots in the form of electric circuits. Then, the resin is cured through a cross-linking chemical reaction, except the area that was exposed to light. When the uncured resin is removed, it exposes the original silicon surface area where the surface was exposed to light. Then it is etched, creating thin channels. Then copper is deposited, which covers the entire wafer. When the wafer is polished using abrasive slurry with polishing pads by the CMP machine, it removes the copper except where the etched channel exists, making a conducting path for electricity (see Fig. 6.2). Then, another layer of semiconducting material is deposited by vapor deposition, which is subjected to similar processes until a semiconductor device is created after the repetition of the above process. The task of the CMP machine is to remove unwanted materials to make the electric circuit layer by layer. Throughout this process, the CMP process must remove materials uniformly to prevent "dishing" of the surface where the center of the wafer is removed more than the edges or removing more materials at the edges of the wafer.

There are many FRs that must be satisfied. To simplify for illustration, we will choose a second-level FR and show how that FR is decomposed to create the next level of FRs and DPs (Melvin 2003a).

FR1.1 = Process wafer;
DP1.1 = Front layer removal.

The next-level FRs will be stated by decomposing FR1.1, which are really the FRs of DP1.1. They may be stated as follows:

FR 1.1.1 = Remove surface material;
FR 1.1.2 = Enable multi-step processes;
FR 1.1.3 = Control remaining thickness;
FR 1.1.4 = Exchange wafers.

The corresponding DPs are as follows:

DP 1.1.1 = Abrasive removal processing;
DP 1.1.2 = Multiple removal station design;
DP 1.1.3 = End point signal;
DP 1.1.4 = Wafer exchange sequence.

It should be noted that another designer might have decomposed it differently, which is equally acceptable if it is done consistently. In the design, there is no uniqueness theorem, but the decomposition must be consistent within the design framework chosen.

---

[6]The MIT Laboratory for Manufacturing and Productivity developed a commercial CMP machine in about 2 years. This example is based on the extensive design work done by Jason Melvin who received his Ph.D. partly based on this work and the work of other students. As discussed in Chap. 4, this project was sponsored by SVG Corporation, which was acquired by ASML. We are grateful to Papken Der Torossian, CEO of SVG, a man with a vision.

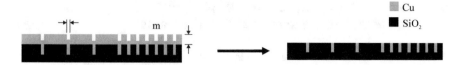

Fig. 6.2 Etched wafer after copper deposition (left) and after removing the copper layer by the CMP process (right). Reproduced with permission from Melvin (2003b)

The design matrix for the above design is given below:

$$\begin{Bmatrix} FR1.1.1 \\ FR1.1.2 \\ FR1.1.3 \\ FR1.1.4 \end{Bmatrix} = \begin{bmatrix} X & O & O & O \\ X & X & O & O \\ X & X & X & O \\ X & O & O & X \end{bmatrix} \begin{Bmatrix} DP1.1.1 \\ DP1.1.2 \\ DP1.1.3 \\ DP1.1.4 \end{Bmatrix}$$

The design is a decoupled design, which satisfies the Independence Axiom.

The above example is a small part of the overall design of the MIT CMP machine, which was presented in Chap. 4 as part of the discussion on the representation of design results, which is shown again in Fig. 6.3.

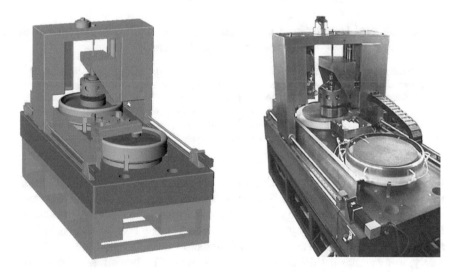

Fig. 6.3 The figure on the left is "Solidworks model" and the picture on the right is the actual fabricated machine. Reproduced with permission from Melvin (2003b)

6.3 Role of Broad Knowledge Base/Data Base in Formulating Functional Requirements

Problem identification is a critical step in the successful execution of the design. In previous chapters, the design was defined as the transformation process of going from domain to domain, e.g., to generate FRs from the problem identified in the customer domain, which is facilitated by "knowledge" and "data." At the beginning of the transformational process, we sometimes do not even know "the question" or "the problem." Initially, we depend on the "knowledge stored in our brain" or the "data stored in some accessible database" to generate questions and ideas to correctly identify the problem we need to solve in the customer domain, which precedes the selection of FRs or DPs or PVs. The generation of DPs and PVs is much easier than the generation of FRs, because we may not have adequately understood the "problem" that resides in the customer domain. Although the computer is powerful with extensive database and increasing intelligence with the use of artificial intelligence (AI), human imagination and the human brain are still the most critical factor in being able to define appropriate FRs.

6.4 On Selection of a Right Set of Functional Requirements—Need to Review Functional Requirements from Time to Time

In 1950, General Motors Company was the largest publically held company in the United States. In 2018, it was no longer. What happened?

> *General Motors dominated the U.S. economy in the 1950s. Since it was founded, it absorbed several companies and under the chairmanship of Alfred P. Sloan, and grew to became the largest automobile company in the world. When President Eisenhower nominated Charles Erwin Wilson, GM Chairman, for defense secretary, he faced the Senate Armed Services Committee in 1953. What he said at the hearing has been quoted widely: "because for years, I thought what was good for our country was good for General Motors, and vice versa."*

Some corporations go through a crisis when they cannot renew themselves in time as the world around them changes. Furthermore, some of the large companies become so bureaucratic that they are no longer creative and competitive. They do not attempt to identify new problems they should solve, establish new FRs, develop new DPs, and deal with resource issues (PVs) to continue to revitalize the business. Fortunately, many companies continue to do well by renewing themselves periodically.

Some universities have problems, too. One of the potential crises facing some of the leading universities is that the cost of operating their universities is exponentially escalating when the number of students and faculty has not changed. They often blame new government regulations, but that may not be the only reason or even the primary reason for the inefficient operation. When governments no longer expand the budget for research and do not guarantee student loans, these universities might have significant problems.

These issues boil down to the following question: how should these institutions renew themselves? The answer is that they should periodically review and re-establish FRs. The right set of FRs is the one that solves the problem identified in the customer domain. Once we select a new set of FRs, we must review the design and attempt to implement new DPs when the changes are required. These institutions are systems that should reinitialize themselves periodically, which is a subject matter discussed in the chapter on complexity.

Selecting the right set of FRs is the most important and the most challenging task in any decision-making process. Anybody can make decisions, but the question is: is the decision the right one? Fortunately, there is not only "one right decision" in that there are equally good equivalent decisions and FRs. Once the FRs are chosen, DPs and PVs must be created or adjusted. Often there are oppositions to institutional changes when they are introduced, especially during the early stages of a new administration.

Example 6.5 "You Should Quit for the Sake of Your Great Department!"

When the head of a distinguished academic department got promoted to a deanship, young faculty members of the department asked the university administration to name a specific senior faculty member of the department to take on the job. The concern was that the department has been living off its past laurels. They thought that it was time to change its direction to be ready for the twenty-first century. Notwithstanding the objections of some senior faculty in one major group of the department, the administration made the appointment as recommended by the search committee. He accepted the appointment because he agreed that the department was now ripe for renewal.

He introduced significant changes, including the renovation of old physical infrastructure, faculty personnel policy, research emphasis, faculty hiring policy, and raised a substantial amount of gifts. The fundamental problem he identified was that the department was dwelling on issues and problems of the late nineteenth-century and early twentieth-century engineering. The department was famous because the many well-known professors had made a fundamental contribution to automotive engineering, macro-scale heat engineering, experience-based instruction of design, and others. These were essential topics to teach, but in terms of research for the future, the department was not in sync with new emerging technologies, e.g., semiconductors, nanotechnology, software systems, biomedical engineering, modern materials, and design theory. The department needed different kinds of professors who can deal with the topics of the twenty-first century and forge a new mechanical engineering department. The department had to change from a discipline that is primarily based on physics into a discipline that is based not only on physics, but also computer science and engineering, biology, information, and modern materials. The department embarked on the task of hiring professors whose doctorate degrees were in disciplines outside of the traditional mechanical engineering to lead the department into a direction that is relevant in the twenty-first century. Also, the old defunct laboratory was demolished to create new updated physical facilities. He worked day and night to bring about these changes because he wanted to move onto other tasks after 3 years of this job. All these changes were conceived in a "solution-neutral environment," which can have unpleasant consequences.

About 5 months into this new task, the chairman of the department's outside advisory committee, who was also a member of the trustees of the university, knocked on the door of the new department head unannounced. They met each other 4 months earlier when the new department head went to see the chairman of the visiting committee at his home in the Midwest of the United States, hoping to raise money for the renovation project underway in the department. Unlike the last time the department head met him, he was not smiling and looked very serious. For a good reason!

He said that he met with the senior faculty members of the department at their request. He said that they had many complaints about the new direction the department was headed. Some of the senior faculty stated to the chairman of the visiting committee: "We must have been doing something right to be so highly ranked all these years. Then, why change?" He stated that 50% of those present at the meeting voted to have the department head removed. That was not a pleasant message. The top administration of the university met and asked the department head to appear and explain. The initial reaction of the department head was to step down for the sake of the department. However, others advised him against the idea, stating that "if you step down, no one else will be able to make unpopular changes, because the idea that faculty opposition can stop any changes can become a part of department legend." The fact that at least 50% of the senior faculty did not join the revolting group gave enough courage to continue the reform process.

The lessons of this story are the following: (1). Changes are hard to make, especially when they affect people. (2). Before making changes, one should clearly define FRs and DPs in a solution-neutral environment. (3). If one wants to be popular and have friends, do not make significant changes that will tilt the apple cart! (4) Be willing to sacrifice personally for the sake of the institution. It should be noted that if the new FRs were not conceived in a "solution-neutral environment," it would have been more challenging to go through a difficult period.

He stayed on the job for a long time to be sure that some of the younger professors brought in from other disciplines into mechanical engineering get tenure and sustain the changing culture of the department. It took about 10 years for this process! Indeed these "young" professors have become the leaders of the department and the new mechanical engineering field worldwide during the period. His contributions to the department and the university were later widely recognized because of the contributions of these "young" professors.

Factors that affect our ability to choose a right set of FRs:

There may be many factors that may affect decision-making ability, such as the following:

1. board and relevant knowledge that applies to the issue in hand;
2. in the case of innovation of technologies, a strong base in engineering and science disciplines;
3. relevant experience in the industry, government, universities, technology development, and other related fields;
4. for organizational design, experience in establishing and administering systems;
5. actual design experience for any systems;
6. innate creativity;
7. deep perspective in design thinking;
8. ability to think out of the box;

9. intense curiosity;
10. questioning mind;
11. asking "why" five consecutive times until the root cause is clearly explained;
12. ability to learn new subjects on one's own;
13. willingness to collaborate with others;
14. an open mind to listen to opposing viewpoints;
15. ability to tolerate criticisms;
16. confidence in one's knowledge and belief;
17. honesty with high ethical standards;
18. ability to admit mistakes made;
19. ability to listen to viewpoints of others;
20. abundant imagination.

The above list is long. No one person may have all those qualities, but they are personal characteristics that should be cultivated.

6.5 On Reverse Engineering to Determine the Functional Requirements of Existing Products

Some companies also try to determine the FRs of the competitor's products through reverse engineering, which is difficult or impossible to do. For example, if someone gives you a hammer and ask you to determine its FRs, you, like most people, would describe one of its FRs as "drive a nail into wood." However, your answer might be wrong if it is used primarily as a paperweight. In other words, it is possible to reverse engineer DPs because they can be measured, tested, and evaluated, but FRs can only be guessed.

Every manufacturer, especially those in consumer products, tries to learn about their competitors' products. They break down or tear down their competitors' products to learn about the merits and demerits of the competitor's product. However, reverse engineering has significant limitations. Although it is possible to measure the geometric shape of the product and determine specific properties through measurements and testing, it is difficult to decide on the FRs of these products through reverse engineering.

Equally challenging is the determination of tolerances associated with the product, although the nominal dimensions can readily be measured, their tolerances cannot be measured. Although we have not covered the Information Axiom in detail yet, the information contents of a product are also difficult to determine through reverse engineering, since information content is a function of the tolerance and the nominal dimensions.

6.6 Minimum Number of Functional Requirements

The Information Axiom states that information content should be minimized. Consistent with this axiom, experienced designers try to satisfy a minimum number of FRs at any given level of design. It may be challenging to deal with many FRs at any level of decision-making, since as the number of FRs increases, it may become more challenging to satisfy the Independence Axiom.

Through the decomposition process, we can develop detailed designs. It is easier to come up with good design ideas and robust designs when we try to limit the number of FRs we have to satisfy at any given level of design hierarchy. If there is only one FR, it is always independent.

When we design large systems with many FRs and many decomposition branches, at any given node of FR and DP, it is better to minimize the number of FRs.

6.7 No Relative Ranking of the Importance of Functional Requirements

When we specify FRs, they are all *equally* important. However, the Information Axiom determines their robustness and the relative importance in terms of the information content, which will be further discussed in Chap. 7.

6.8 Interdisciplinary Background and Choice of Functional Requirements

Every designer is likely to choose a different set of FRs and DPs. People with broader disciplinary or multidisciplinary backgrounds may select better sets of FRs, because they may be able to access their information base for more appropriate FRs. For instance, the knowledge acquired on the mixing of liquids through the impingement of two streams of liquids enabled the creation of mixalloy. Similarly, if Crick and Watson did not get the information that DNA structure has a helical shape by visiting the laboratory of Dr. Rosalind Franklin, they might not have designed and discovered the structure of DNA molecule.

In the future, we will depend more on the database stored in computers to acquire knowledge on FRs and DPs. In some cases, access to the information will be facilitated by the use of AI.

6.9 Importance of Design Matrix and the System Architecture

In the early stage of the design process, it is easy to change FRs without incurring much cost and time. However, if we discover that we have chosen a wrong FR, we may end up redesigning the system from the beginning, incurring a higher cost and delayed implementation. Then, the designer should change it until the design adequately addresses the original problem. It is much easier to make changes before the design is committed to hardware or software development.

Like the example of the CMP machine design indicated, we have to construct the design matrix to be sure that we do not have coupled design. When a large project is undertaken, someone or a group of outstanding designers should be designated as the system architect to make sure that during the decomposition and design process, a coupled design is not introduced. The responsibility of the system architect is to construct the design matrix for the entire project to be sure that some of the decisions made by various participants have not created coupling of FRs.

6.10 Conclusions

Defining FRs is an essential step in design. If a wrong set of FRs is identified, one has to discard the whole design process and embark on a new process.

This chapter presented different means of defining FRs based on the problem statement. Sometimes FRs must be defined as part of the decomposition process, which was briefly reviewed.

The best way of learning how to define FRs is to practice it. By asking the right questions and by practicing the decomposition process correctly, designers learn how to decompose an FR and identify children-level FRs.

Once FRs are defined, we need to identify DPs. This process is where the designer's creativity may make a difference.

Problem

Six (6) exercise problems are given in the text of this chapter. Choose even-numbered exercise problems if your last name begins with an alphabet letter between "a" and "m." If your last name begins with the letter "n" to "z," answer the odd-numbered exercise problems.

Bibliography

Jones HW (2017) Axiomatic design of space life support systems. In: Proceedings of the 47th International Conference on Environmental Systems, South Carolina, USA, p 12. https://ttu-ir. tdl.org/handle/2346/72908

Melvin JW (2003a) Axiomatic system design: chemical mechanical polishing machine case study. Doctor of Philosophy in Mechanical Engineering, Massachusetts Institute of Technology, Massachusetts Ave., Cambridge, MA, 02139, USA

Melvin JW (2003b) Axiomatic system design: chemical mechanical polishing machine case study, Ph.D. Defense Presentation Slides

Tim J (2020) Self-driving intelligent driverless car goes through the city with happy passenger relaxing. Photo licensed from Shutterstock, ID: 383436070

Wong A, Guo H, Kumar V, Park CB, Suh NP (2016) Microcellular plastics. Wiley, pp 1–57. https://onlinelibrary.wiley.com/doi/pdf/10.1002/0471440264

Further Reading

Suh NP (2001) Axiomatic design—advances and applications. Oxford University Press

How Should We Select Design Parameters?

7

Nam Pyo Suh

Abstract

Previous chapters emphasized that the first step in the design process is the identification of the problem(s) after establishing the goal of the design. Then, we define the functional requirements (FRs) the design must satisfy to deal with the problem. Once FRs are determined, we conceptualize a design by selecting DPs that can satisfy the FRs.

Unlike FRs, design parameters {DPs} are problem-specific, i.e., some deal with material things, while others may deal with software or a combination of hardware and software. The DPs dealing with organizations and economic activities are substantially different from those related to the design of technology. For DPs that are physical things, their physical integration or packaging should consider geometric proximity. For those DPs that depend on information and communication exchange, system integration is done through software systems.

Each DP should affect only one FR to generate an uncoupled design. The next acceptable design is a decoupled design, where the relationship between FRs and DPs results in a triangular design matrix. All other designs are not acceptable because they violate the Independence Axiom. The selected DP should not compromise the independence of FRs.

The theorems that govern the design process are given in this chapter. For example, Theorem 4 states that in an ideal design, the number of FRs and the number of DPs must be equal to each other. The number of DPs should never be less than the number of FRs because the design will be a coupled design, which is not acceptable. When the number of DPs is greater than the number of FRs, the design is a redundant design.

N. P. Suh (✉)
M.I.T., Cambridge, MA, USA
e-mail: npsuh@mit.edu

© Springer Nature Switzerland AG 2021
N. P. Suh et al. (eds.), *Design Engineering and Science*,
https://doi.org/10.1007/978-3-030-49232-8_7

In developing a large system with many layers of decomposition, there can be many layers of FRs and DPs, i.e., children-level FRs and DPs, and grandchildren-level FRs and DPs. In executing a large project, there may be many layers of decomposition. Thus, to monitor the selection of DPs by all participants, a Master Design Matrix should be created and monitored by a system architect to be sure that no coupling is introduced by some of the participants in the design project.

The task of selecting the right set of DPs to create an uncoupled or decoupled design is not a trivial task for a complicated system. One way of dealing with this issue is to mine an extensive database available to come up with a design matrix that is either diagonal or triangular. Now with the availability of powerful computers, we may be able to keep searching the database until we find a set of DPs that yield uncoupled or decoupled designs. In the future, this process may be assisted through the use of artificial intelligence (AI) and powerful computers.

The coupling of FRs by chosen DPs in any system is the source of many failures in the field.

7.1 Introduction

The selection of FRs was the topic covered in Chap. 6. In this chapter, we discuss the selection of DPs to satisfy FRs.

The history of modern science and technology is only about 350 years old (about ten generations), although humans existed millions of years before that. Since the Industrial Revolution, people began to use mechanized power. They used their creativity and ingenuity to make things, mostly through trial-and-error processes. Then, the idea that they have to define the problem in terms of FRs and conceive DPs to satisfy FRs would have been a foreign concept. They solved problems by jumping into making things (i.e., DPs) through trial-and-error processes without stating the FRs formally. This empirical approach has been highly successful. Even today, many people create innovative technologies successfully through this brute force approach. Similar things happened in many other fields, but eventually, logical, rational, and science-based methods and theories have gradually replaced empirical approaches, because these trial-and-error processes cost too much, both in financial and human terms, with unpredictable results.

A Unique Lesson for a Young Engineer! Experience has its limitations.

A young student who just finished his third year at an S&T university in the United States was very fortunate. He got a summer job in the industry as an engineer in a small company that manufactured disposable plastic products such as cups, dishes, and the like! When he joined the company, he thought that he would be designing new automatic machines, because the job was advertised as such. The company assigned him to work for the "chief engineer," a creative, experienced, and hardworking head of the machine shop, among other things. The "chief engineer" did not have formal engineering education, but learned to engineer through many years of practical experience and have made many things intuitively even without any drawings. The "chief engineer" and his crew made many new things: vacuum forming molds, the press for punching out vacuum-formed cups, and also other related machines needed for the production of plastic products. The young engineer also worked with the foreman of the production line when a new manufacturing system had to be installed to manufacture various new products. He learned a lot from these experienced people. None of them had gone to colleges for formal engineering education, but they were smart people who had acquired technical skills in the jobs they had over their careers. The young engineer learned a great deal about the "real world" from these craftsmen that he would not have learned in classrooms.

The fantastic thing about the chief engineer was that he did everything without any drawings or written plans! Everything came out of his head! He also conveyed his ideas verbally, and his design was done intuitively. He did not verbalize his thoughts in terms of FRs. The chief engineer made things similar to what had been made before and, therefore, did not worry about FRs. He mostly replicated DPs he saw earlier. He built a small steam locomotive at home from photographs of a locomotive had taken! The young engineer was impressed to see the pictures of the train he constructed without any drawings!

The primary job of the young "engineer" was to go around and measure the dimensions of machines, parts, and molds retroactively that the chief engineer had already built. He then drew the part on paper, mostly for record-keeping. It was not an easy task, because, although the nominal dimensions could be measured, it was impossible to discern the tolerances of those nominal dimensions. Furthermore, it was impossible to state FRs based on DPs.[1]

Then, things got worse. One day, the "chief engineer" bought an old press frame made of solid cast iron in the form of "yoke" to convert it into an automated punching press. His rationale was that it was thick and, therefore, would not deform and damp out vibration during the punching process. Then, he asked the young engineer to use the old machine frame and design a stamping press! This idea of making a new punching press out of the old cast iron part was a costly way of making a press without any FRs and DPs for anyone to see or read because only the chief engineer knew what he had in mind! After a great deal of discussion, the top management decided to abandon this project. This invaluable experience taught this young engineer a lesson of his life! Experience is essential but has its limitations.

A couple of months later, the young engineer got promoted (i.e., became independent of the chief engineer). He ended up inventing and patenting a method of making laminated foam/straight plastic cups and dishes for the company, which was a hugely successful product sold worldwide.

Many years later, back at his university, he encountered a similar but entirely different issue in the field of design. A famous design professor in his department articulated his view on the design that reinforced what the "chief engineer" in the small company practiced. He advocated that design is an "experientially based subject," and thus, it can only be learned through experience. Based on that view, he opposed offering graduate courses in design. However, this engineer, now also a professor in the same department, had learned in the industry that an "intuitive and clever" approach to design might lead to failures that could have been avoided and certainly not the best way to teach design to aspiring young students. Experience is useful and valuable, but the experience-based

---

[1]Sometimes, we use the term "*reverse engineering*" when someone tries to reproduce a well-designed product, typically that of a competitor by taking it apart and make a similar product by coping its components. The *reverse engineering* can reproduce the physical shape, but it is difficult to know the FRs of the original product. Some companies tried to catch up in technology development through reverse engineering of their competitors.

intuitive design is not the most effective way of designing products, machines, and systems. Such a design practice without a theoretical foundation would likely lead to wrong ideas and inferior designs, wasting time and money. The haphazard way of doing engineering design based purely on experience without a theoretical basis is highly risky, leading to high expenses and frequent failures. We read about these failures often in newspapers.

The story of the young engineer in the small company was told to emphasize the importance of starting the design with a clear definition of FRs, followed by DPs that satisfy the FRs. There are still many designers who jump right into DPs before defining the FRs, costing his employer both in time and money.

In this chapter, we will discuss many issues related to DPs. Consider the questions listed below:

1. Given a set of FRs, how do we develop a right set of DPs?
2. In an ideal design, how many DPs should there be when there are n FRs to be satisfied?
3. What happens if there are more DPs than FRs?
4. Can the number of DPs be less than the number of FRs?
5. In designing a large system, there may be many layers of decomposition. How do we make sure that the system is correctly designed?
6. How do constraints affect the choice of DPs?

7.2 Criteria for Selection of Design Parameters

As articulated many times in previous chapters, the design process begins with the identification of the problem in the customer domain that we need to solve through design. From the problem identified, we establish a set of the highest level FRs that the design must satisfy. FRs must be selected in a solution-neutral environment. Then we search for DPs that can satisfy each FR of the highest level FR set without violating the Independence Axiom. Choosing the highest level DPs is most important because all subsequent design decisions are affected by the highest level choices.

The selection of DPs depends very much on the knowledge of the designer(s). The more the designer knows about the problem and FRs, it is the more likely that the designer can come up with a good DP. There is no criterion for selecting the best DP at the highest level of the design process unless a similar design had been done before. However, there are some general criteria for not selecting particular DPs. Some of those criteria are as follows:

1. violation of law;
2. hazardous to humans;
3. harmful to the environment;
4. morally and ethically unacceptable;
5. violation of social norms;

6. an affront to commonly accepted religious and social standards;
7. government regulations;
8. unacceptable cost of the final product;
9. extensive use of rare materials that are difficult to acquire, e.g., rare earth elements.

The criteria for selecting *acceptable DPs* are as follows:

1. each DP selected must satisfy a corresponding FR;
2. DP must not violate the laws of nature;
3. DP must be compatible with the constitutive relationships of matter;
4. DP should not be expensive;
5. DP should be easily manufacture-able;
6. well-known DP is preferable;
7. when DP is a person, the person must be ethical, trustworthy, and knowledgeable;
8. when DP is an organization, it is preferred if the past track record is outstanding;
9. DP should be conceptually simple.

Case Study 7.1: Plastic Cup

A company that has been manufacturing paper cups decided to manufacture plastic cups for the rapidly expanding market for hot coffee. The product has to satisfy the following three FRs:

FR1 = Contain hot beverage such as coffee;
FR2 = Must be stiff enough at 90 C to be held by hand;
FR3 = Have low thermal conductivity to be held by bare hands with hot coffee inside.

We may choose the following as the DPs that can satisfy the FRs:

DP1 = Container in the shape of a cup;
DP2 = Wall thickness of the cup;
DP3 = Foamed plastic.

The design matrix that relates the FRs and DPs is shown below:

	DP1	DP2	DP3
FR1	X	0	0
FR2	0	X	X
FR3	0	X	X

The above design matrix indicates that the proposed design is a coupled design. It violates the Independence Axiom. In this design, if we try to make the cup stiffer, it also affects the heat transfer rate through the wall. This design is a coupled design, i.e., the functions of providing stiffness and thermal insulation are coupled. That is, if we increase the wall thickness to make the cup more rigid when held in hand, it also decreases the heat transfer rate through the wall.

Is there any other way we can uncouple FR2 and FR3 of this design?

One possible way is to vary the density of the foamed plastic to satisfy FR3 and the wall thickness to satisfy FR2. It may not be the best solution because the density variation may also affect both the stiffness and the thermal conductivity.

Is there another way? Perhaps a more effective way is to laminate the foamed plastic sheet with a straight unfoamed plastic sheet to control the stiffness, i.e., FR2. This second solution was patented through the U.S. Patent Office. The company did very well with these laminated products. The inventor got a small bonus for the laminated "composite" product and also for the manufacturing processes and the machine that automatically made the product. The president of the company identified the need for such a product, i.e., thin-walled cup with high thermal insulation.

Whichever DP the designer selects, it has to be executed to the lower level detailed designs through decomposition until the design is completed. Even before the design is fully implemented, the design may encounter insurmountable and unanticipated obstacles in terms of satisfying the FRs within the constraints given such as cost, government regulations, hazardous to human health, performance, and others. Otherwise, one proceeds with the design to completion and then compares the final design with the primary criteria in terms of initial customer expectation, cost, reliability, and competitiveness. Sometimes, the project must be halted in the middle of the project if one discovers that it has been pursuing the wrong DPs.

At each level of decomposition, the FRs and DPs at that level are the children-level FRs and DPs of the higher level FRs and DPs that were chosen earlier. When we select children-level FR and DP, the process of selecting rational and sound FRs and DPs is repeated. When the project is relatively small in scale, the designer can make many decisions without involving others. However, as the project is large involving many people and many FRs, the project management team must make sure that all design decisions are made well by selecting the right sets of DPs for a given set of higher level FRs.

Ultimately, a large design project depends on the decision of many designers. The decisions made by so many designers at all levels may not be acceptable because they violate the Independence Axiom. In that case, there must be a "system architect," who monitors all the decisions made by constructing the design matrix at the system level. When the coupling is introduced inadvertently, the design decision has to be replaced by another that is acceptable.

In conducting a large project involving a sizable number of staff members and engineers, it is good to hold group meetings at least once a week. Everyone working on the project should share information to identify any wrong decisions made by anyone in the project group. The following two case studies illustrate the process:

Case Study 7.2: CO_2 Level in Atmosphere

Suppose the FR is: "Reduce the CO_2 level in the atmosphere?" One or more DPs could be chosen from among the following possibilities as well as many others:

1. *electric cars in place of automobiles with internal combustion engines;*
2. *reduction of the number of automobiles with IC engines in cities;*
3. *replacement of coal-burning electric power plants with solar panels;*
4. *using human-powered automobiles;*
5. *elimination of the use of automobiles in cities;*
6. *storage of CO_2 underwater;*
7. *conversion of CO_2 into CH_4 and useful compounds.*

One or a combination of the above DPs may satisfy the FR of reducing CO_2 concentration in the atmosphere. Depending on which one of the above potential DPs is chosen, we may end up having different designs to achieve the same FR. Once we choose a DP for a given FR, we will end up with an entirely different design, because we will follow different decomposition processes depending on which first-level DP solution we choose. As resources must be expended to implement the design, we may end up having very different design embodiments, depending on how much resources are available for the task. The first decision we have to make as a designer is: "Which DP shall I choose?".

The above example deals mostly with DPs in technology-related fields. How about DPs in non-technology-related fields? For example, suppose the FR is: "Improve high school education in science and mathematics." The possible DPs might include:

1. allocation of more time for instruction of science and mathematics;
2. better teachers of mathematics and science;
3. development of computer games that teach mathematics and science;
4. more homework related to mathematics;
5. summer "math" camp for primary school children;
6. interactive computer software for teaching mathematics and science.

Although these DPs are not physical, we can treat them like the technology-related case to design the system. The design process is the same, although the contents are different.

Exercise 7.1: The P–V Diagram

You are assigned to design a compressor with a cylinder and reciprocating piston connected to a crank mechanism. In order to determine its performance, you wish to measure the pressure–volume relationship of the CO_2 gas that will be compressed in the cylinder. One way of determining the P–V relationship is to attach a sensor to the cylinder to monitor the pressure as a function of the piston position. Your design assignment is to develop the sensor that can automatically generate the P–V trace as the machine operates. What are your FRs? What are your corresponding DPs?

7.3   Ideal Design

The minimum requirement for an ideal design is that it is consistent with the Independence Axiom and the Information Axiom. The Independence Axiom states that FRs must be independent of each other. The information states that the design must be simple to design and operate by minimizing the information content of the design.

Question Raised at a Seminar at a Leading University:

A young professor who was working on Axiomatic Design (AD) was invited to give a seminar on design at a leading university in upstate New York. He went there despite the bad weather. It was windy and cold. After learning about the Independence Axiom, a distinguished professor in the audience, raised his hand to ask the following question: "Isn't it a good idea to have a functional coupling. For example, if I turn on the electric switch to turn the light on for illumination and at the same time, heat the room with the thermal energy emitted by the light bulbs, isn't that a good idea? What is wrong with that design?" The lecturer, in turn, asked the questioner, "What would you do during the summertime when the temperature is high? Teach in a room without light?".

Exercise 7.2:

Consider a design that must satisfy three FRs, i.e., FR1, FR2, and FR3. To satisfy these three FRs, how many DPs do we need?

Suppose we have a design that has three FRs and two DPs. We may express the relationship between FRs and DPs as follows:

$$\begin{aligned}
FR1 &= f1(DP1, \ DP2) \\
FR2 &= f2(DP1, \ DP2) \\
FR3 &= f3(DP1, \ DP2)
\end{aligned} \tag{7.1}$$

In this case, it is easy to see that, all three FRs cannot be independent of each other.

Now suppose that we have four DPs to satisfy three FRs as follows:

$$\begin{aligned}
FR1 &= f1(DP1, \ DP2, \ DP3, \ DP4) \\
FR2 &= f2(DP1, \ DP2, \ DP3, \ DP4) \\
FR3 &= f3(DP1, \ DP2, \ DP3, \ DP4)
\end{aligned} \tag{7.2}$$

In this case, we have a redundancy of having an extra DP for three FRs we need to satisfy. This kind of design where the number of DPs is larger than FRs is called the redundant design. (It is a theorem.)

In an ideal design, the number of DPs must be equal to the number of FRs. (It is a theorem.)

The best design would be the following:

$$
\begin{aligned}
FR1 &= f1(DP1) \\
FR2 &= f2(DP2) \\
FR3 &= f3(DP3)
\end{aligned}
\tag{7.3}
$$

In this case, each FR is controlled and satisfied by one DP. It is an uncoupled design. It satisfies the Independence Axiom. The design matrix is diagonal as shown below[2]:

	DP1	DP2	DP3
FR1	A_{11}	0	0
FR2	0	A_{22}	0
FR3	0	0	A_{33}

If we have three DPs for three FRs that have the following three special relationships exist, we can satisfy the Independence Axiom:

$$
\begin{aligned}
FR1 &= f1(DP1) \\
FR2 &= f2(DP1,\ DP2) \\
FR3 &= f3(DP1,\ DP2,\ DP3)
\end{aligned}
\tag{7.4}
$$

In this special case, we must vary DPs in a particular order to satisfy the Independence Axiom. In the design given by Eq. (7.4), we need to vary DP1 first to satisfy FR1, followed by DP2 and DP3, in that order. Then, the independence of the FRs can be satisfied. This kind of design is called a decoupled design.

It should be noted that the beauty of satisfying the Independence Axiom becomes apparent by examining Eq. (7.4). Although the system represented by Eq. (7.4) involves three inputs and three outputs, the system behaves as a one-input and one-output system, making it easy to control and satisfy. A coupled system with n outputs and n inputs is complicated to operate or control.

---

[2]In terms of indices notation, the relationship between FR_i and DP_j may be written as.
$FR_i = \sum A_{ij} DP_i$,
  where i and j are 1, 2, or 3. FRi and DPj are vectors, and Aij is a second-order tensor, like the stress tensor $_{ij}$ and the strain $_{ij}$ tensor in solid mechanics. In mathematics, we learned to transform the second-order tensor to find the eigenvalues or characteristic values through coordinate transformation. That is how we determine the maximum principle stress and the minimum principle stress. That is, there are only normal stresses and no shear stresses along a certain coordinate axes in a solid body under load. Unfortunately, we cannot do the coordinate transformation in the case of design, because the resulting DP's become something that do not have any physical significance. In design, we choose DPs so as to make the design to "have eigenvalues" through proper choice of DPs. That is, we cannot do mathematical transformation of a design to search for DPs that will give a diagonal matrix (i.e., equivalent to eigenvalues) through proper choice of DPs that will yield a diagonal or triangular matrix.

The following theorems are useful to remember:

Theorem on Rational Ideal Design:

In an ideal design, the number of FRs and DPs is the same.

Theorem on Coupled Design:

When a design cannot satisfy each one of the n FRs independently from each other, the design is a coupled design.

Theorem on Decoupled Design:

When the design can satisfy the independence of FRs by varying DPs in a specific sequence, the design is a decoupled design.

Theorem on Related FRs:

If FR1 is related to FR2 as FR1 = f(FR2), the design has only one independent FR.

Question 7.1:

Can we manufacture PVC parts faster with plastisol?

One way of manufacturing thin PVC plastic parts such as children's boots and PVC-coated tools is to use plastisol. Plastisol is a slurry of PVC (polyvinyl chloride) powder suspended in a viscous liquid called polyol (an organic compound containing multiple hydroxyl groups). Plastisol is a highly viscous liquid. When plastisol is poured into a mold and heated in the mold, polyol diffuses into solid PVC particles at an elevated temperature. PVC swells up and softens, finally fusing, forming a substantial flexible part in the shape of the mold.

Many PVC parts are made from plastisol. The final property of the solidified part is a function of the ratio of the resin to the polyol. The productivity of this plastisol processing is low because it takes a long time to raise the temperature of the slurry in the mold due to the low thermal diffusivity of plastisol. Therefore, the problem with plastisol processing is its slow processing speed.

A young engineer had a bright idea for curing plastisol parts quickly. His brilliant idea: eliminating the need to heat polyol in the mold. The idea was to pre-heat about 75% of the polyol separately to a temperature higher than the average processing temperature of plastisol and then quickly mix it with the remainder of unheated PVC-rich plastisol, which has the PVC resin powder and remaining 25% of the polyol that has not yet been heated. Then the mixture would quickly reach the fusion temperature of plastisol due to the physical mixing of hot polyol and plastisol, shortening the processing time. However, his "great" idea for rapid plastisol processing was not accepted for commercialization.

Exercise 7.3:

What is wrong with this new idea? Is it a coupled design? Why is it a coupled design?

7.4 Generation and Selection of Design Parameters

Given an FR, we must choose an appropriate DP that does not violate the Independence Axiom. Are there fundamental theories that can guide us in this process of transforming FR into DP? Are there algorithms that can lead us to the right DP?

In the absence of a simple way of sorting all possible DPs and choosing the very best DP for a given FR and constraints, we choose DPs based on our understanding of natural laws, materials, and other databases, which are typically stored in designer's head, i.e., "knowledge of the designer matters!" As of now, there is no ideal way of developing ideas that can lead to the selection of the best DP for a given FR. However, when there are many FRs we have to satisfy at a given level of the design hierarchy, it is possible to choose the best set of DPs among a given set of acceptable DPs by constructing the design matrix to check for coupling. This observation can be stated as theorems:

Theorem 1 on Selection of DPs for a given Set of FRs:

In system design, when there are n FRs at a given level of the design hierarchy, an acceptable set of n DPs is those that yield either diagonal or triangular design matrix.

Theorem 2 on Selection of DPs for a given set of FRs:

In many cases, when a specific DP that satisfies a given FR cannot be identified, select a conceptual DP that only satisfies the FR and decompose the FRs and DPs.

Theorem 1 above states that when human designers are given the task of selecting DPs for a given FR, the designer should use the existing knowledge accumulated in the database to create an uncoupled or decoupled design. However, when such a DP cannot be readily identified, Theorem 2 given above states that we should select a conceptual DP that satisfies the FR intending to decompose the FR and the DP further until all the details of the design emerge.

Given the rapid advances made in AI, in the foreseeable future, we should be able to create generalized search tools for finding the best DPs and PVs for a given FR. However, it may be still best for human designers to decompose FRs and DPs to limit the search space of AI.

Notwithstanding the limitations of the current knowledge and database on the FR, DP, and P–V relationships, the following guidelines may aid in developing ideas for DPs and selecting the most appropriate DPs:

For *technology*-related fields (in random order):

1. think of the implication of all basic concepts used in science and technology such as conservation laws, Fick's laws, Newton's laws, electromagnetism, thermodynamic laws, and others;
2. try to ignore the current technologies to avoid becoming mental slaves of current technologies and the thinking that goes with them;
3. review or acquire the fundamental knowledge in subjects related to FR by reviewing the basics of the related fields, e.g., physics, chemistry, and biology;
4. keep reviewing the original problem identified: what are the shortcomings;
5. the best place to start may be introductory textbooks!
6. attend and listen to lectures in fields that may be closely or remotely related to the topic;
7. remember, good ideas are simple!

8. great ideas may be generated by similitude based on developments in other fields;
9. establish the upper and lower bounds of the FR, i.e., the allowable variation of the chosen FR;
10. do something else, such as walking on a treadmill, in order to divert the thought process from time-to-time;
11. think out aloud by talking to other colleagues and friends about the problem. It may force you to organize your thoughts;
12. think of analogies;
13. do not let others belittle your ideas;
14. remember the principle of similitude;
15. if no specific DP can be identified, just put down a conceptual DP, based on which the next level FRs can be selected and subsequently, the corresponding DPs;
16. think!

For *non-technology* fields:

Some of the ideas listed above for technical fields apply here as well. In addition, the following may be useful:

1. understand the history of the organization, including past efforts made to deal with the FR;
2. review the primary objectives of the organizational goals;
3. listen to people who have been working in the field or the organization;
4. understand the fundamental theories or laws or rules that govern the field or the organization;
5. be able to state the goals of the organization succinctly;
6. gather existing opinions of the leaders of the organization or the field;
7. identify who is going to benefit and who is going get hurt if the current organization is changed;
8. have a detailed understanding of the subject matter, à la Warren Buffett;
9. develop a competitive strategy for the operation of companies;
10. do not believe everything you hear;
11. think!

The designer should remember that it may take a while to come up with good DPs, but it is better to take time and think to select appropriate DPs than rushing in with half-baked ideas, ending up with a wrong set of DPs. Otherwise, one might not develop a design that solves the original problem identified in the customer domain.

Role of Constraints in Choosing Design Parameters

In design, it is essential that the constraints imposed on design be stated. The cost of finding out the existence of constraints after the design is completed can be substantial. Some of the constraints on design are generated in the customer domain. Also, during the design process, some constraints are generated due to the design decisions made during decomposition. One of the typical constraints is the cost of the product.

There may be many constraints that eliminate specific DPs from consideration. For example, in choosing DPs that can reduce the CO_2 emission, suppose that the following constraints are imposed:

1. the cost of reducing CO_2 should be equal to economic gains generated by CO_2 reduction in 10 years;
2. the measures undertaken to reduce CO_2 in the atmosphere should not affect the sulfur content of the atmosphere;
3. the measures used to reduce CO_2 should not adversely affect the safety of people;
4. the technology adopted to reduce anthropogenic CO_2 should not increase the average temperature of the ocean.

These constraints may eliminate some of the DPs from further consideration.

Exercise 7.4:

We are charged with developing national health policies. The highest level FR for healthcare is stated as "Provide healthcare for all citizens." Design the next level FRs and DPs. List possible DPs for this FR for healthcare. Also, list Cs (constraints).

Exercise 7.5:

Driverless autonomous electric vehicles (DAEV) are being introduced in urban areas. If the vehicle malfunctions, injuring pedestrians, and damaging properties, we will need to develop insurance policies to pay for the loss of lives and properties. The FR may be stated as: "Develop insurance policies for damages done by DAEV." Design the insurance policy in terms of FRs and DPs by decomposing the highest level FR and DP. Also list constraints.

Exercise 7.6:

The use of social networks (SN) has spread worldwide. One of the significant problems with SN is "fake news" that some people spread for political and other illegitimate purposes. Define FRs and DPs, as well as constraints that can eliminate the intentional misuse of SN.

7.5 Integration of Design Parameters in a System

The DPs generated through the design process discussed in the preceding sections must be integrated into a system. The methodology used in the integration of DPs into a system depends on what the DPs are, i.e., physical things, personnel, software, organization, a combination of these "things."

When DPs are organizational entities that depend on communications between DPs, system integration is done through software and communications systems. In the pre-modern communications era, co-workers were placed in close physical proximity, but with the availability of modern communications tools, many companies are depending on interconnections through the Internet, telephones, and software systems. Even in the case of organizations, it is more efficient and, thus, cheaper to operate even substantial entities without having to have everyone in close geographic proximity. Many large companies operate globally and, therefore, and it is not realistic to depend on close physical proximity. Many large companies allow their employees to work at home, which reduces the need for physical space at one location for everyone.

When the DPs are tangible things such as parts in automobiles, physical location, and physical integration of DPs can be critical. It is better to have certain DPs close together through physical integration if they have to interact in the system. In that case, it is useful to create DP to DP map, using a DP versus DP matrix to identify which DPs interact frequently and thus, need to be in close geometric proximity.

7.6 Case Studies

Case Study 7.3: Identification of DPs Based on Physics and Engineering Science

The goal of this case study is to illustrate how DPs and PVs were conceived to satisfy FRs based on physics.

a. **Design Problem:**

In Example 2.1, the design of the molding process for the manufacture of shoe soles was discussed.

We will review the steps involved in conceiving the process variables (PVs) to create the DPs that satisfy the three FRs in order to illustrate how the design was conceived. In Chap. 2, the FRs, DPs, and PVs for the shoe sole were listed, which is repeated below:

The highest level FR may be decomposed as:

FR1 = Mold the entire shoe sole onto the upper;
FR2 = Make the sole flexible, i.e., pliable;
FR3 = Make the sole wear-resistant;
FR4 = Control the weight (i.e., density) of the sole.

The corresponding DPs in the physical domain may be chosen as:

DP1 = Injection molding of PVC against the upper mounted on last;
DP2 = Density of foamed PVC;
DP3 = Solid skin layer for wear resistance;
DP4 = Total weight of the PVC injected into the mold.

The PVs that enabled the achievement of DPs are given as:

PV1 = Injection of PVC with a chemical blowing agent in pre-determined space;
PV2 = Expansion of the mold volume by moving the bottom plate;
PV3 = Temperature of the mold that comes into contact with the bottom of the shoe sole;
PV4 = Injection volume.

The company tried various approaches without success before this young engineer joined the company. One of the methods tried in the past was to melt PVC (polyvinyl chloride) resins with a chemical blowing agent (that decomposes at the decomposition temperature) in the plasticating screw pump of the injection molding machine. The mixture of the molten gas/polymer is then injected into the mold. The mold cavity was shaped like a shoe sole enclosed on the top by the stitched upper mounted on a last. When the mixture is injected into the mold, the plastic/gas mixture forms gas bubbles and expands as it flows into the mold. This process creates a polymer/bubble structure that is inhomogeneous because the gas bubbles at the flow front expand more than the plastic/gas mixture near the gate. This poor density distribution, a result of the flow front of the molten plastic is subject to low pressure, while the pressure at the gate is high. Therefore, the material distribution is uneven throughout the mold. The density of the polymer/bubble mixture is highest near the gate with small bubbles, while the plastic at the leading edge of the flow has the lowest density. Thus, the material distribution is not uniform throughout the part. Furthermore, this process does not create the wear-resistant skin layer at the bottom of the shoe sole.

b. **Conceptualization of the Process Based on Basic Physics:**

If we look at this problem, the physics tell us the following:

1. We must distribute the material evenly in order to have the right amount of material in the right place throughout the mold.
2. To achieve (1), we cannot allow much expansion of plastic through foaming while it flows into the mold.
3. To achieve (2), we need high pressure while the plastic is being injected into the mold to minimize foaming.
4. To achieve (1) and (3), we need to raise the pressure by narrowing the flow channel in the mold between the last (where the upper is mounted) and the bottom mold plate.
5. (4) can be achieved if we make the bottom of the mold movable to make the flow channel very narrow during the injection.
6. After the injection is completed, if we move back the bottom plate of the mold outward, the plastic with the foaming agent (now gaseous state) will expand with bubbles, filling the mold.
7. To make the wear-resistant skin layer at the bottom of the shoe sole, we keep the bottom mold plate, which is in contact with the hot plastic cold. The plastic in contact with the cold plate cannot foam due to its low temperature, thus creating an unfoamed skin layer.

Case Study 7.4: Identification of DP Based on Tribo-Physics for Electric Connector

a. **Design Problem:**

The use of electrical connectors is ubiquitous. They are used wherever an electrical connection must be made. They consist of male and female parts, which can slide against each other under normal pressure for good electrical contact with a contact resistance of less than 20 milliohms. One type of commercial connector is shown in Fig. 7.1. There are many different kinds of connectors made for many applications ranging from printed circuit boards and simple circuit breakers. In order to have acceptable electric contacts, high normal pressure is applied to the contact area through tight tolerances and sometimes applying elastic "spring" loading. The contact area is plated with gold to prevent oxidation of the contact area, which increases electric contact resistance. Depending on applications, the current density at the contact area can be high, which leads to heating of the connector.

After the extended use of these connectors, the gold plating gradually wears off, exposing substrate metal. When the substrate metal wears off and form a loose wear particle, it can oxidize. These oxide particles may be lodged between two rigid sliding surfaces, separating the two electrodes. Under further sliding, they may cause abrasive wear creating more particles and disrupting the electrical contact. The question here is what are the DPs and how we create them.

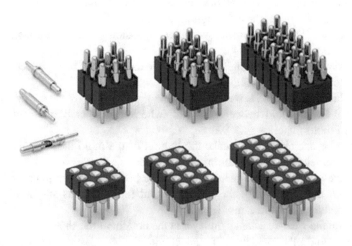

Fig. 7.1 Triple row spring-pin connectors and mating target connectors. (Reproduced with permission from Mill-Max Mfg Corp. 2020)

b. **Design Solution:**

To prevent the wear and disruption of electrical contacts between the pin and the receptor, we need to satisfy the following FRs:

FR1 = Provide good electrical contacts between the pin and the receptor;
FR2 = Allow sliding action between the electrodes.

How shall we now determine two DPs for these two FRs?

AD does not provide domain-specific expert knowledge needed to determine DPs, other than providing the general framework, i.e., the fact that we need two DPs to come up with an ideal design.

Unfortunately, there is no magic in determining DPs. One has to know the basics of tribology[3]; in this case, mostly tribo-physics. One can read introductory reference books on tribology or ask someone who knows the basics of tribology. It is not too difficult to learn the subject and come up with right solutions to this problem. Before we present DPs for these FRs, the following story may shed light on the challenges associated with changing pre-conceived notions.

The DPs for the two FRs for electric connectors may be stated as follows:

FR1 = Provide good electrical contacts between the pin and the receptor;
FR2 = Allow sliding action between the electrodes.

DP1 = Good contact areas for continuous flow of electric current;
DP2 = Sliding interface

FR1 and DP1 may be decomposed as follows:

FR11 = Prevent oxidation of the contact area;
FR12 = Large number of contact areas at the interface for maximum current flow;
FR13 = Provide constant normal load;

FR21 = Modulate the contact forces for ease of sliding;
FR22 = Remove any entrapped wear particles from the sliding interface.

The corresponding DPs are chosen as follows:

DP11 = Gold plating of contact areas;
DP12 = Woven conductor structure;
DP13 = Spring force to limit the maximum load.

---

[3]Tribology refers to the field of science and engineering of friction, wear, and lubrication.

DP21 = Tensioning fiber;
DP22 = Open space between fibers for wear particles to escape.

There can be many different designs that can accommodate the above three DPs. Two of the physical embodiments that satisfy the above DPs is shown in Figs. 7.2 and 7.3.

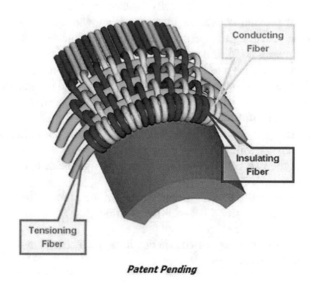

Fig. 7.2 One embodiment of the design. Pin is gold-plated copper. The conducting fibers are wrapped around the tensioning fiber

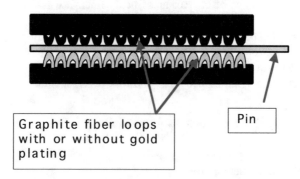

Fig. 7.3 The pin is made of gold-plated metal rods. The female part of the connector is made up of a flexible, bristle-like material held together by a substrate, similar to a velvet-like fabric structure. The fibers are plated with a highly conductive metal such as gold

The insertion force should be extremely low in both cases. The normal load between the pin and the bristle during the insertion is controlled by either the tensioning fiber (Fig. 7.2) or stiffness of the bristle (Fig. 7.3). Therefore, the wear of the pins and the strips should be negligible, allowing an "infinite" number of insertions.

Too Simple to Be True! (Stories About the Visit of a Professor of Practice,[4] AD, and Korean Alphabet).

One of the engineering professors with extensive industrial experience could not believe that some of the technological innovations he heard about were done based on AD! He paid a special visit to a colleague to discuss his misgivings about design axioms. His point was that it is not the AD theory but rather the ingenious inventor who came up with his various inventions mentioned in the literature. It was apparent that he was not prepared to accept the Independence Axiom. His thinking might have been: "Can such a simple statement as the Independence Axiom be the basis for all these creative designs?".

In some ways, this story is not so unique when so many theories, including Newton's, had so many skeptics. About 600 years ago, King Sejong, the third king of the Lee Dynasty of Korea, invented the Korean alphabet, which consists of 24 letters. Most people can read and write Korean words within a day. The Korean alphabet, HanGeul, is so simple that one can learn to write them in a few hours. That was the reason Korean scholars refused to use it, writing poems, poetry, and prose in Chinese for more than 500 years after King Sejong invented HanGeul.

Until about 100 years ago, educated Korean people would not write poems and books in Korean, because the Korean alphabet was so easy to learn that scholars could not distinguish themselves from the peasant, (so they might have thought). Korean scholars spent their lifetime memorizing Chinese characters, which was used as a measure of scholarly achievements. During the Lee dynasty, government civil service examinations consisted of composing poems and poetry in Chinese rather than in Korean! The one who could compose a better poem in Chinese became government officials. Even Korean family books were written in Chinese! The tragedy is that now most Koreans cannot read their family book, because they are written in Chinese characters.

We may have a similar problem in the field of design. Some still say: "How can it be so simple when people spent decades to learn to design by acquiring years of experience." It is time to change because the old way of designing is costly and not reliable.

Exercise 7.7:

Construct the design matrix and write down the design equation, i.e., FRs as a function of DPs for the connectors shown in Fig. 7.3.

Case Study 7.5: Identification of DP in Organizational Design

a. Design Problem:

In designing organizations, we have to decide the FRs of an organization first before we do anything else. Since there are many people involved in large organizations, it is essential that one develop a consensus on the selection of FRs, if

---

[4]This title of Professor of Practice is typically given to people who made important contributions in industry and joined universities to teach students based on their industrial experience.

possible. FRs are the goals of the organization, and DPs are simply the organizational units to fulfill the FRs. In some organizations, FRs are stated under the heading of a "mission statement." However, in many organizations, FRs are not explicitly stated and go directly into selecting DPs, which are often named as "department" or "divisions." There can be more than one DP for a given FR if the task is immense.

The design of an organization is only as good as the people who are in charge of various FRs. When a new person inherits an existing organization, it is necessary to work with the people who have been in the organization. It is more effective to work with these people rather than replacing them with newly hired people unless it is absolutely necessary.

An intricate part of organizational design is the selection of "people in charge" of a given task. One needs to talk to many people to identify the best people already in the organization. However, one should remember that the performance of a person depends on the clarity of the mission given by FRs of the organization, the freedom to execute the task within broad guidelines, and budgetary support.

In many organizations, the interaction with the outside world is essential, because their support can be critical in securing the financial support, in coalescing the support of inside people and implementing the internal programs. In a sense, no organization exists in isolation. It is a part of a continuum of society or a larger organization.

In selecting people who can run different parts of the organization (i.e., PVs), it takes a finite time to assess the performance of a person in a given position. Initially, one has to wait and see what the person does, but it can take a year or more to be able to assess the performance. Some people may occupy a position not doing much, only looking for the next promotion or position. By the time one realizes the situation, one's tenure in that position may be up!

In many organizations, the new leader just appointed to the position must work with available financial resources. The budget was already set 2 or so years beforehand because the budgetary process in public institutions goes through a lengthy decision-making process. Typically, it may take up to 2 years to get the new budget through the system.

In the private sector, things can move faster if the right people back the effort. Often the private sector operates based on personal trust and past performance record. If someone at the top of an organization selects a person for a "fast track" career path, one can become an executive of a large company in a relatively short time. It is partly "luck" for this to happen. An equally able person may never get the promotion if a person is at the wrong place, at the wrong time, working for the wrong people. In this situation, it may be best for the person to leave the organization and seek new opportunities. However, one has to remember that there is no guarantee of success.

Note on Importance of the Reputation of a Person

A new high-tech company established based on a technology developed at a university was struggling. Things were not going well. The young people he hired to run the company and commercialize the invention were using up the initial fund raised from the friends of the founder. They could not raise new money to bring technology to a commercial-stage and find customers. In desperation, the founder of the company asked his acquaintance, who was the CEO of a successful high-tech company, if he would be able to help this struggling company by becoming a member of the board of directors. His answer was immediate: "No." He said that he was too busy with so many activities. The answer was not unexpected.

Surprisingly, the following day, early in the morning, the founder of the company received a telephone call from the CEO, who turned down the request for help less than 24 h ago. He said that he thought about the proposal overnight and changed his mind. He said that he would become a member of the board if he can also invest money into this struggling company. The founder was more than grateful! He then asked the CEO to be the chairman of the board of the company and oversee the management of the company.

Once he assumed the chairmanship, several things happened. Many people wanted to invest money in this struggling company! He could also recruit an experienced business person to be the CEO of the company. Under his leadership, the technology was commercialized successfully in the market place.

The lesson learned is that the impeccable reputation of the industry leader was the key to his success. He was extremely ethical, creative in his thinking, willing to take risks, and dedicated to the public good. He treats people fairly and equally, including the same size cubicle for office for everyone, including the CEO himself, the same class airplane ticket, and the like. He is an exceptional person. Fortunately, people like him make the world a better place for everyone.

b. **Design Solution:**

Again, the design of organizations follows the same sequence as the design of technologies, i.e., the Problem–FR–DP–PV transformation. First, one has to determine the problem the organization has vis-à-vis its mission and goals. Then the FRs must be established, followed by DPs and PVs. In this process, one must realize that there will be criticisms coming from all directions since any change will hurt those who have been the beneficiaries of the old system. Such a controversy should be avoided, but it may be difficult to avoid them if one wants to solve the problem identified through the design of a new organization. However, the compensating feature of such an effort is the advancements made by these transformed organizations. Sometimes, one has to be patient and nurture the newly changed organizations.

Case Study 7.6: Identification of DP Based on Material and Mechanics

a. **Design Problem:**

In materials science, it is assumed that one cannot have both high strength and high toughness at the same time. That is, if one chooses a DP to make the metal stronger, then one has to accept the decrease in the toughness (i.e., the energy the material can absorb before fracturing) of the material. Therefore, it has been a challenge in the materials field, to be able to gain in both toughness and strength at the same time.

One way of increasing strength is through dispersion hardening. It is a simple idea. Metals deform plastically because crystal defects called "dislocations" move along the crystal plane when stress is applied. One way of making the metal stronger is to block the motion of these dislocations or make it harder to slide on the slip plane, which can be done by various metallurgical means. In the case of steel, we add carbon in iron to form iron carbides "particles," which are harder than the iron matrix. When these particles are present, the dislocations cannot go through them and must be "extruded" between the hard particles, which require higher stress. However, these particles must be microscopic, around 100 nm, to increase the strength. When these particles are large, they fracture and crack, lowering the toughness. In the case of copper, it is done by diffusing oxygen slowly into the copper matrix that has a small amount of aluminum dissolved in it. The oxygen then oxidizes aluminum, forming oxide particles in the copper matrix. The problem with this oxidation process is that it is slow and expensive.

Hard and tough copper alloy is needed in many applications. One of the applications is in making electrodes for spot welding guns used in the automotive industry. In this application, a copper rod of about 1–2 cm in length and diameter is forged into a conical electrode shape. Two of these "welding tips" are attached to robot arms. They are then pressed against each other through the two steel sheets to be welded. When a high electric current is sent through the electrodes, the temperature of the compressed junction of the steel sheets increases to the melting temperature, forming spot-welds which join the sheets. Through this welding process, we assemble car bodies. If pure copper is used, the tips deform right away because they do not have the strength to withstand the compressive load.

b. **Design Solution:**

The new design solution of getting both the toughness and high strength in copper was proposed. It consists of the following steps:

1. Prepare two copper solutions in two separate crucibles. In one of the crucibles, dissolve about 5% of titanium (Ti) in molten copper and the other dissolve boron(B) in molten copper. When these two hot streams of copper are quickly mixed, they form tiny titanium boride (TiB2) particles in molten copper to lower the free energy of the two solutions. Then, if the molten copper is quickly solidified, the particles do not have time to grow, forming sub-micron-scale hard particles in the copper solution. Such dispersion-strengthened copper is both strong and tough. The matrix phase must be pure copper without any solutes to maintain the high thermal and electrical conductivity.

The FRs of this dispersion-strengthened copper are the following:

FR1 = Increase the strength of copper;
FR2 = Increase the toughness of copper;
FR3 = Maintain the thermal conductivity of copper.

The DPs are the following:

DP1 = Number of titanium boride particles;
DP2 = Diameter of titanium boride particle;
DP3 = Purity of the copper matrix.

The manufacturing process for making this dispersion-strengthened copper was also designed and developed from scratch. Three brand new Ph.D.s built a factory to manufacture the alloy. In 3 years or so, the alloy was manufactured using newly developed manufacturing processes and sold to car manufacturers. This alloy is given the name Mixalloy.

The remarkable feat of this project was that the manufacturing process could not be tried out in small-scale tests in the laboratory because of the scale of molten copper required to reach a steady-state flow. Therefore, a full-scale production machine was built *from scratch* without the benefit of small-scale experiments. The electrodes produced by this Mixalloy process, using the production machine built from scratch, were shipped to automotive companies in Detroit, Japan, and Korea in 3 years from the date the company was established. This actual case shows the power of AD and is a testimony for hard-working able and smart engineers and technicians.

Exercise 7.8:

Construct the design matrix for the proposed design of the Mixalloy.

Case Study 7.7: Identification of FRs and DPs Based on Fluid Mechanics.[5]

a. **Design Problem:**

Automotive parts such as bumpers and fenders are made of a polymer called polyurethane because of its lightweight, resistance to damage, and low manufacturing cost. Polyurethane parts are made by mixing two chemical components, polyol (viscous resin) and the other is diisocyanate. Trial-and-error processes developed the industrial process of mixing these two chemicals. The problem is how to design the impingement mixing process.

The obvious way of mixing these two liquids is to stir them using a mechanical impala. However, for these fast-reacting liquid systems, it is too slow to mix them before they partially react. Another way of mixing them is by "impingement mixing," which collides two liquid components by shooting them against each other

---

[5]This design problem was partially discussed in Sect. 2.1.1.

at high speeds in a small mixing chamber. This process, which is known as Reaction Injection Molding (RIM), was developed in industry empirically and widely used.

b. **Design Solution:**

The FRs can be stated as follows:

FR1 = Inject polyol and diisocyanate into a mixing chamber;
FR2 = Keep the ratio of the two-fluid components the same;
FR3 = Create turbulent mixing in the chamber;
FR4 = Make the mixing chamber to be free of the dead area;
FR5 = Discharge the mixture of polyol and diisocyanate into a mold;
FR6 = Control temperature of the monomers.

To achieve the above stated FRs, we have to pump the two fluid components at the same rate at any instant. The mixing chamber should be small to be sure that all the fluid in the chamber at any instant undergoes turbulent mixing, i.e., no dead pocket of stagnant fluids. We have to make sure that the turbulent eddy size must be of the order of magnitude to promote the instant reaction of the two-fluid components. Thens the mixture must be discharged continuously. The mixing chamber and the overall system are sketched (Fig. 7.4).

The DPs may be stated as follows:

DP1 = Injection nozzle;
DP2 = Positive displacement pumps in synchronous motion.

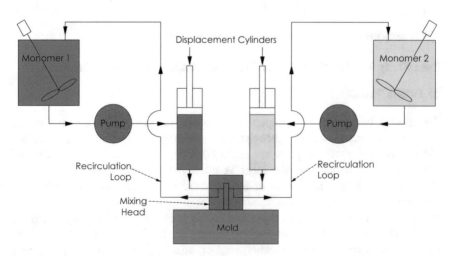

Fig. 7.4 A Typical RIM machine and the mixing chamber

DP3 = Turbulent eddy size;
DP4 = Small mixing chamber;
DP5 = Discharge port;
DP6 = Heat exchanger.

A brilliant student[6] showed, through dimensional analysis, that the turbulent eddy size, δ, is proportional to the Reynolds' number (Re) as follows:

$$\delta \propto (\text{Re})^{-3/4} = (\rho V D / \mu)^{-3/4,}$$

where V is the velocity of the fluid, ρ is the mass density of the fluid, μ is the viscosity of the fluid. Since the polyol has a higher viscosity, its velocity must be high enough in order to be sure that the turbulent eddy size is sufficiently small to provide a complete chemical reaction of polyol and diisocyanate.

The design matrix for the proposed design is as follows:

	DP1	DP2	DP3	DP4	DP5
FR1	X	X	0	0	0
FR2	0	X	0	0	0
FR3	X	X	X	0	0
FR4	0	0	0	X	0
FR5	0	0	0	0	X

The design matrix indicates that the design is a decoupled design. We need to set DP2 first and then DP1, followed by DP3, DP5, and DP4 in any order.

Although this turbulent mixing analysis was done for highly viscous fluids, this technology has been applied to make Mixalloys with molten metals to create nano-scale ceramic particles to produce dispersion-strengthened copper with titanium di-boride as the dispersoids.

7.7   Use of Artificial Intelligence (AI) in Axiomatic Design

Suppose a design task has five FRs. Then, we know that we need to find five DPs. The design matrix that relates FRs to DPs is as shown below:

---

[6]Charles L. Tucker, III, who later became a professor and Associate Provost at the University of Illinois.

	DP1	DP2	DP3	DP4	DP5
FR1	A11	A12	A13	A14	A15
FR2	A21	A22	A23	A24	A25
FR3	A31	A32	A33	A34	A35
FR4	A41	A42	A43	A44	A45
FR5	A51	A52	A53	A54	A55

The design that satisfies the Independence Axiom is the one with a diagonal matrix, i.e., all none diagonal elements in the design matrix such as A12, A34, etc., are zero and all diagonal elements such as A22, etc., are non-zero quantities. That is, find a DP1 that does not affect any other FRs than FR1. Similarly, DP2 does not affect all FRs but FR2. And so on. Sometimes we may be so fortunate that we can readily choose the five DPs that will yield either a diagonal matrix or a triangular matrix based on the knowledge we have in our brain. If that is not possible, we may have to resort to the computational power of a computer. One of the techniques of searching the database may be the use of AI techniques in order to search the database and look for the right DPs to come up with the following design:

	DP1	DP2	DP3	DP4	DP5
FR1	A11	0	0	0	0
FR2	0	A22	0	0	0
FR3	0	0	A33	0	0
FR4	0	0	0	A44	0
FR5	0	0	0	0	A55

The search routine may be stated as

a. search for DP1 that affects FR1 but does not affect FR2, FR3, FR4, and FR5;
b. if (a) is not possible, search for DP1 that affects only FR1 and then search for DP2 that affects FR2 and FR1 but no other FRs;
c. then search for DP3 that affects FR3, FR1, and FR2 but no other FRS;
d. continue this process until a triangular matrix is obtained as follows:

	DP1	DP2	DP3	DP4	DP5
FR1	A11	A12	A13	A14	A15
FR2	0	A22	A23	A24	A25
FR3	0	0	A33	A34	A35
FR4	0	0	0	A44	A45
FR5	0	0	0	0	A55

e. often, a neat triangular matrix as shown may not result, although DPs chosen satisfy the conditions outlined in (a)–(d), requiring the re-arrangement of FRs and DPs until a triangular matrix is obtained.

In some design tasks, there may be a large number of FRs at the highest level. It may also be a result of many layers of decomposition of FRs and DPs. As the number of layers of decomposition increases and as the number of FRs increases, the task of coming up with a set of DPs that can assure either a diagonal design matrix of an uncoupled system design or a triangular design matrix for a decoupled design may become an onerous task and sometimes perhaps beyond human capability without the help of computational and information storage capability of computers. We need to use the capability of large computers that can deal with extensive database and computational issues in comparing various combinations of FRs and DPs.

One way of searching for DPs is to use the computational power to try many combinations and seek a set of DPs for a given set of FRs that yield acceptable designs. Some people have done this using AI, which has created a new business boom in AI-based technologies. This new approach to AI—rather than the old paradigm of "if…, then…" logic—is based on neural network and by using fast learning algorithms.[7] This new AI approach has become feasible, in part, because of the computational power of computers that can accumulate a vast database and compute at a rapid computational speed. There are many industrial firms, IBM, Amazon, Google, and others, that have developed computational machines for dealing with a vast database and means of extracting the desired information. Such a technique is used in self-driving cars, drug discoveries, stock market analysis, and many others. In many of these fields, the highest-level FRs are often known a priori under a prescribed set of conditions and the task is to come up with lower-level FRs and DPs, using the available database, the computational power of computers, and inputs from sensors. Often the challenge is to create an extensive database from the available information and manage it in a cost-effective and timely manner. Such a machine that can generate is named the Thinking Design Machine (TDM).

7.7.1 Thinking Design Machine (TDM)

A TDM is defined as an intelligent machine that can generate creative designs. The concept for TDM is based on the Independence Axiom and the Information Axiom. As presented in preceding chapters, the first thing we need to do in design is to identify the PROBLEM that we need to solve or address. Based on this problem definition in the customer domain, we identify the FRs the designed system should satisfy. Once the highest level FRs are defined, we find a set of DPs that can satisfy

---

[7]Recently, Yann LeCun, Geoffrey Hinton and Yoshuua Bengio received the 2018 Turing award for their contributions to AI.

the FRs, satisfying the Independence Axiom, as discussed in preceding paragraphs in (7.7). This search process can be taken over by the TDM, which can search the database stored in TDM or any other machines, perhaps using the cloud computing system. This task can be complicated if the number of FRs is large at any level of decomposition hierarchy. If we cannot satisfy the highest-level FRs because the selected DPs cannot be implemented for lack of specific details, we must decompose the highest FRs and DPs further, which then creates the next level FR-DP hierarchies. This decomposition process must continue until the DPs have been decomposed to the lowest level that can be implemented. As the layer of FR–DP decomposition hierarchy increases, the database we have to search for the right set of DPs that will not create coupling at the highest level can be vast.

When the search is done without the benefit of AD, the search process for the right design that satisfies the FRs can be quite complicated, because one has to search for a right set without the benefit of the Independence Axiom and the Information Axiom where the universe of the search space can be vast. One may use AI techniques to facilitate this search process. Now that the computational power of computers is immense, and the cost of computation has significantly come down, it is possible to search for the right FR–DP sets in a well-defined universe such as in the synthesis of drugs for various illness such as cancer, self-steering automobiles with many ©sensors, pilot-less air transport planes, and many others.

The power of TDM is that it can deal with many design tasks more effectively than purely AI-based machines since TDM starts with a well-defined FRs and deal with clear FR–DP structure, and follow the logic dictated by the Independence Axiom and the Information Axiom, following the clearly defined decomposition process. TDM can also use a search engine when it searches the FR–DP database to find the right DP for a given FR.

7.7.2 Physical Laws and Thinking Design Machine

In searching for the right DPs for a given FR, we should always make sure that our decision is consistent with the laws of nature and proven theories. TDM must check if the selection of a DP for a given FR satisfies or consistent with the laws of nature. Fortunately, there are a limited number of natural laws we must consider. In engineering, we often deal with Newton's laws, thermodynamic laws, thermal and mass diffusion laws, Ohmic laws, mass and charge conservation laws, thermal radiation laws, and Boltzmann's relationship.

7.8 Guidelines for Choosing Design Parameters and Process Variables

Once we define the FRs to be satisfied, we have to select DPs. This is a challenging task. There are some guidelines that can be helpful in identifying DPs.

Guideline #1
Out of all these potential DPs, which one should I pick as the DP?
Create the Design Matrix to identify and eliminate DPs that can potentially cause coupling!

In searching for the right DPs for a given FR, we should always make sure that our decision is consistent with the laws of nature and proven theories. TDM must check if the selection of a DP for a given FR satisfies or consistent with the laws of nature. Fortunately, there are a limited number of natural laws we must consider. In engineering, we often deal with Newton's laws, thermodynamic laws, thermal and mass diffusion laws, Ohmic laws, mass and charge conservation laws, thermal radiation laws, and Boltzmann's relationship.

Guideline #2 Depend on Knowledge base.
Ultimately, the quality of design depends on the basic knowledge of the designer.

An aspiring designer should learn the laws of Nature, i.e., physics, chemistry, mathematics, biology, etc. If one is more interested in the non-technical aspect, one should learn the common laws (that govern organizations, national laws, local laws, etc.).

In fields where the government regulations (environment, safety, health, etc.) are relevant in decision-making, the designer should work with people who are familiar with these regulatory issues. Sometimes, the regulations may appear to be irrational, but one cannot avoid the reality (or fragility) of human society.

Guideline #3 Create a Database.
Database of important ideas should be maintained.

Data provides a quick path to the final decision. One should compile a database by writing down useful ideas and systems.

Guideline #4 Past experience.
Experience—good or bad—can be valuable. It will be good to remember them.

Many things people do are based on their experience. Good experience and the context that led to an excellent experience should be remembered. However, one should not become a mental slave of the experience.

Guideline #5 Design cannot violate constraints.
It may be good to remove as many constraints as possible to give more room for creativity.

There are many different kinds of constraints. Some are created during the design process because of the decisions made during the design. It is essential to have a complete list of constraints during the design process.

Guideline #6 Do Not Choose DP that Violates Ethics.

The importance of personal ethics cannot be over-emphasized in any field, especially the design field, which deals with the creation of new things that have not been done in the past.

7.9 Conclusions

The quality of design depends on the selection of appropriate DPs, which is the third step in the AD process after the problem is defined, and FRs are selected.

There are a few simple rules that govern the DP selection process. One of the essential rules is that in an ideal design, the number of FRs and DPs is the same. If the number of DPs is less than that of FRs, we always have a coupled design, violating the Independence Axiom. When there are more DPs and FRs, we have a redundant design.

We can create a database on DP for a given FR, but there are no general governing principles that guide the designer to choose the best DPs. We have to invoke the Information Axiom to select the best DPs for a given set of FRs.

We can use the computational power of computers in searching for the best of the set of FRs and DPs, although nothing can replace human capability to select and manage FRs and DPs.

Examples from diverse fields are given to illustrate how DPs should be chosen.

Problems

1. Students should choose three of the exercise problems given in the main text of this chapter and work on them.
2. Engineers at the Technical Center of Nissan Motor Company of Japan published a paper with the following abstract (Reference: "Technical Papers of the Automobile Technology Association", Vol. 50, No. 6, November 2019):

"The automotive industry continues to develop new power plant technologies such as downsizing, rapid combustion for fuel efficiency. But engine excitation force will be increased by those, it's very important to improve the isolation of engine mount. This paper proposes a new active torque rod by using AD which can be a simple design methodology against conflicting requirements. Our technology principle consists of big improvement of the isolation level by lowering the resonance of torque rod and applying the damping force by inertial mass actuator. We successfully achieved a good NVH level on L4 downsizing engine as same as V6 engine."

If you were the designer of this engine mount, what would you choose as the FRs of the engine mount. What would you pick as the DPs that satisfy the FRs?

Appendix 7.1 Algorithm for Changing the Order of {FRs} and {DPs}[8]

The uncoupled design is obvious, because each DP affects by only one FR, regardless of how many FRs and DPs we have in the design. However, when we have many FRs and DPs, and some DPs affect more than one FRs, we need to re-arrange the order of FRs and DPs to determine if the design matrix is a triangular matrix and thus, satisfy the Independence Axiom. Then, it is helpful to have an algorithm for re-arranging the order of FRs and DPs to determine if the design is a decoupled design with a triangular matrix.

The algorithm is as follows:

Find the row which contains one non-zero element. Rearrange the order of {FRs} and {DPs} by putting the row and the column which contains the non-zero element first (i.e., if i-th row contains one non-zero element at j-th column, then put the i-th component of {FR} first and put j-th column of {DP} first. For example, the design matrix for a new design is given below:

	DP_1	DP_2	DP_3	DP_4
FR_1	A11	A12	0	A14
FR_2	0	A22	A32	0
FR_3	0	0	A33	0
FR_4	0	A442	A43	A44

The above matrix may be changed to

	DP_3	DP_1	DP_2	DP_4
FR_3	A33	0	0	0
FR_1	0	A11	A12	A14
FR_2	A23	0	A22	0
FR_4	A43	0	A42	A44

Then, excluding the first row and column, find a row which has one non-zero element, and put the row and the column second.

---

[8]From Suh, N.P.: The Principles of Design. ©**Oxford Publishing Limited.** Reproduced with the permission of Licensor through PLSclear.[p 383]

	DP$_3$	DP$_2$	DP$_1$	DP$_4$
FR$_3$	A33	0	0	0
FR$_2$	A23	A22	0	0
FR$_1$	0	A12	A11	A14
FR$_4$	A43	A42	0	A44

Finally, excluding the first and second rows and columns, find a row which has one non-zero element, and put the row and column third.

	DP$_3$	DP$_2$	DP$_4$	DP$_1$
FR$_3$	A33	0	0	0
FR$_2$	A23	A22	0	0
FR$_4$	A43	A42	A44	0
FR$_1$	0	A12	A14	A11

This process can be done automatically by creating a computer algorithm.

References

Mill-Max Mfg Corp. (2020) Triple row spring-pin connectors and mating target connectors. https://www.mill-max.com/products/new/triple-row-spring-pin-connectors-and-mating-target-connectors

Suh NP (1990) The principles of design. Oxford University Press

Further Reading

Suh NP (2001) Axiomatic design—advances and applications. Oxford University Press

How Should We Select Process Variables?

8

Nam Pyo Suh

Abstract

Preceding chapters presented the transformation of customer needs or problems identified in the customer domain into functional requirements (FRs), and then FRs to design parameters (DPs). In this chapter, we consider the issues involved in selecting the process variables (PVs) of the process domain to satisfy DPs. When we are designing a hardware product, PVs are typically manufacturing processes, human resources, and financial support. In organizational design, PVs are primarily human resources. PVs are equally crucial as FRs and DPs in completing a design project; PVs constitute an element in the continuum going from "need" (in the customer domain) to delivery of solutions via FRs and DPs. In dealing with PVs, domain-specific knowledge is required, such as expert knowledge on manufacturing processes and software systems to create complete systems solutions. In organizational design, PVs are typically people who will determine the achievement of the organizational goals. Ultimately, PVs determine the productivity in the manufacturing and operations of organizations.

The steps involved in selecting PVs to satisfy DPs are similar to the transformation of FRs to DPs. A great deal of imagination and creativity is always the necessary and required elements in sound design. Sometimes, it pays to think out of the "mental" box we sometimes create for ourselves! It is often more productive if designers should start with a clean sheet of paper and create a design rather than being constrained by what was done in the past. There is no assurance that what was done in the past is appropriate to the current problem or was a good design!

N. P. Suh (✉)
M.I.T., Cambridge, MA, USA
e-mail: npsuh@mit.edu

© Springer Nature Switzerland AG 2021
N. P. Suh et al. (eds.), *Design Engineering and Science*,
https://doi.org/10.1007/978-3-030-49232-8_8

8.1   Introduction

Process variables (PVs) are the final embodiment of customer needs or solving the problem identified in the customer domain. In the field of product development, the selection of PVs determines manufacturing cost. In the case of organizational design, PVs represent people and other resources of the organization. As the number of FRs increases, the number of DPs and PVs increases as well, which may result in increased complexity and higher cost of manufacturing depending on the quality of design. PVs, the characteristic vectors in the process domain (i.e., the last of the four domains), are the final outputs of the design process, and they determine the manufacturing process, the cost and the quality of manufactured goods when the design involves manufactured goods.

Steering Column of Automobiles: How Much Should It Cost?

Every car must have a steering column to steer the vehicle. A professor who was invited to teach "Axiomatic Design" to engineers at an industrial firm that manufactures steering columns for automobiles was surprised to learn that there were considerable differences in cost, complexity, and weight among the steering columns. (Fig. 8.1) A manual steering column that performs simple steering functions for small cars may cost around a hundred dollars, but the steering column that performs more functions in larger vehicles may cost an order of magnitude more. He also learned that the most expensive part of these products is the component cost rather than the labor cost. Many of the steering columns that had problems were coupled designs. These classes held in industrial firms are beneficial to everyone, including the instructor, because they deal with real issues.

It should be noted that the production cost is a function of the production volume of the product. If each one of the components of an automobile is manufactured one at a time, rather than using mass production technologies, cars would cost an order of magnitude more expensive than mass-produced products. The power of mass production in lowering the cost of various manufactured products has led to the consolidation of the industry.

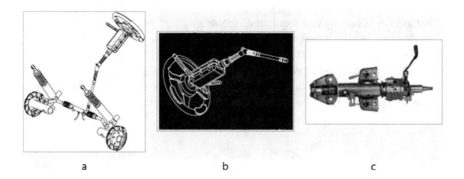

a   b   c

Fig. 8.1 Different steering columns of automobiles (**a** and **b** reproduced with permission from Nikiforov (2019a, b); **c** reproduced with permission from Dmitrii (2019))

Manufacturing is a relevant field for the economic well-being of a nation. Industrial firms engaged in manufacturing strive to improve their productivity to maintain their competitiveness, which depends on how well they deal with the entire transformation process from the customer need to manufacture products. Moreover, the quality of design determines how much they charge for their products. Many companies have developed and adopted specific techniques to be proficient in their manufacturing business, starting from their design operations. Some of these advances made in the industry have influenced academic research as well as teaching. Among the better-known techniques, some universities teach are the "House of Quality" and "Six Sigma." Some of these techniques came out of Toyota Motor Company of Japan. Some companies subscribe to the idea that their products should have coupled FRs so that other companies would not easily be able to replicate the quality of their parts and compete with them. This philosophy, which might have served them well in the past when their traditional business depended on many decades of refinement, may not be the best approach to innovation of new products or developing large, complicated systems that are made in small quantities. Successful companies in highly competitive businesses often owe their success to innovation rather than the mass production of well-developed products. A better approach is to satisfy the Independence Axiom to make it easy to manufacture as well as producing products that perform better.

Replication of PVs versus Innovation

Many developing nations often replicate products that had been made in advanced countries for many decades. That is, without going through the entire transformation process starting from the Customer Domain to PVs, they merely learn to replicate DPs and PVs and sell the product at a lower price. This replication of existing products appears to be a relatively simple process.

Around 1972, an American professor was invited to visit a manufacturing plant in an Asian country that had just decided to industrialize the nation by manufacturing "heavy" products such as machines and automobiles. The new owner of the company, who just had taken over a defunct factory, was to manufacture diesel engines under a license from a German company. The professor was surprised to learn that the executives of this company did not know much about manufacturing (they did not even know the basics of milling machine)! However, in a matter of a year, they were manufacturing diesel engines! This incidence demonstrated that the replication of an existing product is relatively easy if one has an educated workforce and the will to learn and succeed! During the subsequent 20 years, the Asian country has become a prosperous industrialized country, manufacturing sophisticated industrial products for the global market! Such rapid progress was possible because of their emphasis on education. Now their goal is to become innovators of new technologies, which will be much more challenging than becoming proficient in manufacturing existing products. To become innovators, they must execute the transition from the customer domain to the functional domain, to the physical domain, and finally to the process domain most creatively.

In Example 2.1 and Case Study 7.1, the transformation of DPs to PVs in designing and manufacturing shoe soles with three DPs was described. This project illustrated the transformation of customer needs, to FRs, to DPs, and finally, manufacturing processes (PVs). The lesson learned in that example was that once we define FRs based on customer needs, we need specific expert knowledge on the manufacture of such products. We need to develop the right set of PVs to satisfy DPs. Since then, this technology was further developed to manufacture automotive parts, furniture, and many others.

In the design of organizations, the same mapping idea applies between the four domains, although the specific nature of FRs, DPs, and PVs are different from the case of product development. In organizational design, PVs represent the resources, (e.g., people, funds) needed to satisfy DPs. In previous chapters, the design of a government organization was presented to discuss the application of AD to organizations.

"Ban" Axiomatic Design (AD)!?

There once was one of the largest consumer electronics companies in the world. They made good innovative products. Many children from all over the world wanted to have one of their favorite products, a portable radio. The company was, at one point, one of the leading technology innovators in the world. It is no longer. It was speculated that one of the leading causes of their "demise" was the company's insistence on sticking with their "coupled designs"!

The speculative reasoning given to explain what happened to the company is as follows: Before semiconductors were invented, all electrical circuits were made of analog circuits, which makes electric circuits with resistors, capacitors, and inductors. In general, it is difficult to satisfy the Independence Axiom with analog circuits with individual resistors, capacitors, and inductors, especially complicated large circuits! They are mostly coupled designs. Digital circuits with semiconductors do not have this problem! This famous consumer electronics company made most of its products with analog circuits. Even when the entire world is switching to digital systems, this company insisted on analog circuits. This company reasoned that since it is so challenging to develop analog circuits, other companies would not be able to compete with them! So even with the emergence of semiconductors, they refined and improved their products using analog circuits. However, other companies, all relatively new, switched from analog circuits to the digital circuit, which enabled them to create better products that effortlessly satisfy the independence of FRs. Today, these new companies that adopted digital circuits have now become the dominant consumer electronics companies worldwide.

In some cases, it is difficult to satisfy the Independence Axiom with an analog circuit. Digital circuits give the flexibility to meet the independence of FRs.

The lesson to remember: What appears to be a good business strategy, if it violates a good design practice, cannot win!

Exercise 8.1: Battery-Powered Electric Car

Conceptually, the design of battery-powered electric cars (i.e., EVs) is quite simple. It has to deliver the power stored in a set of batteries to the wheel. The most challenging part of EVs is the management of electric energy stored in a large number of cells of lithium batteries to the electric motors that deliver power to the wheels. Unlike cars powered by internal combustion (IC) engines, which have low torque at low speed, EVs do not need a transmission gearbox. The torque and speed of electric motors are proportional to electric power delivered, i.e., current at a constant voltage, to the wheel. Design the electrical power management system for lithium battery-powered cars.

8.2   Precision Engineering

Many mechanical and electronic parts require ultra-precision. These parts are manufactured in a "clean room" with no particles in the atmosphere and an isothermal environment. People who enter the room, including workers, must wear clean garments to be sure that particles from the human body do not contaminate the working environment. All the machines are maintained at the isothermal conditions, and those machines that generate thermal energy due to electrical motors and others must be cooled using cutting fluids and other means. Most of the semiconductor fabrication factories (commonly called the "FAB") and ultra-precision machining facilities belong to this group of "precision manufacturing." Some of the components used in military weapons are made in such a clean environment.

Design Problem faced by those in LLNL of California:

For some applications related to defense and space, we need parts that are atomically smooth and accurate. Can we manufacture such parts by machining?

Design Solution:

Precision engineering was born because of the extremely accurate (to atomic scale) parts needed for U.S. defense applications (e.g., nuclear weapons), X-ray telescope, and laser fusion research. The pioneering research and development for precision engineering were initiated at the Lawrence Livermore National Laboratory (LLNL) of the United States, which is known as the place where the creation of the hydrogen bomb was initiated. The Large Optics Diamond Turning Machine (LODTM) developed at LLNL is the world's most accurate machine tool as of 2019. LODTM can machine metal work-pieces as large as 1.5 m (5 feet) in diameter and 46 cm (18 inches) in height to an accuracy of greater than

Fig. 8.2 Surface generated by the Large Optics Diamond Turning Machine (LODTM). (Courtesy of Lawrence Livermore National Laboratory (Klingmann 2001))

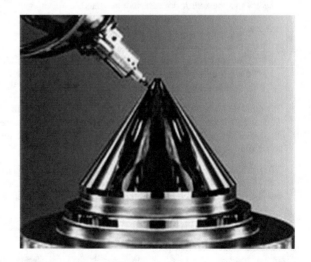

30 nm. It has been used to make optical mirrors for observatory as well as special weapons. One of the surfaces cut by that machine with a diamond-cutting tool is shown in Fig. 8.2. To measure such surfaces, they also developed measurement techniques that measure optical errors to the atomic level while machining.

In cutting atomic-scale precision surfaces and contours, the machine, the work-piece, cutting tools, and cutting fluids must be maintained at absolutely isothermal conditions. Also, the feedback of the surface contour is essential as the surface is cut. In this machine, the contours are monitored continuously, as well as the tool positions during cutting. Although this technology was developed after decades of research in optics and precision engineering without using the AD theory, this technology can be understood by applying the reasoning process of AD.

The problem identified in the customer domain is the manufacture of atomic-scale surfaces and contours on various non-ferrous metal surfaces. The highest FR is the creation of atomically smooth precision surfaces with the diamond-cutting tool (i.e., DP). This highest FR may be decomposed as.

FR1 = Cut surface contours to atomic-scale precision;
FR2 = Monitor the contour of the surface being cut during the cutting operation;
FR3 = Maintain the temperature of the work-piece, cutting tool, machine, and cutting fluids at a constant temperature throughout the manufacturing operation;
FR4 = Provide vibration-free machining of the work-piece;
FR5 = Isolate the building from external vibration.

The DPs may be stated as the following:

DP1 = Precision diamond cutting machine;
DP2 = Laser-based metrology equipment;
DP3 = Temperature controller device;
DP4 = Vibration free machine;
DP5 = Isolation mount for the building.

The PVs in the fourth domain may be stated as follows:

PV1 = Cutting with a diamond tool;
PV2 = Measurement of the surface generated with laser surface profilometer;
PV3 = Constant system temperature, including cutting fluid;
PV4 = Monitoring of machine vibration;
PV5 = Monitoring of building vibration.

It should be noted that in this kind of precision machining, the maintenance of temperature at isothermal conditions is necessary. To achieve this goal, sometimes they pour the cutting fluid over the work-piece to guarantee that it is at the same temperature as the rest of the machining system.

We have to make sure that the FR-DP relationship is diagonal or triangular. Similarly, the DP–PV relationship should be consistent with the Independence Axiom.[1] This was done because they have generated atomically smooth surfaces reliably and repeatedly.

---

[1]They developed the idea of the error budget to delineates how much uncertainty or non-repeatability can be tolerated at each step in the production process. Predictability and repeatability were maximized in these machines with tolerances of fractions of a micrometer.

Exercise 8.2:

Construct the design matrix for FR–DP and DP–PV relationship of the above precision machining process.

8.3   Designing a Manufacturing Process for a Difficult-to-Machine Material

Many parts are manufactured using conventional manufacturing processes. However, sometimes new manufacturing processes must be designed because of either unique features or unusual materials that cannot be machined. The design of manufacturing processes and machines follows the same reasoning process as all other design tasks.

Design Problem:

A major materials company in the United States invented a new composite material consisting of aluminum matrix loaded with silicon carbide (SiC) particles. Such a composite material is expected to be tough, abrasion-resistant, and strong. However, this material is difficult to machine to the desired shape. When ordinary cutting tools are used to cut this composite material, the tools wore out rapidly because of the presence of SiC grits in the composite. Therefore, they chose to grind as the means of removing materials from this composite. However, when they tried to grind it using SiC grinding wheels, the aluminum matrix phase of the composite filled up porous space between the SiC grits of the grinding wheel, stopping abrasive action of the grinding wheel.

How should we process this composite material? This research project was given to a university as a research project. The professor assigned an undergraduate student to work on this project under the supervision of a graduate student.

Design Solution:

The function of removing materials from this composite may be divided into two components: remove carbide particles in the composite with grinding wheel and then removing the aluminum matrix phase electrochemically. This process requires using an electrically conducting grinding wheel.

The FRs may formally be written as

FR1 = Remove SiC particles in the composite with an abrasive grinding wheel;
FR2 = Remove aluminum matrix phase electrochemically.

Then, the DPs may be written as

DP1 = Carbide abrasive grits in the grinding wheel;
DP2 = Electrolysis.

The PVs may be stated as

PV1 = Abrasive action by the grits in the grinding wheel;
PV2 = Electric current flowing from the grinding wheel to the composite.

It was decided to make an electrically conducting grinding wheel by plating a regular commercial SiC grinding wheel with copper. The copper plating was done by flowing electro-less copper plating solution through the grinding wheel at room temperature after the wheel is first catalyzed by passing through a catalytic solution such as palladium chloride solution and hydrochloric acid.

During grinding, an electric potential was applied between the grinding wheel and the workpiece to remove the aluminum phase of the composite electrolytically. Abrasives of the grinding wheel removed silicon carbide particles in the composite. It worked great!

8.4 Mass Production of Microcellular Plastics

Unlike the previous case of removing materials to manufacture discrete mechanical parts by machining, polymeric components are typically processed by melting the polymer for extrusion or injection molding. These mass production processes reduce the cost of manufacturing discrete parts by orders of magnitude when the production volume is significant that we can amortize the cost of tooling over a large number of parts. These things are designed and manufactured using well-established routine processes. However, some cases require innovation of new manufacturing processes and materials. Such is the case with microcellular plastics, which is now used to manufacture automotive parts, among others, worldwide (Wong et al. 2016).

Design Problem:

In Sect. 3.5.5, the creation of microcellular plastics was presented. The idea was to put in tiny bubbles ($\sim$10–30 microns in diameter) in large numbers ($\sim$billion bubbles per cm^3) into plastics to reduce material consumption, enhance the fracture toughness of the plastic, and provide dimensional stability by reducing the residual stress developed in the plastic part. The idea for and design of microcellular plastics were done over a luncheon meeting, but the subsequent design of the manufacturing process took more time.

Initially, to demonstrate the feasibility of introducing bubbles into solid plastics, a technique similar to that used in making popcorns was used, which utilizes the thermodynamic instability phenomenon. The plastic sheet was put into a high-pressure chamber with CO_2 to diffuse and dissolve CO_2 in a solid polymer matrix, creating a polymer/gas solution. At a suitable temperature, if the pressure is suddenly lowered, the dissolved CO_2 in the polymer matrix tries to form a new gas phase by diffusing out of the polymer. However, since they do not have time to diffuse a long distance, they nucleate a large number of tiny bubbles, typically a billion bubbles per cubic cm, i.e., 10^9/cm^3. The bubbles are about 10 microns in diameter.

This batch process demonstrated that microcellular plastic could be made, but the batch process could not be used to manufacture commercial products since it was too slow to be economical. What was needed was a continuous process of making microcellular plastics at a rate that is suitable for industrial production.

Design Solution:

What is needed is the mass production of microcellular plastics. One of the most commonly used processes for thermoplastics is the extrusion using a plasticating screw extruder, which is shown in Fig. 8.3. It consists of a barrel and a screw inside the barrel. Plastic pallets are fed into the extruder through a hopper at one end. The plastic melts in the extruder due to the mechanical work done when it is continuously deformed by the rotational motion of the screw inside the extruder barrel. When the plastic is completely molten, it is extruded through a die to make plastic sheets, tubes, or other profiles.

In extruding microcellular plastics, a conventional extruder such as the one in Fig. 8.2 cannot be used, because to make the microcellular plastic, the following four different functions must be performed independently from each other but in a specific sequence, which conventional extruders cannot satisfy:

FR1 = Melt and mix the polymer to be foamed;
FR2 = Inject CO_2 in a critical state of molten polymer;
FR3 = Dissolve CO_2 in the molten polymer, forming a solution of polymer and CO_2;
FR4 = Extrude the solution of polymer and CO_2 through a die under high pressure;
FR5 = Cause sudden pressure drop to change the thermodynamic state of the solution.

To achieve the FRs stated above, the extruder shown in Fig. 8.3 was modified. The extruder was made longer, and CO_2 at the super-critical state was pumped into the plastic/barrel interface in small quantities continuously at the midsection of the extruder where the polymer is completely molten. After CO_2 dissolves in the molten plastic, the solution of plastic/gas was extruded through a specially designed die. Near the exit of the die, the pressure of the polymer/CO_2 mixture is dropped quickly, which initiates the nucleation of bubbles in large numbers. The nucleation of a large number of bubbles occurs when the pressure is suddenly reduced because the gas in the polymer/gas solution is no longer in thermodynamic equilibrium at the new low pressure. This sudden thermodynamic instability of the polymer/gas solution nucleates bubbles. The die was so designed that the pressure drop occurs over a predetermined distance of the die lip. Then, the extrudate, i.e., plastic sheets, has a plethora of nucleated gas bubbles (about a billion bubbles per cm^3), which

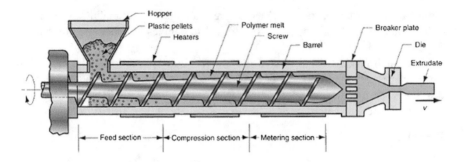

Fig. 8.3 Plasticating extruder for polymers by (Extract from Sukoptfe:ptfe-machinery.com SUKO PTFE Machinery (2017))

Fig. 8.4 Cross section of extruded microcellular plastic (Average cell size ~20 microns) (Courtesy of Trexel, Inc.)

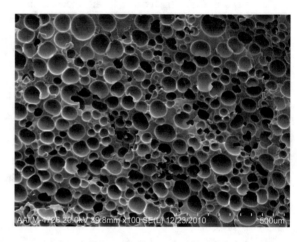

grows until the polymer sheet is cooled. The density reduction could be controlled from a few percent to 90%.

The DPs of this process are as follows:

DP1 = Plasticating section of the extruder;
DP2 = CO_2 injection port;
DP3 = Mixing section of the extruder;
DP4 = Extrusion section of the extruder;
DP5 = Die lip design.

The PVs are the following:

PV1 = Rotation of the screw;
PV2 = Control the pumping rate of the critical CO_2;
PV3 = Length of the extruder after injection of CO_2;

PV4 = Die design;
PV5 = Control of time rate of change of pressure in the die.

Cross section of microcellular plastic is shown in Fig. 8.4.

8.5 3D Printing: Layered Manufacturing[2]

3D Printing has become an essential industrial technology of quickly producing parts from computer graphics into a solid part. There are many different approaches to 3D Printing, but all of them are based on the idea that complicated 3D parts can be manufactured by laying 2D layers of thin materials layer-by-layer. Initially, it was called the "rapid prototyping" technology to meet the needs of the United States defense industry, funded by the U.S. Defense Advanced Research Projects Agency (DARPA), but it has expanded into many sectors of industrial production technology. Some large companies in the United States have established a separate business unit to commercialize the 3D Printing for mass production.

The highest FR of rapid prototyping is

FR = Produce 3D parts rapidly.

The corresponding DP is

DP = Layered manufacturing process.

The PV in the manufacturing domain is

PV = Layered manufacturing process.

Through zigzagging among three domains, (i.e., the functional domain to the physical domain, and finally the process domain), we develop the lower level FRs, DPs, and PVs as follows:

FR1 = Provide 2D information for each layer of a 3D body;
FR2 = Deposit a thin layer of materials;
FR3 = Bond the materials into a continuum;
FR4 = Remove unwanted materials;
FR5 = Build up the body layer by layer.

---

[2]In this section, the materials presented earlier (Suh 2001) are more or less re-produced here.

The DPs are

DP1 = Digitalized 2D information;
DP2 = Thin layer of photoresist (resin);
DP3 = Light beam;
DP4 = Vacuum suction;
DP5 = Table motion.

The product design matrix, i.e., FR/DP matrix, is a diagonal matrix, which indicates that design of the product is acceptable.
The PVs are

PV1 = Computer memory for matrix table of n x m pixels;
PV2 = Resin dispenser and horizontal table;
PV3 = On–off intense light beam that scans in two dimensions;
PV4 = Suction tube that scans in two dimensions;
PV5 = Step motor with ball screw for motion in the vertical direction.

The product and the process conceived by the above FRs, DPs, PVs constitute a layered manufacturing process in which thin photoreactive resin (i.e., photoresist) is deposited on a table that is scanned by a light source to cross-link the resin based on the information supplied by the computer. A vacuum suction tube that also rasters the resin surface after the reaction is completed removes the unreacted resin.
The process design matrix for the DP/PV relationship is

	PV1	PV2	PV3	PV4	PV5
DP1	X	0	0	0	0
DP2	0	X	0	0	0
DP3	X	0	X	0	0
DP4	0	0	0	X	0
DP5	0	0	0	0	X

The process is a decoupled design. Each one of the first-level FRs, DPs, and PVs must now be decomposed.

8.6 Process Variables in Organizational Design

In preceding chapters, we stated that in organizational design, PVs are either people or financial resources. When many people are involved, we need to be concerned about the issues that arise because people are the key elements of the design. For example, the following could be important issues: the accuracy of transmission of information among people, fidelity in the execution of the defined tasks, the ability of human operators to be consistent for an extended period, and assessment of the effectiveness of people in a given job. We need to design the financial and other reward systems for the people in the organization. To deal with these issues, organizations have used compensation and promotion systems as a means of encouraging people to perform the task of PVs as designed.

Perhaps the most challenging systems to design and operate are those that involve humans as PVs. When people are the PVs, we cannot design the person to fit PVs. We can only choose the best people among those available for a given PV. Since human operators have their independent thoughts, different cultural norms, ethical standards, and personal bias, decisions involving humans must be sensitive to these variable factors when a human being is chosen as a PV. All of these characteristics of human operators are strengths, but unlike machines, the input/output relationship of human beings as PVs is less predictable. There can be significant misunderstandings among people because the communication channels among people are imperfect. The situation is worse if the language of communication involves diverse ethnic backgrounds and cultures. Unlike mechanical or electronic components, when people are the PVs, consistency can be a problem; people can change their views, values, and performance. The cultural norms that prescribe how people should behave can help the operation of organizations, but it may take away independent thinking that is the major strength of having people as PVs.

8.7 Conclusions

PVs are a set of vectors that define the process domain. In organizations, PVs are typically performed by humans to satisfy DPs. PVs can also be the financial resources needed to enable the manufacture of products or run an organization. The wise selection of PVs has a significant effect on the quality of products and the cost of manufacturing. It also determines the efficiency of the system designed. In manufacturing firms, PVs are manufacturing processes that determine the cost of their products and their competitiveness.

Problems

1. "3D Printing" is finding many new applications in manufacturing solid parts made of metals, polymers, ceramics, and composite of various materials. The process consists of making 3D parts by depositing 2D layers to build up three-dimensional shapes of all kinds. In "the old days," engineers used to think that solid metallic parts must be worked by forging or deformation to get high strength parts. 3D Printing showed that a large number of parts could be manufactured cheaply when the volume of the manufactured parts is small. The mechanical properties of many 3D parts are acceptable for the intended applications.

Design a manufacturing process for the human knee joints, assuming that you can get the exact shape that has to be manufactured through X-ray scanning of the human joint that has to be replaced. Define FRs, DPs, and PVs. Determine the materials to be used and the sequence of the 3D printing process.

2. You are just appointed to be the new CEO of General Electric Company. Your job is to restore the company to its old eminence. Define FRs. Design your new organization. Clearly, state your DPs and PVs.

3. You just got elected to be the President of the United States. You have only four years to turn the country around. Develop FRs, DPs, and PVs.

4. It appears that BREXIT is going to face many problems. If you just became the Prime Minister of the United Kingdom, what would you do? State your FRs, DPs, and PVs.

5. A country in the Middle East just decided to make all their public universities "semi-private." The government will provide the necessary funding, but each university will have their board of trustees and operate as a private university. If you have the responsibility of running one of these universities, what would you do?

6. You are responsible for designing a software system for the management of hospitals. Describe how you are going to develop the appropriate FRs, DPs, and PVs. Develop the flow diagram to show how the FRs will be administered.

References

Dmitrii B (2019) New car steering column on white background. Photo licensed from Shutterstock, ID: 672174733

Klingmann J (2001) The world's most accurate lathe. Science and Technology Review, Lawrence Livermore National Laboratory, p 13

Nikiforov V (2019a) 3d model of steering column and car suspension on white background. Photo licensed from Shutterstock, ID: 1208610586

Nikiforov V (2019b) 3d model of the steering column on a black background. Drawing. Photo licensed from Shutterstock, ID: 1208610007

Suh NP (2001) Axiomatic design—advances and applications. Oxford University Press

SUKO PTFE Machinery (2017) Polymer screw extruder. https://ptfe-machinery.com/wp-content/uploads/2017/02/Polymer-Screw-Extrusion.gif

Wong A, Guo H, Kumar V, Park CB, Suh NP (2016) Microcellular plastics. Wiley, pp 1–57. https://onlinelibrary.wiley.com/doi/pdf/10.1002/0471440264.pst468.pub2

Mapping in Design

9

Miguel Cavique, António Gabriel-Santos, and António Mourão

Abstract

The preceding chapters presented the basic concept of Axiomatic Design (AD). This chapter takes "MAPPING," one of the important concepts of AD, to deeper understanding. Mapping between the functional and physical domains, and between the physical and process domains, accomplishes a number of important design tasks. First, it enables the designer to decompose functional requirements (FRs), design parameters (DPs), and process variables (PVs) to many branches and levels, in order to advance design solutions while maintaining independence and minimizing information content. Through proper mapping, designers can track the development of large projects. As the number of FRs and DPs increases with many levels and branches of decomposition, and as various participants do mapping, we need to capture the results of the mapping process by creating a master design and process matrices. This chapter also presents some additional hints regarding the best way to define the FRs.

M. Cavique (✉)
UNIDEMI & Escola Naval, Base Naval de Lisboa - Alfeite, 2810-001 Almada, Portugal
e-mail: miguel.cavique@cest.pt

A. Gabriel-Santos · A. Mourão
UNIDEMI & DEMI, NOVA SST, Campus de Caparica, 2829-516 Caparica, Portugal
e-mail: agms@fct.unl.pt

A. Mourão
e-mail: ajfm@fct.unl.pt

© Springer Nature Switzerland AG 2021
N. P. Suh et al. (eds.), *Design Engineering and Science*,
https://doi.org/10.1007/978-3-030-49232-8_9

9.1   Introduction

The four domains of the design—customer, functional, physical, and process—
have already been presented in Chapter 2. They are again shown in Fig. 9.1. The
arrows between the domains show the mapping process between the domains. This
chapter will focus on the mapping process, explaining the zigzagging process
indicated by the arrows between the domains. The design method in AD explicitly
asks what the customer wants and how to satisfy the customers' needs. The method
treats the design as a continuum, from customer needs (CNs) to PVs.

Many engineering approaches to design erroneously jump directly to the
physical domain, based on physical concepts learned in universities or colleges,
while not clearly defining the goals or needs the system must achieve. Designers
often work from their own previous experience and knowledge, using creativity in a
non-structured environment. This working model has a reduced benefit to the
customer. Design solutions for systems or artifacts must compete based on price or
important minor features. Furthermore, such a design practice, jumping to physical
solutions, is more likely to lead to a coupled design that violates the Independence
Axiom. Unnecessary iterations for adjustment and unintended consequences lead to
long development times, continuing modification of the design, higher cost, and
poor performance.

To innovate, the FRs need to be formulated in a *solution neutral environment*
based on problems identified in the customer domain. This chapter provides an
in-depth understanding of the mapping process involved in defining the FRs.

We begin by discussing the use of optimization by experienced designers,
attempting to manage coupled designs, which fail to maintain independence, violating Suh's first axiom. Subsequent sections show the role of the decomposition
process, i.e., zigzagging process, in maintaining independence and minimizing
information.

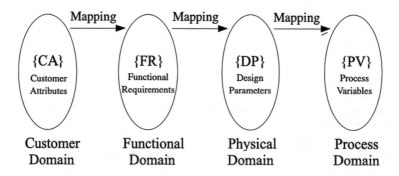

Fig. 9.1 Four Domains of the Design World

9.2 The Role of Optimization

A consequence of not satisfying the Independence Axiom is that when one of the DPs is changed to adjust one of the FRs, other FRs also vary. Therefore, it is difficult to satisfy each specific FR and all the FRs as specified and desired. When such a design is created, many firms and engineers try to "optimize." A typical optimization technique creates an objective function that incorporates most of the DPs and tries to find a set of values that will be as close to the desired performance as possible. Often some FRs must be compromised by establishing relative importance among the FRs. Such an approach involves the creation of an objective function that incorporates the effect of each DP and finds the set of values that maximize the value of an objective function rather than satisfying each FR within an acceptable tolerance. Some call such an approach an "optimization algorithm." For example, in the world of finance, the yield curve is typically "convex," which changes as the interest rate changes. Then, they search for the peak value of the objective function. One of the fundamental goals of AD is to avoid "optimization" by eliminating the coupling of FRs and compromising the satisfaction of each FR.

In many engineering and management schools, optimization is taught as a typical way of solving problems. Optimization implies sacrificing some FRs for the best compromise operation of the system. Many engineers and managers attempt to improve products and processes by optimizing what they have in the time and the budget available for the project. They might improve the performance of a system by five or ten percent in terms of cost, energy, weight, or any other selection criterion through optimization. Regrettably, many times the system might be performing at a fraction of what it could have achieved if each FR were satisfied exactly as specified. The deficient performance is usually the result of choosing a coupled design that does not satisfy axiom one.

Under the heading of "optimization," which is so prevalent in the "real world," they attempt to improve features or cost, rather than satisfying all specified FRs. Therefore, we explore three questions: "What made the optimization so common?" "When might we use optimization?" and "What is the role of optimization in design?".

The optimization in animal feed

George Dantzig developed the simplex method for optimization just after World War II, inspired by the methods he used previously for the US Army. The method can find the best solution in a convex region of hyper-planes studied in operation research (OR). In the 1960s, the simplex produced a revolution in the animal feed industry. The animal feed used dozens of foods, including corn, wheat, oat, vegetables, forage, barley, fruit, and vitamins. Animal food might have certain amounts of calories, vitamins, proteins, fat, the quantity of food to eat, and many other requirements. Creating a mixture that can fulfill the animal needs was a difficult task, which was only achieved by a laborious trial and error method. In those days, it was virtually impossible to create the right mix at the minimum cost when grain prices change constantly. The simplex method made it possible, not only providing a solution but the best solution.

The question is how we should deal with this problem if we are to design the system based on AD. First, we define FRs, which may include the following:

FR₁ = Provide 3,000 cal per day;
FR₂ = Supply the necessary Vitamin A, B, and C;
FR₃ = Provide water;
FR₄ = Provide 300 cal of protein.

Constraint or optimization criterion (OC, Thompson 2013): Minimum cost.

Then for DPs, we can select the following:

DP₁ = grains with the highest calorie per Euro;
DP₂ = Supplementary vitamins;
DP₃ = Water supply;
DP₄ = 100 g of soybeans.

The design matrix for this design is as follows:

	DP_1	DP_2	DP_3	DP_4
FR_1	X	0	0	x
FR_2	0	X	0	x
FR_3	0	0	X	0
FR_4	x	0	0	X

In the above design, FR₄ and DP₄ create a coupled design. One easy solution, if it is acceptable, is to eliminate FR₄ and DP₄. Then, it becomes an uncoupled design. Another possible solution is to give a large tolerance on protein intake, then the relationship between FR₄ and DP₁ becomes zero.

This last example shows two approaches to the same problem. Some animal food requires a difficult balance between the amounts of products for the animal feed. In such a case, the design is coupled, and the inclusion of an optimization criterion f for cost allows for an optimization process to define the best solution. However, if protein is not a requirement, or has a large tolerance, the design problem is uncoupled.

Writing the design equation (DE) and defining the minimum number of FRs that characterize the solution are keys to any design.

Exercise 9.1: Define FRs for Animal Feed

Create the DE for a horse feed using the products given in the example. Discuss the type of design you get and the way to solve the quantity of food a horse needs to eat every day in order not to feel hunger.

Many problems in engineering and management use analysis approaches. In many cases, the problems have couplings, and universities tend to like to handle these types of problems. After graduation, the engineer or manager wants to use the same tools of analysis to address design problems. Many tools apply optimization algorithms. These types of algorithms usually need a starting point, benefiting from being a first attempt for the solution. If an optimization algorithm finds a better solution than the previous attempts, then the user feels like it is a good solution. However, the user just accepted a trade-off between requirements and got a poor design.

The optimization approach forgets how difficult it will be to maintain the system working in slightly different circumstances, how narrow the tolerances will be for the DPs, and what will happen if tolerances change overtime. Optimization is a way to find a trade-off point of operation, therefore achieving a balance between the influences of different DPs on the desired FRs. In other words, optimization applies to coupled designs.

According to AD theory, good design solutions are decoupled or uncoupled. Usually, these ask for tuning the DPs so that the system ranges of all FRs are within the design ranges. Tuning is the process of setting the values of the leaf, or low level, DPs. Tuning applies to decoupled or uncoupled designs to define the DPs within their tolerances. In audio equipment, you may want to enhance bass or treble, or change the balance between the right and left speakers. You can use independent knobs to set the volume, the pitch, and the balance. Tuning a design is like using different knobs to set each of the DPs and fulfill the FRs.

A design achieves its target if the FRs are fulfilled, or in other words, the design provides values of FRs in their acceptable ranges. An acceptable range for an FR in a certain design might be different than the range of the same FR in another design. Students should understand how difficult it can be to make a coupled design work in acceptable ranges for all FRs, and how easy it would be when the design is uncoupled.

Optimization and tuning are part of the design process, but not the design solution itself. Therefore, designers first might find a good design solution and tune it afterward. If the design solution is coupled, it could need to be optimized. However, it is best to seek uncoupled or decoupled designs rather than optimize a coupled design.

This discussion brings us back to explain in further detail the role of the FRs, what an FR is, and how to express it. This consideration is important, as designers are keen on defining the physical parts of the design, i.e., the DPs, but many times, they do not explicitly express what they want to achieve, i.e., FRs.

9.3 Hints for Defining the Functional Requirements

FRs define good designs that solve problems articulated in the customer domain. In other words, the design solution cannot be better than its FRs. This section provides some hints on how to develop FRs in a solution neutral environment. Many designers pass directly from "what they want" to "how they can" do it, based on their experience or market standards in the area of the design. This way, designers copy what already exists, i.e., the physical parts, supposing the DPs expresses reality.

The allegory of the cave

The allegory of the cave is a metaphor of the Greek philosopher Plato who places Socrates telling a story of a group of prisoners that lives in a cave. The prisoners see shadows moving in the walls of the cave and suppose it is the reality. One of them leaves the cave and learns that those shadows come from what passes in front of the cave, interfering with the entrance of the sunlight. He got enthusiastic about the discovery and came back to the cave to explain the new reality. Entering the cave, he cannot see because he had gotten used to the outside sunlight. It made the others suppose that going out would make them blind. The story ends by creating a group rule to kill anyone who wants to drag them out of the cave.

Applying this interesting metaphor to the field of design, make us ask what the reality in the design is. The reality is what we see in the physical parts or something equivalent. Are physical parts the shadows of reality? We live in a world of functions. We seek for functionalities, and the physical parts are the way to achieve the functionalities.

Lawrence D. Miles introduced the idea of "functions" in design when he worked at the General Electric Company. During World War II, GE felt shortages of certain parts, forcing Miles to seek for replacement parts that performed the same functions. The parts used were physically different from the originals but attained the same requirements. It made Miles develop a new methodology of design, the so-called "Value Analysis." Sometimes, it was possible to use new parts that were cheaper and could improve the performance of the system.

The following exercise is an example of what can happen if a design team copies what they see, rather than understanding what the FRS are:

Exercise 9.2: Define the FRs of a Tram

A team of engineers from an electrical tram company is developing a new tram for a hilly city. They decide to visit another city that had installed a new tram system recently. In that city, they saw the tram equipment, and then submitted a technical report on the design. They reported that each tram had two wagons, which was able to transport about 200 passengers. The report also described the number of trams in operation, the number of persons transported per tram, average and maximum velocity of the tram, power and voltage, accessibility, etc. The tram company agreed to create a similar concept for their city, realizing immediately that the new tram restricts its use in the flat part of the city.

Furthermore, the new trams had excess capacity. Therefore, the company started to use fewer trams and increased the time between operations, which made the passengers wait longer to catch a tram. As a result, the customers used the new trams less and less, reducing the number of trams in operation.

Question 9.1:

State what the customers want. Establish the main FR of this project that can address the customers' needs.

This section provides some hints to help the students define the FRs. We first go into the ontology of what a *function* is in design. Assuming that students are familiar with physical and economic functions that describe natural and sociologic phenomena, the question proposed in this section is, "what is the difference between a function of a natural phenomenon and a function in design". The following is an example of a physical function described by Pascal:

The Pascal experiment

Blaise Pascal allegedly made the barrel experiment in 1646 to prove that the pressure a fluid exerts depends on the hydraulic head, not on the mass of the fluid. Opponents said the larger the mass, the higher the pressure would be. To prove his ideas, Pascal inserted a long thin tube into a barrel and started pouring water into the barrel. At a particular moment, the barrel started bursting. Was Pascal concerned about the material of the tube, or the number of wood staves? No! His concern was about the function: what made the pressure increase? For a fluid, water in this experiment, pressure depends on the head.

Students can repeat the barrel experiment many times in different ways to verify the validity of the Pascal equation. Experimenting intends to check the function, not the physical parts of the experiment. Therefore, functions in nature are abstractions of the physical domain.

Science claims to be objective because anyone who uses the correct apparatus can verify the natural laws under observation. Objectivity in Design has a slightly different meaning. Different projects can perform the same functions, so repeatability in design occurs in the functional domain. In this sense, functional repeatability in Design Science is not so different from the objectivity in science.

So, what is the main difference between Natural Sciences and Design Science?

In natural sciences, the function is checked by the experiment, or the experiment is given, and the function is verified. In design, the functions are given, and the physical concretization allows for checking if the DPs can fulfill the functions. In natural science, a theory, or a function can be rejected if it fails the verification of an experiment; in design science, one rejects the artifact if it fails to perform the functions.

These opposite checking directions between natural science and design science have an expression in the use of DEs. DEs relate the FRs to the DPs, the same way a function relates independent variables to dependent variables. However, in a function, the independent variables are known, and we want to obtain the value of the function; in design, we know the function, the FRs, and want to discover what the DPs are! First and Second axioms help to analyze solutions and can deny a solution, but the application of the axioms does not lead to the solution.

The reader already saw in Chapter 5 that a FR is a verbalized action. Examples of FRs are, regulate the water flow, maintain the indoor temperature, cut the beam, or any other phrase with a verb that involves action. The FRs and from DPs submit to the bounds defined by the constraints (Cs). The Cs are derived from CNs, laws, and regulations, arise from physics, or are derived from parent FRs or DPs.

FRs are developed by considering "what we want to achieve?". The "what?" or "what do we want to achieve?" are how to develop the FRs. On the other hand, "how to attain it" locates elements in the physical domain that fulfill FRs. Therefore, the dialogue, or mapping, between the "what" (FRs) and the "how" (DPs) is the basis of the design solution.

The linguistic structure of an FR is a verb and noun implying an action. Therefore, "adjust temperature," or "control airflow" are examples of FRs. Moreover, FRs need to have a target value and a range of acceptance, i.e., a tolerance that can be used for computing the information content of the design. Instead of "adjust the temperature," an FR should be "adjust the temperature to $24 \pm 1\ °C$."

Mistakes of novices and ontological incongruences that can be encountered when developing FRs are discussed below. The following three types of mistakes are common from novice applicants:

- non-designs, "negative FRs";
- mixing FRs with DPs;
- mixing FRs of the artifact with FRs of the design process.

Stakeholders sometimes warn designers that they do not want things that previously had a negative impact on the system. Novice AD users might respond to these warnings with negative FRs. These are formally incorrect. Because the complement of any element is everything else, not creating anything is a non-design. Examples are: "should not be dangerous"; "must not have lead"; "must not create legionella." Design teams still must take these warnings into account in formulating design solutions because they can express important needs of the stakeholders.

Another common novice mistake is to define FRs by a DP the designer intends to use. Instead of "adjust the temperature in a room," the novice designer may describe the FR as "use a fan-coil system." In this design, the DP is the "fan-coil system." Anytime the FR has a syntax "to use + noun" or "to have + noun," and the DP is the noun, the FR is in a non-neutral environment, and should be avoided.

Another class of mistakes is to mix the FRs of an artifact with the FRs or Cs of the design process. The designer knows that "deliver the design solution in two months," or the Cs "budget available," are important constraints on developing a new artifact. Therefore, FRs and Cs of the design process can apply just to the process, and not to the artifact.

Ontological incongruences, inconsistencies in the nature of the AD process, are more difficult to handle. AD users should know these incongruences, avoid them, if possible, and make use of them, if necessary, to solve design problems. Incongruences can be of the following types (Thompson 2013 ICAD):

- mixing FRs with Cs;
- the b-FRs;
- mix FRs with selection criteria (SC) or optimization criteria (OC).

Cs might sound like FRs, although Cs have no tolerance and need not be independent of other Cs or FRs. Cs create boundaries for the design. Usual examples of Cs are limits on cost, or weight, like "maximum cost," or "maximum weight." Nevertheless, an FR can have a range of acceptance with a lower bound but no upper limit, which is a common concept in engineering and management.

In the design of an air conditioning system, the CN "delivery of outdoor airflow greater than…" is often used. However, no one cares about having a huge amount of air, except for fulfilling another requirement regarding energy use. Similarly, in the enterprise field, financial ratios have lower or upper bounds. A high-level requirement for an enterprise design may be "maintaining a financial autonomy greater than 0.5," meaning the enterprise will have financial strength.

Additionally, it is possible to transform some common Cs into FRs, as long as the FR has a target and a range of acceptance. In the example of the cost, changing "maximum cost" to "control the budget of the artifact to a certain amount in a range of" allows one to define cost as an FR and computing its information content.

The b-FRs usually express an emotion about the product with a semantic "be + adjective" or similar. Examples are "be aesthetic," "smell good," or "look like a." Strictly speaking, the b-FRs are not FRs, as there is not a defined target value and a range of acceptance. Moreover, "be something" or "like something" can mix an FR with a DP. Anyway, AD experts should not forget that the b-FRs describe decision criteria for many customers. The designer should then create empirical or emotive scales for those FRs.

Selection criteria and optimization criteria are often used as FRs, a common use being in the energy design processes. "Minimize energy use" may be an FR expressed in different ways along the decomposition process. Ontologically the minimum has no defined target, nor a range, so the information content is not possible to compute. However, an expert in AD might realize that an FR relating to energy use exists. This FR needs to be reworded and specified appropriately, not eliminated.

9.4 The Decomposition Process

The decomposition process runs over all four domains of the design representation, from the highest level CNs to the lowest level PVs. The decomposition works in all the domains, at each level of decomposition, finding DPs and PVs to formulate the best solution by following Suh's two design axioms.

As explained in Chapter 2, CNs are the reverse side of the declaration of a problem, so that CNs usually relate to high-level FRs. It is wise to check all along the decomposition process to see if the FRs are consistent with the CNs. Many times, there is no need to decompose the CNs to lower levels.

Figure 9.2 shows the domains and the zigzagging between adjacent domains. The mapping between CNs and FRs is conceptual design. Product design is mapping between FRs and DPs. Most applications of AD are conceptual and product design. Production, or process, design maps between the physical domains and the process domain, defining the technology and the processes to create the DPs. At the end of this chapter, we introduce "concurrent engineering," where product and production designs occur at the same time.

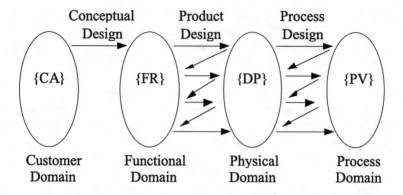

Fig. 9.2 Zigzagging between domains

Figure 9.2 does not show Cs arriving from the CNs, can be legal, and ethical, nor Cs from the FRs and DPs. A common approach for conceptual design is mapping CNs to high-level elements of the functional domain. Concerning product design and production design, Fig. 9.2 shows the zigzagging between FRs and DPs, and between DPs and PVs, along with the various levels of decomposition. However, it may not be necessary to define a PV for high-level DPs when the designer accepts an existing technology and process to manufacture the DPs. In an enterprise of manufacturing home appliances, if the DP is a "washing machine" the designer might not need to describe the PV as being "processes that produce a washing machine." Otherwise, low-level DPs might need to be defined too, including, how to manufacture, install, and dismantle, making it necessary to define the corresponding PVs.

However, the common approach described in the last paragraph may have exceptions. CNs might need to be mapped onto FRs at low levels of decomposition, and high-level PVs might need to be defined. The following example shows the need to define low-level CNs that map onto FRs and DPs at a low level, and the need to consider the high levels PVs:

Play and stop button

On audio recorders, the symbols for play, stop, record, forward, and backward have been used since the sixties. They are low-level DPs concerning the manufacturing of an audio recorder, but as everybody recognizes the symbols, they became a standard in videos, television, and media. The use of symbols became a CN that needs to have a definition on the leaves DPs.

A new fan-coil factory

A European air conditioning enterprise with good local reputation was facing in 2000 competition from the Far East. They wanted to make a new type of fan-coil and decided to consider delocalizing the production. This decision would mean that about a hundred production line workers would lose their jobs, which would cause heavy economic pain in the region. The manager of the enterprise asked for two new equipment designs. One would be manufactured in the Far East by the traditional methods, and another designed for a robotized line. The cost of production plus investment of the second option was 10% higher than the off-shore option, but the manager decided to invest in the robotized line. To off-set the investment in the new production line, he decided to improve sales of those products.

This type of decision benefits from mapping between the four domains and includes an ethics Cs for the manager's decision.

According to Fig. 9.2, design processes are active dialogs between FRs and DPs, the choice of one influencing the other. Zig is the mapping from the functional domain to the physical domain, to find DPs best able to fulfill FRs. Zag operates in the opposite direction coming back from the physical domain to the functional and finding FRs at a lower level. Zigzagging between domains starts at the highest level FRs and develops all the leaf level DPs to complete the solution.

The next example shows the strong interdependency between the FRs and the DPs at higher levels of the abstraction hierarchy.

Thermal comfort design

You are designing a solution for FR_0:"provide thermal comfort to your team". Choosing DP_0 will affect all remaining FRs.

- *The probable DP_0 might be an "air conditioning system". Thus, next FRs will be about adjusting temperature and providing a certain amount of outdoor airflow for indoor air quality purposes.*
- *However, if people are not constrained to work indoors they could lie outside and work with a computer in a hammock, as long as the weather outside is nice.*
- *Another solution might be to take a "metabolism pill," reducing the metabolic rate so that no one will feel hot any longer.*
- *Another solution is to develop a new "thermal suit" that would be able to heat or cool the body according to the metabolism and the indoor temperature.*

Therefore, depending on the choice of DP_0, child FRs will be different. Nevertheless, medical Cs from FR_0 forbid a "metabolism pill", and depending on the context of working, hammocks could be forbidden. Both situations are examples of Cs that arise from FR_0. On the other hand, choosing DP_0, the "air conditioning system", many regulations impose Cs that need to be taken into account.

Design theories can be applied to help achieve a good solution in less time, avoiding trial and error experiments. AD should provide the best solution, at the first attempt, eliminating non-productive iterations. Students might suppose that there are no iterations in the zig process when looking for a DP, or in the zag to attain the FRs, although this is not always the case. AD can avoid iterations between levels of decomposition, and it can avoid ending with solutions that need to be checked again from the beginning. Iterations might happen at each zig and each zag several times until the design team feels comfortable with their solutions. Arrows in Fig. 9.2 are final expressions of design process components.

The following example clarifies what zigzags are while providing some rationale for this design process. The example goes to the second level of decomposition, showing the possible solutions and the reasons for selecting one solution over another. In this example, the experience of the designer helps to choose the solution that has the best probability of success. In seeking a design situation, students might try to understand the probability of success by getting data from examples, talking to experts in the area, making simple models of how the system works, and finally calculating information contents.

Rotate a reel

A manufacturing company uses reels of metal sheet transported in the factory over roller conveyers with the axis vertical. A crane picks up each reel at the end of a conveyor. It needs the roll axes to be horizontal, making it necessary to turn the reel. Figure 9.3 shows the CN that will solve the problem of the factory and, in a box, the new product to design.

The designer translates the CN into FR_0 and then to DP_0 according to.

$FR_0 =$ Rotate steel reel.

And the new product as

$DP_0 =$ Mechanical turning device.

Notice that the decision on DP_0 is crucial for the development of the design. Another DP_0 could create a completely different design, by choosing instead "manpower" or "electromagnetic field" as DP_0. With this DP_0 accepted as a good solution, the zig at the top-level ends, and the process zags back to the functional domain at the next level of the decomposition. Figure 9.4 shows the zag and the corresponding FRs that should be according to DP_1 and at the same time with FR_1.

The figure expresses the FRs in a neutral environment on the second level of decomposition:

$FR_1 =$ Receive the steel reel;

$FR_2 =$ Rotate the reel axis from vertical to horizontal;

$FR_3 =$ Keep the reel axis in a horizontal alignment.

Many DPs are possible for each FR. Figure 9.5 depicts a rationale for the zig, showing possible solutions. Because the transportation system in the factory uses roller conveyors, the receiver can be a roller conveyor (DP_{1-A}). A belt conveyer (DP_{1-B}) is also possible,

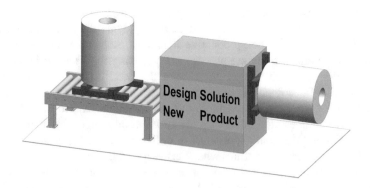

Fig. 9.3 The CN to turn the reel. (Reproduced from Gabriel-Santos et al. (2017), originally published open access under a CC BY 4.0 license: https://doi.org/10.1051/matecconf/201711209010)

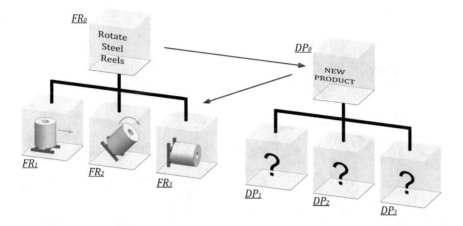

Fig. 9.4 The zag from the first level of decomposition. (Reproduced from Gabriel-Santos et al. (2017), originally published open access under a CC BY 4.0 license: https://doi.org/10.1051/matecconf/201711209010)

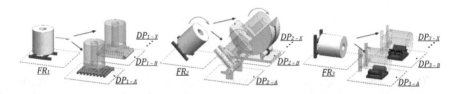

Fig. 9.5 The possible solutions at a zig for the "mechanical turning device". (Reproduced from Gabriel-Santos et al. (2017), originally published open access under a CC BY 4.0 license: https://doi.org/10.1051/matecconf/201711209010)

although less suitable because the surface of the conveyer belt can tear during operation. Similarly, conveyor rollers could get damaged during service, although repairing this implies just changing one or two rolls instead of the entire conveyer belt.

DP_2 can be a handling structure (DP_{2-A}), or a cradle support (DP_{2-B}), or any other solution the student can try to imagine. The handling structure was the choice because it is cheaper than the cradle, and any deformation does not affect the sheet in the reel. Finally, to "keep the reel axis in a horizontal alignment," the options are to use two rolls (DP_{3-A}) or two hinged convex metal supports (DP_{3-B}), the former having the disadvantage of creasing the metal reel.

According to the above rationale, the chosen DPs are

DP_1 = Roller conveyor (DP_{1-A});

DP_2 = Handling structure (DP_{2-A});

DP_3 = Convex metal supports (DP_{3-B}).

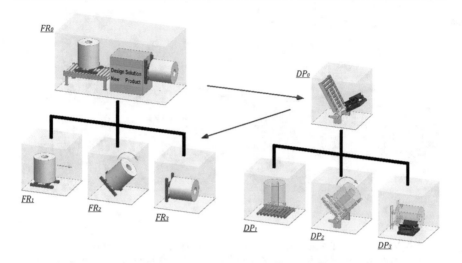

Fig. 9.6 The decomposition process with a solution (Adapted from Gabriel-Santos et al. 2017, originally published open access under a CC BY 4.0 license: https://doi.org/10.1051/matecconf/201711209010)

> *Figure 9.6 shows the decomposition process, integrating into the image of DP_1 the "mechanical turning device."*

The previous example appeals to experience and good sense and shows how to perform the zigzagging, the decisions needed, and the rationale for it. Moreover, it shows on DP_1 the integration of the child DPs.

Next sections formalize each path, the zig, and the zag in deeper detail, using a structured flow chart.

9.5   The Zig

The zig is the mapping between two adjacent domains at the same level of detail, usually expressed by an arrow from left to right. This section focuses on the zig between the functional domain and the physical domain, but it is possible to zig between any two adjacent domains.

The zig arrow can give the student a first impression that making a zig is easy, although it represents the end of a decision process that may have had many iterations, decisions, and counterdecisions. The inputs for the zig are the Cs, FRs, ranges of acceptance of FRs, variation of FRs with time, and tolerances of the DPs. Mapping involves two main tasks:

- "Defining and selecting DPs" and
- "Setting a parameter value for the selected DP."

"Defining and selecting the DPs" is the most important part of the zig because it should be maintain independence and minimize information content for that component of the design solution. If the design is coupled, the design team might try decoupling it or going back to check alternative DPs and FRs. After selecting a physical solution, the design moves to "setting a parameter value for the selected DP." To set the value for a DP may involve an optimization or tuning process that may end with the definitions of the DPs, or in turn, by coming back and starting the zig process again. Optimization and tuning are well-known processes of engineering and management, as explained in the introduction of this chapter. Therefore, we will give special attention to the "Defining and selecting the DPs."

At high levels in designs, an FR may be "machine wash" using as a DP "washing machine." This type of solution for the DP is not completely neutral but defines that the design uses a machine and allows the design to proceed.

For each FR, a DP might be sought, and the design matrix (DM) evaluated by checking the relationships between each DP and the FRs. One way of starting processes at each level is by defining the system at a nominal condition (NC) and obtain a first draft for the DM.

NCs of operation are common in engineering and management. However, final designs must consider all conditions of operation. Otherwise, depending on the condition of operation, the system could fail.

The NC error

A hotel group owning a four stars hotels asked a design team to propose an HVAC (heating, ventilating and air condition) system for a new hotel. The hotel faced West, with a large glass façade on this side. Therefore, during the afternoon, the solar heating load would increase. The solution proposed by the design team can heat and cool at any time. This solution is the so-called "four-pipe system" with two pipes for heating and two other for cooling. However, the owner of the hotel had good experiences in other ones with cheaper two-pipe systems that work in only one mode at a time, cooling or heating. This two-pipe system is less expensive than the four-pipe system. Overriding the advice of the design team, the owner selected two-pipes. He rationalized his argument by saying that the two-pipe solution could fulfill nominal winter and summer conditions.

The hotel opened by November, and the HVAC system was able to fulfill the heating requirements during the winter season. However, in the middle season, there were needs for heating in the morning and cooling in the afternoon in rooms adjacent to the west façade, while just heating all day in the other rooms. Moreover, as the water in the pipes was hot in the morning, the change to cooling requires changing all the water, and it needs more than an hour to start cooling. The hotel had many complaints about uncomfortable temperatures. After a year of operation, they had to change to a four-pipe HVAC system.

The above example shows that the nominal working condition can be a good starting point. However, it is not enough to define a system. The system might work at any actual working conditions. However, all possible working conditions may be hard to define.

In structural engineering, codes define design working conditions. The codes set minimum loads for structures as well as combinations of loads, e.g., wind and snow.

In enterprise management, nominal working conditions can be the target for the core business. However, demands change, and it can be necessary to find temporary ways to increase working capacity, e.g., research for special development needs and lawyers when legal problems arise.

Verifying system performance in all predictable conditions can reveal previously unanticipated coupling between DPs and FRs, missing DPs or FRs. Evaluating all the DPs and FRs lets design teams use the DM to maintain independence in actual working conditions, to direct designers to decoupled or uncoupled solutions. The design team could decide to use DMs that express the behavior of the system as a whole or use different design matrixes for each working state of the system.

Figure 9.7 shows a flowchart of a possible process for "defining and selecting DPs." The top of the figure is about solving the design at NCs, the middle at actual conditions (AC), and the bottom of the figure, checking the information content considering the tolerances of the DPs.

Fig. 9.7 Defining and selecting DP. (Reproduced from Cavique et al. 2017, originally published open access under a CC BY 4.0 license: https://doi.org/10.1051/matecconf/201712701007)

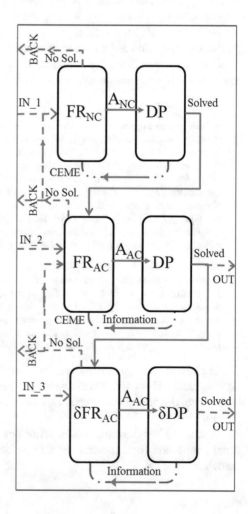

The designer might find one or more DPs that can fulfill an FR. According to AD, good solutions should be uncoupled or decoupled, maintaining the independence of functional elements. To select between DPs that all maintain the independence, choose the one with the least information content, i.e., the greatest chance of success.

Students already know that a 100% probability of success corresponds to zero information. Design teams should compute the information content in ACs. In other words, check if the system performs throughout the intended functional ranges.

Actual working conditions for an artifact are usually easy to define, an example being the earlier case of tilting the steel reel. In engineering systems that depend on nature, ACs are probabilistic, as with weather, wind, earthquakes, and fires. Similar probabilistic approaches happen on security systems, hospital emergency, or enterprise manufacturing, that depend on customer behavior.

Coming back to Fig. 9.7, to define FRs at NC, the inputs IN_1 are the DPs and FRs at the immediately higher level of decomposition and the Cs. Thus, the designer might synthesize the DPs, obtain the DE, and compute or estimate the information content of the design. At high levels in decompositions, the computation of the information content may follow a non-formal way, as expressed in the example of tilting the steel reel. Chapter 11 shows more detail of computing information content.

Besides, it is necessary to check if the child FRs and DPs combine to equal the parent and if the children are independent of each other (collectively exhaustive and mutually exclusive, CEME, Fig. 9.7). Section 9.6 describes the CEME concept in more detail. At the end of a zig, it may be possible to specify values, or preliminary values, and tolerances for the DPs.

Further, we need to understand how systems work under ACs, using DEs, computing the information, and checking again if FRs are CEME. This phase needs additional inputs (IN_2) regarding the DPs, FRs, and Cs. Some designers may proceed directly to the AC phase, using IN_1 and IN_2 to define the DE.

In many engineering or management environments, it is possible to finalize the zig at this stage and proceed to specify DP values and tolerances.

Finally, design teams might want to evaluate ranges of variation of FRs, and corresponding tolerances of the DP, δDP (IN_3). Codes seldom enforce this evaluation in structural engineering, air conditioning design, fire safety, and many building engineering activities, although they are common in machine manufacturing. Once more, if designs fulfill requirements, design teams can proceed to DP specifications at the working level of decomposition and tune them. If design is coupled, an optimization process could be required. Optimization and tuning might not be necessary at the higher levels of decomposition.

Air conditioning design

Variable air volume (VAV) is a common air conditioning system that supplies a variable amount of air at a cold temperature to each room. Figure 9.8 shows spaces 1 and n of n spaces of a building cooled by the VAV system. The figure depicts the air handling unit (AHU), the supply duct (1), and a VAV box (2) controlled by a thermostat (T). The system in the figure is the simplest VAV able to work just in the cooling mode.

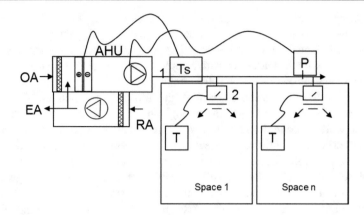

Fig. 9.8 A VAV system. (Reproduced from Cavique et al. (2017), originally published open access under a CC BY 4.0 license: https://doi.org/10.1051/matecconf/201712701007)

When the temperature goes up in any room, the room thermostat asks the regulator in the VAV box (2) to open the damper step-by-step to increase the amount of cooled air entering the room. Thus, the pressure in the duct (1) goes down, and the sensor (P) gives the signal to speed up the fan of the AHU.

The AHU supplies a mixture of outside air (OA) and return-air (RA) throughout duct (1), making the amount of OA delivered at each room to depend on the damper position. Therefore, the amount of OA delivered to each room is a function of the heat removed from the room and all other rooms.

At the higher level of decomposition, FR_0 and DP_0 are

FR_0 = Give comfort to room occupants.

DP_0 = VAV air conditioning system.

The intent of the VAV systems of the middle of the twentieth century is to "achieve indoor thermal comfort," therefore controlling room temperature. In the seventies, the oil crisis forced a reduction in energy use in buildings, and new designs then reduced the usage of outdoor air. Unfortunately, scarce fresh air brings problems of indoor air quality (IAQ), and the latter forced air conditioning systems to include a new function: "provide IAQ." Table 9.1 displays the FRs and DPs for the VAV system, showing that the system has more FRs than DPs.

At NCs, VAV boxes of each room are defined knowing the temperature supply (Ts) and the needs of cooling of each room. The definition of the total airflow of the system and the total cooling requirements can be used for specifying the AHU flow system and cooling systems. Finally, the OA set at the AHU provides the total amount of air needed according to the IAQ of the building.

The OA of each space FR_{21} and FR_{22} depends only on the VAV boxes and OA system of the AHU. Equation 9.1 shows the DE of the VAV system at NCs, which allows specifying the AHU, the VAV boxes, the duct, and the OA system, but not expressing the behavior of the entire system.

Table 9.1 FRs and DPs for the VAV system

FRs	DPs
FR_1- Achieve indoor thermal comfort	DP_1- Temperature control system
FR_2- Provide IAQ	DP_2- Outdoor air control system
FR_{11}- Remove heat from space 1	DP_{11}- 1's VAV box airflow
FR_{12}- Remove heat from space n	DP_{12}- n's VAV box airflow
FR_{13}- Provide total airflow supply	DP_{13}- AHU flow system
FR_{14}- Adjust Ts of the AHU	DP_{14}- AHU cooling coil system
FR_{21}- Provide space 1 OA	
FR_{22}- Provide space n OA	
FR_{23}- Provide building total OA flow	DP_{23}- AHU OA system

$$\begin{Bmatrix} FR_1 \\ FR_2 \\ FR_{11} \\ FR_{12} \\ FR_{13} \\ FR_{14} \\ FR_{23} \\ FR_{21} \\ FR_{22} \end{Bmatrix} = \begin{bmatrix} X & & & & & & \\ X & X & & & & & \\ & & X & & & X & \\ & & & X & & X & \\ & & & & X & X & \\ & & & & & X & \\ & & & & & & X \\ & & X & & & & X \\ & & & X & & & X \end{bmatrix} \cdot \begin{Bmatrix} DP_1 \\ DP_2 \\ DP_{11} \\ DP_{12} \\ DP_{13} \\ DP_{14} \\ DP_{23} \end{Bmatrix} \qquad (9.1)$$

Exercise 9.3: Define the Design Equation of a VAV

In a VAV system, anytime the damper of a VAV box opens, all the system adjusts, as the amount of air delivered in all other boxes changes.

- *Spaces with higher cooling loads receive more supply air, and therefore they receive more OA. Therefore, FR_{21} depends not only on DP_{11} but also on the behavior of all other VAV boxes, creating a coupling between the needs for OA and the cooling load of any space. Try to show this issue by changing the above Eq. 9.1;*
- *The OA airflow is a requirement of the type "the more, the better." Therefore, if the OA airflow delivered in each space is high enough, it can fulfill the needs of any space at any load. Therefore, neglecting the problem of having more FRs than DPs, it might be possible to meet the minimum requirements for OA at each space.*

Explain how this type of coupling can be solved.

After "defining and selecting DPs," design teams need to specify DP values, which can be computed using DEs. DMs, however, usually indicate only non-zero derivative relationships of the DEs with Xs, without showing equations. Normally, it is possible to specify or pre-specify DPs with DEs.

Having the set of DPs, it may help to perform the following tasks to estimate the values of the DPs:

- layout child DPs;
- write parent–child, or decomposition, equations to show how child DPs fulfill and are CEME concerning the parent DP;
- verify DP tolerances and check against the range of the FRs (IN_3 of Fig. 9.7).

Afterward, systems can be studied and tuned or adjusted using specific values of each DP. In case an irreconcilably coupled design results, an optimization process could be applied to get the best possible behavior. On the other hand, it might be possible to tune a coupled design so that it works acceptably through some useful range.

If a design solution fails to comply with the axioms at any phase, go back and redefine the DPs and the DE, or redefine the tolerances of the DPs. If necessary, design teams could need to start the zig again and again. The work already done will help a lot in the following attempt to reach a solution.

The zig arrow is the final representation of many attempts to reach a good solution at a level of decomposition, i.e., selecting a DP for an FR. The experience and knowledge of the design team, as well as their creativity and method, play an important role in attaining a good solution.

The first step in the critical assessment of a zig is to apply the first axiom of AD. If several candidate DPs have equal independence, then the second step is the use of the information axiom to check the probability of success of the design. Finally, the values and tolerances of the DPs need to be specified.

9.6 The Zag

The zag is the process represented by the arrow coming back to the left from a parent level of a domain to a child level of decomposition of the previous domain (Fig. 9.2). The usual task is to come from a DP in the physical domain back to the functional domain. In the functional domain, the new FRs are developed in the context of the upper level DPs. The new FRs must fulfill, i.e., be collectively exhaustive with respect to the parent FR and mutually exclusive to each other.

The next exercise aims to show the role of selecting a DP when zagging back into the functional domain.

Exercise 9.4: Design a Thermal Suit

When a person is in thermal equilibrium, the heat produced by the metabolism is removed from the human body by radiation, convection, conduction, and evaporation. The evaporation accounts for vapor transfer due to respiration and transpiration. To feel comfortable, people need to be in thermal equilibrium while meeting constraints for skin temperature and transpiration.

Therefore, suppose the design starts with the following FR_0 and DP_0:

FR_0 = Achieve indoor thermal comfort.

DP_0 = Thermal suit.

What would be the next level FRs to fulfill FR_0?

The zig synthesizes the DPs that fulfill the FRs by answering "how we achieve it?". The zag comes back to the functional domain and answers, "what we want to achieve?". The new FRs need to be in accordance with the parent FRs and the previous DPs. However, there is no special tool in AD to check if the new FRs are in accordance with the desired design. FRs are derived from the parent DPs and collectively express the parent FR. At the end of a zig, we find a point of consistency in the design.

To help to make the zag, Thompson (2014) introduced the question of "Why did we choose this DP?" the answer is the selection of the child FRs. In addition, child FRs need to be within the Cs. Therefore, the design process using AD theory is a synthesis process to discover the DPs, and it includes a subsequence process of analysis to achieve the child FRs.

Once more, when designers perform the zag, they should not be afraid of coming back to the parent DP at any time, if it seems the design failed. Moreover, if necessary, redo the previous zig. The following steps summarize a way of doing the zag:

- Select an FR–DP pair for decomposition. The DP could have specification or pre-specification values from the previous zig.
- Consider the Cs for FRs and DPs.
- Define child FRs answering to "why did we choose the parent DP?". It can be seen as reverse engineering from the parent DP. Notice that a parent FR needs to have two or more child FRs. Otherwise, the child FR is the parent FR, and no decomposition happens, or there is a missing sibling.
- Check if the proposed FRs align with CNs. If you realize there is a need for a new CN, start the design again from the beginning, from the FR_0.
- Check the FRs for consistency with the parent FR. The set of child FRs needs to be collective exhaustive (CE) regarding the parent FR. Moreover, the FRs need to be independent of each other, so their intersection is nil, and therefore, they are mutual exclusive (ME). Hence, the consistency with the parent FR is CE plus ME, or CEME.
- Make a double check to evaluate if you need all the FRs. The number of FRs should be as low as possible to enable achieving a good design.

Exercise 9.5: Design of a Purchasing Department

The purchasing department of an enterprise needs a redefinition from scratch. The design should develop in these four domains: customer, functional, physical, and process. Services of the department are in the physical domain. Data treat belongs in the process domain.

Most material is purchased locally. Some technical equipment has international orders. There are three major groups of purchased materials:

- *repair and maintenance material, usually purchased in small quantities at low prices;*
- *material for maintenance and manufacture acquired in sets of parts;*
- *technical equipment with detailed specifications.*

Do the mapping between the four domains until you can define the following outcomes for the design solution:

- *define the internal services of the department;*
- *what are the roles of each service?*
- *procedures to implement at each service (define it descriptively);*
- *outline the flow of data between services and external companies;*
- *what are the control and audit operations to implement?*

Students might need to define the operation mode of the department by contacting a real enterprise.

9.7 Decomposition and Concurrent Engineering

The ontological classification of design entities in the four domains helps to define many problems. In designing artifacts, enterprises, management organization, and many other things, identifying the CNs, FRs, DPs, and PVs fosters clear reasoning.

This section presents the Concurrent Engineering approach, which is an important industrial application of the mapping between domains. Concurrent Engineering is intended to integrate all product and process development tasks simultaneously, in the design phase, to develop a product quickly.

The Society of Concurrent Product Development (SCPD) defines (1993): *Integrated product development is a philosophy that systematically employs a teaming of functional disciplines to integrate and concurrently apply all the necessary processes to produce an effective and efficient product that satisfies the CNs.* Moreover, SCPD states Concurrent Engineering *involves the correct interplay of the functional department, including customers and suppliers, and the supporting infrastructure technologies.*

Traditional engineering approaches classify design processes in three sequential stages: conceptual design, product design, and process design. The three stages define the most common way to design. However, this approach depends on the technological or field knowledge of the design team. To overcome the possible lack of field knowledge, the design teams usually have persons with different skills and experiences. The target is always to have a good design that can be constructed, processed, and installed in a short time, so enterprises save money in development and catch the market opportunity.

About 80% of the processing cost can be due to decisions made during the product design phase. Therefore, important product design decisions made without the knowledge of manufacturing, assembly, and inspection, may have extra costs involved. Concurrent Engineering provides rules and techniques for "design for manufacturing" and "design for assembly." In this context, the design process should involve the process domain at the upper levels of the decomposition, unlike the situation when the manufacturing technology is already defined.

Concurrent Engineering provides rules and techniques for "design for manufacturing," and for assembly, hence reducing the total time to market of new products. However, product design by itself might take longer when it interacts with manufacturing design in the full realization of new products. Therefore, Concurrent Engineering can be more difficult to implement in "traditional" enterprises that tend to have new products "designed" in a short time. These shorter "design" times result in iterations at the prototype, production, and test phases and result in a long time to reach the market.

Traditional enterprises accept CAD (computer-aided drafting, or "design") files as representations of completed designs. Typically, these CAD files are grossly inadequate representations of design solutions from an AD perspective. They jump directly to the physical integration phase and include no indication of the design intent (FRs). They lack compliance with Suh's design axioms. Enterprises need to learn to value time spent in rigorous decompositions and physical integrations that produce design solutions that comply with Suh's axioms. Representations of completed design solutions should include decompositions, metrics, design and decomposition equations, design matrices, and physical integration. For Concurrent Engineering solutions, the process domain and process matrix and physical integration of the manufacturing process should be included as well.

Figure 9.9 shows the traditional and Concurrent Engineering approaches. The traditional approach is sequential, knowledge flows from the product design to the process design, and feedback from the process design to the product design is informal or via the marketing information. In contrast, the Concurrent Engineering approach mixes knowledge from product and process designs, and it involves people with different knowledge bases and skills. In Concurrent Engineering environments, the availability of processing knowledge can cause redesigns of the artifact that are problematic from a manufacturing perspective at any phase of the design process.

Fig. 9.9 Engineering approaches to the Product and Process Design

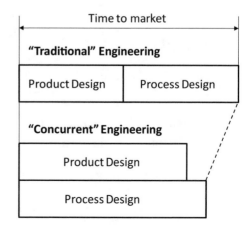

In this context, when the manufacturing technology is not yet known, e.g., large-scale integrated circuits in the early 1960s, then, at high levels of the decomposition, mapping should go from the CNs to the FRs, from the FRs to the DPs, and from the DPs to the PVs. If manufacturing technology is already known, e.g., conventional cars in 2000, the DPs to the PVs can be mapped just at lower levels of decomposition.

Figure 9.10 shows the Concurrent Engineering approach to the zigzag, where the zig to the product design flows to the process design, and the zag to the FRs contains inputs from the process domain.

This approach reduces the subjectivity of decision-making at the early phase of the product development, because it generates viable and cost-effective design solutions, by including the knowledge about the PVs.

Mathematically speaking, the DE for the product design is

$$\{FR\} = [A]\{DP\} \tag{9.2}$$

For the production process design:

$$\{DP\} = [B]\{PV\} \tag{9.3}$$

The combination of Eqs. 9.2 and 9.3 yields

$$\{FR\} = [C]\{PV\} \tag{9.4}$$

where $[C] = [A] \times [B]$ is the design matrix for the concurrent design process. According to the Independence Axiom, in an ideal design, all the three design matrices, [A], [B], and [C], must be square and diagonal or, failing that, triangular.

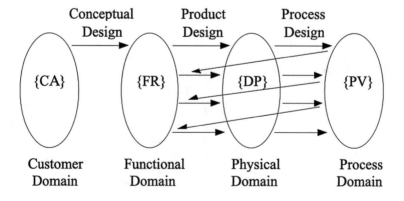

Fig. 9.10 The decomposition process as performed in a Concurrent Engineering environment

Geometric Dimensioning and Tolerancing (GD&T) design to guarantee the assembly of a component

A component (Fig. 9.11) shall be assembled to a machine through a set of four holes and shall be used to attach another component through a set of three holes. The surfaces of the component are previously prepared, and the two sets of holes are analyzed here.

These points are necessary to assure the desired assembly:

(a) *ensure the position of the component in the machine has no ambiguity;*
(b) *the set of four holes must be positioned relative to the structure of the machine;*
(c) *the set of four holes defines the position of the set of three holes;*
(d) *the subsequent assembly, by the set of three holes, must be done with this component laid on the machine;*
(e) *through the set of three holes, a new component will be assembled and must be perpendicular to the plane of the first component.*

The first-level mapping of this case based on the concurrent engineering approach is

FR_1 = *Ensure the position of the component;*
FR_2 = *Ensure holes position.*

DP_1 = *Isostatic support system;*
DP_2 = *Dimensions and geometric tolerances related to holes.*

PV_1 = *Pins in a three-plane datum system;*
PV_2 = *Work-holding solution.*

This mapping between functional, physical, and process domains is represented by these DEs:

$$\begin{Bmatrix} FR_1 \\ FR_2 \end{Bmatrix} = \begin{bmatrix} \times & 0 \\ \times & \times \end{bmatrix} \begin{Bmatrix} DP_1 \\ DP_2 \end{Bmatrix} \tag{9.5}$$

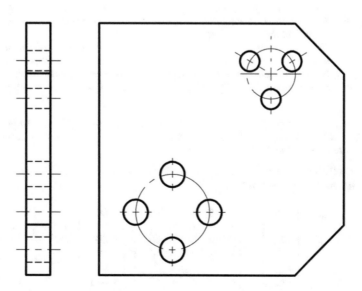

Fig. 9.11 Component used in the exercise: a plate with two sets of holes

$$\left\{ \begin{matrix} DP_1 \\ DP_2 \end{matrix} \right\} = \begin{bmatrix} \times & 0 \\ \times & \times \end{bmatrix} \left\{ \begin{matrix} PV_1 \\ PV_2 \end{matrix} \right\} \tag{9.6}$$

In the second level, the decomposition of FR_1 and FR_2 is a consequence of the previous zig, from functional to process domains.

> FR_{11} = Seat one face of the component on the machine (by three seating points on one reference plane);
> FR_{12} = Guide one edge of the component (by two guiding points another reference plane perpendicular to the first);
> FR_{13} = locate one end of the component (by a single locating point on a third reference plane perpendicular to the first two);
> FR_{21} = Allocate at each one of the four holes a position tolerance at the worst condition to assembly operations, related to the three reference planes;
> FR_{22} = Adopt the set of four holes referenced to the position of the set of 3 holes;
> FR_{23} = Allocate to each of the three holes a position tolerance related to the plane seated on the machine and to the set of four holes, at the worst condition to assembly operations, and at the same condition, this tolerance must be tighter when related to the mentioned plane.

The worst condition to assembly operations occurs when a feature or part has the maximum amount of material (volume/size) within its dimensional tolerance. This situation is the maximum material condition (MMC). The MMC of the shaft would be the maximum diameter; The MMC of the hole would be its minimum diameter. (Georg Henzold 2006).

The set of DPs that satisfy the specified FR are:

> DP_{11} = The face which plane is D;
> DP_{12} = Plane A defines the edge that guides the component;
> DP_{13} = Plane B position the component;
> DP_{21} = The position tolerance at maximum material condition, in any direction, of each hole of the set of four holes, follows the sequence of relationship to faces D–A–B;
> DP_{22} = The geometrical center of the set of four holes is a reference (C) to the position of holes of the set of three;
> DP_{23} = The position tolerance in any direction at maximum material condition, of each hole of the set of three holes, is primarily related to face D, and thus to the four holes as a whole (C) for its worst situation (maximum material condition), and simultaneously has a tight tolerance related to face D at the same material condition.

DPs are depicted in a technical drawing (Fig. 9.12). Letters A, B, C, and D represent datum, and small letters (r, s, and t) represent the value of each tolerance since numerical values are irrelevant for this study.

Equation (9.7) shows the relation between the functional domain and the physical domain and represents the product design:

$$\left\{ \begin{matrix} FR_{11} \\ FR_{12} \\ FR_{13} \\ FR_{21} \\ FR_{22} \\ FR_{23} \end{matrix} \right\} = \begin{bmatrix} \times & 0 & 0 & 0 & 0 & 0 \\ 0 & \times & 0 & 0 & 0 & 0 \\ 0 & 0 & \times & 0 & 0 & 0 \\ \times & \times & \times & \times & 0 & 0 \\ \times & \times & \times & 0 & \times & 0 \\ \times & 0 & 0 & 0 & \times & \times \end{bmatrix} \left\{ \begin{matrix} DP_{11} \\ DP_{12} \\ DP_{13} \\ DP_{21} \\ DP_{22} \\ DP_{23} \end{matrix} \right\} \tag{9.7}$$

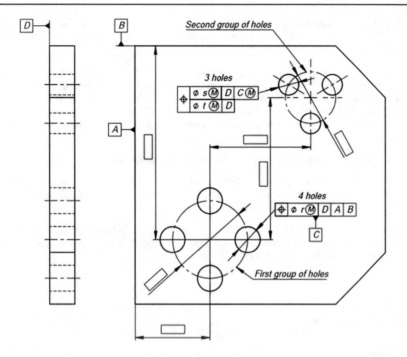

Fig. 9.12 Component with datum system and geometrical tolerances

The set of PVs that characterizes the process that is used to implement the design (achieve or create the DPs), are:

PV_{11} = Define plane D by three seating points;
PV_{12} = Define plane A by two seating (guiding) points;
PV_{13} = Define plane B by one seating (locating) point;
PV_{21} = Clamp the component after positioning according to the sequence D–A–B;
PV_{22} = Determine the geometrical center of the four drilled holes set, which is datum C;
PV_{23} = Support the component on the three seating points (plane D), and use dimensions referred to the center of the four holes set to their production and inspection.

Equation (9.8) shows the relation between the physical domain and the process domain and represents the process design.

$$
\begin{Bmatrix} DP_{11} \\ DP_{12} \\ DP_{13} \\ DP_{21} \\ DP_{22} \\ DP_{23} \end{Bmatrix}
=
\begin{bmatrix}
\times & 0 & 0 & 0 & 0 & 0 \\
0 & \times & 0 & 0 & 0 & 0 \\
0 & 0 & \times & 0 & 0 & 0 \\
\times & \times & \times & \times & 0 & 0 \\
\times & \times & \times & 0 & \times & 0 \\
\times & 0 & 0 & 0 & \times & \times
\end{bmatrix}
\begin{Bmatrix} PV_{11} \\ PV_{12} \\ PV_{13} \\ PV_{21} \\ PV_{22} \\ PV_{23} \end{Bmatrix}
\qquad (9.8)
$$

The ease of manufacturing, assembly, and inspection operations is a consequence of the GD&T specifications (FR) making the DM show the independence between FRs and DPs and between DPs and PVs.

Concurrent Engineering leads to the specification of the functionalities in agreement with the manufacturing, assembly, and inspection operations. This example shows that GD&T is an engineering language that helps the creation of independent solutions, as long as, at each mapping, the DMs are triangular (Eqs. 9.7 and 9.8). Moreover, this example shows that AD domains and mapping give good theoretical support for the foundation of Concurrent Engineering.

Exercise 9.6: A Small Change in the Design of the Component

After designing the component, a factory gets to manufacture it. The manufacturing engineer decides to use the datum A, B, and D on both sets of holes. He argues the dimensions are the same using one datum system or the other.

Discuss the manufacturing engineer's idea by redefining the design matrixes from FRs to DPs and from DPs to PVs at the second level of decomposition. Moreover, discuss the problems the manufacturing process will face.

9.8 Conclusion

AD theory (AD) avoids trial and error, helps to classify a solution as good or poor but does not give the solution by itself. A good design process needs to develop and define good FRs. A design solution can be no better than its FRs. This statement encouraged the authors of this chapter to give extra hints on how to define FRs.

The main message of this chapter is that it can take many attempts to perform good zigs and zags. The design team might not be depressed about starting the mapping process repeatedly. AD is about doing a good design at the first attempt, avoiding trial and errors. However, at each level of decomposition, many attempts might need to finalize a zig. Finalizing a zig with success provides consistency to the design because it makes it possible to apply Suh's two axioms.

The zag requires child FRs that are collectively exhaustive with respect to the parent and mutually exclusive with respect to each other.

Finally, this chapter presents the mapping to help to reason in different domains of design and shows Concurrent Engineering as an example that needs decomposition in all four domains at the same level.

Problems

1. Deploy up to the third level a possible FR and DP zigzag decomposition for a two-stroke internal combustion engine.
2. Comment on the statement: "Decisions at each level have important consequences at lower levels."
3. A manufacturing company works in a traditional industry of shoemaking. A consultant said to the enterprise chair that "there is no such thing as a poor technological market". Discuss what the consultant said:

- the industry needs to map between the physical and process domains;
- the industry needs to map at the same time between the functional, physical, and process domains.

4. An HVAC system has at the first level of decomposition the same FRs and DPs as the ones shown in the air-conditioning example:

FR_1 = Achieve indoor thermal comfort;
FR_2 = Provide IAQ;

and

DP_1 = Temperature control system;
DP_2 = Outdoor air control system.

A system uses an AHU to treat the outdoor-air and a convection-type system to cool the indoor ambiance.

- define the DM for the first level of decomposition;
- decompose the design until the next level.

5. The traditional salt industry harvests a mixture of salt crystals and clay. A possible way to separate salt crystals from clay is by dissolving the clay. The process uses a solvent, called brine, which is a saturated aqueous salt solution. This solution can no longer solve salt but dilutes the clay and maintain the salt crystals. The main FRs of this design are as follows:

FR_1 = Separate clay from salt;
FR_2 = Dilute the clay;
FR_3 = Remove the clay;
FR_4 = Remove the solvent;
FR_5 = Collect the washed salt.

- Define the DPs and PVs while meeting the first Axiom of AD.

References

Cavique M, Fradinho J, Gabriel-Santos A, Gonçalves-Coelho A, Mourão A (2017) The Iterative Nature of the "Zig" and How to Define the "Hows". In: Slătineanu L (ed) 11th International Conference on Axiomatic Design (ICAD), MATEC Web of Conferences, Iasi, Romania. https://doi.org/10.1051/matecconf/201712701007

Gabriel-Santos A, Martinho A, Fradinho J, Cavique M, Gonçalves-Coelho A, , Mourão A (2017) How Axiomatic Design can promote creativity in the design of new products. In: Slătineanu L, Nagit G, Dodun O, Merticaru V, Coteata M, Ripanu M, Mihalache A, Boca M, Ibanescu R, Panait C, Oancea G, Kyratsis P (eds) 21st Innovative Manufacturing Engineering & Energy International Conference—IManE&E 2017, MATEC Web of Conferences, vol 112, p 8. https://doi.org/10.1051/matecconf/201711209010

Further Reading

Cavique M, Gonçalves-Coelho A (2011) Repeatability in Design Science. In: Thompson MK (ed) 6th International Conference on Axiomatic Design (ICAD 2013). KAIST, Axiomatic Design Solutions Inc., Daejeon, Korea, pp 31–34

Dickinson A, Brown CA (2009) Design and Deployment of Axiomatic Design. In: ao de Azevedo Gonçalves Coelho AMFR (ed) Proceedings of the 5th International Conference on Axiomatic Design, Universidade Nova de Lisboa, accessed at Axiomatic Design Solutions, Inc., Lisboa, Portugal

Gonçalves-Coelho A (2004) Axiomatic Design and the concurrent engineering paradigm. Acad J Manufact Eng 2(2):6–15

Henzold G (2006) Geometrical Dimensioning and Tolerancing for Design, Manufacturing and Inspection: A Handbook for Geometrical Product Specification using ISO and ASME standards, 2nd edn. Butterworth-Heinemann

Suh NP (1990) The Principles of Design. Oxford University Press

Tate DE (1999) A roadmap for decomposition : activities, theories, and tools for system design. Doctor of philosophy in mechanical engineering, Massachusetts Institute of Technology, 77 Massachusetts Ave., Cambridge MA 02139, USA

Thompson MK (2013) A classification of procedural errors in the definition of functional requirements in Axiomatic Design theory. In: Thompson MK (ed) 7th International Conference on Axiomatic Design (ICAD 2013), CIRP, accessed at Axiomatic Design Solutions, Inc., Worchester, MA, vol 32, pp 1–6

Thompson MK (2014) Where is the 'Why' in Axiomatic Design? In: Thompson MK (ed) 8th International Conference on Axiomatic Design (ICAD 2014), CIRP, accessed at Axiomatic Design Solutions, Inc., Lisboa, Portugal, vol 33

Redundant Designs

10

Miguel Cavique and António Gonçalves-Coelho

Abstract

The concept of redundancy is common in day-to-day life. In engineering, redundancy allows a system to work safely, often by creating a backup that enters on service if the primary system fails. Redundancy in management may have the meaning of plan-B if the initial plan fails. In nature, redundancy appears in many living organisms, man included. This chapter starts by presenting examples of redundancy in nature, then showing how redundancy applies to many engineered systems, and how redundancy may have different meanings in engineering. According to Axiomatic Design (AD), a redundant design has more design parameters (DPs) than functional requirements (FRs). There are two types of approaches for redundancy: reliability motivated and the functionally motivated approach. These thoughts give room for discussing the ontology of redundant design, allowing the derivation of new theorems on redundancy. One of these theorems helps to decouple coupled designs.

10.1 Introduction

The standard definition of redundancy relates superfluousness or to have surplus resources to perform a specific task. The surplus resources may be required in case part of the system fails. This definition has many applications in engineering as failure happens in computer, energy, and structural engineering. In reliability, redundancy

M. Cavique (✉)
UNIDEMI & Escola Naval, Base Naval de Lisboa – Alfeite, 2810-001 Almada, Portugal
e-mail: cavique.santos@marinha.pt

A. Gonçalves-Coelho
UNIDEMI & DEMI, NOVA SST, Campus de Caparica, 2829-516 Caparica, Portugal

© Springer Nature Switzerland AG 2021
N. P. Suh et al. (eds.), *Design Engineering and Science*,
https://doi.org/10.1007/978-3-030-49232-8_10

helps to maintain the entire system working in case something fails. As an example of the last case, the air-conditioning of a data center may use more indoor units than necessary. A standard solution is to use two more indoor units. Each additional unit switches on in case of failure occurs on any of the working units. In the communications field, redundancy may mean that a message will flow through two different channels that can reach the receptor. Therefore, the system still operates in case one of the channels fails. The system may use two channels of the same kind to deliver the message or two completely different ways to fulfill the same requirement.

Redundancy is common in the day-to-day use of computers, by using back-ups, cloud systems shared by distinct computers, or data storage in separate disks.

RAID

The Redundant Array of Inexpensive Drives (RAID) is a way to store data in separate hard disks. There are many types of architectures for RAID systems, the simplest one consisting of replication of data in two separate disks. Therefore, if a failure occurs in one disk, the system can keep operating without any visible disturbance to the user.

Exercise 10.1: Redundant Design Equation

Wellington sent a message to London regarding the victory at the Waterloo battle, using a semaphore chain and a carrier pigeon. Due to the fog, the pigeon was the first to reach the destination. Define the design equation of this design.

In "education," a message sent by the teacher may not reach the student in the first attempt. Therefore, teachers use redundant techniques to make the message reach the student. One way is to repeat the same subject; another is to use many exercises on the same topic or to observe the occurrence in a lab or videos; or a blend of all these processes that produces an interesting course.

Exercise 10.2: Defining an AD Course

The student read the last nine chapters of an AD course and may have an opinion about the key concepts of the subject. Define the FRs of an introductory course on AD using the action verb "Understand ...". Define the DPs for the FRs identified and check if the design is a redundant design.

This section presents examples of dissimilar concepts of redundancy. Next sections give a closer look at this subject in what concerns reliability and functionally motivated redundancy. At the end of this chapter, the theorems of redundancy are presented.

10.2 Redundancy in Nature

Natural systems depend on many variables that usually make the design redundant. In a lake, the water temperature depends on wind velocity, air temperature, and humidity, solar radiation and absorption of radiation by the plants and soil, the soil temperature, etc. The soil temperature depends on depth, thermal amplitude, radiation, and average outdoor temperature. The number of fishes in the lake, or the photosynthesis of plants, depends in turn on some of these variables. Therefore, Eq. (10.1) may represent a natural phenomenon, where y's represent the outputs and x's are input variables, with m larger than n:

$$y_1 = f_1(x_1, x_2, ..., x_m)$$
$$y_2 = f_2(x_1, x_2, ..., x_m)$$
$$...$$
$$y_n = f_m(x_1, x_2, ..., x_m)$$

(10.1)

In biology, equations are harder to define, but biologists know the way variables interfere in the phenomenon under analysis. In medicine, medical doctors may not be able to quantify all variables in a medical episode, but they know what cross-dependencies exist between the variables and symptoms. To make a decision, medical doctors need to assume some variables as fixed and work with all the others. A similar situation may happen in management practice, on a marketing campaign or at a military theater, making the person in charge of the decision to fix some variables to allow a solution for the set of equations.

The Laplace's demon

Laplace lived in the eighteen century and died at the beginning of the nineteenth century. It that period, Newton's laws were the fundamentals of mechanistic theories that tried to explain all phenomena based on mechanic causalities. Laplace supposed that if it would be possible to write all the equations of all atoms, then the Universe would have a deterministic behavior. Therefore, knowing their present location and momentum, the equations would reveal the future and the past of the universe. This reasoning is known as the Laplace's demon, which would be a mind that can know the past and future.

Calculation algorithms in engineering frequently address redundant designs. Suppose we need to define the diameter of a duct that delivers water in some spots of the line. Topologically, the duct is a sequence of edges in series. The calculation of the diameters of the edges starts by defining the available head loss. Thus, knowing the flow at each edge makes it possible to use many combinations of edge diameters that satisfy the available head loss. Therefore, the design is a redundant design. Duct algorithms use a common parameter or a dimensionless number to define the ducts diameters. It is usual to define as a dimensioning criterion a constant velocity, a constant head loss per unit of length, a constant energy loss, or a minimum investment over a period. In any case, using these parameters, the diameters turn to depend on flow at each edge. This method changes the design from redundant to non-redundant and uncoupled. The following equations help to explain this subject.

Equation (10.2) shows that a set of n branches with diameters D_i and flows Q_i can fulfill the available pressure drop ΔP. In this equation, what we want to achieve (FR) is the pressure drop ΔP, and the DPs are the diameters D_i, for the known flow rates Q_i. Therefore, the equation to solve is:

$$\Delta P = f(D_1, D_2, \ldots, D_n, Q_1, Q_2, \ldots, Q_n) \tag{10.2}$$

The equation may change to an ideal design by using a dimensioning criterion: if the diameters D_i are functions of the flows Q_i. Knowing the flows at each edge allows defining the diameters. According to AD, "what we want to achieve" are the diameters, and the DPs are the known flows Q_i at each branch. Equation (10.3) shows this idea:

$$\begin{bmatrix} D_1 \\ D_2 \\ \vdots \\ D_n \end{bmatrix} = \begin{bmatrix} X & & & \\ & X & & \\ & & \ddots & \\ & & & X \end{bmatrix} \cdot \begin{bmatrix} Q_1 \\ Q_2 \\ \vdots \\ Q_n \end{bmatrix} \tag{10.3}$$

Exercise 10.3: Selection of a Beam

A student wants to select a beam with a uniform rectangular section to support a maximum bending moment M_{max}. For a section with dimensions b and h, the maximum axial stress σ_{max} is $\sigma_{max} = \frac{M_{max} \frac{h}{2}}{I}$, where h is the thickness of the beam, and I is the moment of inertia of the cross section, $I = \frac{bh^3}{12}$. Therefore, the student might be able to:

write the design equation for the FR = "be able to sustain a maximum bending moment M_{max}"; and

define a variable so that the design turns from a redundant to a non-redundant design.

The last examples show that some redundant designs may turn into non-redundant designs using quantified dimensions. In many engineering applications, it is possible to aggregate variables in dimensionless variables and relate the FR, "what we want to achieve," with some dimensionless quantities. In fluid mechanics, the friction coefficient of a pipe, f, is a function of the Reynolds number, Re, and the dimensionless roughness, ε. Moody, after Rouse developments, depicted the diagram that shows the equation $f = f(Re, \varepsilon)$, where f is the friction coefficient. The friction coefficient defined by the Moody diagram applies to most of the engineering fluids.

The advantage of using dimensionless numbers is the possibility of using a smaller number of experiments to find the function between the dimensionless numbers than the number of experiments that would be necessary if all the variables in the dimensionless number were used. Thus the findings can apply to other applications.

Usually, the design team knows what the main variables are, but does not know the dimensionless numbers to use. The Buckingham theorem of dimensionless variables, the so-called π theorem, is very common in engineering but less used in other fields. The authors encourage the reader to study and apply the π theorem as a means to turn redundant designs into uncoupled or decoupled designs.

The student may find more comprehensive approaches to this subject in the theories regarding the design of experiments.

From the aforesaid, redundancy in nature exists. The following section introduces, in a formal way, the concept of redundancy according to the view of AD.

10.3   The Theorem of Redundancy

According to AD, the ideal design is uncoupled (Theorem 4). If there are fewer DPs than FRs, either the design is coupled, or the FRs cannot be simultaneously satisfied (Theorem 1).

Equation (10.4) shows a redundant design with three FRs and four DPs. It is a redundant design because DP_2 and DP_3 are used to fulfill FR_2. This design equation may express two different designs: a design that uses DP_2 and DP_3 at the same time to fulfill FR_2, and a design that uses DP_2 on specific states and DP_3 on other situations.

$$\begin{bmatrix} FR_1 \\ FR_2 \\ FR_3 \end{bmatrix} = \begin{bmatrix} X & & & \\ & X & X & \\ & & & X \end{bmatrix} \cdot \begin{bmatrix} DP_1 \\ DP_2 \\ DP_3 \\ DP_4 \end{bmatrix} \tag{10.4}$$

On the second interpretation, the design equation is the amalgamation of the states the system performs. This concept is similar to the one used on the common-sense definition of redundancy. The hyperstatic structures in civil engineering are examples where all DPs work at the same time. These examples show redundant design of the aforementioned first type. On the other hand, a UPS (uninterruptible power station) enters on service when the main fails, belonging to the second kind of redundant designs.

We may now introduce the 3rd Theorem of AD. This theorem regarding redundant designs states:

– "When there are more DPs than FRs, the design is either redundant or coupled."

In a better assertion, Theorem 3 states:

– "When there are more DPs than FRs, the design is a redundant design, which can be reduced to an uncoupled design or a decoupled design, or a coupled design."

Exercise 10.4: Hybrid or Electric Car

The automotive industry has introduced innovative hybrid and electric cars to solve the environmental problem created by CO_2 emissions. Carbon dioxide (CO_2) has been a pollutant of concern due to the greenhouse effect it causes in the atmosphere. Electric cars do not emit CO_2 directly but increase the needs for electricity, the generation of which releases carbon depending on the energy mix. To define the design equation, we start by defining the following two high-level FRs:

FR_1 = *Move the car;*

FR_2 = *Control emissions.*

Define the design equation for an electric car and a hybrid car and discuss how these solutions fulfill these FRs. Discuss what might be a better solution with a higher probability of success.

The theorem of redundancy may include two different realities: the reliability motivated and the functionally motivated approaches. Section 10.4 shows this reliability approach, classifying the redundancy in two groups: active and passive redundancy. On the other hand, Sect. 10.5 discusses the functionally motivated approach, which covers designs with different DPs to satisfy a range of FR that may change over time.

10.4   Reliability-Motivated Redundancy

Reliability-motivated redundant designs are classified into two types: active and passive redundant. If the design is an active one, then it has two or more states of operation, and the redundant design equation can be split in so many equations as the number of states of operation. Equation (10.410.4) may express a passive or an active redundant design. Case Eq. (10.4) is an *active redundant design* it expresses two states of operation, defined by two different design equations, as per Eq. (10.5).

$$
\begin{bmatrix} FR_1 \\ FR_2 \\ FR_3 \end{bmatrix} = \begin{bmatrix} X & & \\ & X & \\ & & X \end{bmatrix} \cdot \begin{bmatrix} DP_1 \\ DP_2 \\ DP_3 \\ DP_4 \end{bmatrix} \text{ or } \begin{bmatrix} FR_1 \\ FR_2 \\ FR_3 \end{bmatrix} = \begin{bmatrix} X & & \\ & X & \\ & & X \end{bmatrix} \cdot \begin{bmatrix} DP_1 \\ DP_2 \\ DP_3 \\ DP_4 \end{bmatrix}
$$

$$(10.5)$$

Heating and cooling system

Figure 10.1 shows a system that heats a house and produces domestic hot water (DHW). A fan-coil (FC) delivers the heat into the house, and the faucet represents the delivery of DHW. In many countries, it is more cost-effective to use the heat pump rather than the gas boiler. If the heat pump fails, or if it cannot work due to a very low outdoor temperature, then the gas boiler starts, and the heat pump turns off.

This type of redundant designs can fulfill the FRs regardless of the working mode. Active redundant designs are quite common in the energy field.

The designer intends to fulfill the range of acceptance for each FR at any mode of operation.

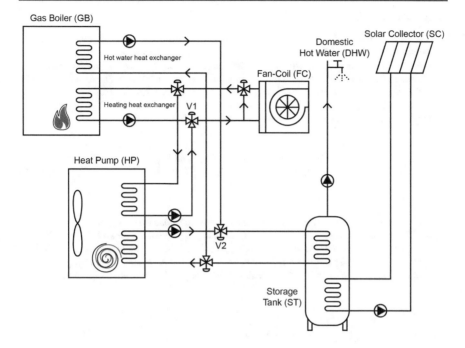

Fig. 10.1 System for heating a room and for delivering domestic hot water

According to the example mentioned above, the FRs of the design are:

FR_1 = *Heat the house;*

FR_2 = *Produce domestic hot water.*

The system has a gas boiler (GB), a heat pump (HP), a solar collector (SC), and a storage tank (ST). The hot water supply of the fan-coil comes from the GB or the HP, according to the position of the three-way valve V_1. Regarding the hot water production, it comes from the ST, where two heat exchangers can heat the water coming from the mains supply. The SC feeds the lower heat exchanger of the ST. Case the solar heat is not enough to heat the water, then the HP or the GB feed the upper heat exchanger depending on the position of the three-way valve V_2.

Exercise 10.5: Design Equation of Fig. 10.1

Regarding Fig. 10.1 and using the above-defined FRs, find a design equation and all states of the functioning of the system. Further, write the design equation of each state of operation. Notice that, concerning the production of domestic hot water, the design may have passive redundancy.

Any security system needs a redundant design. Usually, the security systems are active redundant designs. Case a system fails, another system comes into operation. The following example shows the case of electrical supply to a network operation center:

Electric supply to a data center

The electric power that feeds some data centers comes from an uninterruptible power supply (UPS) that isolates the computers from the grid, the so-called galvanic insulation. Batteries are the heart of the UPS and produce direct current (DC). DC is transformed into alternating current (AC) that supplies the computers in the data center. The batteries have autonomy for a certain period without external energy supply. The external supply comes from the electrical grid (EG) or a diesel generator (DG). Therefore, the design equation of the electrical supply of the data center is according to Eq. (10.6):

$$[ES] = [X \quad X \quad X] \cdot \begin{bmatrix} EG \\ UPS \\ DG \end{bmatrix} \tag{10.6}$$

The system may operate in three modes. The most common mode uses the supply of the EG to the UPS and thus transforms the DC into AC; in case of a grid failure, the DG starts working providing energy to the UPS; during the start-up of the DG the electricity supply comes only from the UPS. In the case of total failure of the EG and DG, the UPS can supply the data-center during a defined period. Equation 10.7 shows the three modes of operation:

$$[ES] = [X \quad X \quad 0] \cdot \begin{bmatrix} EG \\ UPS \\ DG \end{bmatrix} \text{ or}$$

$$[ES] = [0 \quad X \quad X] \cdot \begin{bmatrix} EG \\ UPS \\ DG \end{bmatrix} \text{ or} \tag{10.7}$$

$$[ES] = [0 \quad X \quad 0] \cdot \begin{bmatrix} EG \\ UPS \\ DG \end{bmatrix}$$

Exercise 10.6: Data-Center without Galvanic Isolation

Write the design equation of a data-center that receives electricity directly from the grid or the diesel generator. This system uses UPS as a side supply during transition or total failure. Discuss the fulfillment of energy supply in the three operating modes.

If the design is a passive redundant design, then all DPs are always in operation, and no action changes the operating mode of the system.

For a steel structure to hold specific loads, it is possible to use a topology with a minimum number of bars. However, many structures use more bars than the minimum and distribute the loads through all of them. In such cases, it is necessary to add the equations of displacement to the equations of the sum of forces and sum of bending moments to allow defining the forces at each bar. These structures are hyperstatic and very well known in civil and mechanical engineering. In case a bar fails, the structure does not fail, at least immediately, as it happens in a non-hyperstatic structure, the isostatic ones.

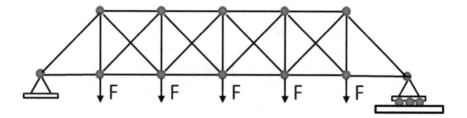

Fig. 10.2 A hyperstatic structure

Hyperstatic structure

Figure 10.2 shows a 2D hyperstatic structure with five loads, F, twelve nodes, an anchoring node on the left, and a sliding node on the right. The loads are applied to the nodes according to the picture so that each bar is subjected to compression or traction loads, but not to bending.

Exercise 10.7: Hyperstatic Structure

Using the example of Fig. 10.2, define the minimum number of bars that allows supporting the loads F. Define the design equation for the structure presented in the figure.

Fluid networks are other examples of redundant passive systems. In many water networks, the ducts, which are topologically edges, form different paths from the injection node to the consumption nodes. Therefore, it makes possible the flow to vary in each edge depending on the consumption flows. Figure 10.3 depicts a topology of a water network, with four nodes, two of them consumption nodes, and one injection node. The network has five edges and forms two loops. The pressure equilibrium in the loops makes the pressure to vary on the nodes depending on their consumption. The pressure equilibrium causes the flow to vary in each duct along the time. The network would need just two edges to supply the two nodes, for example, edge 1 and 2. All other edges make the network to be a redundant design. The student is invited to discuss why this type of networks is so prevalent in real life.

In conclusion, regarding the reliability point of view, the design may be passive or active. If the design has passive redundancy, then:

- all redundant parts are always on duty;
- no special action needed.

Regarding active redundancy, the design meets these characteristics:

- an action puts the redundant parts working;
- the modes of the system change over time.

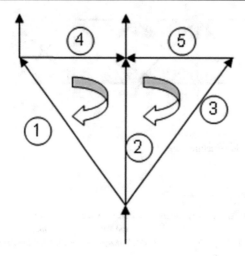

Fig. 10.3 A water network topology

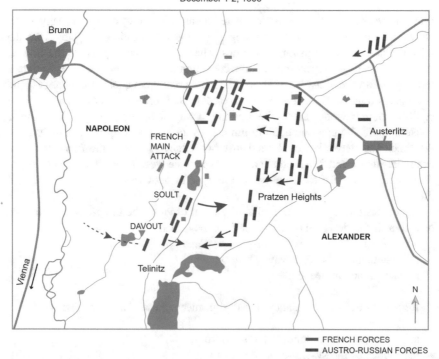

Fig. 10.4 Deployment of forces during the Battle of Austerlitz. Figure sketched from public domain maps of the Department of History Atlas (courtesy of the United States Military Academy Department of History)

In both types of designs, the system aims to fulfill the FRs in the ranges defined in the project. Therefore, the above examples assume that at any time, the range of acceptance of the FRs remain constant.

However, the designer may want to change the FRs range over time. In such a case, the FRs may have more than a target value and more than a range of acceptance. These type of problems belongs to the classification of functionally redundant design.

10.5 Functionally Related Redundancy

According to the AD theory, the acceptance of a solution depends on the fulfillment of the FRs. Therefore, the acceptance of the design occurs in the functional domain.

Intrinsic redundancy, discussed at the beginning of this chapter, is inherently related to the functions and therefore belongs to the functionally related type of redundancy. In such a case, the functions to perform, their target value, and range of acceptance remain.

Other designs need to change their target value and their range of acceptance of the FRs over time, called "alternative redundancy." In this way, an alternative redundant design is always an active redundant design.

Therefore, regarding functional redundancy, the classification of designs is:

- intrinsic redundancy;
- alternative redundancy;
- adaptive, or augmentative, redundancy.

PTO/PTI Marine Engines

When a vessel docks, the main engine usually stops to reduce energy consumption, as well as to reduce pollution in the port. At this working state, the energy supply to the vessel comes from the dock infrastructure. However, for safety reasons, the vessel might need to set sail urgently. As the main engine takes some time to start and cannot drive the propeller in time according to the urgency of the maneuver, a quicker engine needs to start.

Many vessels use the concept of PTO/PTI to maneuver on time. During regular operation, the main engine drives the propeller and supplies energy to a generator by engaging a clutch to move its shaft. In this case, the generator charges a set of electric batteries. This situation is called the power take-off, or PTO mode. The PTI mode, power take in, occurs during an emergency start. Some port regulations enforce the use of PTI mode for safety and pollution reasons. In this case, the electrical batteries power an electric motor that connects to the propeller shaft by another clutch.

The generator and the motor are usually the same device that works as a generator when it receives mechanical energy and works as a motor when it receives electrical energy.

The last example is an alternative redundant design. Based on the classification of Sect. 10.4, it is an active redundant design.

The FR is "produce shaft power," and the DPs are the main engine, usually a Diesel motor (DP_1), the electric motor system (DP_2), and the alternator system (DP_3). The electrical motor system includes the engine, clutch, shaft, electric supply, and all other equipment and control systems needed to make it work. Similarly, the alternator system contains the alternator, clutch, batteries, electrical system, and control.

The design equation is according to the following Eq. (10.8):

$$[FR] = [X \quad X \quad X] \cdot \begin{bmatrix} DP_1 \\ DP_2 \\ DP_3 \end{bmatrix} \tag{10.8}$$

This equation has two states of operation defined in the following equation, where FR_{PTO} regards the propulsion by the diesel engine at PTO mode and FR_{PTI}, the propulsion through the electrical motor. In Eq. (10.9), we suppose FR_{PTO} and FR_{PTI} may have different target values and different ranges of acceptance:

$$[FR_{PTO}] = [X \qquad X] \cdot \begin{bmatrix} DP_1 \\ DP_2 \\ DP_3 \end{bmatrix} \text{ or } [FR_{PTI}] = [\quad X \quad] \cdot \begin{bmatrix} DP_1 \\ DP_2 \\ DP_3 \end{bmatrix} \tag{10.9}$$

The design is a redundant design, classified as alternative regarding functional redundancy, and active regarding the reliability point of view. As FR_{PTO} and FR_{PTI} have different ranges and target values, then the design is adaptive.

The system may also work with the main engine only, FR_D, without delivering energy to the alternator.

In some arrangements, the main engine, as well as the electrical motor, may contribute to the shaft power. In this case, the shaft power may add the Diesel engine and electric power, called combined diesel and electric (CODAE), the design is adaptive. Equation (10.10) shows the four possible states of this arrangement: diesel only, PTO, PTI, and both diesel and electrical motor:

$$[FR_D] = [X \qquad] \cdot \begin{bmatrix} DP_1 \\ DP_2 \\ DP_3 \end{bmatrix} \text{ or }$$

$$[FR_{PTO}] = [X \quad X \quad] \cdot \begin{bmatrix} DP_1 \\ DP_2 \\ DP_3 \end{bmatrix} \text{ or }$$

$$\tag{10.10}$$

$$[FR_{PTI}] = [\qquad X] \cdot \begin{bmatrix} DP_1 \\ DP_2 \\ DP_3 \end{bmatrix} \text{ or }$$

$$[FR_{DE}] = [X \quad X \quad] \cdot \begin{bmatrix} DP_1 \\ DP_2 \\ DP_3 \end{bmatrix}$$

Exercise 10.8: New Definition of the Design Equation for the PTO and PTI Arrangements

Last example shows a redundant design for the FR "produce shaft power." Redo this example by considering an adaptive redundant design, using the following two FRs:

FR_1 = Produce shaft power;

FR_2 = Produce electricity to the service grid.

Using the design equation, discuss the possible working modes and identify the design matrix for each mode of operation.

Blue Angels

The Blue Angels squadron is a flying aerobatic squadron of the United States Marines formed in 1946. One of the planes of the squadron is a Lockheed Hercules C-130 with rock-assisted take-off (RATO) capability. During take-off, the plane uses the four turbo-propellers plus rockets to increase thrust. Therefore, this arrangement is an adaptive redundant design that increases power during take-off.

The last example addresses an adaptive redundant design. To fulfill part of the range of the FR: "produce thrust power" the Blue Angels Lockheed C-130 uses four turboprops, and the extra power needed at take-off comes from rockets. In this situation, the FR definition remains, and more DPs allows the system to be able to fulfill the whole working range.

The student might be aware when facing a redundant design if the design lacks the definition of some FR. Known examples are very important to discuss the application of a theory, but knowing the DPs may cause a misunderstanding of the targets of the system. Next exercise asks the student to discuss this problem.

Exercise 10.9: The Battle of Austerlitz

The Battle of Austerlitz opposed Napoleon Bonaparte to the Austro-Russian coalition commanded by the Russian czar Alexander. This battle is a masterpiece of strategy that offered one of the greatest victories of Napoleon. He could defeat a larger army and affirm the new French empire. On the 1st December 1805, Napoleon had his forces near the Pratzen Heights, which he abandoned some days before to make the enemy feel he was in a weak condition. Moreover, he purposely weakened his right flank at Telinitz.

The Russian commander decided to attack the right flank of Napoleon to roll up the French line and cut the French contact with Vienna. However, Napoleon has ordered Marshal Davout to do a risky and crucial maneuver: to march during 48 h from Vienna to help his right flank. Davout was one of the best French marshals and was able to accomplish this movement, just in time to support General Legrand at the right flank. Meanwhile, the Austro-Russian army has left their forces at the Pratzen Heights, which allowed the French Marshal Soult to make a frontal attack and cut the Austro-Russian forces into two pieces.

Napoleon said: "If the Russian force leaves the Pratzen Heights to go to the right side, it will certainly be defeated."

Napoleon may have had in mind the following two high-level FRs:

– *persuade the Austro-Russian forces to attack the French flank;*
– *attack the center of the Austro-Russian army.*

The DPs were the forces of Legrand, Davout, and Soult.

Is it a redundant design? Define the design equation of Napoleon's strategy.

10.6   More Theorems on Redundancy

AD's Theorem 3 says a redundant design "can be reduced to an uncoupled design or a decoupled design, or a coupled design". This section shows how to classify redundant designs and define new theorems.

Equation (10.11) shows a redundant design with three FRs and five DPs. The subset of the design matrix regarding DP_1, DP_2, and DP_3 shows a coupled design. Anyway, the set of DP_1, DP_2, and DP_3 allows fulfilling FR_1, and then DP_4 can tune FR_2 and DP_5 tunes FR_3. This equation shows the zero elements of the matrix to improve matrix readability:

$$\begin{bmatrix} FR_1 \\ FR_2 \\ FR_3 \end{bmatrix} = \begin{bmatrix} X & X & X & 0 & 0 \\ X & X & X & X & 0 \\ X & X & X & X & X \end{bmatrix} \begin{bmatrix} DP_1 \\ DP_2 \\ DP_3 \\ DP_4 \\ DP_5 \end{bmatrix} \qquad (10.11)$$

The sequence for tuning the FRs is $DP_1 + DP_2 + DP_3$, DP_4, and finally, DP_5, showing it is a decoupled design.

Theorem R1 states:

– All redundant designs with right-trapezoid design matrix are decoupled.

Next section uses this theorem to decouple coupled designs, showing some examples and applications.

If the design matrix has diagonal blocks, then the designs matrixes are similar to Eq. (10.12) and

Theorem R2 applies:

– Redundant designs with design matrices composed by contiguous diagonal blocks are uncoupled.

In this case, $DP_1 + DP_4$ fulfill FR_1; $DP_2 + DP_5$ fulfill FR_2, and DP_3 fulfills FR_3. The sets of DPs can fulfill an FR independently, making the design redundant and uncoupled. Notice that on any column of the matrix appears just one "X".

$$
\begin{bmatrix} FR_1 \\ FR_2 \\ FR_3 \end{bmatrix} = \begin{bmatrix} X & 0 & 0 & X & 0 \\ 0 & X & 0 & 0 & X \\ 0 & 0 & X & 0 & 0 \end{bmatrix} \begin{bmatrix} DP_1 \\ DP_2 \\ DP_3 \\ DP_4 \\ DP_5 \end{bmatrix} \tag{10.12}
$$

If the matrix has triangular blocks, then Theorem R3 applies:

– Redundant designs with design matrices composed by contiguous triangular blocks are decoupled.

Equation (10.13) shows an example of theorem R3, with a redundant design formed by two decoupled designs. In this example, the sequence of tuning is $DP_1 + DP_4$, thus $DP_2 + DP_5$, and lastly, DP_3.

$$
\begin{bmatrix} FR_1 \\ FR_2 \\ FR_3 \end{bmatrix} = \begin{bmatrix} X & 0 & 0 & X & 0 \\ X & X & 0 & X & X \\ X & X & X & 0 & 0 \end{bmatrix} \begin{bmatrix} DP_1 \\ DP_2 \\ DP_3 \\ DP_4 \\ DP_5 \end{bmatrix} \tag{10.13}
$$

Using both triangular and diagonal matrices, Theorem R4 states:

– Redundant designs with design matrices composed by contiguous diagonal and triangular blocks are decoupled.

Equation (10.14) shows an application of Theorem R4. Notice the sequence of tuning of Eqs. (10.13) and (10.14) is the same, but FR_2 does not depend on DP_4, which allows a wider tolerance for DP_4 in the design expressed by Eq. (10.14).

$$
\begin{bmatrix} FR_1 \\ FR_2 \\ FR_3 \end{bmatrix} = \begin{bmatrix} X & 0 & 0 & X & 0 \\ X & X & 0 & 0 & X \\ X & X & X & 0 & 0 \end{bmatrix} \begin{bmatrix} DP_1 \\ DP_2 \\ DP_3 \\ DP_4 \\ DP_5 \end{bmatrix} \tag{10.14}
$$

If it is necessary to create a redundant design, it is easy to use already available systems. On Exercise 10.5, the heat pump, boiler, and solar panel helped to define a redundant new system. We apply this idea in the next theorems that help to synthesize new systems. Therefore, it is possible to raise new in the following paragraphs.

Theorem R5 states:

– The combination of an arbitrary number of uncoupled designs with common FRs and unshared DPs is again an uncoupled design.

As an example, having the following three designs defined by their design equations (10.15), it is possible to create a redundant design according to Eq. (10.16):

$$
\begin{bmatrix} FR_1 \\ FR_2 \\ FR_3 \end{bmatrix} = \begin{bmatrix} X & 0 & 0 \\ 0 & X & 0 \\ 0 & 0 & X \end{bmatrix} \cdot \begin{bmatrix} DP_1 \\ DP_2 \\ DP_3 \end{bmatrix} \text{ and}
$$

$$
\begin{bmatrix} FR_1 \\ FR_2 \end{bmatrix} = \begin{bmatrix} X & 0 \\ 0 & X \end{bmatrix} \cdot \begin{bmatrix} DP_4 \\ DP_5 \end{bmatrix} \text{ and} \tag{10.15}
$$

$$
\begin{bmatrix} FR_2 \\ FR_3 \end{bmatrix} = \begin{bmatrix} X & 0 \\ 0 & X \end{bmatrix} \cdot \begin{bmatrix} DP_6 \\ DP_7 \end{bmatrix}
$$

The three designs create a new redundant design:

$$
\begin{bmatrix} FR_1 \\ FR_2 \\ FR_3 \end{bmatrix} = \begin{bmatrix} X & 0 & 0 & X & 0 & 0 & 0 \\ 0 & X & 0 & 0 & X & X & 0 \\ 0 & 0 & X & 0 & 0 & 0 & X \end{bmatrix} \cdot \begin{bmatrix} DP_1 \\ DP_2 \\ DP_3 \\ DP_4 \\ DP_5 \\ DP_6 \\ DP_7 \end{bmatrix} \tag{10.16}
$$

To fulfill each FR, the new design expressed by Eq. (10.16) has two or more DPs. The designer might be aware of the interconnections of the DPs not to create a coupled design at lower levels of decomposition. In many circumstances, the interconnection couples the systems and may create a coupled design.

Theorem R6 states:

– The combination of an arbitrary number of decoupled designs with common FRs and unshared DPs is again a decoupled design.

Equation (10.17) and (10.18) show an example of matching three existing decoupled designs into a redundant decoupled design:

$$
\begin{bmatrix} FR_1 \\ FR_2 \\ FR_3 \end{bmatrix} = \begin{bmatrix} X & 0 & 0 \\ X & X & 0 \\ X & X & X \end{bmatrix} \cdot \begin{bmatrix} DP_1 \\ DP_2 \\ DP_3 \end{bmatrix} \text{ and}
$$

$$
\begin{bmatrix} FR_1 \\ FR_2 \end{bmatrix} = \begin{bmatrix} X & 0 \\ X & X \end{bmatrix} \cdot \begin{bmatrix} DP_4 \\ DP_5 \end{bmatrix} \text{ and} \tag{10.17}
$$

$$
\begin{bmatrix} FR_2 \\ FR_3 \end{bmatrix} = \begin{bmatrix} X & 0 \\ X & X \end{bmatrix} \cdot \begin{bmatrix} DP_6 \\ DP_7 \end{bmatrix}
$$

Create:

$$
\begin{bmatrix} FR_1 \\ FR_2 \\ FR_3 \end{bmatrix} = \begin{bmatrix} X & 0 & 0 & X & 0 & 0 & 0 \\ X & X & 0 & X & X & X & 0 \\ X & X & X & 0 & 0 & X & X \end{bmatrix} \cdot \begin{bmatrix} DP_1 \\ DP_2 \\ DP_3 \\ DP_4 \\ DP_5 \\ DP_6 \\ DP_7 \end{bmatrix} \qquad (10.18)
$$

Finally, Eqs. (10.19) and (10.20) show the existing designs and the redundant design created by Theorem R7, which states:

– The combination of an arbitrary number of uncoupled and decoupled designs with common FRs and unshared DPs is again a decoupled design.

$$
\begin{bmatrix} FR_1 \\ FR_2 \\ FR_3 \end{bmatrix} = \begin{bmatrix} X & 0 & 0 \\ X & X & 0 \\ X & X & X \end{bmatrix} \cdot \begin{bmatrix} DP_1 \\ DP_2 \\ DP_3 \end{bmatrix} \text{ and}
$$
$$
\begin{bmatrix} FR_1 \\ FR_2 \end{bmatrix} = \begin{bmatrix} X & 0 \\ 0 & X \end{bmatrix} \cdot \begin{bmatrix} DP_4 \\ DP_5 \end{bmatrix} \text{ and} \qquad (10.19)
$$
$$
\begin{bmatrix} FR_2 \\ FR_3 \end{bmatrix} = \begin{bmatrix} X & 0 \\ 0 & X \end{bmatrix} \cdot \begin{bmatrix} DP_6 \\ DP_7 \end{bmatrix}
$$

$$
\begin{bmatrix} FR_1 \\ FR_2 \\ FR_3 \end{bmatrix} = \begin{bmatrix} X & 0 & 0 & X & 0 & 0 & 0 \\ X & X & 0 & 0 & X & X & 0 \\ X & X & X & 0 & 0 & 0 & X \end{bmatrix} \cdot \begin{bmatrix} DP_1 \\ DP_2 \\ DP_3 \\ DP_4 \\ DP_5 \\ DP_6 \\ DP_7 \end{bmatrix} \qquad (10.20)
$$

This section helps the student to classify a redundant design using Theorems R1 to R4. Moreover, it helps synthetizing redundant designs using existing systems by using Theorems R5 to R7. A corollary of Theorem R1 can help to solve coupled systems. Due to the importance of solving coupled design, a complete section concerns this matter. Following section addresses this problem, giving some examples to illustrate the application.

10.7 Solving Coupled Designs

Theorem R1 states that "all redundant designs with right-trapezoid design matrix are decoupled" no matter the classification of the square part of the design matrix. Therefore, it is possible to join a right diagonal or right triangle matrix to any design matrix to create a right-trapezoid matrix.

Thus, Theorem R8 states:

– Any coupled design can be reduced to a redundant decoupled design by joining an upper triangular matrix with unshared DPs.

Therefore, if a design is a coupled design, as shown in the example of Eq. (10.21), then it is possible to reduce it to a decoupled design.

$$\begin{bmatrix} FR_1 \\ FR_2 \\ FR_3 \end{bmatrix} = \begin{bmatrix} X & X & X \\ X & X & X \\ X & X & X \end{bmatrix} \cdot \begin{bmatrix} DP_1 \\ DP_2 \\ DP_3 \end{bmatrix} \qquad (10.21)$$

Knowing "what we want to achieve," the designer may identify new unshared DPs than can fulfill a certain FR. In Eq. (10.22), DP_4 and DP_5, new unshared DPs, fulfill FR_2 and FR_3, respectively. Therefore, knowing a working mode of $DP_1 + DP_2 + DP_3$ that fulfills FR_1 makes it possible to tune the other FRs. Therefore, the sequence of tuning is freezing DP_1, DP_2, and DP_3, and then set the unshared DPs.

$$\begin{bmatrix} FR_1 \\ FR_2 \\ FR_3 \end{bmatrix} = \begin{bmatrix} X & X & X & 0 & 0 \\ X & X & X & X & 0 \\ X & X & X & 0 & X \end{bmatrix} \begin{bmatrix} DP_1 \\ DP_2 \\ DP_3 \\ DP_4 \\ DP_5 \end{bmatrix} \qquad (10.22)$$

The de-carbonization of the world economy

Most of the World countries agreed in the 2015 Conference of Paris to reduce their carbon emissions. Moreover, they decided to apply the best practices to keep global warming "well below 2 °C" of the pre-industrial era. According to the International Panel on Climate Change (IPCC) of the United Nations, the World needs to perform a hard path to reduce carbon in the atmosphere. Many evolutions of future carbon emissions have been studied and cataloged according to the average radiative forcing. The representative concentration path (RCP2.6) allows the temperature of the earth's atmosphere to increase in the range of 0.9 to 2.3 °C until 2100. This RCP requests to reduce human emissions to values well below the ones experienced in 1980. This path needs a substantial increase in the use of renewable energy as well as nuclear energy. To ensure the needs of energy for 2100 while reducing the carbon emissions, the technologies using coal, natural gas, and bio-energy, must be helped by technology for carbon capture and storage (CCS).

In the context of the last example, the thermoelectric generators (TEG) are facing a difficult challenge. There has been a huge effort to increase the efficiency of the TEGs and to substitute them with cleaner technologies. However, according to the RCP2.6, coal TEGs will be necessary for the future, due to the increase in energy demand.

The FRs for a coal thermoelectric power plant are:

- FR_1 = Adjust power production;
- FR_2 = Reduce carbon emissions.

A central power station starts with a certain number of thermoelectric generators of specific power and adjusts the power production at any time by changing the number of generators in operation. The DPs are:

- DP_1 = Power of a thermoelectric generator (P_{TEG});
- DP_2 = Number of thermoelectric generators (n).

Equation (10.23) shows the design equation. The second row harms the reduction of emission, making the "Xs" of this row to be negative.

$$\begin{bmatrix} FR_1 \\ FR_2 \end{bmatrix} = \begin{bmatrix} X & X \\ X & X \end{bmatrix} \cdot \begin{bmatrix} P_{TEG} \\ n \end{bmatrix} \qquad (10.23)$$

The above FRs and DPs solve the demand for energy, but the reduction of carbon emission makes to reduce the number of TEG in a power plant. Therefore, on a given power plant, carbon emission depends strongly on power production. How can the World solve this problem? According to the IPCC, CCS is a solution by changing the design into a redundant design, described by Eq. (10.24). CCS gives an extra possibility to lower the carbon emissions to the atmosphere despite the production of carbon on the power plants.

$$\begin{bmatrix} FR_1 \\ FR_2 \end{bmatrix} = \begin{bmatrix} X & X \\ X & X & X \end{bmatrix} \cdot \begin{bmatrix} P_{TEG} \\ n \\ CCS \end{bmatrix} \qquad (10.24)$$

Exercise 10.10: The Energy-Mix Equation

The RCP2.6 asks for using by 2020 an energy-mix of carbon resources (coal, oil, natural gas), bio-energy, renewable, and nuclear sources. Also, there is a need to use a technology for carbon capture and storage. Write the energy-mix equation using the FRs of the previous example:

- FR_1 = Adjust power production;

- FR_2 = Reduce carbon emissions.

Redundant designs are more common than we may realize. In this chapter, most of the examples considered energy supply or safety, but many situations in the day-to-day work use redundant designs.

The two-visa problem

A person goes to a country where it is necessary to travel with a visa in the passport. However, that person was urgently asked to travel to a second country by the end of the month, requiring a new visa added to the passport. It is necessary to leave the passport to apply for a new visa, but during that month, the person will need it for traveling. However, in such cases, the foreigner affairs services allow a person to have two passports. However, it is necessary to present the booking of the hotel and the flight tickets to receive a second passport. Nevertheless, it is no sense to pay for the hotel and plane without knowing if the passport visa would arrive on time. So, how would you solve this problem?

Exercise 10.11: The Two-Visa Problem

Write down what the requirements of the passenger are and define the design equation. Then, look for a solution using a redundant design.

Managers often use redundant designs to solve organizational problems. With time, organizations tend to slow down the fulfillment of their original stated requirements. High-level decision-makers or managers introduce new requirements in the organization to fulfill new needs or hidden personal agenda. Redirecting the organization to perform the original requirements is often a traumatic experience for many persons. A way to solve this problem is by using a redundant design.

10.8 Conclusions

When there are more DPs than FRs, the design is either a redundant design or a coupled design (as per Theorem 3). Redundant designs are common on energy grids applications, on safety systems, and many applications of real life.

This chapter identifies three kinds of redundancy: adaptive, alternative, and intrinsic.

Moreover, this chapter presents theorems on redundancy: theorems R1 to R8. All redundant designs with a right-trapezoid design matrix are decoupled (as per Theorem R2). Redundant designs with design matrices composed by contiguous diagonal blocks are uncoupled (as per Theorem R2).

Redundant designs with design matrices composed by contiguous triangular blocks are decoupled (as per Theorem R3). Four base theorems (R1 to R4) help to classify uncoupled and decoupled redundant designs. Redundant designs with design matrices composed by contiguous diagonal and triangular blocks are decoupled (as per Theorem R4).

Moreover, Theorems R5 to R8 give a framework for creating redundant designs. Linking two uncoupled or decoupled designs with unshared DPs create new uncoupled or decoupled designs. Finally, theorem R8 helps to solve coupled designs. Therefore, it is a powerful tool for AD applications. It states that case the design is coupled, then it is possible to turn it into a decoupled design by adding DPs so that the design matrix becomes right-trapezoidal.

References

United States Military Academy, Department of History (2020a) The Battle of Austerlitz, 1805—Situation, 0900 h, 2 December. https://www.westpoint.edu/sites/default/files/inline-images/academics/academic_departments/history/Napoleonic%20wars/Nap23.pdf

United States Military Academy, Department of History (2020b) The Battle of Austerlitz, 1805—Situation, 1800 h, 1 December. https://www.westpoint.edu/sites/default/files/inline-images/academics/academic_departments/history/Napoleonic%20wars/Nap22.pdf

Further Reading

Gonçalves-Coelho A, Neştian G, Cavique M, Mourão A (2012) Tackling with redundant designs through axiomatic design. Int J Precis Eng Manuf 13(10):1837–1843

Suh NP (1990) The principles of design. Oxford University Press

Suh NP (2001) Axiomatic design—advances and applications. Oxford University Press

The Information Axiom and Robust Design

11

João Fradinho and António Gonçalves-Coelho

Abstract

In preceding chapters, it was emphasized that the first task in innovative design is the problem definition. The problem is then transformed into functional requirements (FRs), then into design parameters (DPs) and process variables (PVs), the vectors that define the four domains of the design world. Design matrices give the relationship between these vectors. The Independence Axiom states that the FRs must always be independent of other FRs as DPs and PVs are chosen. In this chapter, the role of the Information axiom in creating the best design is presented, including how to measure the information content, how to make a design robust by satisfying the Independence Axiom and the Information Axiom. A coupled design has large information content, in some cases, approaching infinite information content, which implies that the design will never work as intended. An uncoupled design can be made to have zero information content, making the design easy to implement and the resulting design most reliable. The determination of information content is presented in this chapter with many examples.

List of abbreviations

AD Axiomatic Design
FR Functional Requirement (FRs)
DP Design Parameter
PV Process Variable

J. Fradinho (✉) · A. Gonçalves-Coelho
UNIDEMI & DEMI, NOVA SST, Campus de Caparica, 829-516 Caparica, Portugal
e-mail: jmf@fct.unl.pt

© Springer Nature Switzerland AG 2021
N. P. Suh et al. (eds.), *Design Engineering and Science*,
https://doi.org/10.1007/978-3-030-49232-8_11

11.1   Introduction

Axiomatic Design consists of a simple and logical general design framework to deal
with the design of products, services, or organizations. It provides designers with
criteria to support decision-making along with all the steps of the designing process.
Figure 11.1 depicts a simple workflow for the AD framework.

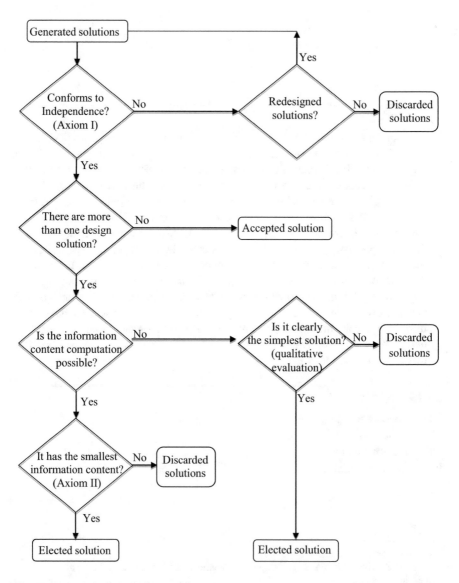

Fig. 11.1 An Axiomatic Design workflow

True Story: "Poor" Ph.D. Candidate!

Sometimes academic research and academic career can be challenging in many different ways, especially to be a graduate student working on what appears to be a simple idea! Sometimes, it can be more challenging to advance "simple ideas" than solve some "complex problems." Appearance can be deceiving in many fields, but especially in academia!

When a young professor was invited to join the faculty of a renowned technological university, he was overjoyed. The only problem was that the salary offer was much less than what he had been receiving at the current university he had been teaching for a few years. Furthermore, the housing cost and the tax on the house in the region where the technical university was located was at least double the cost of where he was. With three small children to educate, the offer was not as attractive as it first appeared. However, his wife thought that it would be a good thing for children's education to go to the more expensive area and suffer financially! She had always been right on these matters, so they left a comfortable place and went to a more challenging environment.

When he got to the new university, there were many prominent professors in the department. Many of them were his professor when he was a student there a few years back. Furthermore, to earn his tenure, he could not offend too many of these senior professors. However, that was the first thing this young professor did! He came up with a view that the design education that had been taught at the university, which had been well recognized throughout the world, needs to be improved! The eminent professor in design and his younger professors in design believed in the notion that "design can be learned only through experience and no lectures and research are needed." Therefore, when this new young professor proposed a contrary view, his new view was not well received, not only at this university but also throughout the national and international community of traditional design professors! Many openly criticized him. Since he had not yet had a tenured appointment, he told his wife that they should be mentally prepared to seek another job. Fortunately, the primary national funding agency for research liked his new idea on design and gave substantial funding to his design research project. Fortunately, he also got his tenure soon after he joined this new university—before the mandatory tenure date. Therefore, he could pursue his idea for a new design approach without worrying about his job!

Four graduate students were hired to work on AD. They all suffered since there was no precedent for the research they were conducting. One Ph.D. student was dealing with the question: "what is INFORMATION?" The second Axiom stated that the information content should be minimized." He and his professor struggled with this question of information content and other related questions. They could not even state clearly the meaning of "information content." They struggled with the question: "Is there more information in a square than in a circle?"

Somehow, this first Ph.D. student put together a doctoral thesis, which his advisor thought was good enough for his doctorate and should get his degree. The fact that he and his wife wanted to raise a family and that he had received an excellent job offer also weighed in on the decision of his advisor.

On the day of his thesis examination, the room was full of design professors. After the presentation, the senior professor in the design section of the department refused to pass him based on what the student presented, although his advisor explained the difficulty of his thesis topic! The objection was more on the research the young professor was conducting than what the graduate student had done! There was a shouting match between the Ph.D. candidate and the traditional design professor.

The faculty vote was against accepting the doctoral thesis by this student. The student stayed another six more months and finally passed the thesis examination. The contribution of his thesis was that it established the problematic questions the group had to answer related to the second axiom, i.e., "Minimize the information content." The notion that the information in design is related to tolerances versus the nominal dimension was advanced, which was a promising beginning in formalizing the second axiom. Also, the idea that the information is related to the "design range" and the "system range" was advanced. Once these ideas were crystallized, much progress has been made, but the first Ph.D. student had to take the brunt of criticisms. Some people compared what this first Ph.D. student had gone through to what happens to the first-born piglet. A pig gives birth to many piglets at the same time, but the first piglet suffers the most to come out of the womb! The professor still thinks that he did a great job! Later many other researchers joined the AD research group and made many important contributions, including visiting professors, Professors H. Nakazawa and Professor G. Solenius.

The length of the Shore Line of Australia!

Sometimes, it is complicated to answer simple questions related to information, especially those related to geometry. For example, what is the length of the shoreline of Australia? How much information do we need to specify the length of the shoreline? Is it difficult to answer it? Why?

The difficulty is that although we draw shorelines around Australia, it is only approximate because what is presented as a straight line is made up of jagged lines. If we look at the jagged lines in higher magnification, they are made of more jagged lines. Mathematicians call it a "fractal," a subset of Euclidean geometry. Fractal appears to be nearly the same at different levels of magnification. However, the area does not change much although the actual length can be much longer. Likewise, when we determine the information content related to FRs and DPs, we have to define the tolerance we need to satisfy within which we define these quantities. That is the functional independence is defined by the tolerance of interference we are willing to tolerate. Similar comments apply to DPs and PVs.

Similarly, when we specify FRs, DPs, and PVs, we have to define the tolerance within which we must satisfy them.

As it was shown in the previous chapter, the functional independence clearly distinguishes the preferred design alternatives. This is the case of the uncoupled and the decoupled design solutions, while coupled solutions shall be discarded or reformulated to attain functional independence. The Independence Axiom is therefore an early acceptance criterion for alternative solutions.

When more than one suitable design alternative exists, then the question that arises is: which solution is the best one? The answer can be found through the Information Axiom.

The process terminates after a number of iterations, according to the designer's criterion.

11.2   The Information Axiom

The Information Axiom provides the last criterion in the choice of the best design solution. It can be stated as (Suh 2005, p. 23):

Minimize the information content of the design;

or, alternatively, as Park (2007, p. 18):

The best design is a functionally uncoupled design that has minimum information content;

or yet as Gonçalves-Coelho et al. (2005):

In a set of designs that satisfy the same FRs and conform to the independence axiom, the best is the one with the minimum information content.

The Information Axiom lays on the information content, similar to that defined by Shannon (1948), which is based on the probability of success of each solution. For a single FR design, the mathematical expression of the information content, I, is:

$$I = -\log_2 p = \log_2\left(\frac{1}{p}\right) \tag{11.1}$$

where p is the probability of success of achieving a given FR.

Therefore, the information content of a design is null when its success is always guaranteed. For any other value of the probability between 0 and 1, the information content will be a positive number.

If the probability density function (pdf) of the existing FR is known, then the probability of accomplishing the FR can be computed by a quotient of areas, as shown in Fig. 11.2.

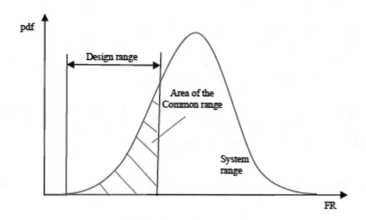

Fig. 11.2 The system range, the design range, and the common range

In Fig. 11.2, the system range represents the whole ability of the system, while the design range represents the working range that the designer is looking for. The common range is the intersection of the system and design ranges.

Most of the designs have a set of FRs that are satisfied by a set of DPs. The information content of those designs is a measure of the probability of the simultaneous success of all the FRs. Then, the information content of a design with m FRs is given by:

$$I_{\text{total}} = \sum_{i=1}^{m} I_i \qquad (11.2)$$

The probability of success, p_i, of satisfying FR_i is expressed by:

$$p_i = \int_{\text{design range}} p(FR_i)dFR_i \qquad (11.3)$$

or, graphically, by:

$$p_i = \frac{\text{Area Common Range}}{\text{Area System Range}} \qquad (11.4)$$

In some cases, a uniform distribution is assumed as an approximation.

11.3 Independence and Information Content

There are two types of designs where independence is fulfilled: uncoupled designs and decoupled designs. Uncoupled designs are always preferable to decoupled designs. Theorems 6 and 7 (Suh 2005, p. 46) relative to path dependency apply.

Theorem 6—*The information content of an uncoupled design is independent of the sequence by which the DPs are changed to satisfy the given set of FRs.*

Theorem 7—*The information contents of coupled and decoupled designs depend on the sequence by which the DPs are changed to satisfy the given set of FRs.*

In uncoupled designs, each DP only affects one FR. As a consequence, the order in which they are attained is irrelevant and the information content of the design I_{total}, is the algebraic sum of the individual information content, I_i, of the m FRs:

$$I_{\text{total}} = \sum_{i=1}^{m} I_i = -\sum_{i=1}^{m} \log_2 p_i = -\log_2 \left(\prod_{i=1}^{m} p_i \right) = -\log_2 p_{\text{total}} \qquad (11.5)$$

Example 11.1

Consider a game that consists of throwing a dice once and withdrawing a card from a 52-card deck. A prize is awarded to anyone who has a "six" in the dice and a "king" in the cards. What is the probability of success? What is the information content of the designed game (in the player viewpoint)?

Solution: The result of the game is made of two independent events which order does not matter. Therefore:

$$p_{\text{total}} = p_1 \times p_2 = \frac{1}{6} \times \frac{4}{52} = \frac{1}{78}$$

and

$$I = -\log_2\left(\frac{1}{78}\right) \simeq 6,29$$

Example 11.2

The owner of a small coffee shop intends to provide customers with a new game consisting of the sequential throwing of two darts on a single target. Players earn a prize when they hit both darts in the center of the target. There are two alternatives (A and B) for the shape of the target, as shown in Fig. 11.3. Considering that the players always hit the target, what is the best game in the owner's viewpoint?

Solution: In both cases, the two events (throwings) are independent. So, their probabilities of success are:

$$\text{Area}_{\text{center } A} = 80^2 = 6400 \quad \text{Area}_{\text{center } B} = \pi \times 50^2 = \pi \times 2500$$

$$\text{Area}_{\text{total } A} = 300^2 = 90000 \quad \text{Area}_{\text{total } B} = \pi \times 200^2 = \pi \times 40000$$

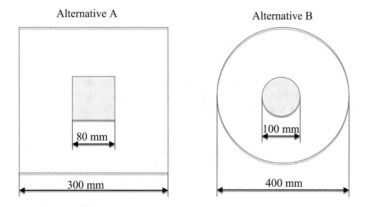

Fig. 11.3 Two alternatives for an arrow launching game

$$p_A = \frac{6400}{90000} \simeq 0,0711 \quad p_B = \frac{\pi \times 2500}{\pi \times 40000} = 0,0625$$

The coffee shop would have better profitability with alternative B because alternative A is easier for the players.

Decoupled designs are designs where independence is also assured, but there is one only order to fulfil the FRs without the need of reiteration. Consider the 2-FR, 2-DP decoupled design equation presented below:

$$\begin{Bmatrix} FR_1 \\ FR_2 \end{Bmatrix} = \begin{bmatrix} \times & 0 \\ \times & \times \end{bmatrix} \begin{Bmatrix} DP_1 \\ DP_2 \end{Bmatrix} \tag{11.6}$$

To satisfy both FRs at the first attempt, one should begin by choosing the value of DP_1 as to satisfy FR_1. The chosen value of DP_1 also affects FR_2, which must be then fulfilled by choosing the value of DP_2. The information content of this design depends on the sequence by which DP_1 and DP_2 are chosen to satisfy FR_1 and FR_2. The satisfaction of FR_1 through DP_1 has a certain probability, p_1, but the satisfaction of FR_2 through DP_2 only occurs after satisfaction of FR_1 trough DP_1. This is a case of conditional probability. The probability of satisfying FR_2 is

$$P_{(2\backslash 1)} = \frac{P_{(1 \cap 2)}}{p_2} \tag{11.7}$$

and the probability of success of the design is

$$p_s = p_1 \times P_{(2\backslash 1)} \tag{11.8}$$

The probability of success of a decoupled design with m FRs and the same number of DPs, is

$$p_s = p_1 \times P_{(2\backslash 1)} \times P_{(3\backslash 2)} \times \ldots \times P_{(m\backslash m-1)} \tag{11.9}$$

It should be noted that in practice, the conditional probability is difficult to determine during the design phase.

Example 11.3

Consider that a given design requires that a body with mass, m, to slide on an inclined plane that makes a θ angle relative to the horizontal. The body should reach certain acceleration, a, and should exert a normal force on the plane, F_N, within the following limits:

$$3\,\text{ms}^{-2} \leq a \leq 5\,\text{ms}^{-2} \tag{11.10}$$

$$0.5\,\text{N} \leq F_N \leq 4\,\text{N} \tag{11.11}$$

The designer has two alternative devices, A and B, embodied by a mass, m, and by a plan with the slope angle θ, within the following ranges:

$$\text{Device A}: \quad 0.1 \text{ kg} \le m_A \le 0.5 \text{ kg} \tag{11.12}$$

$$10° \le \theta_A° \le 30° \tag{11.13}$$

$$\text{Device B}: \quad 0.5 \text{ kg} \le m_B \le 2 \text{ kg} \tag{11.14}$$

$$20° \le \theta_B° \le 60° \tag{11.15}$$

Which device is the preferable one? Which one has the smaller information content?

Solution: In the context of this example, Eqs. (11.10) and (11.11) describe the design range and Eqs. (11.12), (11.13), (11.14), (11.15) denote the system ranges of the two devices. Figure 11.4 depicts the vector diagram of the devices.

The relations between the FRs a and F_N, and the DPs m and θ, are given by

$$a = g \sin \theta \tag{11.16}$$

$$F_N = mg \cos \theta \tag{11.17}$$

where g is the gravitational acceleration. For the sake of simplicity, its value will be considered as 10 ms^{-2}.

If there is no friction, the design equation is

$$\left\{ \begin{array}{c} a \\ F_N \end{array} \right\} = \begin{bmatrix} \times & 0 \\ \times & \times \end{bmatrix} \left\{ \begin{array}{c} \theta \\ m \end{array} \right\} \tag{11.18}$$

Equation (11.18) depicts a decoupled design, where a definite order in the fulfillment of the FRs must be followed by virtue of the independence axiom: First, selecting the value of θ determines a, then selecting the value of m, together with the previously chosen value of θ, determines F_N. Thus, the total probability of success, p_s, is given by

Fig. 11.4 Vector diagram of the devices

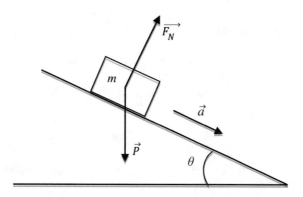

$$p_s = p_1 p_{2\backslash 1} \tag{11.19}$$

For the device A,

$$a_{A\min} = 10 \times \sin 10° \simeq 1.74 \text{ ms}^{-2}$$

$$a_{A\max} = 10 \times \sin 30° = 5 \text{ ms}^{-2}$$

$$p_{1A} = \frac{5 - 3}{5 - 1.74} \simeq 0.613$$

The common range varies between 3 ms^{-2} and 5 ms^{-2}. So, these are the values for a to be considered for the normal force, F_N. An acceleration of 3 ms^{-2} corresponds to an angle of 17.4°.

$$F_{NA\min} = m_{\min}g \cos \theta_{\max} = 0.1 \times 10 \times \cos 30° \simeq 0.866 \text{ N}$$

$$F_{NA\max} = m_{\max}g \cos \theta_{\min} = 0.5 \times 10 \times \cos 17.4° \simeq 0.470 \text{ N}$$

$$p_{2\backslash 1A} = \frac{0.866 - 0.5}{0.866 - 0.470} \simeq 0.924$$

$$p_A = p_{1A}p_{2\backslash 1A} \simeq 0.613 \times 0.924 \simeq 0.566 \quad I_A \simeq 0.82$$

For the device B,

$$a_{B\min} = 10 \times \sin 20° \simeq 3.42 \text{ ms}^{-2}$$

$$a_{B\max} = 10 \times \sin 60° \simeq 8.66 \text{ ms}^{-2}$$

$$p_{1B} = \frac{5 - 3.42}{8.66 - 3.42} \simeq 0.302$$

The common range varies between 3.42 ms^{-2} and 5 ms^{-2}. These are the values for a to be considered for the normal force, F_N. An acceleration of 5 ms^{-2} corresponds to an angle of 30°.

$$F_{NB\min} = m_{\min}g \cos \theta_{\max} = 0.5 \times 10 \times \cos 60° \simeq 2.5 \text{ N}$$

$$F_{NB\max} = m_{\max}g \cos \theta_{\min} = 2 \times 10 \times \cos 30° = 10 \text{ N}$$

$$p_{2\backslash 1B} = \frac{4 - 2.5}{10 - 2.5} = 0.2$$

$$p_B = p_{1B}p_{2\backslash 1B} \simeq 0.302 \times 0.2 \simeq 0.060 \quad I_B \simeq 4.06$$

Device A has a higher probability of success and consequently the smaller information content. Accordingly, device A is the best alternative solution.

11.4   The Computation of Information Content of Decoupled Designs Through Graphical Methods

The computation of the information content of decoupled designs is a hard task. A graphical method to deal with 2-FR, 2-DP decoupled designs with uniform probability density FRs was developed by Suh (2001, p. 528) and Park (2007, p. 38).

For this case, the random variations of the FRs due to the random variations of the DPs are given by

$$\begin{Bmatrix} \delta FR_1 \\ \delta FR_2 \end{Bmatrix} = \begin{bmatrix} A_{11} & 0 \\ A_{21} & A_{22} \end{bmatrix} \begin{Bmatrix} \delta DP_1 \\ \delta DP_2 \end{Bmatrix} \Leftrightarrow \begin{cases} \delta FR_1 = A_{11}\delta DP_1 \\ \delta FR_2 = A_{21}\delta DP_1 + A_{22}\delta DP_2 \end{cases} \quad (11.20)$$

Equation (11.20) shows that δFR_1 is statistically independent, while δFR_2 is statistically dependent with respect to δFR_1.

Let us consider $A_{ij} \geq 0$, as well as the tolerance ranges:

$$-\Delta FR_i \leq \delta FR_i \leq \Delta FR_i \quad (11.21)$$

$$-\Delta DP_i \leq \delta DP_i \leq \Delta DP_i \quad (11.22)$$

Combining Eqs. (11.20), (11.21), and (11.22), we have the limit lines of the system range and of the design range in the physical domain:

$$-\Delta FR_1 \leq A_{11}\delta DP_1 \leq \Delta FR_1 \quad (11.23)$$

$$-\Delta FR_2 \leq A_{21}\delta DP_1 + A_{22}\delta DP_2 \leq \Delta FR_2 \quad (11.24)$$

$$-\Delta DP_1 \leq \delta DP_1 \leq \Delta DP_1 \quad (11.25)$$

$$-\Delta DP_2 \leq \delta DP_2 \leq \Delta DP_2 \quad (11.26)$$

In a similar way, for the functional domain, we have:

$$-\Delta FR_1 \leq \delta FR_1 \leq \Delta FR_1 \quad (11.27)$$

$$-\Delta FR_2 \leq \delta FR_2 \leq \Delta FR_2 \quad (11.28)$$

$$-A_{11}\Delta DP_1 \leq \delta FR_1 \leq A_{11}\Delta DP_1 \quad (11.29)$$

$$-A_{22}\Delta DP_2 \le \delta FR_2 - \frac{A_{21}}{A_{11}}\delta FR_1 \le A_{22}\Delta DP_2 \qquad (11.30)$$

Figure 11.5 depicts Eqs. (11.20)–(11.22) in the physical domain.

The parallelogram [ABCD] of Fig. 11.5 is the system range of the design, while the quadrilateral [EFGH] is the design range and the hexagon [IFJKHL] is the common range. Thus, for the case of uniform pdfs, the information content is given by

$$I = \log_2\left(\frac{1}{p}\right) = \log_2\left(\frac{\text{Area of quadrilateral EFGH}}{\text{Area of hexagon IFJKHL}}\right) \qquad (11.31)$$

The areas of the quadrilateral and of the hexagon can be analytically computed. Those areas can be much more easily evaluated using a 2D CAD system capable of measuring areas of closed polygons.

By the same token, the functional domain of the 2-FR, 2-DP decoupled design of Fig. 11.5 can be depicted in Fig. 11.6, by using Eqs. (11.27)–(11.30).

Notice that this graphical method is valid only for uniform pdfs. The method can be extended to 3-FR, 3-DP decoupled designs with uniform pdfs (Fradinho et al. 2017). The random variation of the generic FRs, δFR_i, due to the random variation of the DPs, δDP_i, is expressed by

$$\begin{Bmatrix} \delta FR_1 \\ \delta FR_2 \\ \delta FR_3 \end{Bmatrix} = \begin{bmatrix} A_{11} & 0 & 0 \\ A_{21} & A_{22} & 0 \\ A_{31} & A_{32} & A_{33} \end{bmatrix}\begin{Bmatrix} \delta DP_1 \\ \delta DP_2 \\ \delta DP_3 \end{Bmatrix}$$
$$\Leftrightarrow \begin{cases} \delta FR_1 = A_{11}\delta DP_1 \\ \delta FR_2 = A_{21}\delta DP_1 + A_{22}\delta DP_2 \\ \delta FR_1 = A_{31}\delta DP_1 + A_{32}\delta DP_2 + A_{33}\delta DP_3 \end{cases} \qquad (11.32)$$

Fig. 11.5 The isogram of a 2-FR, 2-DP decoupled design in the physical domain. (Reproduced from Fradinho et al. (2017), originally published open access under a CC BY 4.0 license: https://doi.org/10.1051/matecconf/201712701004)

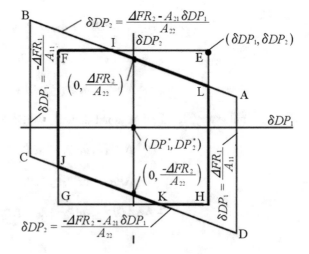

Fig. 11.6 The isogram of a 2-FR, 2-DP decoupled design in the functional domain

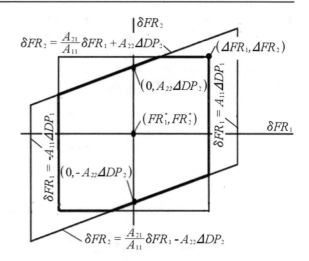

Considering unbiased tolerance ranges, and that

$\Delta FR_i \geq 0$; $\Delta DP_j \geq 0$; $A_{ij} \geq 0$;
δDP_j are statistically independent;
δFR_2 is statistically dependent to δFR_1;
δFR_3 is statistically dependent to δFR_1 and δFR_2.

From Eq. (11.25), one can obtain the shapes of the system range and of the design range in the physical domain:

$$-\Delta FR_1 \leq A_{11}\delta DP_1 \leq \Delta FR_1 \tag{11.33}$$

$$-\Delta FR_2 \leq A_{21}\delta DP_1 + A_{22}\delta DP_2 \leq \Delta FR_2 \tag{11.34}$$

$$-\Delta FR_3 \leq A_{31}\delta DP_1 + A_{32}\delta DP_2 + A_{33}\delta DP_3 \leq \Delta FR_3 \tag{11.35}$$

$$-\Delta DP_1 \leq \delta DP_1 \leq \Delta DP_1 \tag{11.36}$$

$$-\Delta DP_2 \leq \delta DP_2 \leq \Delta DP_2 \tag{11.37}$$

$$-\Delta DP_3 \leq \delta DP_3 \leq \Delta DP_3 \tag{11.38}$$

The first three conditions characterize the system range and the last three denote the design range.

The system range is the intersection of three pairs of semi-spaces. The first condition represents two profile planes that are parallel to the lateral projection plane and orthogonal to the δDP_1 axis; the second one represents two vertical planes that are parallel to δDP_3 axis and orthogonal to the horizontal projection plane; and the third condition represents two planes that are oblique to the three projection planes. The design range is a rectangular parallelepiped that is centered in the origin.

Similarly, the equations of the design range and of the system range in the functional domain are given by

$$-\Delta FR_1 \leq \delta FR_1 \leq \Delta FR_1 \tag{11.39}$$

$$-\Delta FR_2 \leq \delta FR_2 \leq \Delta FR_2 \tag{11.40}$$

$$-\Delta FR_3 \leq \delta FR_3 \leq \Delta FR_3 \tag{11.41}$$

$$-A_{11}\Delta DP_1 \leq \delta FR_1 \leq A_{11}\Delta DP_1 \tag{11.42}$$

$$-A_{22}\Delta DP_2 \leq \delta FR_2 - \frac{A_{21}}{A_{11}}\delta FR_1 \leq A_{22}\Delta DP_2 \tag{11.43}$$

$$-A_{33}\Delta DP_3 \leq \delta FR_3 - \frac{A_{32}}{A_{22}}\delta FR_2 - \left(\frac{A_{31}}{A_{11}} - \frac{A_{21}A_{32}}{A_{11}A_{22}}\right)\delta FR_1 \leq A_{33}\Delta DP_3 \tag{11.44}$$

In the physical domain, the system range is determined by six planes. Figure 11.7 shows the intersections of the six planes with the orthogonal projection planes. The values of A_{ij}, ΔFR_i and ΔDP_j were considered as positive in the graphical representation. Thus, the vertical and the oblique planes are opened to the right.

Figure 11.8 depicts the resulting geometric solid, which is a six-face polyhedron centered in the origin and composed of three pairs of parallel faces. Four of those faces are defined by the profile planes (π and π') and the vertical planes (θ and θ'). All these four planes are orthogonal to the horizontal projection plane. The upper and the lower limits of the polyhedron are the oblique planes (α and α').

The design range is a quadrangular prism that is also centered in the origin.

The system range is the six-face polyhedron [ABCDA'B'C'D'] with two profile faces ([ADA'D'] and [BCB'C']), two vertical faces ([ABA'B'] and [CDC'D']), and two oblique faces ([ABCD] and [A'B'C'D']).

The design range is the quadrangular prism [EFGHE'F'G'H'] with faces that are parallel to the projection planes.

The common range is the ten-face polyhedron [AA'''II'JJ'KL'C''C'MM'NN'PQ'], which is the intersection of those two solids and is made of five pairs of parallel faces.

The coordinates of all the vertices are easily computed because each one results from the intersection of three known planes.

The probability of success of this design, p_s, is given by

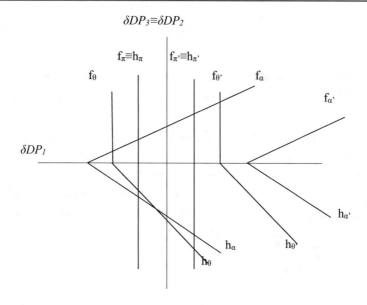

Fig. 11.7 The six planes that determine the system range in the physical domain of a 3-FR, 3-DP decoupled design. (Reproduced from Fradinho et al. (2017), originally published open access under a CC BY 4.0 license: https://doi.org/10.1051/matecconf/201712701004)

Fig. 11.8 The system, the design, and the common ranges in the physical domain of a 3-FR, 3-DP decoupled design. (Reproduced from Fradinho et al. (2017), originally published open access under a CC BY 4.0 license: https://doi.org/10.1051/matecconf/201712701004)

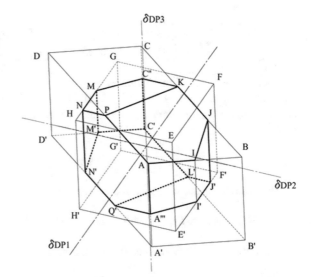

$$p_s = \frac{V_c}{V_{dp}} \tag{11.45}$$

where V_c is the volume of the common range and V_{dp} is the tolerance volume for the DPs, which is the design range.

Example 11.4

The design depicted in Fig. 11.7 will be used as an example, where the following data is assumed:

Profile planes intersect the δDP_1 axis at points 2 and (-2);

Vertical planes intersect the δDP_1 axis at points 3 and (-3) and open $45°$ to the right;

Oblique planes intersect the δDP_1 axis at points 4 and (-4) and open $45°$ to the right;

$\Delta FR_1 = 2$ length units;
$\Delta FR_2 = 3$ length units;
$\Delta FR_3 = 4 \tan 35°$ length units.

$$A_{11} = A_{22} = A_{33} = 1$$

$\Delta DP_1 = \Delta DP_2 = DP_3 = 3$ length units.

As a result, from Eq. (11.32), the design equation of this decoupled design is

$$\begin{Bmatrix} \delta FR_1 \\ \delta FR_2 \\ \delta FR_3 \end{Bmatrix} = \begin{bmatrix} 1 & 0 & 0 \\ 1 & 1 & 0 \\ \tan 35° & 1 & 1 \end{bmatrix} \begin{Bmatrix} \delta DP_1 \\ \delta DP_2 \\ \delta DP_3 \end{Bmatrix} \tag{11.46}$$

Thus, the volume of the common range, V_c, is the volume of the feasible range represented by the polyhedron [AA‴II′JJ′KL′C″C′MM′NN′PQ′]. This volume can be computed, although very hard to attain. Therefore, a 3D solid modeler software was used to evaluate V_c.

$$V_c = 90,31 \text{ volume units} \tag{11.47}$$

The volume of the tolerance region for the DPs, V_{dp}, is

$$V_{dp} = 8 \times \Delta DP_1 \times \Delta DP_2 \times DP_3 = 216,000 \text{ volume units} \tag{11.48}$$

Thus, the probability of success and the information content are given by

$$p_s = \frac{90,31}{216,00} \simeq 0,42 \tag{11.49}$$

$$I = -\log_2 p_s \simeq 1,26 \tag{11.50}$$

If ΔDP_1, ΔDP_2, and ΔDP_3 were sufficiently small, then the whole design range would be contained in the system range and the information content would be null.

11.5 Information Content and Robustness

The Information Axiom states that, among designs that conform to independence, the best is the one with the minimum information content. In Sect. 11.2, it was shown that the information content decreases (or the probability of success increases) when the area of the common range increases. The minimum information content can be achieved by moving the median value of the design range to the median value of the system range. This distance is called bias. Thus, a small or null bias should always be preferred. This may be easy for designs that conform to independence because each FR can be tuned through a DP only.

Another way to increase the area of the common range is to extend the design range. Designs that allow large random variations in the DPs with small response deviation are known as robust designs. One of the possible strategies to increase the robustness of design is to identify the limit values of the largest range of the DP that achieves the looked-for functional tolerance range.

The relationship between a FR and the corresponding DP is either already known or may be experimentally determined. Graphically, it can be represented by a line, as shown in Fig. 11.9.

For a certain ΔFR, $(\Delta DP)_1$ represents the DP limits for a design, between points A and B, while $(\Delta DP)_2$ represents the DP limits between points C and D. Since $(\Delta DP)_2$ is larger than $(\Delta DP)_1$, then $(\Delta DP)_2$ corresponds to a more robust design. The most robust design is the one with the smallest absolute value of the average variation rate between the DP limits. In other words, the preferable situation is the one with the smallest slope modulus of the straight line linking the two points of the curve.

Robust designs have a small information content and large capacity to allow DP random variations with small disturbance of their response.

Fig. 11.9 Different design ranges for the same functional tolerance

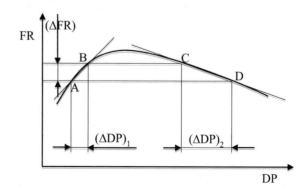

11.6 Summary

This chapter presents the Information Axiom and the meaning of information content. For simple designs it is presented how to make the computation of the information content, and it is shown that it measures the probability of success of the design.

The computation of information content is only possible for designs that conform to independence (uncoupled and decoupled designs). Three simple examples with two FRs were presented.

The computation of the information content of decoupled designs is hard to preform because it involves the use of conditional probability. A graphical method is presented to compute the information content of 2-FR, 2-DP and 3-FR, 3-DP decoupled designs considering uniform probability density for FRs.

Finally, the concept of robust design is discussed, and desirable design ranges withdrawn from the analytical relationships between FRs and DPs are indicated.

Problems

1. Explain the following expression according to the Information Axiom of AD:

$$I_{\text{total}} = -\sum_{i=1}^{n} \log_2 p_i = -\log_2 \prod_{i=1}^{n} p_i = \sum_{i=1}^{n} I_i$$

2. Comment the following statement: "The calculation of the information content of a decoupled design implies the use of conditional probability."
3. The following figure shows the probability density function (pdf) of the system range of a certain FR with a uniform distribution. The figure also shows the limits of the design range and of the common range. Explain how the information content for this FR could be computed (Fig. 11.10).
4. Consider the following equations of two designs. Explain how the information content of each design can be calculated.

$$\begin{Bmatrix} FR_1 \\ FR_2 \end{Bmatrix} = \begin{bmatrix} A_{11} & 0 \\ 0 & A_{22} \end{bmatrix} \begin{Bmatrix} DP_1 \\ DP_2 \end{Bmatrix} \qquad \begin{Bmatrix} FR_1 \\ FR_2 \end{Bmatrix} = \begin{bmatrix} B_{11} & B_{12} \\ 0 & B_{22} \end{bmatrix} \begin{Bmatrix} DP_1 \\ DP_2 \end{Bmatrix}$$

5. The following figure shows the pdf of a design with one only FR. The figure also shows the design range of three possible solutions (A, B, and C). According to AD theory, which solution is the best one? And the worst? Why? (Fig. 11.11)

Fig. 11.10 Pdf of a uniform distribution

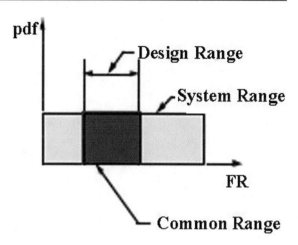

Fig. 11.11 Non-uniform pdf of a design

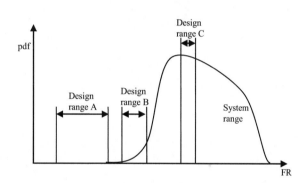

References

Fradinho J, Cavique M, Gabriel-Santos A, Mourão, A, Gonçalves-Coelho A (2017) How to compute the information content of 3-FR, 3-DP decoupled designs with uniform probability density functions for their FRs. In: MATEC web of conferences, vol 127, no. 01004, The 11th International Conference on Axiomatic Design (ICAD 2017). https://doi.org/10.1051/matecconf/201712701004

Gonçalves-Coelho A, Mourão A, Pereira ZL (2005) Improving the use of QFD with axiomatic design. Concur Eng Res Appl 13(3):233–239. https://doi.org/10.1177/1063293X05056787

Park GJ (2007) Analytic methods for design practice. Springer-Verlag, London

Shannon CE (1948) A mathematical theory of communication. Bell Syst Techn J 27(3):279–423, 623–656

Suh NP (2001) Axiomatic design—advances and applications. Oxford University Press, NY

Suh NP (2005) Complexity. Oxford University Press, NY

Complexity in Axiomatic Design

12

Erik Christian Nicolaas Puik

Abstract

In the previous chapter, the concept of information in design was introduced. It was shown how the Information Axiom could be applied to increase the robustness of processes. It was also shown that the axioms in Axiomatic Design (AD) should be addressed in a distinct order.

In this chapter, four different kinds of complexity in AD are explained that can be applied for typical situations. Also, a way to visualize complexity in design is introduced; the "Functionality Diagram."

After studying this chapter, the reader should know the following:
The reader will understand the particular but powerful definition complexity of in AD, which kinds of complexity in AD have been defined, and how they can be applied. The reader will also learn how to apply complexity in functionality diagrams, that offers a powerful way to visualize the design process as it evolves over time.

12.1 Motivation for the Complexity Theory in Axiomatic Design

So far, this book has been focusing on two axioms: (i) the Independence Axiom and (ii) the Information Axiom. In this chapter, a third axiom will be introduced and explained: The "Complexity Axiom."

E. C. N. Puik (✉)
Knowledge Centre for Healthy and Sustainable Living, HU University op Applied Sciences Utrecht, Postbus 182 Padualaan 99, Utrecht 3584 CH, The Netherlands
e-mail: erik.puik@hu.nl

© Springer Nature Switzerland AG 2021
N. P. Suh et al. (eds.), *Design Engineering and Science*,
https://doi.org/10.1007/978-3-030-49232-8_12

12.1.1 Applying a Complexity Theory to Real Problems

After the AD methodology was refined for over 20 years, it appeared still difficult to explain simple things such as "How do we control the semiconductor processing machines such as the track machine to maximize productivity?", "Why is the control of job shops (i.e., machine shops) so difficult?", "How does mitosis work so well?", "Why did the GM ignition key fail, killing several people?", and, "Why did it take so long to build the new Berlin airport?", etc. These systems appear to have high complexity. Trying to understand why some commercial and industrial systems have so many problems, Professor Nam Suh started to study Shannon's information theory that was also invoked by many others to investigate complexity in scientific literature. After spending quite some time trying to understand what they had done, he concluded that there wasn't a practical and accurate definition of the concept of "complexity." All variations in literature defined complexity as a mathematical issue but that approach does not seem suitable for AD that is focusing to solve real problems. The conclusion was that complexity is a design issue.

If a task cannot be achieved, it looks complex. For instance, even a short computer software program appears to be complex when it is a coupled design. It is not the length of the program that creates the complexity of a software system, but the coupling of FRs. Some computer scientists unsuccessfully tried to explain complexity in terms of the length of the software code.

If we cannot solve real problems, the theory is not useful in the field of design and engineering. The complexity theory on AD tries to change this and apply the concept of complexity in a practical manner, enabling the capability to address real problems in practice.

12.1.2 What is Complexity

There is not a single explanation for the term "Complexity", though everyone will have a certain interpretation of the general concept. Also, from a scientific perspective, there are many interpretations of complexity or complex systems. Many of these concepts were inventoried and explained by Suh in the context of AD (Suh 1999). Some interpretations of complexity as were mentioned by him are the following ones:

- Gallagher and Appenzeller define complex systems as systems whose properties are not fully explained by an understanding of its component parts (Gallagher and Appenzeller 1999);
- Goldenfield and Kadanoff state that complexity means that we have a structure with variations. Thus, a living organism is complex because it has many different working parts, each formed by variation in the working out of the same genetic coding (Goldenfeld and Kadanoff 1999);
- Whiteside and Ismagilov state that a complex system is one whose evolution is (i) very sensitive to initial conditions or to small perturbations, one in which the

number of independent interacting components is large, or one in which there are multiple pathways by which the system can evolve and (ii) the system is complicated by some subjective judgment and is not amenable to exact description, analytical, or otherwise (Whitesides and Ismagilov 1999);

- Weng, Bhalla, and Iyengar state that complexity arises from a large number of components, many with isoforms that have partially overlapping functions, from the connections among components; and from the spatial relationship between components (Weng et al. 1999);
- Shannon and Weaver, as well as Gellmann and Lloyd equate complexity with the number of bits of information it takes to describe an object or a message (Shannon and Weaver 1949). Gellmann and Lloyd introduce the concept of "Irregularities" that describes that elements are not organized well and therefore should be considered complex.

In order to be able to imagine what complexity is in daily life, here are some examples of complex systems. It concerns systems that are really difficult to comprehend:

- weather forecasting;
- understanding the interactions in a rainforest;
- understanding the dynamics of social media;
- governing a country;
- understanding and prediction of global warming.

12.2 Theory of Complexity, Periodicity, and the Design Axioms

Among the definitions of complexity, AD has a generic though particular approach of complexity. Where many definitions define complex systems in the physical domain, AD defines the complexity in the functional domain. This means that complexity in AD is not determined by what a system is or what it looks like, but it is determined by the functional behavior of the system. A complex system does not automatically have the capability to perform as it should according to its functional requirements (FRs) and as such its complexity should be reduced. Therefore, the definition of complexity in AD is

- the Complexity Axiom: "Reduce the complexity of a system";
- in which complexity is defined as "A measure of uncertainty in satisfying the FRs".

The Complexity Axiom is also referred to as the "Third Axiom," "Axiom 3," or the "Main Axiom." The Complexity Axiom is directly related to the Independence Axiom and the Information Axiom since their goal is to make sure that the FRs are satisfied accordingly. To be more precise: the Independence and the Information Axioms appear to be a subset of the Complexity Axiom (Puik and Ceglarek 2014a). However, this relation is still being investigated and as such the Independence and the Information Axioms are maintained as unbound axioms for the benefit of the designer.

If we want to deal with complexity, understand and eventually eliminate it, it is essential to perceive what the fundamental cause is of complexity in a system. To understand this cause, it helps to have a closer look at some complex systems:

(1) Let's say the challenge is to replace the front wheel of a car. Even someone who never has done this may understand that the car needs to be lifted by use of the jack. When this task is successfully completed, the next step is to remove the bolts from the wheel. When trying to exceed the torque needed to unscrew the bolts from the wheel hub, it appears that the wheel freely rotates in the air when a torque is applied to the bolts. The bolts needed to be loosened first when the car was still standing on the ground.

   This first example shows a decoupled system. With the right knowledge of the design matrix, it would have been possible to determine the right order to address the DPs on forehand in order to satisfy the FRs. However, without this knowledge, the person resorts to trial and error methods of evaluation trying the possible sequences of addressing the DPs to satisfy the FRs. As long as he has not found the right sequence, the design shows an unwanted response to his actions. This fairly simple problem is uncertain to succeed for people that miss the knowledge and therefore, for them it is a complex task.

(2) A second example is that of a combination lock (Suh 2005a; Foley et al. 2016). A combination lock is hard to open without the right knowledge of the sequence of numbers we have to activate. Using trial and error it is extremely laborious and time-consuming to try all combinations of the lock since the lock was designed to be complex. However, with the knowledge of the right numbers and the instruction manual at hand, the lock is easy to open. Without the right knowledge, opening the lock is quite complex. When the right knowledge is available, opening the lock is not complex at all.

(3) A space shuttle consists of over 2 million parts. A vast majority of these parts should perform within the tolerance window of their FRs to enable safe launch and return. This means that the error margin per part is incredibly low. To satisfy over 2 million FRs with their respective DPs is very complex.

(4) If a designer is sloppy when decomposing the FRs of a system, it can happen that one of FRs with lower hierarchy is forgotten. As the design process continues, there will not be a matching DP appointed for the forgotten FR. As a result, the main FRs (at higher hierarchical levels) will not be satisfied under all conditions. Since it is not known that the FR and DP are missing, the system is misunderstood and seems complex.

All these examples have a common feature and that is that the designer lacks knowledge about the system he is working on. Because of that, it is not possible to fully understand all constituent elements of the system. This lack of knowledge leads to uncertainty in satisfying the FRs, leads to failing systems, and makes a system complex.

If we zoom in further to Complexity in AD, it appears that we have to make a distinction regarding how complexity develops over time. Some kinds of complexity do not change with time, others do strongly depend on time as will be shown in the next sections.

12.2.1 Time-Independent Complexity in Axiomatic Design

This section deals with "Time-Independent" Complexity. This means that the complexity basically does not change with time. It changes due to the involvement of the designer and his environment.

Time-independent complexity consists of two components: "Real" and "Imaginary" time-independent complexity, further to be referred to as real complexity and imaginary complexity (C_R and C_{Im}).

Real Complexity
Real complexity is inversely related to the probability of success that the associated FRs are satisfied according to one of the following relations:

$$C_R = -\sum_{i=1}^{m} \log_b P_i \tag{12.1}$$

$$C_R = -\sum_{i=1}^{m} \log_b P_{i|\{j\}} \quad \text{for } \{j\} = \{1, 2, \ldots, i-1\} \tag{12.2}$$

depending if the system is uncoupled (12.1) or decoupled (12.2). Relation (12.1) is under the reservation that the total probability P_i is the "joint probability of processes that are statistically independent" so the different processes that are summarized do not influence each other. Relation (12.2), for decoupled systems, is modified to correct for dependencies in the probabilistic function (Suh 2005a). "b" Is in both cases the base of the logarithm, usually in bits ($b = 2$) or nats ($b = 2.718$) depending on the preferred definition. Given (12.1) and (12.2), C_R can be related to the information content in AD, which was defined in terms of the probability of success of achieving the desired set of FRs (Suh 1990), as

$$C_{Real} = I \tag{12.3}$$

in which C_R is the real complexity and I being information as defined by the Information Axiom.

C_R is by definition addressed by the Information Axiom. It is addressed by matching the design and system ranges of the product design.

Examples of systems with C_R are

- tolerances of a manufacturing process;
- a paint job of a car with color difference;
- sloppy work of a shoemaker;
- people continuously crossing road markings while driving a car;
- being too late for a job interview.

These examples describe systems that need (constant) attention to be executed well, but when procedures are closely followed they will deliver good results.

Imaginary Complexity

"Imaginary Complexity" is a little harder to understand. Suh defines it as "uncertainty that is no real uncertainty" and "it arises because of the designer's lack of knowledge and understanding" (Suh 2005b). When a design is uncoupled or decoupled, the imaginary component of complexity is equal to zero (Suh 2005b). Note that for a decoupled design this is only guaranteed if the optimization order of the design relations is known. This makes C_{Im} inversely related to the satisfaction of the Independence Axiom; an uncoupled system is a system with no C_{Im}. Vice versa, a coupled system is a complex system.

To illustrate C_{Im}, Suh describes a designer trying to optimize a system without writing down the design equations (Suh 2005a). Even if this design is a decoupled design, the designer will have to resort to trial-and-error methods of evaluation. The design will tend to behave erratically and not conforming his (limited) understanding. He will have to try many different sequences of DP adjustments to see if the FRs get satisfied. There are $n!$ distinct sequences of DPs, of which only one is correct. The probability of finding the right sequence n DPs to find the entire set of m FRs is given by

$$P = \frac{1}{n!} \tag{12.4}$$

The probability of finding the right sequence through a random trial-and-error process goes down rapidly with an increase in the number of DPs, as shown in the table below:

n	n!	P = 1/n!
1	1	1.000
2	2	0.500
3	6	0.1667
4	24	0.04167
5	120	0.8333×10^{-2}
6	720	0.1389×10^{-2}
7	5,040	0.1984×10^{-3}

When $n = 5$, the probability of finding the right sequence is 0.008 per try which is very low. Therefore, this design appears to be quite complex because the uncertainty that a solution is found and the FRs will be satisfied is large. This kind of complexity is typical for C_{Im} and it resides in the designer's head due to a lack of knowledge of the system. C_{Im} is a kind of complexity that is caused by a lack of fundamental understanding of the AD theory and its application. To the designer, a system may look complex, although it may not be when the right knowledge is present.

Examples of systems with C_{Im} are

- you get an assignment on the first day of a new job that requires an understanding of the organization;
- finding your way without a map or GPS in a foreign city;
- cooking without a recipe;
- opening a combination lock without the code;
- you offer a friend to help moving to a new house without knowing how much stuff he owns.

Complex Versus Complicated Systems in AD

We have been elaborating about complex systems. However, in many other complexity theories distinction is made between complex and complicated systems (Snowden 2000; Kurtz and Snowden 2003; Boone and Snowden 2007). These are not the same and for those readers that have experience with other definitions the differences are explained here:

- For complex systems, cause and effect relations are not (yet) understood. This the traditional domain of complexity theories, which study how patterns emerge through the interaction of many elements. It is not that everything in this context is unknown or unsure. However, emerging cause and effect relations that are still fuzzy and the number of elements are too mind-boggling to oversee the situation and analyze it. Emergent patterns can be perceived but not predicted. In the work of Snowden and Boone, this phenomenon is called "retrospective coherence" (Boone and Snowden 2007); things become clear in retrospect, but could not be predicted on forehand. As such, the designer can expect to be surprised as his design is not fully understood yet;
- Complicated systems however, deal with knowable cause and effect relations. Complicated systems, unlike simple ones, may contain multiple right answers, and although there is a clear relationship between cause and effect, not everyone can see it. The fact is that problems can be solved by bringing in the right team of experts, however, the issue is whether we can afford the time and resources to reduce complicated systems to simple systems with clear and documented cause and effect relations. In general, this is not possible and, instead, it relies on expert opinion, which in turn creates a key dependency on trust between expert advisor and decision-maker. Complicated systems need systems thinkers, learning

organizations, and the adaptive enterprise, all of which are too often confused with true complex systems.

By this definition complex systems are systems without a cause and effect relation. Complicated systems are systems that do have a causality but not everyone can see it.

There is an important difference how AD approaches complexity. Due to its definition "A measure of uncertainty in satisfying the FRs," it defines **complexity as an issue that compromises functionality**. This means that any system that lacks the capability to meet the FRs is a complex system. Here emerges a discrepancy in comparison to most complexity theories as described above. A system that is considered "complicated" in other complexity theories may appear to be "complex" in the complexity definition of AD. This is because complexity is considered from the perspective of functionality. If a designer is not able to gather the required knowledge to understand and solve the problem, a system is considered complex according to the definition in AD (note that "the designer" may represent a group of designers with various expertise). Even if the designer would have some understanding of the problem but he is not given enough time to adequately address all issues of the system, it is considered a complex system. Complexity in AD focuses on functional performance, not on implementation, nor on a solution that could be realized by engineers that cannot be mobilized, nor what Einstein could do if he were here.

In summary, the distinction of complex and complicated systems is not made in AD. Both are referred to as C_{Im} and they exist because the designer does not have the knowledge to fully understand the design. Complexity in AD is inversely related to the capability of the designer to address problems well. The result is assessed in the functional domain and depends if the system actually does what it should do.

12.2.2 Time-Dependent Complexity

Sometimes, complexity changes with time. Even if no involvement with a system takes place, it still tends to become more complex. Time-dependent complexity occurs because future events occur in unpredictable ways and therefore the nature of these events also is unpredictable (Suh 2005b). This is caused by a system range that moves away from the design range. The overlap of system and design range will become smaller and the certainty that the FRs will be satisfied by the DPs decreases. This is shown in Fig. 12.1.

There are two kinds of time-dependent complexity:

- combinatorial Complexity;
- periodic Complexity.

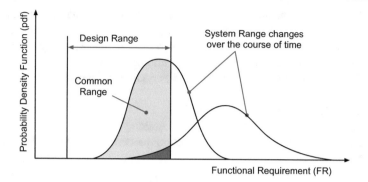

Fig. 12.1 If the system range moves away from the design range in time, the overlap between design range and system range will decrease. Chances that the FRs are successfully satisfied by their DPs is negatively affected

Time-Dependent Combinatorial Complexity

Time-dependent Combinatorial Complexity is defined as the complexity that increases as a function of time due to a continued expansion of the number of combinations with time, which may eventually lead to a chaotic state (Suh 2005a). An example is the airline scheduling problem. When there is a major storm in Chicago, the airplanes that were to arrive in and leave from Chicago cannot operate according to their schedules. In fact, some flights may be canceled. Eventually, this weather in Chicago affects the flight schedules at all the airports that are connected to Chicago either directly or indirectly. As a result, there will be increasing uncertainty in dispatching aircraft as a function of time. This is an example of time-dependent Combinatorial Complexity. When a system is affected by time-dependent Combinatorial Complexity, it eventually breaks down because it will go into a chaotic state.

Examples of systems of time-dependent Combinatorial Complexity are

- a computer that operates slower when active for a longer time;
- a developing traffic jam during traffic hours;
- an increasing failure rate of a production process due to tool wear;
- search for exact and exhausting information on the internet;
- brexit discussions in the UK House of Commons.

Time-Dependent Periodic Complexity

Time-dependent Periodic Complexity can be understood if we go back to the airline scheduling problem caused by a major snowstorm in Chicago. Typically, the airline scheduling problem continues to worsen throughout the day because of the cascading effect of airlines having to make decisions on the deployment of available airplanes. However, since the airline schedule is periodic each day, all of the uncertainties introduced during the course of the day terminate at the end of a 24-h cycle, and hence this Combinatorial Complexity does not extend to the following day. Each day, the schedule starts over again (Suh 2005a). The periodic nature of the airline schedule resets between periods and the uncertainties created during the prior period are irrelevant. Within the same period, complexity may be combinatorial, but over many periods we speak of Periodic Complexity.

Examples of systems of time-dependent Periodic Complexity are

- rebooting your computer every morning;
- a traffic jam that disappears during evening hours;
- a decreasing failure rate of a production process when tools are regularly replaced;
- daily life and its worries;
- even in the UK House of Commons, brexit discussions have ended at some point.

One important conclusion of the complexity theory is that complexity is greatly reduced when a system with time-dependent Combinatorial Complexity is transformed to a system with time-dependent Periodical Complexity. The period is the functional period, not necessarily temporal period, where the same set of functions repeats, i.e., the periodicity does not necessarily have a constant time period. Where Combinatorial Complexity tends to keep emerging further and further till something goes horribly wrong, Periodic Complexity is reset from time to time and because of that it is far more manageable.

Combinatorial- and Periodic Complexity are mostly time-dependent forms of C_R due to the fact that they deal with a changing overlap between system range and design range. In theory, it is possible to distinguish "time-dependent Imaginary Complexity," where even the FRs may change over time, and though they are referred to in literature (Lee 2003) they are extremely hard to deal with since a fix would require conceptual changes of the system.

12.2.3 Limiting Behavioral Options by Banning Irregularities from the Design

A practical view on dealing with Complexity in a design and the uncertainties that arise from it was described by Gell-Mann and Lloyd (1996). As they state, the cause of uncertainties is found in a "Lack of Regularities" of the considered system (in our case a product or system design). The lack of regularities, which may be seen as a missing structure in the design, will be reduced as the knowledge of the designer increases. While the designer is working on his design, the lack of regularities will be reduced as much as the knowledge of the designer permits. It works two ways, (i) a designer that has no knowledge of the design cannot be expected to deliver a well-structured design, and (ii) the irregularities in this ill-structured design will not be addressed (Puik and Ceglarek 2015). As a result, the design will not be regulated well and, at some point, it will show unexpected behavior.

This makes Complexity inversely related to the knowledge of the designer. In a situation where the designer has unlimited time and resources to acquire and implement the right knowledge, the product design will be fully regulated and therefore it will have no freedom of choice in its operation other than the envisioned way by the designer; as a result, all complexity is eliminated from the system and it will behave exactly the way it should; all FRs of the product design satisfied by their DPs.

Summarized, it can be said that the way of looking to a design as proposed by Gell-Mann and Lloyd, leads to an accessible way to deal with complexity in design. Complexity in AD is a measure for the lack of regularities in a product design and it leads to uncontrolled behavior of the system.

12.2.4 Known and Unknown Kinds of Time-Independent Complexity

A problem with complexity in general is that lacking knowledge does not automatically come to the surface. Complexity may show that it is present but may also remain hidden. These are called "Known" and "Unknown" kinds of complexity.

Known and Unknown Kinds of Imaginary Complexity

C_{Im} also has known and unknown variants. In a lucky situation, C_{Im} in the design plays up at some point and warns the designer that he does not yet fully understand his design. A perceptive designer will be alarmed and try to replicate the situation till he learns what irregularities cause unexpected behavior. In the less lucky situation, the designer is not confronted with the system's misbehavior, or he does not acknowledge it. In this case, the C_{Im} stays hidden in the system for some time longer. Note that this is virtually always of a temporary nature; in a later stage, the irregularities in design will play up and need to be restricted by an appropriate design solution.

Based on these examples, two specific kinds of C_{Im} may be recognized:

The first one is "*Unrecognized Imaginary Complexity*," the subset of C_{Im} that is not recognized by the designer and therefore remains hidden in the system. It may be addressed by the determination of the right FRs, DPs, and PVs. However, this will typically not happen because the designer is not aware of its existence.

Examples of Unrecognized C_{Im} are

- a cook trying to copy a recipe, however, without exactly knowing what the right ingredients are;
- partial modelling of a system (when elemental parts were forgotten);
- a DP that was not recognized that changes an FR.

Second, "*Recognized, Imaginary Complexity*" is the subset on C_{Im} that indeed is recognized by the designer, however, the knowledge to address the problem is lacking. Because of this, it cannot yet be eliminated from the design. It is addressed by definition of the right design matrix and successively decoupling it.

Examples of Recognized C_{Im} are

- during the design process, it appears that a conceptual error was made and the design matrix needs repair but this has far-reaching consequences;
- insufficient means or time to address a problem, or the problem needs to be solved by an external party;
- the back-log in a Scrum session.

Known and Unknown Kinds of Real Complexity

Analog to C_{Im}, it is also possible to decompose C_R one step further.

Comparable to the definition above, "*Unrecognized, Real Complexity*" is the subset of C_R that is not recognized by the designer and therefore remains hidden in the system. It is addressed by the knowledge how the DPs satisfy the FRs.

Examples of Unrecognized C_R are

- A German car manufacturer was suddenly confronted with the problem that the windshields showed large cracks within hours after completion of the manufacturing process. It appeared to be a problem with the material properties of the glass material. It took 6 weeks to find the cause and understand the problem and another four weeks to fix the problem;
- A manufacturing process that runs out of its operating window without the cause being known;
- A redundant situation where drifting DP's compensate for each other's deviations. The related FR will remain satisfied but the system might be operating out of their design ranges.

And second "*Recognized, Real Complexity*" is the subset of C_R that indeed is recognized by the designer but cannot yet be eliminated from the design. It is addressed by understanding how the system ranges and their tolerances satisfy the design ranges (and their tolerances).

Examples of Recognized C_R are

- when the German car manufacturer understood the cause of cracking windows, it was largely dependent on a supplier to fix the problem;
- basically, all situations where well-engineered systems fail and a diagnosis has not yet be executed;
- a traffic situation where traffic is slowing down and a car is driving at too high velocity while keeping insufficient distance to the car ahead.

12.2.5 Overview of All Kinds of Time-Independent Complexity

To complete this explanation of complexity in AD, now follows an overview of the all definitions that were described. Figure 12.2 shows a graphical overview:

- Complexity Axiom; complexity related to the Complexity Axiom based on information in design according to the definition of Shannon and that affects the FRs.
- C_{Im}; a specific kind of useful information due to a discrepancy in design ranges and system ranges according to the Information Axiom.
- C_R; Information in design as defined by the Information Axiom. It is caused by insufficient overlap between the design and system ranges.
- Unrecognized C_{Im}; the part of C_{Im} that is not recognized by the designer and therefore remains unaddressed. It should, when eventually discovered, be addressed by all relevant FRs and DPs of the design matrix. Once this kind of complexity is recognized, it instantly changes to Recognized C_{Im}.
- Recognized C_{Im}; the part of C_{Im} that is recognized by the designer but the knowledge to address the problem in an appropriate manner is still lacking. Recognized information is addressed by decoupling of the design matrix.
- Unrecognized C_R is eliminated by understanding how the DPs satisfy the FRs, knowing all relevant parameters (decomposition of the DPs).
- Recognized C_R is eliminated by optimizing the system and design ranges.

12.3 Graphical Representation of Complexity

In this section, complexity in AD from the former section will be applied to visualize the design process as it develops during the execution of the design process.

12.3.1 The Functionality Diagram

The "Functionality Diagram," also referred to in literature as "Axiomatic Maturity Diagram" or "AMD" visualizes complexity of a product design (Puik and Ceglarek 2014b). As complexity in AD is related to the satisfaction of the FRs, it plots the extent to which functionality of a system is met. The diagram, shown in Fig. 12.3, uses two axes, one for each axiom, plotting the degree in which the axioms are satisfied.

The horizontal axis is the "axis of conceptual organization" starting at "No Organisation" and ending with "Proof of Concept." Proof of concept indicates that the product design is a viable design; the design matrix is decoupled and therefore

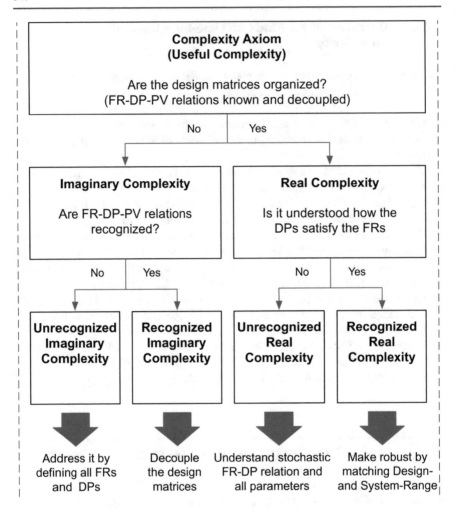

Fig. 12.2 Breakdown of complexity starting with the complexity axiom in AD

C_{Im} has become equal to zero. This implies that both Unrecognized C_{Im} and Recognized C_{Im} have been eliminated. The vertical axis represents robustness of the design from "Not Robust" to "Fully Robust."

Note that both axes have a continuous measure. Irregularities in design can have all sizes and therefore the progression on the axes can have any intermediate value. For the horizontal axis, that plots C_{Im} (related to the Independence Axiom) this contains; (i) the definitions of the right FRs, (ii) the according DPs, including all DPs that need to be fixed during the process of conceptual validation, and (iii) the process of decoupling the FRs and DPs one by one. Removing irregularities to guarantee independence is much more than just decoupling the design matrix.

Fig. 12.3 The functionality diagram. The horizontal axis plots the independence axiom, the vertical axis plots the information axiom. Together they plot complexity. The development path is arbitrary. (Reproduced with permission from Puik and Ceglarek (2014b))

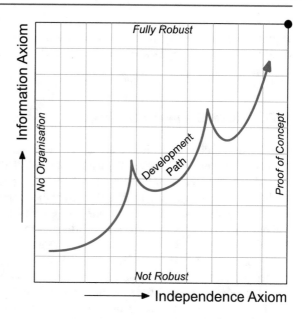

The lower left-hand corner in the functionality diagram indicates a high level of ignorance and high complexity accordingly; the designer has little knowledge of how to satisfy FRs with his DPs and therefore the functionality is low. The upper right-hand corner shows low complexity and maximum probability of FRs being satisfied. Therefore, this is the area of high functionality. Development of products starts in the lower left-hand side and moves to the upper right-hand side. Products are fully mature when they reach the upper right-hand corner of the functionality diagram, as marked with a dot (Fig. 12.3).

12.3.2 Presumed and Legitimate Position in the Functionality Diagram

At any moment of development, the designer may presume an actual position in the diagram according to the current status of the design, but this position may differ from the real and legitimate position of the design; the presumed and legitimate positions may have discrepancies. A discrepancy is caused by a lack of knowledge of the designer because he has missed some essential design artefacts. As a result, the designer rates the level of engineering of the current product design higher than it actually is good for. When he finds the design error that causes the discrepancy, the problem can be addressed. However, if it is not discovered, the discrepancy will present itself at some point in the remaining part of the development process or after market introduction as a surprise to the engineers. The presumed position in the diagram needs to be corrected and that may lead to a project delay. Discrepancies between the presumed and legitimate position in the functionality diagram are the result of Unrecognized C_{Im} and due to its disruptive character, it may have a large impact on the remaining product development process. Therefore, the goal is to discover discrepancies between presumed and legitimate positions as early as possible.

12.3.3 Ideal Development Path for Product Design

Product development, as indicated above, will start somewhere at the lower left-hand side and will move diagonally upward. The exact starting point will depend on the difficulty of the project. A high-tech project that is new to the world might start with a high amount of ignorance in the deep lower left corner. A project that aims to develop according to the Right-First-Time philosophy should start without Unrecognized C_{Im} and starts further to the lower right-hand side of the diagram.

The chosen path may be dependent on the amount of risk that is acceptable to the company, e.g., the most efficient development path in terms of investment (SME), a path that reduces the lead time (semiconductor industry), or a path that minimizes development errors (medical or avionics). As explained in Chap. 11, it is preferred to start with the Independence Axiom followed by the Information Axiom due to the disruptive character of Unrecognized C_{Im}, thus:

- define FRs and find all relevant DPs to address Unrecognized C_{Im};
- decouple the design matrix to address Recognized C_{Im};
- learn about all parameters that influence the FRS to address Unrecognized C_R;
- tune the design ranges and system ranges to guarantee an adequate common range to address Recognized C_R.

This leads to a preferred path that first moves to the right and then angles upward. It is plotted in the left-hand graph of Fig. 12.4.

Depending on the preferred project strategy, a more or less risky path could be followed. In case of the rather conservative and slow but safe path of the Waterfall Model, (Royce 1970) the procedure of following Independence and Information Axioms in that order would be persistent (Fig. 12.4, right-hand graph). A slightly more risky path that in practice enhances the development speed of projects is the path of "Simultaneous Engineering" (Bullinger and Warschat 2012). This gives the designer more room to start early work on robustness, process technology, and other life cycle elements. This merges the work on Independence and Information Axioms and possibly shortens project lead time.

12.3.4 Examples of Typical Errors

Unexpected errors in the development process are mostly related to the discovery of Unrecognized C_{Im}. This reveals the discrepancy between the presumed and

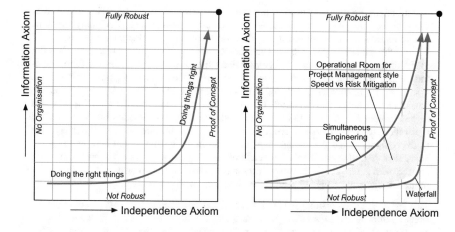

Fig. 12.4 Left; preferred development path through the functionality diagram, as indicated in literature, first moves to the right to satisfy Axiom 1. After this, Axiom 2 is satisfied in an upward direction. (Reproduced with permission from Puik and Ceglarek (2014b)). Right; depending on the nature of the project, a different strategy may be followed. The right lower curve would represent a waterfall management approach, while the upper would represent the path in case of a simultaneous engineering strategy

legitimate position. It will divert the development path in the functionality diagram. Depending on the kind of error, a discontinuity will appear. This discontinuity is the result of the conversion of Unrecognized C_{Im} to Recognized C_{Im}. It may show as a kink in the development path or a jump to a different position in the diagram, depending on

- availability of a solution to address the problem;
- robustness of the current design being affected or not.

The following typical design errors could occur:

Example 12.1 Dealing with Coupling of the Design Matrices

The first example that will be analyzed with the functionality diagram is that of coupling in a system. As many examples in this book already have explained the problem of coupling, a different kind of example is chosen; the problem of repairing a defective system.

Let's say we want to repair an old radio that produces bad quality sound. The problem could be that it just needs to be adjusted by trimming the various potentiometers, capacitors, and inductors. However, it is also possible that one of the electronic components is defective and needs to be replaced. A repairman will typically start asking questions, e.g.: When did the sound degrade, did it occur all of a sudden or did it occur gradually, what was the temperature and maybe humidity when the problem occurred for the first time. All these questions will help the repairman to understand the problem. Now let's say the radio still produces some sound and repairman does not understand that a problem is caused by a defective component. He chooses to repair the radio by readjusting some of the components of the radio. Since this is an old radio, and system ranges may have drifted away from their design ranges, he might succeed in improving the functionality of the radio. However, at some point, this process stops because the defective component structurally prohibits further improvement. As shown in Fig. 12.5 (left diagram, left blue line), it is possible to readjust the radio to a higher level. The process does unfortunately not reach the black dot of the diagram since the defective component causes a structural barrier for further optimization. In this situation, C_R is eliminated, however, Unrecognized C_{Im} still resides in the system as the repairman is not aware of the defective component. At some point, the repairman will notice that his efforts do not sort the effect he was aiming for. He will start digging deeper into the design till his knowledge increases and enables him to locate and repair the defective component. From this point, there are two possibilities; (i) Replacement of the component and the tolerances it introduces in the system require him to repeat the adjustment procedure, or (ii) the tolerances of the component do not affect his earlier work and the radio is repaired. The former of these two possibilities is shown with the dotted line in the left diagram of Fig. 12.5, the latter is shown in the right diagram.

This last observation is comparable with a designer developing a new system of which he starts optimizing the DPs before he is sure that the conceptual design is stable. Further optimizations of the conceptual design may eliminate the optimized DP causing earlier optimization efforts to be spent in vain.

Example 12.2 Wrongly Chosen DP

A wrongly chosen DP leads to the situation that this DP does not actually satisfy the related FR. It will seem to the designer that the design matrix is understood and decoupled, but in fact, this is not the case. In our radio repair example, this would mean that the repairman closely has located the circuit that is malfunctioning, however, he is not 100% sure which part to replace and from a limited number of options he guesses wrong. The efforts to repair the radio do not reduce Unrecognized C_{Im} and the position in the functionality diagram does not advance to the right. There may even be a fallback in C_R due to the added tolerances of the new part. The right diagram of Fig. 12.6 plots the possible discontinuities when the right part in the radio is replaced.

Example 12.3 Non-Matching System and Design Ranges

In Chap. 11, the example was given how to determine the length of the shoreline of Australia. The difficulty was that although shorelines around Australia are drawn, they are only approximate because what is presented as a straight line is made up of jagged lines. If we look at the jagged lines in higher magnification, they are made of more jagged lines. It was explained that the shoreline may be described by a fractal and that it has a mathematical basis. When zoomed in on the fractal, it appears that at a smaller scale the shape of the shoreline remains the same, and when zoomed further this happens again. The determination is a complex problem because every time the level of accuracy is increased, there is the challenge to go a level deeper and increase the accuracy; it is impossible to completely match the system and the design range for this problem.

A non-matching system and design range for one or more of the design relations between FRs and DPs leads to the situation that the Information Axiom cannot be fully satisfied. Note that the definition of C_R is based on joint probability or the sum of all information in the design relations. Therefore, the mature state is only reached if all system- and design-ranges are matched (Fig. 12.7). In this case, there is no discrepancy between presumed and legitimate positions. Problems with non-matching systems and design ranges can be the result of Unrecognized C_R. However, when this is discovered Unrecognized C_R is changed in Recognized C_R but an infinitely accurate determination cannot be made.

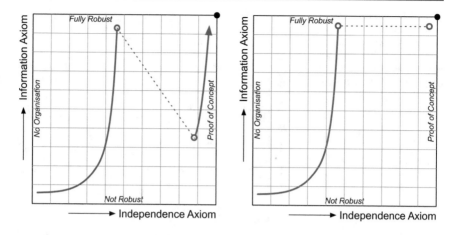

Fig. 12.5 Irregularities in the design matrix do not necessarily conflict with satisfaction of the information axiom. However, if decoupling of the matrix needs replacement of DPs, the information axiom is not automatically satisfied for the new DPs and efforts may be lost (left). The second option shows a luckier situation that the DPs can be maintained. In this case the impact on the design is minimal (right)

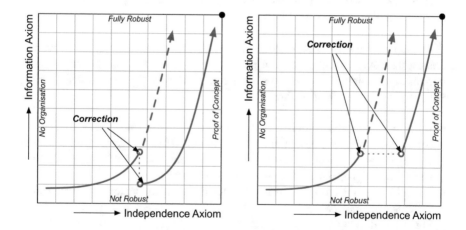

Fig. 12.6 Discovery of a wrong DP leads to a discontinuity in the development process. In the unlucky situation that an obsolete DP was already optimized, efforts are lost and the new DP again needs optimization and a correction takes place (left). In a lucky situation, the problem can be solved with minor efforts. In this case, the related unrecognized as well the Unrecognized Imaginary Complexity disappears (right)

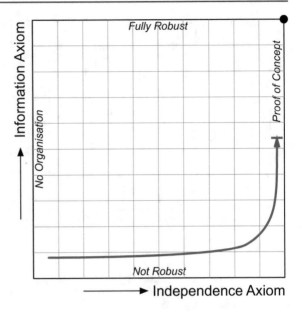

Fig. 12.7 Non-matching system- and design ranges prevent the mature state from being reached. The design will not become robust. (Reproduced with permission from Puik and Ceglarek (2014b))

12.3.5 Summary of the Application of Complexity in Functionality Diagrams

The complexity theory of AD, plotted in functionality diagrams can be applied to monitor the development process of products and systems. It has the capability to monitor if complexity and the axioms are addressed in the right order. Typical patterns that were defined so far:

- If the designer starts optimizing the design according to the Information Axiom, before decoupling the design, the horizontal axis will start rising early. It may to discrepancies in presumed and legitimate positions in the functionality diagram since the designer is not always aware of this problem.
- The different development paths for SMEs, semiconductor industry, safety systems, or medical industry, follow different trajectories as indicated in Fig. 12.4. It is up to the designer or his organization which path is the most optimal path for each situation.
- It was shown what errors can occur, how to recover from it, and what the consequence is in terms of work that needs to be redone in Figs. 12.5 and 12.6.
- If the designer does not succeed in making the design robust it will not reach the fully robust status marked with the dot Fig. 12.7.

In learning organizations like universities but as well as companies, the functionality diagram can serve as a tool to explain the origin of errors made in projects to students and novice designers. Causes and consequences become clear lessons for future design projects and it will contribute to the learning experience of the designer (design team). Communication, supported by these visual means, could function as a universal language to widen the scope of personnel, increasingly being capable of understanding what went wrong, for students, engineers, but also managers, and executives.

12.4 Conclusions of This Chapter

This chapter has explained how complexity in AD is defined and how it can be applied. Complexity in AD is defined as "a measure of uncertainty in achieving the specified FRs." Four main kinds of complexity in AD are defined:

- real Complexity;
- imaginary Complexity;
- combinatorial Complexity;
- periodic Complexity.

The first two kinds of complexity are Time-Independent: these kinds do not change with time. The last two are Time-Dependent and they indeed do change with time. There are two kinds of C_R and C_{Im}; complexity that is recognized or is not unrecognized by the designer.

Second, it is shown that complexity in AD being defined in the functional domain, is very applicable for engineers. As Gell-Mann and Lloyd state it, complexity is the result of a "lack of regularities in the design." If these regularities are either; (i) not recognized, or (ii) ignored they will reside in the system and, as a result, the system will behave in a stochastic manner outside its specifications. On the other hand, if all irregularities are removed from the system, it will thereafter behave fully according to expectations and the designer has made a good design.

Third, when complexity in AD is visualized in a functionality diagram, it becomes a valuable tool to monitor the design as it evolves over time. This diagram reveals the design consequences of errors in the development process when the Independence Axiom and Information Axiom are not fully satisfied or if they are not applied in the right order. A number of typical situations have been analyzed and the causes of their risks are explained. The acceptable amount of risk differs per project as lead times, budget, and available resources are not the same. The diagram can be used to estimate remaining development risks and create awareness of how to best deal with them.

References

Boone ME, Snowden DJ (2007) A leader's framework for decision making. Harvard Bus Rev 85 (11):68–76

Bullinger HJ, Warschat J (2012) Concurrent simultaneous engineering systems. Springer Science & Business Media, Berlin/Heidelberg, Germany

Foley JT, Puik ECN, Cochran DS (2016) Desirable complexity. In: Presented at the 10th international conference on axiomatic design ICAD2014, Xi'an, 2016, p 6

Gallagher R, Appenzeller T (1999) Beyond reductionism. Science 284(5411):79–80

Gell-Mann M, Lloyd S (1996) Information measures, effective complexity, and total information. Complexity 2(1):44–52

Goldenfeld N, Kadanoff LP (1999) Simple lessons from complexity. Science 284(5411):87–89

Kurtz CF, Snowden D (2003) The new dynamics of strategy: sense-making in a complex and complicated world. IBM Syst J 42(3):462–483

Lee T (2003) Complexity theory in axiomatic design. Massachusetts Institute of Technology, Cambridge, U.S

Puik ECN, Ceglarek D (2014a) A review on information in design. In: Presented at the 10th international conference on axiomatic design ICAD2014, Lisbon, 2014, 1st ed, pp 59–64

Puik ECN, Ceglarek D (2014b) A theory of maturity. In: Presented at the 10th international conference on axiomatic design ICAD2014, Lisbon, 2014, 1st ed, pp 115–120

Puik ECN, Ceglarek D (2015) The quality of a design will not exceed the knowledge of its designer; an analysis based on axiomatic information and the cynefin framework. Procedia CIRP 34:19–24

Royce WW (1970) Managing the development of large software systems. In: Proceedings of IEEE WESCON, pp 328–338

Shannon CE, Weaver W (1949) The mathematical theory of communication. The University of Illinois Press, Chicago

Snowden D (2000) Cynefin: a sense of time and space, the social ecology of knowledge management

Suh NP (1990) The principles of design (Oxford series on advanced manufacturing). Oxford University Press on Demand, Oxford, England, U.K.

Suh NP (1999) A theory of complexity, periodicity and the design axioms. Res Eng Design 11 (2):116–132

Suh NP (2005a) Complexity: theory and applications. Oxford University Press, Oxford, England, U.K.

Suh NP (2005b) Complexity in engineering. CIRP Ann 54(2):46–63

Weng G, Bhalla US, Iyengar R (1999) Complexity in biological signaling systems. Science 284 (5411):92–96

Whitesides GM, Ismagilov RF (1999) Complexity in chemistry. Science 284(5411):89–92

Axiomatic Design Application to Product Family Design

13

Masayuki Nakao and Kenji Iino

Abstract

The basic concepts and the framework of Axiomatic Design (AD) provide powerful tools in the design of products and product families, especially for visualizing the design goals and improving the design process. When learning how to apply AD, however, nearly a half of the uninitiated designers like students may need to devote much effort to advance a sufficient number of different design concepts in terms of functional requirements (FRs) and/or design parameters (DPs), which is often done in abstract phrases like the first step in AD. The instructors must encourage them to think freely and squeeze out all the FRs and DPs they have in their minds and must guide them to integrate FRs functionally and DPs physically to obtain the desired design matrix.

13.1 Axiomatic Design Application for Product Family Design

13.1.1 Design Concept Description as the First Step in Axiomatic Design

The idea of AD shows powerful effects in designing product families.

By "product family," we mean a group of interacting or interrelated entities that form a unified entirety. In other words, a product family is a unified whole whose structural elements have effects on one another, thus, applying Independence

M. Nakao (✉) · K. Iino
The University of Tokyo, Tokyo, Japan
e-mail: nakao@hnl.t.u-tokyo.ac.jp

© Springer Nature Switzerland AG 2021
N. P. Suh et al. (eds.), *Design Engineering and Science*,
https://doi.org/10.1007/978-3-030-49232-8_13

Axiom for decoupling such interference of FRs increases the possibility of satisfying all FRs; that is good design.

AD is a universal conceptual enabler without any constraints (Cs) of the design objects, thus, we can apply it to subjects including engineering designs of mechanical, electrical, buildings, or chemical processes, as well as such social demands as planning of structuring organizations, proposing policies, developing new products, or improving lifestyles; we can apply the method in any creation. AD, in other words, is a set of general axioms that can effectively support design no matter what the subject is.

In learning how to apply AD, one can read the methods described in detail in the earlier chapters. Just reading AD methods, however, may lead only half of the readers, to quickly acquire the skills in applying them, because they need to describe the design concept in a natural language as the first step in AD.

When learning AD with Suh's textbook (Suh 2001), half of the uninitiated designers like students may not even reach the stage of an axiom application. The reason is the difficulty for such designers in describing design concepts of FRs or DPs in abstract phrases instead of actual shapes laid out in drawings. Suh introduced a teaching method to list the FRs and DPs of a beverage can. The can has only three parts of the body, top lid, and the bottom, but it has more than 12 FRs. These three parts are physically integrated from more than 12 DPs. For example, about half of the students missed the FRs of the cylindrical body, the size of the pull tab, or the beautiful body print showing images about the beverage.

Another useful design example is an ongoing research topic for a bachelor's or master's degree (see problem 2). The students have to list up, at least, ten FRs and DPs related to arcs to construct the FR–DP charts, and identify the critical DP that signifies the novelty of the research. Although the students are always concerned about this requirement, only about half of the students may complete this task (Nakao and Iino 2018). A half dropped primary FRs or DPs that the instructor could recognize or made the mistakes of "mixing the FRs of the designer (the project budget, the project deadline, or so)" as pointed out by Thompson (2013). Without establishing the FRs and DPs that construct the design, the students cannot proceed to the next step of applying AD.

To guide the students, as we will describe with case studies in Sect. 13.2, we have them squeeze out all the FRs and DPs from their brains as a preparatory step for AD. General methods of mind mapping or work breakdown structure (Fig. 13.1) will work just fine.

13.1.2 Axiomatic Design Application with Proper Functional Requirements

For the next step, the students group the design concepts they generated into FRs and DPs, then connect related FRs and DPs with arcs to produce FR–DP charts. Next is a key technique in applying AD of listing up an equal number of FRs and DPs (Nakao and Iino 2018). This step leads to a regular design matrix (regular: invertible square matrix with a non-zero determinant) that can be decoupled into a diagonal or triangular one with proper row operations.

Failing to list up proper FRs and DPs blocks the students from reaching the entrance to AD application. Many students can describe DPs that are visible, however, they often cannot spell out the FRs that are hard to visualize. We have to loudly emphasize "FR first!" or "set FRs under a solution-neutral condition," otherwise, they will end up with smaller numbers of FRs compared to those of DPs.

The AD textbook (Suh 2001) teaches that zigzag thinking is effective in setting FRs and DPs. The zigzagging starts from an abstract high-level concept toward low-level ones that are easier to picture and alternates between the functional and physical spaces going FR, DP, FR, DP, and so on. The method leads to an equal number of FRs and DPs, and at the same time, avoids describing multiple FRs with combinations of the same DPs. Therefore, the design matrix becomes regular, and its determinant is non-zero. The situation with students in the early stage, however, lacks efficient numbers of FRs and DPs in their minds. Thus, even with zigzag thinking, they overlook important aspects. It is just like an excellent recipe without the right materials, failing to produce a good dinner. Proper FRs are necessary for AD application.

The instructors twist the students' arms to list up FRs and DPs, and they tend to list FRs chronologically and DPs spatially (Nakao and Iino 2018). The way they work comes from imagining how they would use the product, i.e., the sequence of work, to list up the FRs, and next referencing the bill of material (BOM) of similar existing products to list up the DPs. Listing up FRs and DPs in separate mindsets against the zigzag thinking process naturally leads to discrepancies in their numbers. Once the students produce their imperfect FR and DP lists, the instructors and teaching assistants (TAs) guide the students to integrate FRs functionally and DPs physically. This step is a grouping of low-level concepts of FRs and DPs, and it can rearrange the FR and DP vectors to have the same dimension. After this integration, retrying the above mentioned zigzag thinking can operate perfectly. The students have enough numbers of the right materials now.

Management professors teach the need for skills in setting the problem in a "mutually exclusive and collectively exhaustive (MECE)" manner if one wants to be a business consultant. The first part of mutual exclusiveness is the same as the Independence Axiom in AD, and engineering students can manage to set mutually independent FRs by avoiding trade-offs. The second part, collective exhaustiveness, is more challenging for the students who always have some mind slips. After a one-semester-long design class or seminar, for any objective designs, half of the young participants can directly build the design equations by tacitly setting FRs/DPs and integrating them in the brain.

13.1.3 Axiomatic Design Application with Many Functional Requirements

Generally, real product family design in industries have so many FRs that the designers cannot easily check the trade-offs or interferences with their brains or hands. In later chapters, however, AD shows positive and effective work for large or complex systems.

A software system design starts by listing up the FRs. This process, with a business consultant, describes what the customer wants to happen in natural language. Then a computer scientist translates the FRs into detailed specification, and programmers map the specifications to programs to realize the functions. A typical number of FRs, for these cases, easily exceeds 1,000 and the number of steps of checking for interferences among them turns out huge to reach 1 million cases, i.e., the square of the number of FRs. Testing in software design is said to take about the same number of days as designing takes, e.g., if the design took one year, its testing will take another 1 year because checking the interferences takes huge manpower.

AD can split the FRs into explicit ones FR_e and implicit ones FR_i as shown later in Fig. 13.8a. The former are those that the customer wants with the design, i.e., FRs that AD explained up to the previous chapters. The latter, on the other hand, are those without customer voices. If the design cannot meet the voice of the customer, the customer may file claims, and so the makers prepare those FRs to prevent some risks of future claims. For example, large-scale programs like one for an automatic teller machine (ATM) in banking is said to have 70% of its program lines to realize implicit FRs. Examples of these implicit FRs include operation schedules, future development plans, recovery plans upon problems, transition plans for new systems in the future, prevention of unauthorized access, aseismic reinforcement, installation weight, electrical power consumption, and so on. These problems will arise in situations like; a 24 h a day, 365 days a year operation without not even a minute of margin for update to program modifications; expanding the capacity to eight times after a successful operation caused congestion due to narrow data bus; or loss of electrical power following an earthquake caused loss of live data, and thus, the makers have to prepare against such emergency states.

AD often teaches to set these requirements into Cs, such as cost, safety, physical proximity, durability, and so on, as shown later in Fig. 13.8b. It is adequate if narrowing the tolerable ranges for DPs alone can satisfy Cs, however, if the narrowing lowers the probability of realizing FRs, the solution is not desirable. A different method, frequent in practice, is to prepare a separate DP for satisfying an implicit FR. For example, in preparation against the above problems; halt the operation for 10 min every day starting at 2 o'clock in the middle of the night; design the system in advance with a high data transfer frequency to allow 16 times the expected information transfer volume, or place a mirror server in a city located 1,000 km away. In general, describing the FR_i gives better chances of finding interferences with other FRs, as shown in Fig. 13.8a. For example, security and electric power consumption relate to all programs, and they result in rows with all Xs meaning interference with everything.

13.1.4 Creating New Design Using Axiomatic Design

Design assignments of creating new designs, instead of improving existing ones are now globally common, especially in the information business. This type of new assignment, however, gives further hurdles in listing up all the FRs and DPs, especially the FRs. The problem is not in the lack of linguistic ability to express concepts but in the overlooking of FRs that will surface later. The main cause is not recognizing the values of customer attributes (CAs). Some examples are; a change in a rival organization disturbing the designer, a competitor filing suit on a patent issue, a customer applying the product in ways the designer did not expect, a sudden change in regulation that prohibits using the product, or a workers' strike unrelated to the designer's responsibility. In such cases, the designer has to set a new set of CAs and FRs, and creation is always faced with such changes in reaching a successful design.

To find what element is missing from the formation, relying on imagination while sitting in the office will never lead to discovery. One will have to quickly go through the cycle of the first prototype, testing, improvement, the second prototype, testing, improvement, and so on, to find what concepts are missing from the formation. Mark Zuckerberg said, "Done is better than perfect."

The design solution is not necessarily unique. The FR itself, changes with the customer and situations that surround the society, forcing changes in the optimum DP. This transformation makes the design different from mathematics that has a single unique and eternal solution, and that is what gives compelling attraction to the act of designing. One of the most effective design methods is AD when we want to teach the philosophy of design to young designers visually.

13.2 Product and Product Family Design Cases Using Axiomatic Design

13.2.1 Automatic Driving

Figure 13.1 shows the method for exhausting design concepts with the example of designing an automatic driving system. Figure 13.1a is the result of applying mind mapping, and (b), work breakdown structure. Both methods start from a single concept and reach multiple concepts following the association game method. They also allow grouping of concepts so the player can exhaust all concepts without leaving out any. In the end, the designer separates the FRs and DPs, for example, by collecting verbs for FRs and nouns for DPs, and in step (c), they are aligned in the FR–DP chart with arcs connecting related FRs and DPs. As noted with gray balloons in (c), the discrepancy in the counts of FRs and DPs is evident, as well as design interference indicated with intersecting arcs.

When a designer is at the stage in (c), the design matrix is irregular and coupled, and advancing to the decoupling phase is quite discouraging. These problems look complicated in design. We thus tried concept integration. As the dotted boxes of stage (d) shows, for example, "shoulder, pedestrians, and vehicles" are all obstacles and can form a single group FR, and "GPS + map, steering, brake, and gas pedal" are all in constant use to form a single group DP. The resulting design equation for

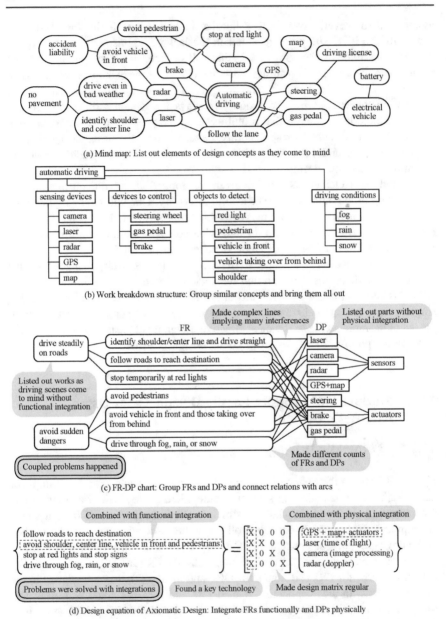

(a) Mind map: List out elements of design concepts as they come to mind

(b) Work breakdown structure: Group similar concepts and bring them all out

(c) FR-DP chart: Group FRs and DPs and connect relations with arcs

(d) Design equation of Axiomatic Design: Integrate FRs functionally and DPs physically

Fig. 13.1 Design of automatic driving. (Reproduced from Nakao and Iino (2018), originally published open access under a CC BY 4.0 license: https://doi.org/10.1051/matecconf/201822301011)

(d) is 4D and is easy to understand the design definition. An interference is seen in the column in the dotted box for DP1, "GPS + map + actuators." Without them, no matter how sophisticated the sensors may be, there is no way to accomplish automatic driving. In other words, they are the key technologies. The design equation in (d) solved these problems, and now we can use the axioms of AD for decoupling.

13.2.2 Fan Design

Automatic driving we saw in Fig. 13.1, with a great deal of attention from the society and a large number of articles about it in a variety of journals and magazines, allows the students to search the internet and easily collect articles and pick up concepts of FRs and DPs from them. A fan design in Fig. 13.2, on the other hand, is a mature product, and there are no articles that discuss it. The students have to think for themselves. Figure 13.2a is a typical FR–DP chart by a student who visualizes a fan in the air and sets the FRs following the process of activating one, while on the other hand, the student virtually disassembles one and sets the DPs following the BOM. Naturally, the two methods force different mental processes. Thus, the numbers of FRs and DPs do not match with intersecting arcs for related FRs and DPs. In this unstructured situation, zigzag thinking does not work well, either.

To escape the situation, we rearrange the breakdown by integrating multiple lower level FRs into a single FR at a higher level like "set airflow power" or "stop upon falling asleep," or combine related DPs into a higher level module DP like "motor + fan" or "motor + knob." For the DP "cover" without a corresponding FR in (a), we add the hidden FR of "injury-free finger poking" in (b). A hidden FR is one unnoticed during the early stage of design. The DP with influences on all FRs, shown with a corresponding column with all Xs is "motor + fan." This interference shows that this DP is the key technology for the product fan.

Figure (c) shows the design equation for the bladeless fan that was a recent hit product. Its shape is clearly different from a conventional model, but it only has an additional attractive FR of "hide blades." All the remaining FRs are carried over from a conventional model. The attractive FR, however, was so effective. The FR brought the large value of being "bladeless," and led consumers to purchase them at $300 even though a conventional model would only cost $50. Within the set of DPs, the novel technologies are "ring-shaped blower" and "place blades inside the base." The key technology remained with "motor + fan," but a new small synchronized motor with rare-earth magnets hid the motor in the base.

13.2.3 Entrance Exam Administration

Figure 13.3 shows the case of "Planning administration of admission exam." Shown in (a) is the first FR–DP chart. A student listed up the FRs following the schedule and wrote down the DPs looking at the list of stakeholders. Naturally, the

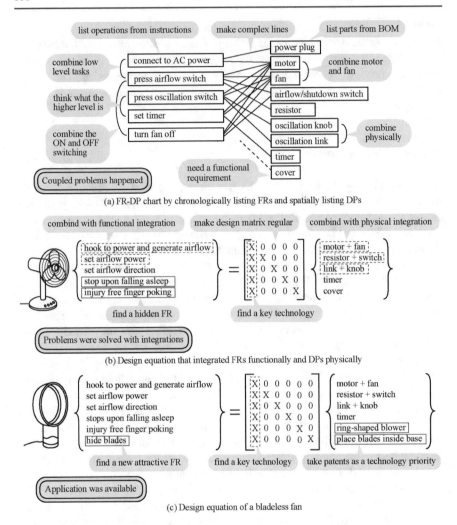

(a) FR-DP chart by chronologically listing FRs and spatially listing DPs

(b) Design equation that integrated FRs functionally and DPs physically

(c) Design equation of a bladeless fan

Fig. 13.2 Fan design. (Reproduced from Nakao and Iino (2018), originally published open access under a CC BY 4.0 license: https://doi.org/10.1051/matecconf/201822301011)

FR and DP counts did not match, and intersections were there among their relations. Applying the integration techniques, respectively, to the FRs and DPs led to a 4D design equation in (b). In the end, a column with all Xs in the design matrix that influenced all FRs was the DP of "exam committee." The committee takes the leading role in all aspects with the responsibility to all the FRs. As shown in (c), a flaw in the exam questions one year was found after the exam was over, and the university received social blame. For the following year's exam, a hidden FR of "eliminate errors in questions" was added with a corresponding DP of "exam review committee" consisting of young teaching staff tackling the exam questions in advance of the real exam. The DP of "exam committee" appears to also have influence on this FR, however, such an influence would discourage the young staff to point out errors by tenured professors. Thus, this exam review committee alone was kept independent on purpose.

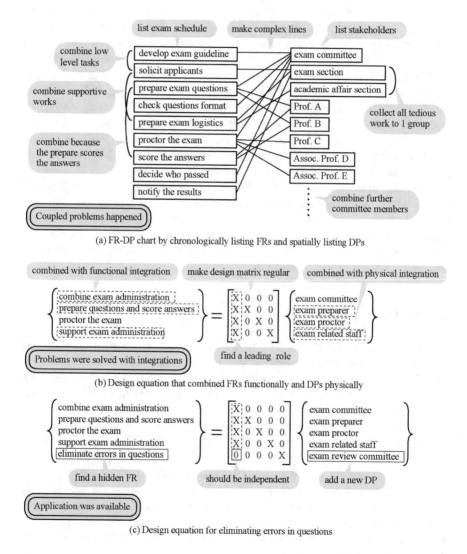

(a) FR-DP chart by chronologically listing FRs and spatially listing DPs

(b) Design equation that combined FRs functionally and DPs physically

(c) Design equation for eliminating errors in questions

Fig. 13.3 Planning administration of admission exam. (Reproduced from Nakao and Iino (2018), originally published open access under a CC BY 4.0 license: https://doi.org/10.1051/matecconf/201822301011)

13.2.4 Umbrella that Follows the Owner

Figure 13.4 is the design of an "Umbrella that follows the owner." It was a student creation in a design exercise class. The first idea was to mount an umbrella on a drone. However, that resulted in a noisy follower like a mosquito above the head. The next design iteration was a helium-filled balloon to counter the weight of the umbrella and a pair of propellers mounted on the two sides to control forward/backward, and left/right turns. A camera mounted on the umbrella balloon recognized a red hat and controlled the propellers to follow its motion. The test session resulted in the balloon flying away after 20 s or so following the hat, and the testers had to pull the balloon back with the "emergency string." The designers had failed to recognize the FRs of controlling rolling and pitching. Only two propellers were insufficient to control rolling and pitching additionally. Looking into an airplane design led the team to find the need for a tail wing. Also, the camera had a narrow view angle and would easily lose sight of the red hat. The students placed a fish-eye lens on the camera to counter this problem.

What improvements to make are easy to find through quick prototyping and testing. Many large-sized corporations like to "start with a perfect solution" and extend the development period. However, they often lose their business chances. Startups like to quickly place products still under evaluation into the market and have the market tell them what improvements to make. The latter attitude is needed for creative design to find hidden FRs.

13.2.5 Stirling Engine

Figure 13.5 shows two sets of FRs of a Stirling engine, one when they are set following the chronological operation, and the other following functional evaluation of laws of thermodynamics. The former referenced the case of setting FRs for a steam engine in Suh's textbook (Suh 2001). Four FRs of producing hot air, raising the piston, producing cold air, and lowering the piston form a lower triangular matrix. The latter FR set, on the other hand, from the point, that the difference in injection and extraction of heat produces work, sets four FRs of injecting heat, extracting heat, doing work, and repeating the cycle. The two designs are physically different from different sets of FRs and DPs. Both design matrices, however, are also lower triangular ones. In other words, both approaches lead to correct answers for decoupling. The difference in their descriptions comes from matrix multiplication, just like performing a coordinate transformation to FR and DP. The burner also heated the air cooler; the difference between hot and cold temperatures became zero; the engine eventually stopped.

This discussion showed that there are cases of describing FRs and DPs of the same machine in design equations with different concepts, but both descriptions are correct.

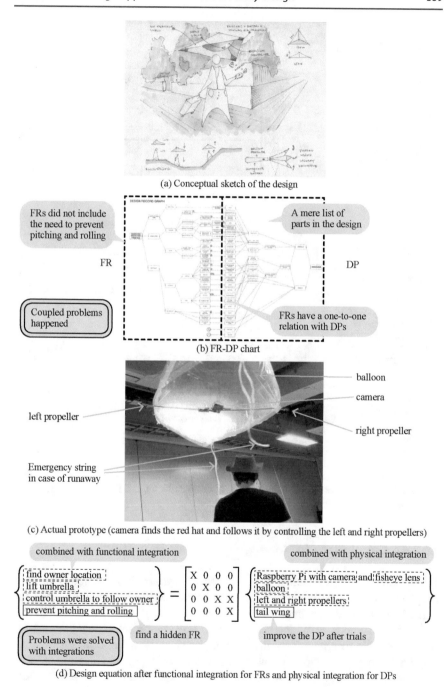

(a) Conceptual sketch of the design

FRs did not include the need to prevent pitching and rolling

A mere list of parts in the design

FR   DP

Coupled problems happened

FRs have a one-to-one relation with DPs

(b) FR-DP chart

balloon

camera

left propeller

right propeller

Emergency string in case of runaway

(c) Actual prototype (camera finds the red hat and follows it by controlling the left and right propellers)

combined with functional integration   combined with physical integration

$$
\left\{ \begin{array}{l} \text{find owner location} \\ \text{lift umbrella} \\ \text{control umbrella to follow owner} \\ \text{prevent pitching and rolling} \end{array} \right\} = \begin{bmatrix} X & 0 & 0 & 0 \\ 0 & X & 0 & 0 \\ 0 & 0 & X & X \\ 0 & 0 & 0 & X \end{bmatrix} \left\{ \begin{array}{l} \text{Raspberry Pi with camera and fisheye lens} \\ \text{balloon} \\ \text{left and right propellers} \\ \text{tail wing} \end{array} \right\}
$$

Problems were solved with integrations

find a hidden FR

improve the DP after trials

(d) Design equation after functional integration for FRs and physical integration for DPs

Fig. 13.4 Design of umbrella that follows the owner. (Reproduced from Nakao and Iino (2018), originally published open access under a CC BY 4.0 license: https://doi.org/10.1051/matecconf/201822301011)

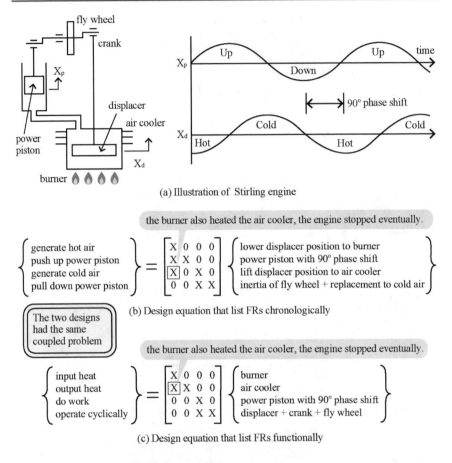

(a) Illustration of Stirling engine

the burner also heated the air cooler, the engine stopped eventually.

$$
\begin{Bmatrix}
\text{generate hot air} \\
\text{push up power piston} \\
\text{generate cold air} \\
\text{pull down power piston}
\end{Bmatrix}
=
\begin{bmatrix}
X & 0 & 0 & 0 \\
X & X & 0 & 0 \\
X & 0 & X & 0 \\
0 & 0 & X & X
\end{bmatrix}
\begin{Bmatrix}
\text{lower displacer position to burner} \\
\text{power piston with } 90° \text{ phase shift} \\
\text{lift displacer position to air cooler} \\
\text{inertia of fly wheel + replacement to cold air}
\end{Bmatrix}
$$

(b) Design equation that list FRs chronologically

The two designs had the same coupled problem

the burner also heated the air cooler, the engine stopped eventually.

$$
\begin{Bmatrix}
\text{input heat} \\
\text{output heat} \\
\text{do work} \\
\text{operate cyclically}
\end{Bmatrix}
=
\begin{bmatrix}
X & 0 & 0 & 0 \\
X & X & 0 & 0 \\
0 & 0 & X & 0 \\
0 & 0 & X & X
\end{bmatrix}
\begin{Bmatrix}
\text{burner} \\
\text{air cooler} \\
\text{power piston with } 90° \text{ phase shift} \\
\text{displacer + crank + fly wheel}
\end{Bmatrix}
$$

(c) Design equation that list FRs functionally

Fig. 13.5 FRs of Stirling engine that are listed chronologically or functionally. (Reproduced from Nakao and Iino (2018), originally published open access under a CC BY 4.0 license: https://doi.org/10.1051/matecconf/201822301011)

13.2.6 CurcurPlate for Managing Peoples in a Building

This section introduces "curcurPlate," a software system designed for monitoring people's whereabouts. Implicit FRs, mentioned in Sect. 13.1.3, are introduced and Fig. 13.6a illustrates the implicit FRs (FR$_i$s), compared with Cs. Although AD allows both methods, preparing new solutions (DP$_i$s) for a set of new FR$_i$s usually is more feasible than narrowing the DP ranges against new Cs. Both FR$_i$s and Cs may have many couplings with other DPs as shown in FR$_{i1}$ or C$_1$ in Fig. 13.6.

Figure 13.7a shows the presence display panel, a hardware system placed at our office entrance that lab members can flip their nameplates to show their presence and absence (FR$_1$). If one is running an experiment in a lab other than the office, a little magnetic sticker with the name of the lab placed on the steel nameplate shows

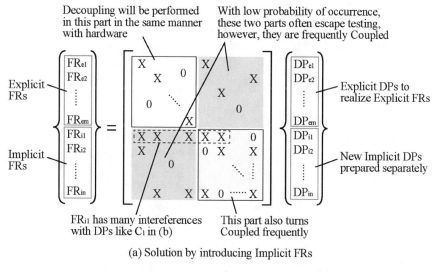

Decoupling will be performed in this part in the same manner with hardware

With low probability of occurrence, these two parts often escape testing, however, they are frequently Coupled

Explicit FRs

Implicit FRs

Explicit DPs to realize Explicit FRs

New Implicit DPs prepared separately

FR_{i1} has many intereferences with DPs like C_1 in (b)

This part also turns Coupled frequently

(a) Solution by introducing Implicit FRs

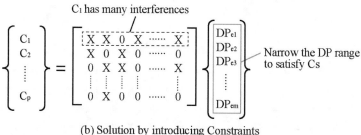

C_1 has many interferences

Narrow the DP range to satisfy Cs

(b) Solution by introducing Constraints

Fig. 13.6 Implicit FRs versus constraints for preventing the future trouble

the whereabouts (FR_2). Further, in case of an emergency like an earthquake or fire, any lab member can take the entire frame to the evacuation site and if someone present is not around at the site, others can head out for rescue (FR_3).

Figure 13.7b is "curcurPlate" the tablet version of this tool. The phrase "kurukuru (curcur)" is the onomatopoeic word for flipping a nameplate. DP_{e1} and DP_{e2} are input by tapping, and DP_{e3} is to store the data in a remote server so one can output the data in case of evacuation. The structure is simple and free of interference even with 200 laboratories using it.

When put in practice, however, everyone trying to update their whereabouts information caused a delay in the server response, and an increased number of labs further pushed back the response and the system needed to counter this problem (FR_{i1}). Moreover, if an earthquake or fire shuts down the server, data immediately before the evacuation are unavailable as well as the state of evacuation (FR_{i2}). Another requirement rose to register the whereabouts information from off-campus

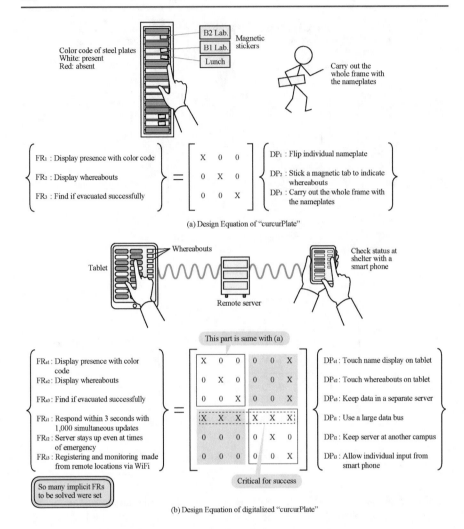

Fig. 13.7 "CurcurPlate" design with implicit FRs

locations (FR_{i3}). These implicit FRs greatly affected the success of the tool, especially "FR_{i1}: Respond within 3 s with 1000 simultaneous updates" led to its acceptance.

13.2.7 Tool for Brushing the Back of Teeth

This section discusses a tool for brushing the back of teeth with some constraints. The target is to design a tool that allows brushing the back of teeth for elderlies that cannot open their mouths widely and avoid aspiration pneumonia at the same time. The conventional solution has a caregiver insert a thin toothbrush into a gap of only about 1 cm and blindly brush the back of teeth as Fig. 13.8a shows. FR_1 is "brush the back of teeth after meal" and FR_2 "insert the brushing tool through a 1 cm gap between the upper and lower teeth." The conventional method used a toothbrush (DP_1) and a small brush head (DP_2) to insert it. However, the small brush head failed to give a good thorough brushing and interfered with FR_1. We set the third

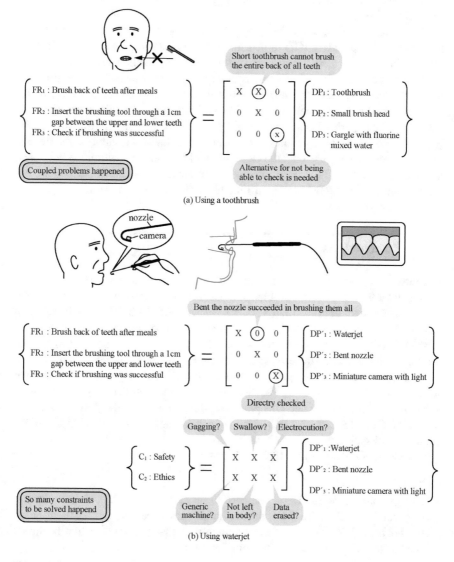

Fig. 13.8 A tool for brushing the back of teeth

requirement FR_3, "check if the brushing was successful," however, there was no way of looking at the back of the teeth so the third parameter DP_3 "gargle with fluorine mixed water" did not satisfy FR_3. In the end, sniffing the mouth was the method for judging how good the brushing was.

We then replaced the toothbrush with water jet (DP'_1), as Fig. 13.8b shows. After the nozzle was inserted past the teeth, waterjet squirted out through a bent nozzle (DP'_2), and the tool successfully cleaned the entire back of teeth without interference with FR_1. We even attached an LED mounted miniature camera (DP'_3) by the nozzle to directly check if there is still food debris left especially between teeth. So far, so good.

When we, however, wanted to apply the solution to visitors that cannot open their mouths wide, safety (C_1) turned into a large obstacle. We claimed that "it is just brushing of the teeth," however, if a dentist or hygienist uses the tool, it is a medical procedure. We had to demonstrate through experiments that the user will not gag with water, and the nozzle will not come off to choke the user, or the electricity to the camera with illumination will not electrocute the user. Next, we had to run the experiments against a variety of people, mandatorily thinking, ethics (C_2). We had to repeat explaining that waterjet is a device available to the general public and anyone can use one, the cleansing tool will not stay within the body, and that we will not keep the private information of teeth data and will erase them, but the ethics committee gave us a hard time to reach approval to use it.

13.3 Conclusions

The idea of AD shows powerful effects, especially for visualizing the design definition and improving design problems in product family design no matter what the subject is as shown in Figs. 13.1, 13.2, 13.3, 13.4, 13.5, 13.6, 13.7 and 13.8. When learning how to apply AD, half of the beginner designers, however, fail to describe enough numbers of design concepts of FRs or DPs in abstract phrases. The instructors have them squeeze out all the FRs and DPs in their minds as a preparatory step for AD with general methods of mind mapping or work breakdown structure as Fig. 13.1 shows. For the next step, the instructors guide them to integrate FRs functionally and DPs physically for getting a regular design matrix, as shown in Figs. 13.1, 13.2, 13.3, 13.4. We also discussed further applications. Finally, some tacit requests which customers do not claim should be set as implicit FRs or Cs, as shown in Figs. 13.6, 13.7 and 13.8.

Problems

1. Design your future life. Here, you need to set money as FR, DP, or C: the dream to become a millionaire (FR), the inevitable tool to eat enough meals or enjoy the hobbies (DP), or one of the minimum necessary resources like health or academic background to realize your FRs (C).

2. Make the design equation on your current research or your job. You should clarify the purpose (FR) and the method (DP), at least. Do not mix the FR of the designers, that is, the project budget, the project deadline, the promotion, the thesis, and so on.

References

Nakao M, Iino K (2018) Students list FRs chronologically and DPs spatially, and need to integrate FRs functionally and DPs physically. In: Puik E, Foley JT, Cochran D, Betasolo M (eds) 12th international conference on axiomatic design (ICAD). MATEC web of conferences, Reykjavík, Iceland

Suh NP (2001) Axiomatic design—advances and applications. Oxford University Press

Thompson MK (2013) Improving the requirements process in axiomatic design theory. In: Annals of the CIRP, 1, vol 62, pp 115–118 (2013)

Design of Large Engineering Systems

14

Gyung-Jin Park and Amro M. Farid

Abstract

One defining characteristic of twenty-first-century engineering challenges is the breadth of their scope. The National Academy of Engineering (NAE) has identified 14 "game-changing goals." At first glance, each of these aspirational engineering goals is so large and complex in its own right that it might seem entirely intractable. Fortunately, design science provides a continually advancing perspective built upon a meta-problem-solving skill set. This chapter introduces the design engineer to the world of large complex systems from an Axiomatic Design (AD) perspective. In particular, the chapter focuses on two critical "systems-thinking" design skills that help the designer manage the inherent and abstract complexity of large systems. They are (1) system decomposition and (2) the allocation of function to form. The chapter also practically demonstrates these design skills in several design stories and case studies. The chapter discusses why and how these design skills are used differently when the system has a fixed versus flexible structure. Finally, the chapter concludes with several avenues for further investigation.

G.-J. Park (✉)
Hanyang University, Ansan, South Korea
e-mail: gjpark@hanyang.ac.kr

A. M. Farid
Dartmouth College, Hanover, NH 03755, USA
e-mail: amfarid@dartmouth.edu; amfarid@mit.edu

A. M. Farid
Massachusetts Institute of Technology, 77 Massachusetts Ave, Cambridge, MA, USA

© Springer Nature Switzerland AG 2021
N. P. Suh et al. (eds.), *Design Engineering and Science*,
https://doi.org/10.1007/978-3-030-49232-8_14

14.1   Introduction

There are two kinds of large systems. The first kind is a tree-like large system. It starts with a limited number of functional requirements (FRs) and design parameters (DPs) at the highest level but requires many layers of decomposition for actual implementation, involving a large number of lower level FRs to satisfy the limited number of the highest level FRs. For example, the original idea for making a dispersion-strengthened copper alloy had only a limited number of FRs at the highest level. The central idea was to manufacture a dispersion-strengthened copper alloy that consists of a pure copper matrix phase with a plethora of nanoscale titanium di-boride particles dispersed throughout the copper matrix as dispersoids to strengthen the alloy. The process designed involved high-speed impingement mixing of Cu/Ti solution with Cu/B solution. The mixed liquid was then rapidly quenched to create an alloy with copper matrix phase with nanoscale titanium di-boride particles dispersed throughout the matrix.

To satisfy the high-level FRs, they had to be decomposed, creating many lower level FRs and DPs. For example, the mixture of Cu/TiB_2 solution had to be quickly solidified on a cold spinning copper disk to prevent the coagulation of the ceramic TiB_2 particles. Then, the liquid mixture of Cu and TiB_2 alloy was rapidly quenched on the rotating copper disk. Then, the ribbon of the Cu/TiB_2 alloy was shredded. The shredded chips of Cu/TiB_2 alloy were then compacted into a solid rod using a high-pressure hydrostatic compaction/extrusion process.

In this case, the number of FRs at the highest level was relatively small. However, when the design of the process was finalized, the entire manufacturing system became quite large. The final system designed had many FR, DPs, and PVs with many layers of decomposition, making the system large with many lower level FRs and DPs.

The second kind of a large system has a large number of FRs at the highest level from the beginning. For example, if we are designing an airport for a major hub, there are many highest level FRs that must be satisfied. These FRs, in turn, generate many lower level FRs, making the system very large. The materials presented in this chapter are equally applicable to any large systems design.

14.1.1   Motivation

One defining characteristic of twenty-first-century engineering challenges is the breadth of their scope. The National Academy of Engineering (NAE) has identified 14 "game-changing goals":

1. advance personalized learning;
2. make solar energy economical;
3. enhance virtual reality;
4. reverse engineer the brain;
5. engineer better medicines;

6. advance health informatics;
7. restore and improve urban infrastructure;
8. secure cyberspace;
9. provide access to clean water;
10. provide energy from fusion;
11. prevent nuclear terror;
12. manage the nitrogen cycle;
13. develop carbon sequestration methods;
14. engineer the tools of scientific discovery.

At first glance, each of these aspirational engineering goals is so large and complex in its own right that each might seem entirely intractable. Furthermore, each goal might appear so different from the next that an aspiring engineer might easily conclude that the skills needed to solve one challenge are entirely distinct from those of another. Consequently, our engineering education system would have to turn "on a dime," orient itself toward each of these 14 challenges, and ask our first-year engineering students to commit themselves to one of these challenges; never to change direction again. And in the unlikely event that we are successful on such a course, the engineering education system would have to pivot again years later to address the newly cropped up grand challenges.

Fortunately, design science provides an alternative and continually advancing perspective. While each of these aspirational NAE goals might seem entirely different, in reality, they exhibit many common characteristics which can be integrated into a consistent design framework. In time, this design framework increasingly spans individual engineering disciplines and real-life problem domains. It also increasingly sets aside limiting paradigms and assumptions in its quest toward a refined meta-problem-solving skill set.

Design Story 14.1:

The design engineer reconsiders the 14 NAE challenges in the context of the four AD engineering domains shown in Fig. 14.1.

- First, they recognize that the "design solution" to each of the grand challenges can be viewed as a newly designed *large complex system* that is very much a refined version of the large complex system that exists in its place today.
- Second, they realize that unlike "traditional products," these systems have not just one "customer" in the stakeholder requirements (SRs) domain but rather a *diversity of internal and external stakeholders*. These stakeholders impose a wide variety of hard and soft requirements which must ultimately be resolved into the FRs and constraints (Cs) of the functional architecture domain.
- There, the aspiring design engineer finds that large complex systems are characterized by a large *number* of FRs. Managing such a large number is a psychological and organizational challenge in its own right.
- Beyond just number, the design solution is complicated by the *heterogeneity* (or diversity) of the FRs. Functions are closely tied to siloed engineering disciplines.

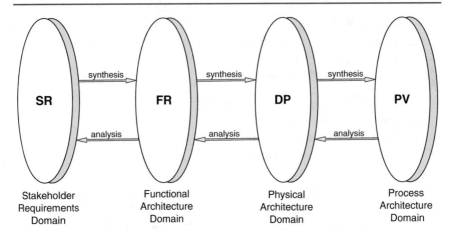

Fig. 14.1 Four domains in the engineering design of systems—an Axiomatic Design perspective

At their simplest, an electrical engineer knows electricity, a chemical engineer knows chemical reactions, and a mechanical engineer knows classical mechanics. A diversity of function means that the design engineer must either absorb the functions associated with other disciplines themselves or work effectively with other design engineers who have.

- It is at this point, when the design engineer crosses the synthesis path from the functional architecture domain to the physical architecture domain and its associated DPs that they face their greatest challenge: *creativity*. The word strikes fear in the hearts of many young designers. As young designers ourselves, we recall being perpetually in awe of how our design professors seemed to magically come up with design solutions from "thin air." And yet, creativity is not a binary characteristic encoded in DNA. Rather, it is cultivated by a willingness to loosen and expand one's established mental constructs, whether by picking up new books or immersing oneself amongst and appreciating the perspectives of a broad diversity of people. Each person, their field, and personal set of experiences can be characterized by a set of "mental constructs" that serve as "meta-design-parameters" that the design engineer deploys creatively in the moment of synthesis. The design engineer soon recognizes that the 14 NAE goals are indeed challenges for the specific reason that they require a broad number and diversity of such "meta-design-parameters." No single design engineer will have them all, but design teams can produce maximally effective large complex systems by fostering an environment where new ideas are encouraged and easily communicated.
- As the design engineer implements their solution and crosses over to the process architecture domain, they find that the large complex system has already been implemented—at a cost of millions, billions, or even trillions of dollars—poorly no less—in the form of the *legacy system*! The likelihood of implementing their

"forward-engineering design" is low. Despair can set in. But with newfound energy, the design engineer sets off in the reverse direction; now along the "analytical path," "reverse-engineering" the legacy system. They task themselves with modeling the PVs, DPs, FRs, and SRs of the legacy system; knowing full well that they will have to make a sequence of meaningful piecewise transformations toward an "ideal" design solution that reconciles their forward design with the existing system all while it remains operational.

14.1.2 Chapter Contribution

This chapter introduces the design engineer to the world of large complex systems from an AD perspective. It would be entirely intractable to try to address *all* of the specific challenges mentioned in the large complex system design story relayed above. Rather, this chapter focuses on two critical "systems-thinking" design skills that help the designer manage the inherent and abstract complexity of large systems. They are (1) system decomposition and (2) the allocation of function to form. The chapter also practically demonstrates these design skills in several tractable design case studies. The chapter also discusses why and how these design skills are used differently when the system has a fixed versus a flexible structure. The chapter concludes with a discussion of several open challenges in the design of large complex systems.

14.1.3 Chapter Outline

The remainder of the chapter is organized as follows: Section 14.2 treats the AD of large fixed systems. Section 14.3 then provides several design stories of large fixed systems. Finally, Sect. 14.4 discusses large flexible systems and contrasts them with the large fixed systems discussed earlier in the chapter.

14.2 Axiomatic Design of Large Fixed Engineering Systems

14.2.1 What Are Large Fixed Engineering Systems?

The previous section used the examples of the 14 NAE challenges to motivate the topic of large complex systems. This section addresses an important subset of these called "large fixed engineering systems (Farid and Suh 2016)." To gain insight, the term must be deconstructed into its constituent words.

There is no shortage of definitions in the literature for the term "system." This chapter adopts the definition below:

Definition 14.1. System: A set of components (subsystems, segments) acting together to achieve a set of common objectives via the accomplishment of a set of tasks.

Note that the mere definition of the term requires the definition of three more abstract systems thinking concepts:

Definition 14.2. System Boundary: The delineation between the system and its environment or context.

Definition 14.3. System Form: What a system "is." It includes a description of

1. all the system's components (or DPs);
2. how the components are interconnected;
3. what portion of the total system behavior/function is carried out by each component.

Definition 14.4. System Function/Behavior: What a system "does." It is its reason for existence. A set of subfunctions (or FRs) that must be performed to achieve a specific objective.

Returning to the AD framework shown in Fig. 14.1, the system form constitutes the physical architecture domain and the system function constitutes the functional architecture domain.

"Large systems" are referred to as such because they have a "large" number of system elements; be they FRs or DPs. How large is a "large number"? For all practical purposes, the answer is driven by the psychological limitations of the human mind as it attempts to design the system. In 1956, Miller recognized that human beings can typically recall 7 ± 2 numerical digits in short term memory. Consequently, as a rule of thumb, the literature refers to systems with approximately 7 elements as "small-sized," $7^2 \approx 50$ elements as "medium-sized," and $7^3 \approx 300$ elements as "large-sized." Interestingly, at $7^4 \approx 2500$ elements or greater, the system can no longer be designed practically by a single designer (or system architect). Instead, multiple designers or design teams with their respective responsibilities must cooperate to produce a well-functioning large system.

The mere existence of multiple designers implies that they must manage the interdependencies between the systems' elements. The term "complex system" is often used to refer to systems with a large number of interdependencies between its constituent elements. For clarity, it is useful to distinguish between two types of such interdependencies:

Definition 14.5. Interactions: An interdependency is caused by the sequence of one FR followed by another.

Definition 14.6. Interfaces: An interdependency is caused by the relationship between one DP and another. For example, there may exist a flow of matter between two components.

One can imagine that a system with N elements can have up to N^2 interdependencies. Consequently, a large system by virtue of its number of elements is likely to be complex as well by virtue of the interdependencies between these elements.

As the large complex system grows in size, potentially over many years, it is likely that its elements and their interdependencies will change. Consequently, AD distinguishes between "large fixed engineering systems" and "large flexible engineering systems."

Definition 14.7. Large Fixed Engineering System: An engineering system with a large set of FRs which do not evolve over time and whose components (DPs) also do not change over time.

Definition 14.8. Large Flexible Engineering System: An engineering system with many FRs that not only evolve over time but also can be fulfilled by one or more DPs.

Finally, this book is devoted to "engineering systems" rather than "systems" broadly; in that the latter includes (natural) systems (e.g., the solar system, the human body) that are not engineered but still adhere to the three minimal requirements of being a system stated above.

14.2.2 Divide and Conquer: Decomposition of System Hierarchy

The first critical "systems-thinking" design skill is decomposition of the system hierarchy. Here, the engineer must use a "divide and conquer" mentality to manage the design of the large system. In brief, the system's elements; be they FRs or DPs must be decomposed into their constituent parts (Park 2007).

For the moment, let's assume a large fixed engineering system. By Definition 14.7, it has many FRs. Following Fig. 14.1, these were identified in a requirement engineering process where the requirements of the SRs domain were transformed into the high-level FRs of the functional architecture domain.

To recall, the FRs describe what the system must do, and sometimes they are simply referred to as the systems' functions to describe what the system does. Said differently, they are a mutually exclusive and collectively exhaustive set that describes the system functionally. Each FR must be defined in a solution-neutral way that doesn't presuppose the technologies of the design solution. By convention, each function is defined as a transitive verb stated in the third person singular followed by its associated object/operand. For example, in a home design, one FR may be:

FR1 = Protect Internal Climate.

There is a lot packed into such a "high-level" FR. For this reason, it is often necessary to *decompose* each function into a number of lower level of functions that *aggregate* to achieve the same end. In decomposing a given FR, the designer must be careful to keep the lower level FRs mutually exclusive and collectively exhaustive. For example, FR1 can be decomposed into:

FR1.1 = Keep out Moisture;
FR1.2 = Damp out Hot/Cold Fluctuations in the External Environment;
FR1.3 = Heat and Cool Interior Area to desired temperature;
FR1.4 = Redirect falling rain away from the house;
FR1.5 = Admit natural light;
FR1.6 = Protect from Insects;
FR1.7 = Allow entry/exit of inhabitants;
FR1.8 = Protect from Intruders.

The designer can further decompose each of these FRs into even lower level FRs until the large system has sufficient functional detail to be fully realized. In an abstract and general sense, this iterative process generates a functional hierarchy as shown in Fig. 14.2. Furthermore, in many cases, it is useful to explicitly identify the functional interactions between each system function at each level of functional decomposition. At such a point, the functional hierarchy becomes a complete functional architecture.

In an analogous fashion, a large system also has a physical hierarchy composed of multiple decompositions of DPs; be they systems, subsystems, components, or single numerical parameters. At the highest level of hierarchy, the large system is a single DP. For example, in-home design:

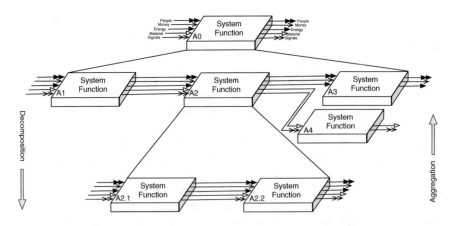

Fig. 14.2 A functional architecture that has been decomposed two levels. Parallel and serial interactions are shown between each function

DP1: House's External Barrier.

This high-level DP can be decomposed into several lower level DPs (as subsystems):

DP1.1 = Waterproof Shell;
DP1.2 = Insulation layer;
DP1.3 = Air-source heat pump;
DP1.4 = Gutter system;
DP1.5 = Window;
DP1.6 = Window screens;
DP1.7 = Doors;
DP1.8 = Door locks.

Finally, when the physical hierarchy is depicted with the physical interactions between each DP, it becomes the physical architecture. At such a point, it resembles the functional architecture in Fig. 14.2; but with the functions replaced with components (or DPs).

Functional and physical decomposition create the AD dual hierarchy shown in Fig. 14.3. It serves as the primary means by which a designer tackles the inherently large number of elements (i.e., FRs and DPs) in the system. Rather than view the large system as a loose collection of functions and components, these sets are organized methodically in a tree-like structure. The primary advantage is to reduce the "mental-load" of the designer so that they are only thinking of the elements that are directly related within the associated hierarchy.

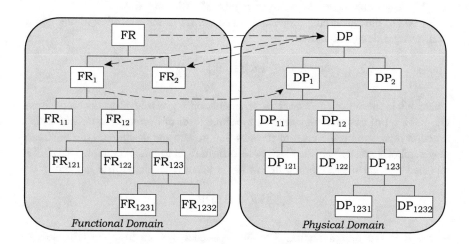

Fig. 14.3 The Axiomatic Design dual hierarchy: Functional decomposition, physical decomposition, and the allocation of function to form in a "Zigzagging" process

One question that often arises is how to organize the functional and physical hierarchies. One may imagine that a given FR or DP can be decomposed all at once into many (potentially hundreds) of elements. Alternatively, one may imagine that the designer organizes these elements into many decomposition layers. In theory, the choice of the number of decomposition steps is arbitrary. In practice, it matters tremendously. For example, the physical hierarchy may be organized into assemblies and subassemblies that have real manufacturing significance. Similarly, design teams may have certain functional expertise that drives how we may think of the FRs. Finally, the 7 ± 2 rule mentioned above provides a practical "design rule of thumb" from which designers should not depart too far.

14.2.3   Allocation of Function to form—the Zigzagging Process

The second critical "systems-thinking" design skill is the allocation of function to form in what is called the "zigzagging process." In the previous section, functional and physical decomposition were presented independently. In reality, a given FR can rarely be decomposed without first assuming some technological solution that fulfills it. In the meantime, decomposing a given DP has little meaning without understanding the FRs that the decomposed DPs fulfill. Consequently, in forward-design, the designer considers a given FR, conceives a DP to fulfill it, and then allocates the function to this new element of form. At that point, the designer decomposes the FR while assuming the newly conceived DP. In such a way, the two critical design skills of decomposition and function-to-form allocation are used in an alternating fashion. A single designer can handle several zigzagging processes to accommodate several hundred DPs. Beyond that, a design team can work together to accommodate a system of potentially arbitrary size.

As part of the zigzagging process, AD keeps track of the allocation of function to form using a design equation:

$$FR \, \$ \, f(DP)$$

where FR is the set of functional requirements on a given level of decomposition, DP is the set of design parameters on the same level of decomposition, and f() is a function representing the laws of physics that govern the design and the relatively new symbol $ means "satisfies" when read from right to left. When the $ symbol is replaced with an = and the first derivative is taken it yields a linear equation:

$$\Delta FR = B \Delta DP$$

where B is the design matrix. The Independence Axiom instructs designers to ensure that this design matrix is square and diagonal to reach an uncoupled design, and if not then square and lower triangular to reach a decoupled design. When the

	1.1	1.2	1.3	1.4	1.5	1.6	1.7	1.8
1.1	X							
1.2	X	X						
1.3	X	X	X					
1.4	X			X				
1.5	X				X			
1.6					X	X		
1.7	X						X	
1.8							X	X

Fig. 14.4 Axiomatic Design matrix of a house's external barrier

design matrix is anything else, the design is said to be coupled and it violates the Independence Axiom. For example, the decomposed FRs and DPs mentioned in the previous section yield the design matrix below (Fig. 14.4).

One important consequence of the Independence Axiom is that it affects the project management of the design or the design workflow. A designer's task is to complete the selection of all the DPs that fulfill the FRs. The design matrix shows the selection of DPs must be taken in groups. The group of DPs that fulfill a given FR is called a *module*. The design matrix also shows that there is a specific order in which to design each module. In the case of an uncoupled design, the modules can be designed entirely independently in parallel. As shown in Fig. 14.5, in a design flow diagram, such a case is defined by a summation (Ⓢ) junction of two or modules. In the case of decoupled design, Fig. 14.5 shows a control (ⓒ) junction to indicate the design of one module must follow another sequentially. Finally, in the case of a coupled design, Fig. 14.5 shows a feedback (Ⓕ) junction to indicate that the design of one module is in an iterative feedback loop with another module. The problem with such feedback loops is that it is not always clear how many design iterations will be required to escape the design feedback! In the design of large systems, such design feedback loops can be entirely debilitating and ultimately bring design progress to a screeching halt! In short, the Independence Axiom does not just facilitate good designs, it also facilitates efficient design workflows.

To summarize, the forward-design zigzagging process follows several rules. The designer must:

1. Conceive the DPs associated with the FRs in the same level.
2. Respect the Independence Axiom when allocating function to form. The design is ideally uncoupled and otherwise decoupled. If necessary, draw a design workflow diagram to operationalize the sequence of design task amongst the design team.
3. Decompose the FRs of the subsequent level based upon the choice of DPs in the level immediately above.

Fig. 14.5 Elements and
junctions in a design
workflow diagram. Summing,
control, and feedback
junctions correspond to
uncoupled, decoupled, and
coupled designs, respectively

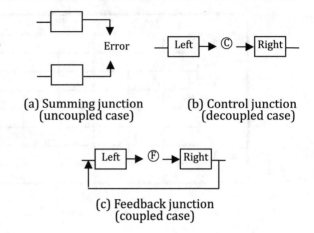

(a) Summing junction
(uncoupled case)

(b) Control junction
(decoupled case)

(c) Feedback junction
(coupled case)

4. Ensure that the FRs and DPs in a lower level are a mutually exclusive and
   collectively representation of the FRs and DPs in the level immediately above.
5. Continue the zigzagging process until the AD dual hierarchy includes sufficient
   detail to implement the design solution.

Zigzagging in reverse-engineering simply runs in reverse. The designer must
start from the individual components (or DPs) and then deduce the associated FRs.
From there, the designer proceeds to a higher level of aggregation in the DPs and
then deduces the associated FRs on that level. Such a reverse-engineering approach
is necessary when a part or a whole of the system has already been built and the
development of the functional architecture is required to determine how to "evolve"
the system forwards to a more advanced stage of development. In some cases, the
deduction of the associated FR is straight forward. Many tried-and-true physical
solutions have well-known functions. For example, I-beams in buildings support
weight and railways transport trains.

14.3 Examples

The two critical "systems-thinking" design skills of system decomposition and the
allocation of function to form are surprisingly powerful tools in the engineer's
armament toward the design of large complex systems. This section presents case
studies where these two skills are applied practically. The provided examples have
been chosen for their manageable size so as to facilitate learning.

14.3.1 Axiomatic Design of the Mount Type Air Conditioning System

The mount type air conditioning system is a type of heating, ventilating, and air conditioning (HVAC) control system that is installed between a ceiling and the ceiling boards of a room to control room temperature. Such a product is investigated from AD point of view (Lee et al. 2009). The overall decomposition of the system hierarchy is established down to the "atomic" level components. Some coupled aspects are found, but ultimately kept at the request of the design sponsor. The sponsor wants to keep some of the existing component-level parts, and so the coupled aspects of the design are reported as warnings in the design process.

The basic operating principle of the mount type air conditioning system is to absorb heat in a room and emit it to the exterior. Figure 14.6 illustrates the components of the mount type air conditioning system which consists of indoor and outdoor machines. Most of the air conditioning systems employ the refrigeration cycle using a refrigerant to generate cool air in a room. Figure 14.7 presents the refrigeration cycle using the refrigerant. In the outdoor part, a compressor generates the flow of refrigerant and a condenser releases heat. The indoor part consists of a capillary tube to control the flow of the refrigerant and an evaporator to absorb the heat in the room. The refrigerant periodically circulates between the two sides so that the indoor heat is absorbed and released outside. Currently, the design is carried out based on the conventional process illustrated in Fig. 14.8. Since the machine is not a new one, most of the design components are already known. Therefore, the designer selects appropriate components and sets the values of the associated DPs. Performance tests are then conducted to meet the requirements. The designer iteratively redesigns the components until the performance requirements are satisfied. The associated workflow is illustrated in Fig. 14.9.

Each customer presents a new set of performance requirements. In such a case, the product should be re-designed and re-manufactured each time to satisfy the new conditions. The conventional design method relies on a trial-and-error approach to

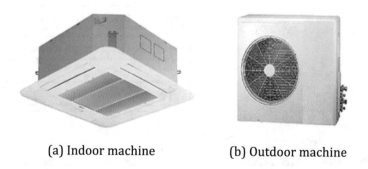

(a) Indoor machine   (b) Outdoor machine

Fig. 14.6 Indoor and outdoor machines. (Reproduced with permission from Lee et al. 2009)

Fig. 14.7 Composition of an air conditioning system. (Reproduced with permission from Lee et al. 2009)

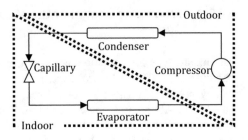

Fig. 14.8 The conventional design process for an overall air conditioning system. (Reproduced with permission from Lee et al. 2009)

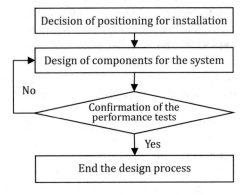

Fig. 14.9 The conventional design process for the design of a part of an air conditioning system. (Reproduced with permission from Lee et al. 2009)

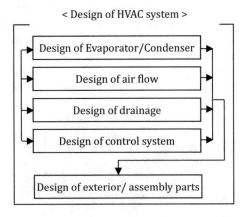

meet the new set of requirements because it is not easy to identify the relationships between the components and their characteristic DPs. Furthermore, the designer may find it difficult to follow a rational design process that converges toward

Table 14.1 Customer needs for a mount type HVAC control system

Customer needs from general users	Customer needs from design engineers
People should feel cool	Dust or bad smell should be eliminated
The room should be cooled as soon as possible	The maintenance and management of the system should be easy
The cool air must sufficiently circulate	The system should need a small space and have an aesthetic shape
Uniform temperature is required	Regulations must be satisfied
Each vane should be controlled separately	Production costs should be minimized
Temperature control should be easy	
Control from a distance is required	
The machine should operate quietly	
Energy consumption should be minimized	

satisfied FRs. Along the way, the designer may exercise engineering judgment that relies on tacit knowledge. Such knowledge is neither written nor systematic and consequently is difficult to transfer to junior designers. All of these challenges make the conventional design process costly and slow.

In contrast, a new AD approach is demonstrated. Customer needs (*CNs*)—a subset of the SRs described in Sect. 14.1—are gathered first based on customer surveys and customer interviews with design engineers. The *CNs* are shown in Table 14.1. *FRs* are then identified based on the *CNs*, and *DPs* are selected to satisfy the independence of the *FRs*. The *FR–DP* relationship is made by the design matrix and the dual hierarchy of the design process is established. Again, the decomposition of the functional and physical hierarchies is made by the zigzagging approach. *CNs* are defined from the customer survey and interviews with design engineers.

Based on the *CNs* in Table 14.1, the *FRs* and *Cs* are defined at the top level.

FR1 = Minimize a possessed space of the mount type air conditioning system;
FR2 = Generate appropriate air current in the room;
FR3 = Make enough cold air;
FR4 = Minimize the vibration/noise of the mount type air conditioning system;
FR5 = Maintain purity of the air quality in the room;
FR6 = Control the temperature under user's directions.

Note that the FRs are stated in a solution-neutral language. All of the nouns in the FRs either (1) refer to the higher level DP of the "mount-type air conditioning system" or (2) refer to nouns in the design context (e.g., air space, air current, cold air, noise, air purity, temperature). Cs are defined as well. They provide bounds on acceptable design solutions and differ from the *FRs* in that they do not have to be independent.

$C1$ = Satisfy the first-grade for energy efficiency;
$C2$ = Satisfy related standards;
$C3$ = Satisfy the product size to sufficiently insert the air conditioning system between the ceiling and ceiling board;
$C4$ = Minimize production cost;
$C5$ = Make maintenance and repair of the system easy.

To meet the FRs, an appropriate set of DPs are defined.

$DP1$ = Ceiling type structure;
$DP2$ = Air current formation system;
$DP3$ = Mutual assistance system;
$DP4$ = Vibration/noise reduction system;
$DP5$ = Air cleaner system;
$DP6$ = Temperature control system.

Then the allocation of function to form is captured in the design matrix:

	DP1	DP2	DP3	DP4	DP5	DP6
FR1	X	0	0	0	0	0
FR2	X	X	0	0	0	0
FR3	0	X	X	0	0	0
FR4	0	X	X	X	0	0
FR5	0	0	0	0	X	0
FR6	0	X	X	0	X	X

where X represents where the FR is being fulfilled by one or more DPs and O represents otherwise. At the top level of decomposition, the design is decoupled, and the design matrix is lower triangular. Therefore, the independence of FRs (in the Independence Axiom) is guaranteed if the DPs are determined in increasing numerical order from FR1 to FR6.

The FRs and DPs at the top level are then iteratively decomposed using the zigzagging process described in the previous section until the bottom or "atomic" level components are reached. For the sake of brevity, a full explanation of the system decomposition is omitted here. The complete design matrix, however, is presented in Fig. 14.10. The left column of the table represents the FRs and the upper row includes the corresponding DPs. The mount type air conditioning system has a decoupled design at the top level as shown in Eq. (14.1). The entire design matrix at its lowest level of decomposition is, however, non-square and the resulting product design is classified as redundant and coupled. This situation is the direct result of the sponsor's request to keep the existing component-level parts.

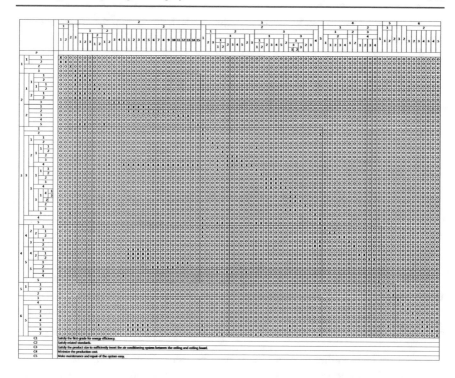

Fig. 14.10 Complete design matrix for mount type air conditioning system. (Reproduced with permission from Lee et al. 2009)

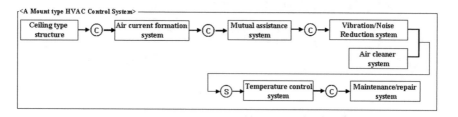

Fig. 14.11 Design flow of a mount type air conditioning system. (Reproduced with permission from Lee et al. 2009)

The coupled aspects are explained. The entire matrix in Fig. 14.11 is a non-square and consequently, some *FR–DP* relationships are coupled at some points of the hierarchy. For example, consider *FR*2.2.2.

*FR*2.2.2 = Generate the air flow in the perpendicular direction using a rotary motion.

The existing system has five corresponding *DP*s that make up the components of the turbofan.

DP2.2.6 = The number of blades;
DP2.2.7 = Ratio of the inside/external diameters;
DP2.2.8 = The angle among blades;
DP2.2.9 = Shape of the blade;
DP2.2.10 = Ratio of pitch/chord.

Consequently, the relationship between *FR2.2.2* and its *DP*s is:

	DP2.2.6	DP2.2.7	DP2.2.8	DP2.2.9	DP2.2.10
FR2.2.2	X	X	X	X	X

Obviously, it is a redundant design and a lot of feedback is required. The redundancy is also found in other components such as the motor, the orifice, the fin of the evaporator, and the condenser.

Several subsystems within this detailed design warrant further discussion. The *FR*s and *DP*s for the compressor system are defined as:

FR3.1 = Generate the pressure to change the state of the refrigerant;
FR3.2 = Generate the air-flow for the ability of air conditioning to sufficiently cool the room;
DP3.1 = Compressor system.

The associate portion of the design matrix is:

	DP3.1
FR3.1	X
FR3.2	X

In this case, the compressor system has an insufficient number of DPs, and its design matrix is full and therefore the compressor subsystem constitutes a coupled design. The capillary tube subsystem suffers from the same problem.

The heat exchanger system has an equal number of FRs and DPs but they are fully coupled.

FR3.3.2 = Change refrigerant from gas to liquid;
FR3.3.3 = Change refrigerant from liquid to gas;
DP3.2.2 = Evaporator system;
DP3.2.3 = Condenser system.

	DP3.2.2	DP3.2.3
FR3.3.2	X	X
FR3.3.3	X	X

Because the refrigerator cycle consists of the compressor system, the capillary tube, and the heat exchanger system, the refrigerator cycle as a whole also constitutes a coupled design. Note that only one coupled subsystem is required for the system as a whole to be classified as coupled. In an ideal situation, the DPs of the coupled design should be modified or replaced with a set that yields either an uncoupled or decoupled design. In this case, the firm decided to flag the coupled characteristics to alert designers to the potential for iterative feedback loops in the design process.

Returning back up to the top level of design decomposition, the associated design flow diagram is illustrated in Fig. 14.11. Because it is a decoupled design at the top level of hierarchy, the design flow links the modules sequentially. That said, if the design workflow were detailed further, feedback loops would appear within each of the system's modules.

In summary, this example has served to apply AD for large fixed systems to a mount type air conditioning system. AD demonstrates a rational and effective design process that decomposes the FRs and DPs at each level of hierarchy and then allocates function to form using the design matrix. These two systems thinking techniques allow the design team to manage the complexity of the design. Finally, the design flow diagram organizes the design's project management and is established from the design matrix.

The AD approach highlighted some differences between the existing conventional approach. In the conventional approach, each module was designed in parallel and then later integrated into a larger system; resolving inconsistencies in the design all at once. In contrast, AD highlighted the need for a sequential approach to the design of the high-level modules; thus avoiding the need to resolve downstream design inconsistencies. The improved design process is more effective for designers to not only understand the overall design process but also to meet the diversity of customer demands. Finally, the AD approach highlights the presence of coupled design feedback in lower levels of the dual hierarchy. These are fairly inefficient and time-consuming and have the potential to derail the design of the system as a whole. These coupled aspects are identified and flagged for management attention without eliminating them from the design as a whole.

14.3.2 Automobile Cooling System

We consider the design of a cooling system for a hybrid vehicle as illustrated in Fig. 14.12 (Park 2018). Coolant material is circulated in a cooling system to expel the generated heat from the engine. The circulation is illustrated in Fig. 14.13. Some of the heat is reused for heating the inside of the car.

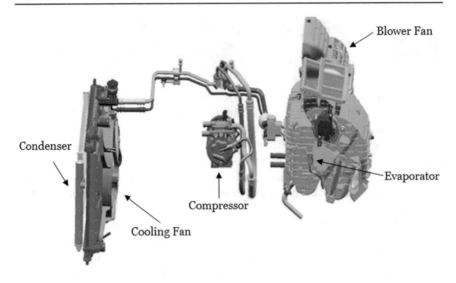

Fig. 14.12 An automobile cooling system

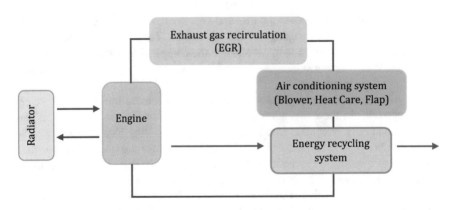

Fig. 14.13 Circuit of coolant and air in the cooling system

The *CN*s of the system are defined as:

CN1: The inside temperature should be kept within a certain range;
CN2: Environmental pollution is undesired;
CN3: The vehicle fuel economy should be high.

The top-level *FR* is defined based on the *CN*s: Increase the energy efficiency of a hybrid car while maintaining the inside temperature.

From the top-level *FR*, the next level *FR*s, *DP*s, and design matrix are

FR1 = Maintain the temperature of the air inside the vehicle;
FR2 = Reduce the emission of hazardous substances during operation;
FR3 = Control fuel consumption within acceptable bounds;

DP1 = Air conditioning system;
DP2 = Hazardous material reduction system;
DP3 = Energy management system.

	DP1	DP2	DP3
FR1	X	x	x
FR2	0	X	0
FR3	x	0	X

Note that FR1 and FR3 have a coupled design with respect to DP1 and DP3. This coupling is discussed in greater detail at lower levels of decomposition. *DP1* and *FR1* are decomposed to:

FR1.1 = Decrease room temperature;
FR1.2 = Increase room temperature;
DP1.1 = Air cooling system;
DP1.2 = Air heating system.

	DP1.1	DP1.2
FR1.1	X	0
FR1.2	0	X

The air cooling system is not considered further in this example. *FR1.2* and *DP1.2* are then decomposed to:

FR1.2.1 = Generate a heat source;
FR1.2.2 = Generate additional heat;
FR1.2.3 = Absorb the generated heat;
FR1.2.4 = Deliver the heat;
FR1.2.5 = Heat the air;
FR1.2.6 = Move the heated air;
FR1.2.7 = Adjust the air direction;
DP1.2.1 = Engine operation request logic;
DP1.2.2 = Positive temperature coefficient (PTC) system;
DP1.2.3 = Coolant;
DP1.2.4 = Coolant circuit;
DP1.2.5 = Heat core;
DP1.2.6 = Blower;
DP1.2.7 = Flap.

The associated design matrix is:

	DP1.2.1	DP1.2.2	DP1.2.3	DP1.2.4	DP1.2.5	DP1.2.6	DP1.2.7
FR1.2.1	X	0	0	0	0	0	0
FR1.2.2	0	X	0	0	0	0	0
FR1.2.3	0	0	X	0	0	0	0
FR1.2.4	0	0	0	X	0	0	0
FR1.2.5	0	0	x	0	X	0	0
FR1.2.6	0	0	0	0	x	X	x
FR1.2.7	0	0	0	0	0	x	X

FR2 and *DP2* can be decomposed to:

FR21 = Reduce the hazardous material before the combustion;
FR22 = Reduce the hazardous material after the combustion;
FR23 = Reduce the hazardous material during the combustion;
DP21 = Evaporative gas reduction system;
DP22 = Engine emission reduction system;
DP23 = Catalyst system.

The associated design matrix is:

	DP21	DP22	DP23
FR21	X	0	0
FR22	0	X	0
FR23	0	0	X

FR3 and *DP3* are decomposed as well. Figure 14.14 presents the entire design matrix after several more decomposition and zigzagging steps.

At first glance, the design of the automobile cooling system *appears* to be highly coupled. There are filled *X* elements in both the upper and lower triangles of the design matrix. Recall that FR1 and FR3 have a coupled design by virtue of DP1 and DP3 at the highest level of decomposition. These coupled elements manifest themselves in lower levels of decomposition as well. The situation, however, is not as bleak as one might think. The high-level coupling between FR1, FR3, DP1, and DP3 does not mean that *all* of the low-level FRs and DPs are coupled. Quite a bit of sparsity is introduced into the design matrix with each subsequent decomposition. After careful inspection, the designer finds that many of the filled elements in the upper triangle of the design matrix do not have their associated filled elements in the lower triangle. Indeed, a minimum condition of a truly coupled design is that there exist two DPs that are coupled to two FRs. Or mathematically, there exists at

	1.1	1.2.1	1.2.2	1.2.3	1.2.4	1.2.5	1.2.6	1.2.7	2.1.1	2.1.2	2.2.1	2.2.2.1	2.2.2.2	2.3.1	2.3.2	2.3.3	3.1.1	3.1.2	3.2.1.1	3.2.1.2	3.2.2.1	3.2.2.2
1.1	X	O	O	O	O	O	O	O	O	O	O	O	O	O	O	O	O	O	O	O	O	O
1.2.1	O	X	O	O	O	O	O	O	O	O	O	O	O	O	O	O	O	O	O	O	O	O
1.2.2	O	O	X	O	O	O	O	O	O	O	O	O	O	O	O	O	O	O	O	O	O	x
1.2.3	O	O	O	X	O	O	O	O	O	O	O	O	O	O	O	O	O	O	O	O	O	O
1.2.4	O	O	O	O	X	O	O	O	O	O	O	O	x	O	O	O	O	O	O	O	O	x
1.2.5	O	O	O	x	O	X	O	O	O	O	O	O	O	O	O	O	O	O	O	O	O	O
1.2.6	O	O	O	O	O	x	X	x	O	O	O	O	O	O	O	O	O	O	O	O	O	O
1.2.7	O	O	O	O	O	O	x	X	O	O	O	O	O	O	O	O	O	O	O	O	O	O
2.1.1	O	O	O	O	O	O	O	O	X	O	O	O	O	O	O	O	O	O	O	O	O	O
2.1.2	O	O	O	O	O	O	O	O	O	X	O	O	O	O	O	O	O	O	O	O	O	O
2.2.1	O	O	O	O	O	O	O	O	O	O	X	O	O	O	O	O	O	O	O	O	O	O
2.2.2.1	O	O	O	O	O	O	O	O	O	O	O	X	x	O	O	O	O	O	O	O	O	O
2.2.2.2	O	O	O	O	O	O	O	O	O	O	O	O	X	O	O	O	O	O	O	O	O	O
2.3.1	O	O	O	O	O	O	O	O	O	O	O	O	O	X	O	O	O	O	O	O	O	O
2.3.2	O	O	O	O	O	O	O	O	O	O	O	O	O	O	X	O	O	O	O	O	O	O
2.3.3	O	O	O	O	O	O	O	O	O	O	O	O	O	O	O	X	O	O	O	O	O	O
3.1.1	O	O	O	O	O	O	O	O	O	O	O	O	O	O	O	O	X	O	O	O	O	x
3.1.2	O	O	O	O	O	O	O	O	O	O	O	O	O	O	O	O	O	X	O	O	O	x
3.2.1.1	O	O	O	O	O	O	O	O	O	O	O	O	O	O	O	O	O	O	X	O	x	O
3.2.1.2	O	x	O	O	O	O	O	O	O	O	O	O	O	O	O	O	O	O	O	X	O	O
3.2.2.1	O	O	O	O	O	O	O	O	O	O	O	O	O	O	O	O	O	O	O	O	X	O
3.2.2.2	O	O	O	O	O	O	O	O	O	O	O	O	O	O	O	O	O	O	O	O	O	X

Fig. 14.14 Complete design matrix of an automobile cooling system prior to resorting FRs and DPs

least one pair of elements in the design matrix DM such that $DM(i, j) = DM(j, i)$, where $i \neq j$. Such a condition occurs in exactly one place above: FR1.2.6 and FR1.2.7 are coupled with DP1.2.6 and DP1.2.7. All of the other filled elements in the design matrix are asymmetric and indicate a decoupled design for the remainder of the automobile cooling system. To emphasize this point, the rows and the columns of the design matrix can be sorted in such a way as to bring all of the off-diagonal terms to either the matrix's upper or lower triangle. Figure 14.15 shows the complete design matrix of the same automobile cooling system after the FRs and DPs have been sorted. It reveals clearly the original conclusion that only FR1.2.6 and FR1.2.7 are coupled. This example illustrates that a high-level coupled

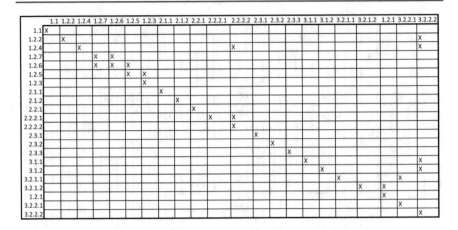

	1.1	1.2.2	1.2.4	1.2.7	1.2.6	1.2.5	1.2.3	2.1.1	2.1.2	2.2.1	2.2.2.1	2.2.2.2	2.3.1	2.3.2	2.3.3	3.1.1	3.1.2	3.2.1.1	3.2.1.2	1.2.1	3.2.2.1	3.2.2.2
1.1	X																					
1.2.2		X																				X
1.2.4			X									X										X
1.2.7				X	X																	
1.2.6				X	X	X																
1.2.5						X	X															
1.2.3							X															
2.1.1								X														
2.1.2									X													
2.2.1										X												
2.2.2.1											X	X										
2.2.2.2												X										
2.3.1													X									
2.3.2														X								
2.3.3															X							
3.1.1																X						X
3.1.2																	X					X
3.2.1.1																		X		X		
3.2.1.2																			X	X		
1.2.1																				X		
3.2.2.1																					X	
3.2.2.2																						X

Fig. 14.15 Complete design matrix of automobile cooling system after resorting FRs and DPs

design can be "rescued" with respect to the Independence Axiom to become a decoupled design in lower levels of decomposition if the nature of the coupling is reflected in an asymmetric design matrix! Fortunately, a creative designer can often find clever ways to introduce such asymmetry into the design.

14.3.3 Automobile Suspension System

The Independence Axiom is used to design the automobile suspension system shown in Fig. 14.16 (Park 2018). It connects the wheels and the body to make the automobile move. There are two suspension subsystems; one for the front wheels and the other for the rear wheels.

The *CN*s are:

CN1 = The vehicle must have a driving capability;
CN2 = Safety must be provided to the vehicle when driving.

From the *CN*s, the top-level *FR* is:

FR = Suspend the vehicle with stability while driving (*CN1* + *CN2*).

which is in turn decomposed into six *FR*s:

FR1 = Generate forward thrust from transmission system torque;
FR2 = Permit wheel rotation;
FR3 = Secure the car body;
FR4 = Suspend the vehicle with stability while driving on rugged roads;

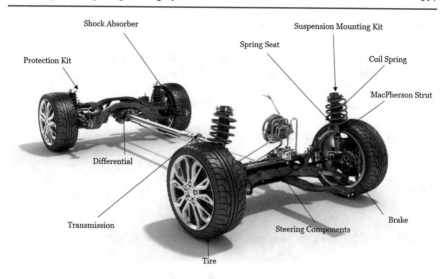

Fig. 14.16 An automobile suspension system. (Reproduced with permission from Nosorog 2019)

FR5 = Suspend the vehicle with stability while turning;
FR6 = Provide turning ability.

To meet *FR*s, an appropriate set of *DP*s are defined as follows:

DP1 = Wheel system;
DP2 = Knuckle and bearing;
DP3 = Mounting system;
DP4 = Independent link system;
DP5 = Stabilizer bar and shock absorber;
DP6 = Tie rod and ball joint.

The associated design matrix shows a decoupled design at the highest level of decomposition.

	DP1	DP2	DP3	DP4	DP5	DP6
FR1	X	0	0	0	0	0
FR2	x	X	0	0	0	0
FR3	0	0	X	X	0	0
FR4	0	x	x	X	x	0
FR5	x	0	x	x	X	0
FR6	0	x	0	0	x	X

FR1 and *DP1* are then decomposed.

FR11 = Generate friction force from transmission system torque;
FR12 = Deliver forward thrust from friction force;
DP11 = Tire;
DP12 = Wheel.

The associated design matrix shows a decoupled subsystem.

	DP11	DP12
FR11	X	0
FR12	x	X

FR2 and *DP2* are then decomposed and the corresponding design matrix is defined.

FR21 = Impede the motion of the wheel system through five coordinates (3 translation and 2 rotation);
FR22 = Permit the rotation of the wheel system about its axis;
DP21 = Knuckle;
DP22 = Bearing.

	DP21	DP22
FR21	X	x
FR22	x	X

FR3 and *DP3* are then decomposed and the corresponding design matrix is defined.

FR31 = Absorb vibration in mounting;
FR32 = Connect the car body;
DP31 = Mounting bush;
DP32 = Mounting bolt.

	DP31	DP32
FR31	X	0
FR32	x	X

FR4 and *DP4* are then decomposed and the corresponding design matrix is defined.

FR41 = Absorb vibration and noise at the junctions;
FR42 = Connect the mounting and wheel system;

FR43 = Allow the wheel system to move independently;
DP41 = A,G bush;
DP42 = Sub-frame;
DP43 = Lower arm.

	DP41	DP42	DP43
FR41	X	0	0
FR42	x	X	x
FR43	x	x	X

FR5 and *DP5* are then decomposed and the corresponding design matrix is defined.

FR51 = Provide rigidity for roll mode;
FR52 = Provide rigidity for the ride mode;
FR53 = Decrease in vertical energy;
FR54 = Limit the vertical distance of motion;
DP51 = Stabilizer bar;
DP52 = Spring;
DP53 = Damper;
DP54 = Bump stopper.

	DP51	DP52	DP53	DP54
FR51	X	x	0	0
FR52	x	X	0	0
FR53	0	x	X	0
FR54	0	x	x	X

FR6 *and* *DP6* are then decomposed and the corresponding design matrix is defined.

FR61 = Restrain the wheel system to turn;
FR62 = Provide a turning input;
DP61 = Ball joint;
DP62 = Tie rod.

	DP61	DP62
FR61	X	0
FR62	x	X

	1.1	1.2	2.1	2.2	3.1	3.2	4.1	4.2	4.3	5.1	5.2	5.3	5.4	6.1	6.2
1.1	X														
1.2	X	X													
2.1		X	X	X											
2.2			X	X											
3.1				X											
3.2				X	X		X					X			
4.1		X		X	X										
4.2					X			X	X						
4.3					X		X	X	X						
5.1					X					X	X				
5.2	X			X	X					X	X				
5.3					X							X			
5.4										X	X	X			
6.1		X										X	X		
6.2													X	X	

Fig. 14.17 Complete design matrix of an automobile suspension system

The entire design matrix is illustrated in Fig. 14.17. Although the suspension system has received many design iterations over a long period of time, there are many and more importantly non-negligible points of coupling between the FRs and the DPs. In the early stage of product development, the suspension system had relatively few and simple *FRs*. Over time, more *FRs* were added, and the design became quite complex with many non-zero off-diagonal terms in the design matrix. Despite this large number, only three pairs of DPs (shown in red above) have coupled designs. They are DP2.1 and DP2.2, DP4.2 and 4.3, and DP5.1 and 5.2. Although these pairs of DPs formally violate the Independence Axiom, the situation is quite manageable. These three pairs of DPs can be treated as three DPs, with each pair being treated as a single entity. Furthermore, the DPs appear at the bottom of the AD dual hierarchy, and so their coupled nature does not "ripple" across the design of the rest of the suspension system. Finally, product design companies can find it beneficial to have highly coupled components at the bottom of the dual hierarchy because they effectively embody proprietary and potentially secret design know-how that is not easily reproduced. That said, this special condition should not be interpreted as a license to ignore the Independence Axiom. The product's overall dual-hierarchy should remain uncoupled or decoupled (as above) and only if necessary introduce coupled DPs at the very bottom of the hierarchy.

14.3.4 Mobile Harbor

As the worldwide volume container shipments increases and very large container ships emerge as a dominant player in the maritime cargo transport market, the functional capabilities of container ports need to be greatly enhanced. For example, large container ships with streamline hulls lack maneuverability in tight and highly suggested maritime ports and often require tug boats which may in and of themselves be otherwise occupied. To address this problem, the Korea Advanced Institute of Science and Technology (KAIST) is undertaking a project to design a novel container transport system called Mobile Harbor (MH). A conceptual illustration of the MH is presented in Figs. 14.18 and 14.19 (Lee and Park 2010). MH refers to a system that can go out to a large container ship, anchor in the open sea, load and unload containers between itself and the container ship, and transport them to their destination. It has a flat bottom design so that it is maneuverable in narrow shipping lanes and stable enough to handle a wide variety of ocean-going cargo. Like many other large-scale engineering projects, the design of MH presents a number of challenges at the beginning stages of the project. In the conceptual

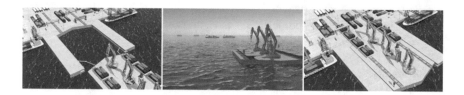

Fig. 14.18 Illustration of a revised mobile harbor concept (approved for funding by a national R&D program)

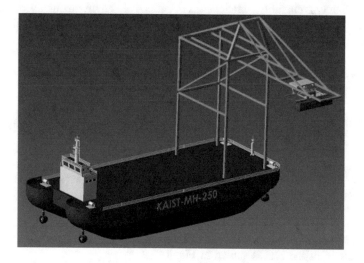

Fig. 14.19 The mobile harbor as conceptualized by Axiomatic Design (republished with permission of SAE international, from managing system design processusing Axiomatic Design: a case on KAIST mobile harbor Project, Lee and Park, 3, 1, 2010; permission conveyed through Copyright Clearance Center, Inc.)

design phase of the project, the design team must properly define and disseminate FRs, clarify interface requirements between its subsystems, identify and reconcile potential design conflicts like functional coupling.

To begin the AD, the top-level *FRs*, *DPs*, and Cs are defined.

FR = Transfer containers from ships anchoring in the sea to a harbor;
FR1 = Load/unload the containers;
FR2 = Keep the containers in MH (Mobile Harbor);
FR3 = Let MH float on the sea;
FR4 = Let MH navigate on the sea;
FR5 = Dock MH against the container ship in the open sea.

DP = Mobile harbor (MH);
DP1 = Crane system;
DP2 = Deck system for loading the containers;
DP3 = Floating body structure;
DP4 = Driving system <propulsion + navigation>;
DP5 = Mooring system + Docking system.

Constraints

C1 = The capacity of the power generator should be large enough to cover the needed energy (Generate a certain power for operating.);
C2 = The total weight should be less than a specified value;
C3 = The MH carries the containers up to 250 TEU;
C4 = Safety, reliability, efficiency, cost-effective, environmentally acceptable, automation, the satisfaction of standard and shipping registration or other rules.

According to the relationship between *FRs* and *DPs*, the design matrix is defined as follows:

	DP1	DP2	DP3	DP4	DP5
FR1	X	x	0	0	0
FR2	x	X	X	0	0
FR3	x	x	X	0	0
FR4	x	0	x	X	0
FR5	x	0	x	x	X

For illustrative purposes, the AD of DP1 is presented in detail and the completed design matrix of the MH is shown in Fig. 14.19.

Decomposition of FR1 (DP1: Crane system)

FR11 = Translocate the containers between MH and a container ship in the open sea or a harbor;

FR12 = Load and unload the containers, while MH is on the sea;
DP11 = Container crane;
DP12 = Dynamic control system of MH movement.

	DP11	DP12
FR11	X	0
FR12	X	X

Decomposition of FR11 (DP11: Container crane)

FR111 = Let the container crane of MH approach to the containers in a container ship or open sea;
FR112 = Hold the container;
FR113 = Move the container;
DP111 = The size and shape of the container crane and moving system of the container;
DP112 = An appropriate configuration of the crane structure to have sufficient strength;
DP113 = The hoist device including a trolley.

Decomposition of FR12 (DP12: Dynamic control system of MH movement)

FR121 = Minimize the movement of the container due to the vibration of the boom while working on the sea;
FR122 = Minimize the movement of the container due to the vibration of the hoist while working on the sea;
DP121 = Zero moment point (ZMP) system for stability control;
DP122 = Dynamic control system of the trolley;
Cs = The condition of sea state 3 (a wave level) should be satisfied.

	DP121	DP122
FR121	X	0
FR122	x	X

The MH constitutes an entirely novel large complex product. It is able to go out to a ship anchored in the open sea to load and unload cargo from it without occupying a pier of a land-based harbor. Such a functionality relieves the cargo ship from having to come into a stationary harbor to unload and load its cargo. Furthermore, the increasing size of container ships means that fewer and fewer harbors have a sufficiently large pier and are sufficiently deep. The MH is also capable of loading and unloading cargo to and from a large ship to the stationary land-based harbor without a container quay by pre-loading the cargo in freight cars placed on the MH which themselves can be moved onto and removed from the MH. The MH was designed so that it can approach both sides of a cargo ship and attach itself securely; further reducing the time to load and unload cargo. In addition to these us cases, the MH can be used inland within a canal to allow the crossing of transport containers and goods. One integral part of the design is positioning. Not only must the MH control horizontal translation on the sea and vertical height alignment but it also uses a large gyroscopic apparatus to stabilize rotation even in the presence of large waves.

The final design matrix is illustrated in Fig. 14.20. It is almost entirely decoupled. FR2 is weakly coupled with FR1 and FR3. Keeping the containers in the MH has the potential to impact their loading/unloading as well as the overall floating functionality of the MH. Over most conditions, these coupling are quite weak. They only represent a few DPs and can be given sufficient design attention upfront so as to allow the remainder of the design to proceed. Nevertheless, one must recognize that as the designers pursue ever-more "aggressive" MH designs with an ever-larger number of increasingly heavy containers, the coupling will strengthen and eventually lead to design infeasibility. Indeed, the presence of such coupling is entirely inherent to the mobile application and is predicted by AD theory. The "Design Range and Coupling" theorem in AD theory states:

> Theorem 20. Design Range and Coupling: If the design ranges of uncoupled or decoupled designs are tightened, they may become coupled designs. Conversely, if the design ranges of some coupled designs are relaxed, the designs may become either uncoupled or decoupled.

Many mobile applications ultimately suffer from such coupling because the mobility of the application effectively places hard Cs on the design range for space, energy, and functionality. The energy and power capabilities of many robots and drones are limited by their size and weight. Sea-faring vessels must also ensure flotation, and aerospace applications must ensure flight. Finally, the most recent smart city research demonstrates that as an urban population expands, and the demands for water, energy, mobility, and other infrastructure services grow, the design and planning of the city's infrastructure systems become increasingly interdependent within the city's confined geography. Whereas such couplings can provide the integrated delivery of infrastructure services, they are also susceptible to failures propagating from one subsystem to another. Alternatively, the city's confined geography can be loosened to avoid such a situation; at which point urban sprawl becomes the concern.

14.3.5   The Online Electrical Vehicle

The On-Line Electrical Vehicle (OLEV) is a type of electric vehicle that was developed at KAIST to overcome many of the problems posed by conventional electric vehicles: limited driving range on a single charge, the battery's heavy weight, and its high cost. The conceptual configuration is illustrated in Fig. 14.21 (Hong and Park 2010). The OLEV design team is composed of many designers from many engineering disciplines including automobile engineering and electromagnetics.

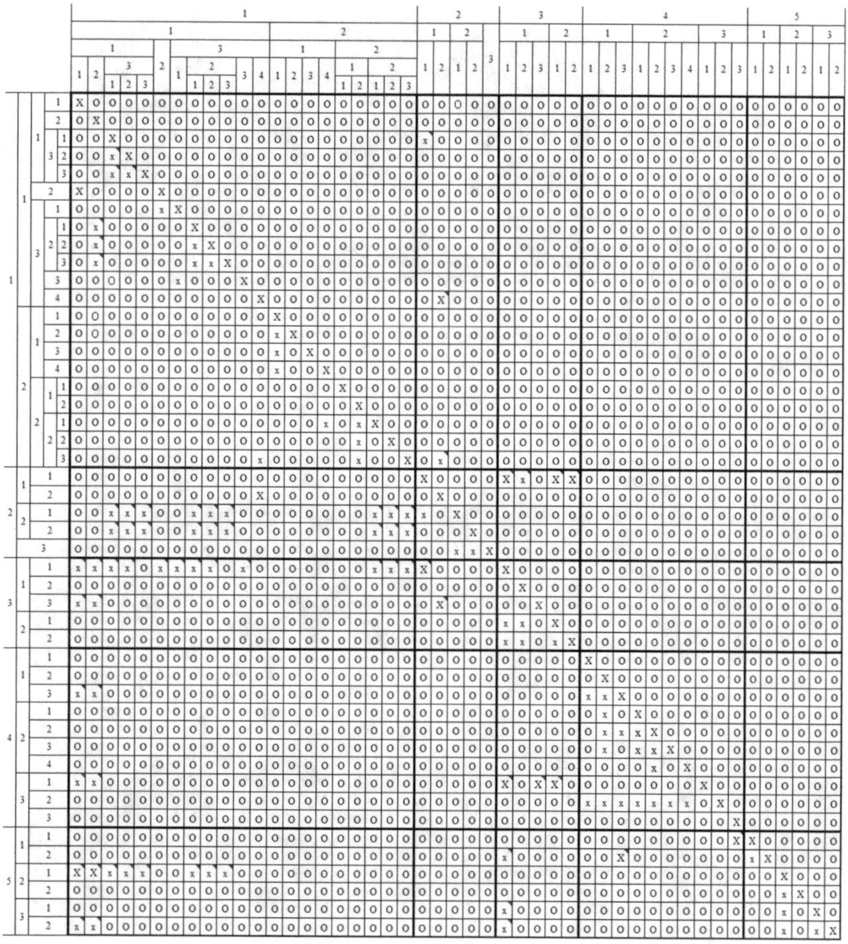

Fig. 14.20 Complete design matrix of the mobile harbor

The integration of these multiple fields presents a significant design challenge. Consequently, the design was conducted by a "design team" and an "integration team." Their roles and workflows are illustrated in Fig. 14.22. The integration team defines the FRs, at which point, the design team defines the DPs, at which point the integration team defines the design matrix and defines the new set of decomposed FRs. This alternation between the two teams realizes the zigzagging process on the fly and prevents the inadvertent introduction of design coupling.

The FRs and DPs at the top level are

$FR1$ = Import electric power;
$FR2$ = Transmit electric power to the vehicle;

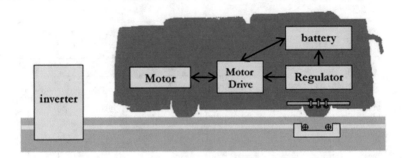

Fig. 14.21 Conceptual organization of the OLEV (approved for funding by a national R&D program)

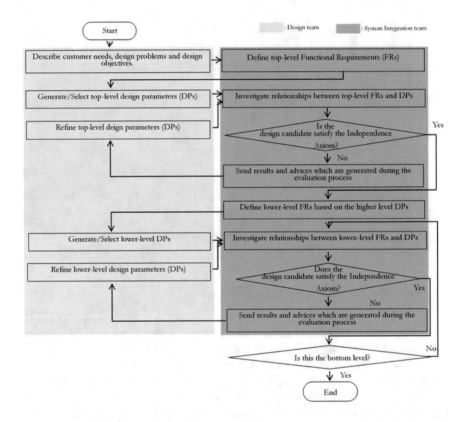

Fig. 14.22 Design process of the OLEV. (Republished with permission of SAE International, from Design Information Management of an On-Line Electric Vehicle Using Axiomatic Design, Hong and Park, 3, 1, 2010; permission conveyed through Copyright Clearance Center, Inc.)

FR3 = Operate the vehicle using electric power;
FR4 = Protect systems from external loads;

DP1 = Three phase AC 370-440 V;
DP2 = Induction Coupling System;
DP3 = Electric Vehicle;
DP4 = System protection devices.

From the *FR-DP* relationship, the design matrix is defined.

	DP1	DP2	DP3	DP4
FR1	*X*	*0*	*0*	*0*
FR2	*X*	*X*	*0*	*X*
FR3	*0*	*X*	*X*	*0*
FR4	*0*	*X*	*0*	*X*

Throughout the design process, much effort was exerted to maintain a decoupled design. Nevertheless, the design matrix above shows a high-level coupling by virtue of the FR2–DP4 coupling. Investigating further, this coupling arises because the system protection devices are coupled to the transmission of electric power to the vehicle. This coupling is ultimately inevitable because the safety considerations of transferring many kilowatts of electricity inductively through an air gap require a highly integrated design between the induction coupling and the protection devices. From this high-level design matrix, the zigzagging process is carried out until the bottom level is reached. The final design matrix is presented in Fig. 14.23. The FR2–DP4 coupling is highlighted to alert the design and integration teams to the potential for design iterations.

This design example, much like the MH example before it, serve to demonstrate the utility of AD in large systems of unprecedented function. The engineers on the project cannot rely on other products or large systems for inspiration. Rather, they must deeply reflect on what the system must achieve and consequently synthesize the associated FRs and DPs. From there, the two critical systems thinking skills detailed at the beginning of the chapter become the guiding principles of forward-design: decomposition of the functional and physical hierarchy and the allocation of function to form through the zigzagging process. When used in concert, they serve as the primary means by which a designer or design team can tackle the design of large fixed engineering systems.

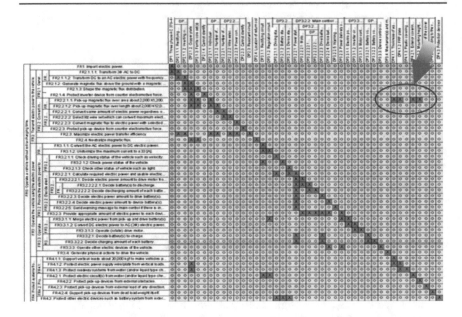

Fig. 14.23 Complete design matrix of the OLEV (Republished with permission of SAE International, from design information management of an On-Line Electric Vehicle using Axiomatic Design, Hong and Park, 3, 1, 2010; permission conveyed through Copyright Clearance Center, Inc.)

14.4 Axiomatic Design of Large Flexible Engineering Systems

Thus far, the chapter has motivated the role of design science as a means by which engineers can tackle the 14 grand challenges identified by the National Academy of Engineers. It recognized that design science provides engineers with a meta-problem-solving skill set composed of several systems-thinking design skills. The chapter focused on two of these: decomposition of the system function and form as a means to "divide-and-conquer" and the allocation of function to form in a manner consistent with the Independence Axiom. These two design skills were demonstrated on a half-dozen design examples and in so doing demonstrated their salience to a wide variety of large fixed engineering systems in many application domains.

A curious engineering design student may naturally ask: "What if we wished to design a large flexible engineering system?" (see Definition 14.8 at the beginning of the chapter.). Indeed, many of the NAE grand challenges identified at the beginning of the chapter will require enduring engineering solutions that respond to the changing needs of society. Furthermore, they are likely to require such large investments that it would be entirely cost prohibitive to design systems from scratch. These design solutions will need to build upon existing legacy systems and will need to continually evolve their functionality over and over again. Unfortunately, the answer to the curious student's question cannot be answered comprehensively in a single book chapter, or perhaps even book, because in many ways it presents a relatively open frontier for the development of design science as an engineering discipline. The literature on the AD of large flexible engineering systems has expanded over the years and has developed to now be called hetero-functional graph theory; given its heavy reliance on graph theoretic concepts. Nevertheless, this chapter can serve to open the door to this fascinating realm of design science and systems engineering.

The AD of large flexible engineering systems was first mentioned by Suh in his 2001 text. He presented the following abstract example of a large flexible engineering system *knowledge base*:

$$FR_1 \$ (DP_1^a, \; DP_{1,...,}^b DP_1^r)$$

$$FR_2 \$ (DP_2^a, \; DP_{2,...,}^b DP_2^q)$$

$$FR_3 \$ (DP_3^a, \; DP_{3,...,}^b DP_3^w)$$

$$\cdots$$

$$FR_m \$ \left(DP_m^a, \; DP_{m,...,}^b DP_m^s\right)$$

where the first line means that FR1 (as indicated by the $) can be satisfied by DP_1^a *or* DP_1^b *or* DP_1^r, etc. These few lines are remarkably profound. First, note that the knowledge base does *not* say that DP_1^a *and* DP_1^b *and* ... *and* DP_1^r satisfy FR1. If it did, it would become the design matrix used throughout the earlier parts of this chapter, and DP_1^a *and* DP_1^b *and* ... *and* DP_1^r would form either a decoupled or coupled engineering system. Instead, the focus is on the word "or." In other words, at a given moment in time, DP_1^a *alone* satisfies FR_1. Such a statement is simply another way of stating adherence to the Independence Axiom. Consequently, the knowledge base above (as presented in the Suh 2001 text) did not allow for decoupled and uncoupled designs. In so doing, it implicitly reached a profound conclusion: large flexible engineering systems *must* adhere to the Independence Axiom if they are to maintain their ability to evolve their FRs and DPs over time.

We offer a logical proof by contradiction. In the case of an ideal uncoupled design (with an identity design matrix), the engineer would remove a DP from a functioning system, and an entire FR would be removed at the same time. The system would then continue to function with reduced functionality. In contrast, if a given FR demonstrated a decoupled design and was coupled to multiple DPs, or if the FR demonstrated a couple design and was coupled to other FRs, then when one of the associated DPs were removed, the system would demonstrate broken functionality! Furthermore, removing additional DPs to remove an entire module and its associated FR would lead to downstream effects on other FRs. By Definition 14.8, such a condition contradicts a functioning large flexible engineering system. Indeed, large flexible engineering systems demonstrate a "plug-and-play" functionality similar to that found in modern computers where functional and physical elements can be added or removed at will.

The knowledge base above also serves the design of large flexible engineering systems for two other reasons. First, by Definition 14.8, large flexible engineering systems have FRs that can be fulfilled by potentially many DPs. An identity design matrix does not show this. Therefore, in order to reveal this functional redundancy,[1] the set of FRs *instances* **FR** must be distinguished from the set of functional requirement *classes* $\mathbb{FR}$.[2] Second, the knowledge base allows a single DP to fulfill more than functional requirement class $\mathbb{FR}$. The importance of doing so is discussed later in the context of hierarchy in large flexible engineering systems. In brief, the knowledge base becomes the single most important concept in the design of large flexible engineering systems, in much the same way that the design matrix is important to the design of large fixed engineering systems.

As the AD of large flexible engineering systems developed into hetero-functional graph theory, the knowledge base was given an explicitly quantitative definition.

Definition 14.9 System Knowledge Base : A binary matrix **J** of size $\sigma(\mathbb{FR}) \times \sigma(\mathbf{DP})$ whose element $J(w,v) \in \{0,1\}$ is equal to one when an action e_{wv} (in the SysML sense) exists as a FR class $\mathbb{FR}_w$ being executed by a design parameter DP_v. These actions represent the "capabilities" in the engineering system.

Consequently, the design equation of the large flexible engineering system can be written in terms of the system knowledge base.

$$\mathbb{FR} = J \odot DP$$

where $\odot$ represents matrix Boolean multiplication.

Definition 14.10 Matrix Boolean Multiplication $\odot$. Given sets or Boolean matrices **B** and **C** and Boolean matrix **A**, **C** = **A**⊙**B** is equivalent to

$$C(i,k) = \bigvee_j A(i,j) \wedge B(j,k)$$

where $\wedge$ refers to the scalar "AND" operation and $\bigvee_j$ is an "OR" operation over j elements much like the well-known sigma sum Σ.

---

[1]Note that functional redundancy refers to having the same functional requirement repeated. For example, FR1 = generate electric power and FR2 = generate (backup) electric power. Functional redundancy should not be confused with "redundant designs" in the AD of large fixed systems were the number of DPs exceeds the number of FRs.

[2]The terms class and instance are drawn from the fields of software/systems engineering. Note that many works on AD do not make this distinction between functional requirement instances and functional requirement classes because it is rarely needed within a single design work. Here, the distinction is made in order to maintain the conceptual link between large fixed and large flexible engineering systems and the universality of the Independence Axiom in both cases.

The design equation of the large flexible engineering system stated above in no way replaces the design matrix B. In fact, the design equation stated at the beginning of the chapter can be written in a set-theoretic expression as well.

$$FR = B \circledast DP$$

where the aggregation operation $\circledast$ is defined as:

Definition 14.11 Aggregation Operator $\circledast$: Given Boolean matrix **A** and sets **B** and **C**, $C = A \circledast B$ is equivalent to

$$C(i) = \bigcup_j a(i,j) \wedge b(j)$$

where the $\bigcup_j$ operation is a union operation of j elements much like the well-known sigma sum Σ.

The engineering design student must recognize that these two statements of the design equation are equivalent in meaning, but must absolutely be distinguished from each other. They simply express the allocation of function to form in terms of the system knowledge base **J** or the design matrix **B**. The fine mathematical distinctions between the aggregation operator $\circledast$ and matrix Boolean multiplication $\odot$ and the set of functional requirement instances FR and the set of functional requirement classes $\mathbb{FR}$ facilitates the analysis of large flexible engineering systems in complementary ways.

Example 14.1

To solidify these large flexible engineering systems, consider the example of the simple manufacturing system depicted in Fig. 14.24. It consists of a drill press and milling machine. The former is able to drill a hole and the latter is able to do the same and mill surfaces. Each contains its respective fixture. The manufacturing system also has two one-way conveyors between them.

A quick analysis of the system yields:

FR = drill hole, drill hole, mill surface, store the part at point A, transport part from point A to point B, transport part from point B to point A, store the part at B.

DP = {drill press, milling machine drill, milling machine end mill, drill press fixture, conveyor 1, conveyor 2, milling machine fixture}.

Consequently, the design matrix $\mathbf{B} = \mathbf{I}^{7 \times 7}$. As expected, the system is uncoupled, and the Independence Axiom is satisfied. To continue the analysis, the FR classes are viewed instead of their instances.

$\mathbb{FR}$ = drill hole, mill surface, store the part at A, transport part from point A to point B, transport part from point B to point A, store the part at B}. Rather than viewing the DPs at the very lowest level of aggregation, it is often useful to

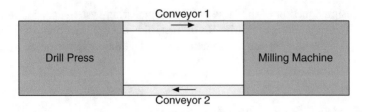

Fig. 14.24 A simple manufacturing system that consists of one drill press, one milling machine and two conveyors

aggregate the DPs to a higher level of abstraction. In this case, a logical aggregation yields:

$\overline{DP}$ ={drill press, milling machine, conveyor system}

At this level of physical aggregation, the system knowledge base J is defined.

$$
J = \begin{bmatrix} 1 & 1 & 0 \\ 0 & 1 & 0 \\ 1 & 0 & 0 \\ 0 & 0 & 1 \\ 0 & 0 & 1 \\ 0 & 1 & 0 \end{bmatrix}
$$

Note that the first column of the knowledge denotes that the drill press is cable of both drilling holes as well as storing the part. The second column shows that the milling machine is cable of doing both of those functions as well as also milling surfaces. The third column shows that the conveyor system is capable of transporting parts back and forth between the two machines. In all three cases, the columns assigned to each of these aggregated DPs, (often called resources in hetero-functional graph theory), was greater than one because each was capable of more than one function. Conversely, the first row has a sum greater than one to reflect that the function "drill hole" has two instances in the system. In short, the design matrix and the system knowledge base give complementary insights into how function is allocated to form in large flexible engineering systems.

Returning to the original exposition of large flexible engineering systems in the 2001 Suh text, the *flexible* nature was emphasized by a set of FRs that changed in time.

$$
\begin{aligned}
@t = 0 \qquad & \{FR\}_0 = \{FR_1, \ FR_5, \ FR_7, \ FR_m\} \\
@t = T_1 \qquad & \{FR\}_1 = \{FR_3, \ FR_5, \ FR_8, \ FR_z\} \\
@t = T_2 \qquad & \{FR\}_2 = \{FR_3, \ FR_9, \ FR_{10}, \ FR_m\}
\end{aligned}
$$

As the AD of large flexible engineering systems developed into hetero-functional graph theory, this time-dependent system functionality was quantified using a system Cs matrix.

Definition 14.12 System Cs Matrix: A binary matrix **K** of size $\mathbb{FR} \times DP$ whose element B(w,v) $\in \{0,1\}$ is equal to one when a constraint eliminates action e_{wv} from the action set.

A *reconfiguration process* is said to change the value of the system Cs matrix. Therefore, the system knowledge base contains information on the **existence** of capabilities in the engineering system. Meanwhile, the Cs matrix contains information on their **availability**. Quantitatively keeping track of these capabilities is done via the system's structural degrees of freedom as a quantitative measure.

Definition 14.13 Structural Degrees of Freedom[3]: The set of independent actions E_S that completely defines the available capabilities in a large flexible engineering system. Their number is given by

$$DOF = \sigma(\varepsilon) = \sum_{w}^{\sigma(FR)} \sum_{v}^{\sigma(DP)} [\mathbf{J} \odot \mathbf{K}](w, v)$$

Perhaps the last necessary topic in this introductory discussion of large flexible engineering systems is that of the AD dual hierarchy. When a functional or physical element is added or removed, it has the potential to disrupt their respective hierarchies as well. Simply speaking, a plane ceases to be one if it were to lose a wing. And its high-level function of flight would be impossible if it loses propulsion. Nevertheless, the designer can proceed cautiously.

Developing the AD dual hierarchy for large flexible engineering systems , downward in the direction of design synthesis, proceeds in the same way as for large fixed engineering systems. The system is viewed in terms of FR instances rather than classes. Because the Independence Axiom has been strictly maintained, each structural degree of freedom can be designed as previously described as if it were its own system. The engineering design problem is separable. Therefore, the addition or removal of a structural degree of freedom adds or removes all of the associated lower branches in the dual hierarchy .

It is also useful to consider the dual hierarchy of a large flexible engineering system upward in the direction of design analysis. Here, it is no longer required to aggregate the physical and functional hierarchies simultaneously. It is particularly common in bottom-up design to aggregate only the physical hierarchy into higher level DPs (or resources). A corresponding functional aggregation does not need to occur. Such was the case of the manufacturing system example above. This is because, in bottom-up design synthesis and analysis, physical aggregation and functional aggregation do not have the same meaning and do not necessarily imply

---

[3]The term structural degrees of freedom is appropriately named. Previous works on hetero-functional graph theory have shown that it is a generalization of the well-known concept of degrees of freedom in mechanical systems.

each other. Consider, for example, five tasks as FRs and five individuals as DPs; each of whom completes one task. This a large flexible engineering system that fulfills the Independence Axiom. The five individuals may be aggregated into a resource called a team without making any statement about the five tasks. They may not be related in any way (i.e., share any functional interaction). Similarly, the five tasks may be aggregated into a project without making any statement about the five individuals who complete them. They may have never met (i.e., share any physical interface). Physical aggregation is particularly interesting because it yields resources with many capabilities. An addition or removal of a DP yields the corresponding change in a resource's capabilities. In contrast, the functional aggregation of a large flexible engineering system may result in a rigid top-down structure. Any time the set of FRs changes, the functional hierarchy would need to change as well. In a project, the elimination of a single task causes the elimination of the project as a whole.

14.5 Conclusion

This chapter has introduced the design engineer to the world of large complex systems from an AD perspective and motivated the pressing need for such design skills in terms of the 14 grand challenges of the NAEs. The chapter focused on two critical systems-thinking design skills that help the designer manage the inherent and abstract complexity of large systems. They are (1) system decomposition as a means to "divide-and-conquer," and the allocation of function to form in what is often called the "zigzagging" process. These two skills were demonstrated in several tractable design case studies of large fixed engineering systems. The chapter also discusses why and how these design skills are used differently when the system has a fixed versus a flexible structure.

In distinguishing between large fixed and flexible engineering systems, this chapter has also opened the door to a fascinating realm of design science and systems engineering; one that remains a very open frontier for methodological development. Three broad directions of enquiry are worthy of note here:

- a quantitative understanding of life cycle properties;
- the treatment of cyber-physical systems;
- hetero-functional networks in large flexible engineering systems.

First, the field of systems engineering is increasingly concerned with developing a quantitative understanding of life cycle properties which can be deployed within engineering design. Many life cycle properties are called "ilities" because they end with that suffix. Flexibility, sustainability, reconfigurability, maintainability, and interoperability are but a few that follow this grammatical pattern. In the meantime, research into safety, quality, and even stability is well established in many engineering curriculums as independent design methods. Still, other life cycle properties like resilience are relatively new and garner active research interest. These "ilities" are usually classified as non-FRs; which are further classified as Cs in AD theory. Nevertheless, most of these life-cycle properties have a highly integrative nature and consequently, their integration into formal engineering design approaches like AD theory presents a significant intellectual challenge.

Second, most large complex systems have a cyber-physical nature. In addition to the underlying engineering physics, the system as a whole deploys control, automation, and decision-making components that make the system operate efficiently, reliably, and stably. These components can be entirely automated as in the case of PID controllers, or entirely manual as in the case of aircraft pilots. Furthermore, the control, automation, or decision-making system can have centralized, distributed, or decentralized algorithms. Figure 14.25 contrasts four types of cyber-physical systems: (a) open-loop physical systems, (b) closed-loop cyber-physical systems, (c) closed-loop cyber-physical systems a centralized controller, and (d) closed-loop cyber-physical systems with a distributed control architecture. Each of these can be modeled as a SysML block diagram, analyzed for its system behavior, or inspected in terms of its underlying system structure. The challenge, here, is that many closed-loop control systems end up creating cyber-physical systems with coupled designs. Consequently, the design workflows develop feedback loops that are not easily managed and prone to design error; particularly for large complex systems with demanding engineering physics. One can perhaps speculate whether the recent news about the Boeing 737 MAX airplanes is the result of the feedback design loops caused by the plane's underlying cyber-physical nature. In any case, we must recognize that as the modern world continues to automate its technologies, it designs cyber-physical systems that are increasingly safety–critical. Developing engineering design approaches that target the closed-loop nature of cyber-physical systems is imperative.

Finally, the study of large flexible engineering systems must continue to develop through hetero-functional graph theory. Three broad communities are actively working to develop the methods to tackle the types of systems that sit at the heart of the NAE's grand challenges. The network science community has deployed graph theory as a means to analyze the *form* of large flexible engineering systems. These works, however, are relatively divorced from the established understanding of function within the engineering design field. Furthermore, many of the large-scale architectural transformations of the twenty-first century appear within the functional architecture or in the system knowledge base, but not in the physical architecture alone. In the meantime, model-based system engineering has established graphical modeling techniques like SysML to approach systems of arbitrary size and complexity. However, the quantitative understanding of the underlying system structure has remained elusive. In the meantime, much of the AD community focuses on the quantification of such a system structure, but most investigations have been limited to large fixed engineering systems. To the network science community, hetero-functional networks present a new view as to how to construct graphs with fundamentally different meanings and insight. To the systems engineering community, hetero-functional graph theory may come to be viewed as quantification of

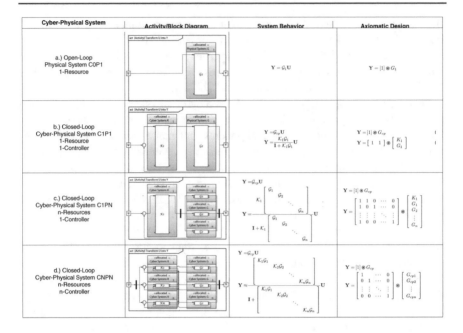

Fig. 14.25 Cyber-physical systems from the perspectives of SysML, transfer functions, and Axiomatic Design

many of the structural concepts in model-based systems engineering. Finally, to the engineering design student interested in large flexible engineering systems, hetero-functional graph theory presents itself as a natural extension of AD theory where the Independence Axiom is applied to study systems of flexible structure.

Problems

1. Former mayor of Atlanta in the state of Georgia and the U.S. Ambassador to the United Nations learned about the MH project at KAIST. He thought the MH offers an ideal solution to the problem he has been concerned about for years. His idea was to make the state of Georgia a hub for cargo transportation, just as he made the city of Atlanta the hub of air transportation by enlarging the Atlanta airport, which had made a significant impact on Georgia's economy.

   His new idea was as follows: When large containerships come through the Panama Canal from Asia, there are no large harbors that can accommodate these large ships that require ports with deep waters. One solution is to moor these ships off the Georgia coast and then let MHs unload containers from the large container ships in the open sea about 35 miles offshore from the Georgia coast. Then, these MHs can transport the containers from the containership in the open sea to Savannah, Georgia, or Jacksonville, Florida, as well as other harbors in the Florida Pan-Handle. The containers transported to the Savannah harbor from the containerships by the MH can then be transported to the East Coast cities as well as the Mid-West cities of the United States by the railroad system that is already there.

This proposed system can solve the current problems. There are no harbors with deep enough waters along the Eastern seaboard of the United States to accommodate these large containerships. Therefore, most of the containers from Asia are unloaded at harbors at Long Beach, or Los Angeles, California. They are then transported by rail to the East Coast or the Mid-West region of the United States.

Design a platform that can be anchored in the open sea with the capability of supplying fuel and water to the large containership moored in the open sea.

2. One of the goals of automobile companies is to manufacture driverless automobiles that will take passengers to new destinations without the intervention of drivers. The idea is to use sensors of many different kinds, computational power, information storage systems, GPS (ground positioning system), AI (artificial intelligence), automated steering system, telecommunications system, and intelligent engines.

    Propose your approach in developing such vehicles, identify potential problems, define FRs, and select DPs and PVs.

    Based on the FRs, DPs, and PVs selected, develop the design matrix for your vehicle.

3. Many universities are large systems. Typical research universities have teaching staff (i.e., professors, research staff, technical staff), administrative staff, undergraduate students, and graduate students. They must have the right and adequate physical facilities for teaching, research, housing for students, and sports facilities. Your job as its president is to make this university one of the best research universities in the world. The university has 4,000 undergraduate students and 6,000 graduate students. It receives an annual budget from the government, which can meet roughly 50% of its budget. All of its students do not pay any tuition, which is covered by the budget allocated by the government. Define the highest level FRs, DPs, and PVs after identifying the potential problems that must be overcome to make it into one of the leading universities in the world. Develop a strategic plan for the next 5 years.

4. Boeing 737 MAX, the new airplane introduced by Boeing Airplane Company, developed flight control problems during take-off. Two of these planes crashed soon after take-off during ascending. The speculation is that the computer control system, which was installed to prevent the potential stalling problem during ascending, failed to do its function. When the airplane stalls, it loses its lifting force and can fall. The control system was so designed that the pilot did

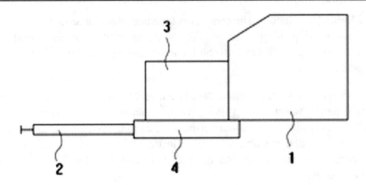

Fig. 14.26 Schematic view of the front part of a train

not have any control over the computer system. Define the first three-levels of FRs and DPs for this airplane, if you are in charge of the development of this airplane. What caused this plane to crash?

5. Analyze the design of your cell phone using AD. The functions of the cell phone do not have to be considered. Define the hierarchies of FRs and DPs only for physical parts of the phone.

6. A schematic view of the front part of a train is illustrated in Fig. 14.26. The figure indicates (1) train structure, (2) coupler, (3) honeycomb structure, (4) headstock. The train is going leftward. The front part is composed of (2), (3), and (4), and it absorbs the impact energy in a crash event. Generally, the coupler absorbs the impact energy first and the headstock and honeycomb structure

Fig. 14.27 The airbag in the steering system

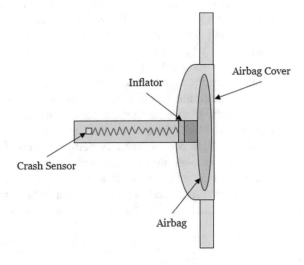

absorb the rest of the energy. The patent KR20090059520A can be referred for a detailed explanation. Design the front part of the train using AD.

7. An automobile airbag system is illustrated in Fig. 14.27. The airbag is for a driver and is installed inside of the steering system. Design the airbag using AD.

Various drones are being sold in the market due to an increase in demand. Design a drone according to the following steps:

(1) define the purpose of your own drone (FRs);
(2) define the design specifications based on your environment and conditions (Cs);
(3) design a product (DPs).

Using a hierarchy of FRs and DPs is recommended. You can pick a drone in the market and modify it according to your definition.

14.8 Recently, pedestrian protection is a hot issue in the automotive industry. Some engineers are studying the installation of a pedestrian protection airbag system as illustrated in Fig. 14.28. When the car impacts a pedestrian, the airbag is deployed according to the following process:

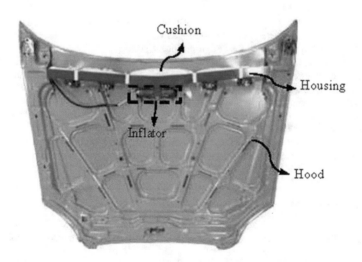

Fig. 14.28 A pedestrian protection airbag system (Hyun-Ik Yang, Yong-Won Yun, and Gyung-Jin Park, Design of a pedestrian protection airbag system using experiments, Proceedings of the Institution of Mechanical Engineers, Part D: Journal of Automobile Engineering (230.9) pp. 1182–1195. Copyright © 2016 (Sage Publishing). https://doi.org/10.1177/0954407015603854)

(1) a sensor in the bumper detects the collision;
(2) an actuator opens the hood a little. The actuator is equipped at the hinge that connects the main body and the hood;
(3) the inflator generates gas to inflate the airbag cushion;
(4) the head of the pedestrian is impacted by the airbag.

The pedestrian airbag is installed in the housing at the back of the hood. The airbag has a disadvantage that it can block the driver's sight. Design the pedestrian protection airbag using AD. Refer to Yang et al. (2016) for further information.

References

Farid A, Suh NP (eds) (2016) Axiomatic design in large systems. Springer, Cham, Switzerland

Hong EP, Park GJ (2010) Design information management of an on-line electric vehicle using axiomatic design. SAE Int J Mater Manufactur 3(1):133–141. https://saemobilus.sae.org/content/2010-01-0279/

Lee S, Hong E, Park GJ (2009) Analysis of a mount type HVAC control system using axiomatic design. In: Coelho AG (ed) Proceedings of the 5th international conference on axiomatic design, Universidade Nova de Lisboa, accessed at Axiomatic Design Solutions, Inc., Lisboa, Portugal

Lee T, Park GJ (2010) Managing system design process using axiomatic design: a case on KAIST mobile harbor project. SAE Int J Mater Manufact (1):125–132. https://saemobilus.sae.org/content/2010-01-0278/

Nosorog UA (2019) Car suspension separately from the car isolated on white 3D illustration. Photo licensed from Shutterstock, ID: 415090513

Park GJ (2007) Analytic methods for design practice. Springer

Park GJ (2018) Application of axiomatic design to the design of automobile parts (keynote speech). In: Puik E, Foley JT, Cochran D, Betasolo M (eds) 12th international conference on axiomatic design (ICAD), MATEC web of conferences, Reykjavík, Iceland, contained proprietary data, contact author for details

Suh NP (2001) Axiomatic design—advances and applications. Oxford University Press

Yang HI, Yun YW, Park GJ (2016) Design of a pedestrian protection airbag system using experiments. In: Proceedings of the institution of mechanical engineers, Part D: journal of automobile engineering, vol 230.9, pp 1182–1195

Further Reading

Buede DM (2009) The Engineering Design of Systems: Models and Methods. Hoboken, N.J.: John Wiley & Sons, 2nd Ed.

Crawley E, Cameron B, Selva D (2015) System Architecture: Strategy and Product Development for Complex Systems. Upper Saddle River, N.J.: Prentice Hall Press

Farid AM, Suh NP (2016) Axiomatic Design in Large Systems: Complex Products, Buildings and Manufacturing Systems. Berlin, Heidelberg: Springer

National Academy of Engineering (2019) "NAE Grand Challenges for Engineering," https://www.engineeringchallenges.org/challenges.aspx

Schoonenberg WC, Khayal IS, Farid AM (2018) A Hetero-functional Graph Theory for Modeling Interdependent Smart City Infrastructure. Berlin, Heidelberg: Springer

Suh NP (2001) Axiomatic design—advances and applications. Oxford University Press

Complexity in the Kitchen

15

Joseph T. Foley, Erik Puik, Lindy Puik, Joseph Smith, and David S. Cochran

Abstract

Axiomatic Design (AD) and Complexity Theory are often applied to highly complex and technological systems that provide educators with many engineering examples and case studies. The use of AD is applicable outside of these areas. However, there are not many examples outside of these areas. As a result, students often have trouble understanding the breadth and impact of Axiomatic Design's application to problem-solving. One large complex system that is often

Author's Note: This chapter is an adaptation of the paper "Complexity in the Kitchen" presented by the same authors at ICAD2019 in Sydney Australia (Foley et al. 2019) . This paper was published open access at https://doi.org/10.1051/matecconf/201930100007 under a CC BY 4.0 license.

J. T. Foley (✉)
Reykjavík University, Menntavegur 1, Reykjavík, Iceland
e-mail: foley@ru.is; foley@MIT.EDU

Massachusetts Institute of Technology, 77 Massachusetts Ave, Cambridge, MA, USA

E. Puik
HU Utrecht, Hudsondreef 32, 3565 AV Utrecht, The Netherlands
e-mail: erik.puik@hu.nl

L. Puik
Eindhoven, The Netherlands
e-mail: lindy@puik.com

J. Smith
Purdue University—Fort Wayne, 2101 E. Coliseum Blvd, ETCS233, Fort Wayne, IN, USA
e-mail: smitjj09@pfw.edu

D. S. Cochran
Purdue University—Fort Wayne, 2101 E. Coliseum Blvd, ETCS229B, Fort Wayne, IN, USA
e-mail: dscochran@pfw.edu

© Springer Nature Switzerland AG 2021
N. P. Suh et al. (eds.), *Design Engineering and Science*,
https://doi.org/10.1007/978-3-030-49232-8_15

417

overlooked is that of the kitchen. In this chapter, we present different food-related preparation tasks that are inherently complex: cooking a turkey, baking an apple pie, reverse engineering a recipe, and designing ecologically minded food packaging while also discussing the impact of prepared food's packaging approaches on the environment. The authors believe such examples demonstrate Axiomatic Design's applicability in a new aspect that is approachable to a wide audience.

15.1 Introduction

Axiomatic Design (AD) has been already shown to be effective in highly technical realms and creative areas. Technical applications include Shape Memory Allow actuator testing (Pétursson et al. 2017), Industry 4.0 Human–Robot interfacing (Gualtieri et al. 2018), industrial safety practices (Iino and Nakao 2018), and reconfigurable manufacturing system design at Mercedes-Benz (Kujawa et al. 2018). Nontechnical interest comes in the areas of football[1] (Rolli et al. 2018), diabetes treatment (Smith et al. 2018), university department organization (Suh 2001, 2015), special education curricula (Wettasinghe and Koh 2008) and interactive art (Foley and Harðardóttir 2016).

These articles provide case studies and analogies that are relevant to engineering students and the technically literate. Unfortunately, for those who wish to use AD outside of those fields, educators are left with examples that resonate with engineering students, but not with the design and student community at large. The nontechnical analogy most commonly used by educators is that of designing a water faucet that is easy to use. This example was initially published by Suh (2001) and further expanded and revised by Foley et al. (2017).

One area that contains highly technical challenges that are approachable by a large audience is that of food preparation. The ubiquity and success of cooking show clearly indicate large interest from the viewing public. In the latest edition of "On Food and Cooking," Harold McGee celebrates that the worlds of science and culinary arts have become tightly integrated and collaborative since he first wrote the work that has brought him fame (McGee 2007). The authors agree that this indicates that it is an excellent area to exploit for interdisciplinary research while also providing rich examples to use in teaching design. The idea of using food preparation as a design exercise is not unique: Slocum (2008) uses cooking dinner as one of his common examples in his modified AD method called FRDPARRC. Cooking itself is a transformative process, which fits well within the functional requirement (FRs) mapping to the physical requirement aspect of AD.

---

[1] Also known in the United States as Soccer, which is distrinct from what some might call "hand-egg."

15.1.1 Axiomatic Design in Other Words

The reader should be now familiar with the two axioms: (Suh, 2001).

Independence Axiom (1):   "Maintain the independence of the FRs"
Information Axiom (2):   "Minimize the information content of the design"

The authors have found that the axioms are often confusing to beginning practitioners of the design discipline and non-technical parties of interest. Joe Foley presented these at the ICAD2017 tutorials in a zen koan riddle (Foley 2017):

Independence Axiom (1):   Find harmony in conflict
Information Axiom (2):   Prepare for the unexpected

One might clarify this explanation further:

Independence Axiom (1):   Modularize
Information Axiom (2):   Choose robust elements and their combinations

To go into the creative realms, (Foley and Harðardóttir 2016) changed "Functional Requirement" into a "*Feeling Requirement*". The axioms also changed focus

Independence Axiom (1):   Ensure the chosen emotions or interactions can be separately adjusted
Information Axiom (2):   Choose implementations that reach the largest audience with the highest impact

We have considered AD through multiple lenses to apply the same core concepts into different disciplines. Now, we will quickly review the concept of Suh's complexity.

? AD in other disciplines

Think of other disciplines, technical or not, and augment the two Axioms to be appropriate for that area. Are two axioms sufficient? Do you need more or less?

15.1.2 Complexity Theory

To simplify the understanding of how many reliability (primarily Axiom 2) issues can be addressed, Suh's later focus combines the AD concepts into a singular complexity Theory (Suh 2005).

He explores the meaning of complexity, finally settling on "Complexity is defined as a measure of uncertainty in achieving the specified FRs" (Suh 2005, p.58). Vossebeld et al. (2018) summarizes the four different types succinctly:

- **Time-independent real complexity** which is simply the information content of a design: $C_R = I$, where $I_i = -\log_2 P_i$ and P_i is the probability of meeting satisfying FR_i. For uncoupled designs, the total information of the system is simply the sum $I = \sum_i I_i$. For other cases, we refer the reader to Suh's deeper discussion in Suh (2005).
- **Time-independent imaginary complexity** arises in coupled or path-dependent solutions where the order in which DPs should be addressed is unclear or improperly ordered.
- **Time-dependent combinatorial complexity** develops in systems in which operation has a higher probability of going out of specification due to "continued expansion in the number of possible combinations with time." In short, time-dependent combinatorial complexity describes systems that progress toward chaotic states over some time.
- **Time-dependent periodic complexity** is similar to combinatorial complexity except that a functional period has been identified over which the system can be reset before it enters an unpredictable state.

15.1.3 Cooking Science

Harold McGee wrote one of the seminal works in trying to bridge the gap between cooking and science in his work "On Food and Cooking" in 1984 later revised in 2004 (Donovan 2006; McGee 2007). This book is considered one of the required texts for those interested in the science behind food and the cooking processes considered commonplace today. When the book was first introduced, technical terms such as "emulsified" and "denatured" were foreign to chefs except perhaps those previously schooled in chemistry (Donovan 2006). McGee's book is highly relevant to this article due to its focus on a deeper understanding of how food and cooking processes interact. To AD practitioners, the word "interact" should instantly remind us of the concept of "coupling" and for good reason.

? Definition

What is the definition of cooking? Must it involve heat? Does your definition fit dishes such as kimchee,[2] lutefisk,[3] salami, and ceviche?[4]

---

[2]Spicy Korean-style fermented cabbage often started with a raw oyster to begin fermentation.
[3]Norwegian whitefish preserved in lye.
[4]South American raw fish dish where the fish is cured in fresh citrus juices.

15.2 Cooking Axioms

We believe the AD axioms can be easily translated to cooking:

Independence Axiom (1): Reduce interaction between ingredients and processes to only the ones desired

Information Axiom (2): Produce the desired food aspect reliably

Of note, there is one fast food chain that is famous for mastering Axiom 2 on a global basis: the McDonald's corporation. It is well known to the point of an adage that "A McDonald's hamburger is the same no matter where you are." The unspoken secondary part is that they are consistent, but not considered high quality, i.e., "consistent mediocrity" (Bramlett 2018); they could be considered high precision, but low accuracy. In Sect. 15.5, we examine a structured way to evaluate the quality of a cooking result, particularly for "complex" recipes. Perhaps we need to consider this in terms of a quality definition heuristic (Cochran et al. 2016) shown in Eq. 15.1:

$$\text{quality} = \frac{\text{Satisfaction of Needs}}{\text{Resources consumed}} \qquad (15.1)$$

? Evaluation of food

When you last ate food prepared by another person, how would you rate its quality? Can you state a set of FRs and measure how many resources were consumed? How would a McDonald's hamburger rate in the quality heuristic you developed?

To demonstrate how these axioms can direct cooking to a more desirable result reliably, we will now present challenging recipes in the next sections.

15.3 Cooking a Turkey

In the United States, the holiday known as Thanksgiving is associated with roasting a turkey in modern times (Fig. 15.1). How this came to be is a fascinating story which we will explain in brief.[5]

---

[5] An excellent resource on Thanksgiving's turkey tradition is Davis's "More than a Meal" (Davis 2001) which provided much of our historical resources and may convince some readers to go vegan.

Fig. 15.1 The annual US Thanksgiving tradition of roasting a turkey. (Reproduced with permission from Weinersmith (2011))

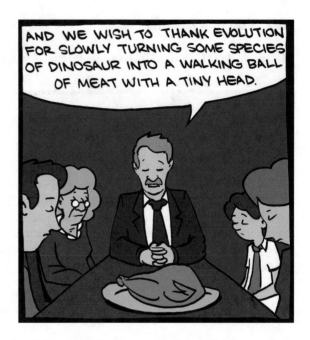

> **? Holiday Gobble Gobble**

If you eat turkey during the holidays, what was your favorite part and why? If you don't, what is your favorite alternative and why? If you were the one to prepare the turkey, how happy were you with the result last time?

15.3.1 Why Does US Thanksgiving Mean Eating a Turkey?

The word turkey for the bird we know came into use during the Middle Ages. Its origins are best explained as being associated with the Turkish Empire being the main European trade route from which exotic birds such as the peafowl were arriving (Davis 2001, p.28).

> Three centuries before any actual turkeys appeared in sixteenth-century Europe, the word *turkey* was being used to describe exotic birds from Asia (Schorger 1966, p. 16).

The choice of it being a roasted bird (Fig. 15.1) in the United States are clear due to it being plentiful, especially in the New England area where the Puritan settlers arrived (Davis 2001, p. 33). That said, records of the feast from the first Thanksgiving mention a large variety of birds but no specific mention of turkey (Bradford 1981, p. 100). Thanksgiving was not a significant national holiday in the United States until 1863 when President Abraham Lincoln used it as a mechanism to promote unity (Davis 2001, p. 53). Alexander Hamilton, the first secretary of the Treasury is perhaps the earliest proponent of turkey being critical to Thanksgiving, saying "[n]o citizen of the United States should refrain from turkey on Thanksgiving Day" in 1805 (Schorger 1966, p. 369; Davis 2001, p. 53). By 1857, it had become a traditional part of Thanksgiving in New England. The English had an even earlier introduction to Turkey in 1573, being referred to as "Christmas husbandlie fare" (Wright 1914, p. 338; Davis 2001, p. 54). The bird had been shipped there from Mexico by Spanish explorers in the sixteenth century and became commonly bread during Renaissance England (Davis 2001, p. 54). Strangely enough, the breeds that made their way there were then brought back to the United States to become the forerunner of modern domesticated turkey breeds (Davis 2001, p. 54). In short, the patriotic United States holiday Thanksgiving, strangely enough, is all about devouring a Latin American repatriated bird species!

15.3.2 Bringing the Bird to the Table

The challenge of cooking a turkey consistently was deeply considered in November 1993 by the cooking journal Cooks Illustrated.[6]

Anyone who has tried to cook a frozen turkey in any reasonable amount of time has run into the problem of having the meat cooked thoroughly while also remaining juicy. The problem stems from a few factors:

- a frozen turkey requires a huge amount of energy to heat the center;
- a large turkey has a large amount of thermal mass. (16 kg or greater);
- the turkey is not homogeneous, so the various parts cook at different rates;
- the US Department of Agriculture recommends an internal temperature of at least 165 °F (73.9 °C) to "destroy bacteria and prevent food-borne illness" (United Stated Department of Agriculture 2015).

Rather than focus on the details of meat thermal models which have already been explored in Papasidero et al. (2015), McGee et al. (1999), and Chang et al. (1998), we place our attention on the overall design aspect. McGee[7] discusses the challenge of roasting whole birds including chickens and turkeys (McGee 2007). He agrees that the challenge is that the meats are "best cooked differently." Breast meat becomes an unpleasantly chewy and tough texture to the palate if cooked much over 68 °C. Conversely, the leg and other dark meat have significant connective tissue that is chewy at temperatures below 72 °C. We have a contradiction, similar to what the Russian design methodology TRIZ (Atshuller 1994) delights in; what is a cook to do?

---

[6]The first reference to analyzing turkey storage and cooking the authors were able to find was from 1962 in Goodwin et al. (1962).

[7]Who is a co-author on one of the meat thermal models.

? TRIZ Turkey

Read about TRIZ:"Theory of the resolution of invention-related tasks". What kind of approaches would TRIZ suggest for cooking a frozen turkey?

Rather than be further distracted by TRIZ's enthusiasm, let us consider the problem in an axiomatic framework:

- FR_1 = Heat breast meat to a maximum 68 °C;
- FR_2 = Heat thigh meat to a minimum 72 °C.

Traditionally, cooks have tried to solve this with a single DP, which results in the design matrix shown in Eq. 15.2.

- DP_1 = Heated enclosure at 180 °C for X minutes per kg.

$$\begin{Bmatrix} FR_1 \\ FR_2 \end{Bmatrix} = \begin{bmatrix} X \\ X \end{bmatrix} \{DP_1\} \tag{15.2}$$

? TV Dinners

Frozen pre-compiled meals on included trays i.e. "TV dinners"[8] must include instructions for preparation. Previously, these instructions were simply to place them into an oven of the correct temperature for a set amount of time. In the modern era, instructions for a microwave oven of a "given wattage" are also included. What mechanisms have the manufacturers done to ensure that the food is consistently cooked according to these instructions? What are the failure cases for under-cooking and over-cooking?

This will clearly have issues: There is a single DP for 2 FRs, so it is inherently coupled. Besides, the chances of meeting both FRs are very low since breasts and thighs are both at the surface and have varying thicknesses. Perhaps we could change the thickness of the meat, choosing turkeys with thicker breasts and following the thermal transfer model derived by Chang et al. (1998). Unfortunately, measuring the exact size of the turkey breast without removing it is rather challenging, so this approach is abandoned.

One other thought is to compress our FRs:

- FR_1 = Heat breast and thigh meat to a individual optimal temperatures.

---

[8]Probably because people would often prepare them quickly to eat while watching a television program.

Which does not show unreasonable coupling due to it being a 1FR1DP design (Eq. 15.3), but has a large information content because the two temperatures are different.

$$\{FR_1\} = [X]\{DP_1\} \tag{15.3}$$

An obvious improvement is to add feedback:

- DP_1 = Heated enclosure at 180 °C;
- DP_2 = Thermometer.

Unfortunately, this still won't work because of the contradiction. Clearly, we need to uncouple the two FRs somehow. One answer is to physically uncouple them with a kitchen knife as shown in Fig. 15.2:

- FR_1 = Separate meat pieces according to dark vs. light meat;
- FR_2 = Heat each type of meat to the optimal temperature:

  - $FR_{2.1}$ = Heat breast meat to a maximum of 68 °C;
  - $FR_{2.2}$ = Heat thigh meat to a minimum 72 °C.

- DP_1 = Knife and knowledge of turkey anatomy;
- DP_2 = Heated enclosure at 180 °C and thermometer probe in meat.

The resulting design matrix in Eq. 15.4 is de-coupled or "path-dependent" indicating that we must do things in the correct order. Clearly, we have to cut the turkey before we can put it into the oven.

$$\begin{Bmatrix} FR_1 \\ FR_2 \end{Bmatrix} = \begin{bmatrix} X & 0 \\ X & X \end{bmatrix} \begin{Bmatrix} DP_1 \\ DP_2 \end{Bmatrix} \tag{15.4}$$

Fig. 15.2 Joseph T. Foley's interpretation of un-coupling a turkey's anatomy to reduce the cooking complexity. (Reproduced from Foley et al. (2019), originally published open access under a CC BY 4.0 license: https://doi.org/10.1051/matecconf/201930100007)

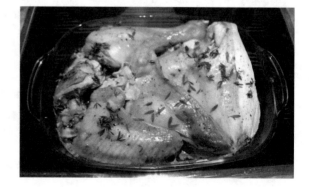

Fig. 15.3 The Spidurky: a novel method of increasing drumstick availability. (Reproduced with permission from Weinersmith (2018))

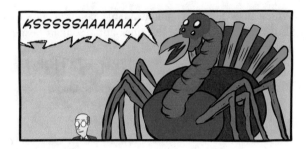

This new configuration greatly reduces the information content (Axiom 2) because the temperature of each type of meat can be carefully controlled. Seeing that people seem to prefer some parts of the turkey more than others, this seems like a very simple way to uncouple. Unfortunately, such desirability of a particular type or part of the meat such as the often desired drumstick can result in decisions that lead to the terrifying implications supposed in Fig. 15.3.

Joseph T. Foley's grandfather often told the story of having to do KP[9] while on a large naval vessel during the Second World War:

Design Story 15.1:

The ship had an impressive kitchen, which made sense since it had to feed a few hundred seamen. It had a steam-heated cooking pot that took up much of the room and was as deep as a man. To make it easy to get ingredients in, the top was accessible from an upper floor. You had to be careful with that thing; any leaking steam would cook you instantly and that's how you cleaned it.

The head of the kitchen once came to me and said "Foley, today you're making chicken soup. The crates of frozen chicken are over in the freezer. Get 10 of them out and put 'em in the pot. Get to it!"

Well, I dragged a couple of those crates from the freezer (which was also something to see) and brought them into the room. I was pretty tired at that point because they were heavy, but food needed to be made. I got a crowbar and started levering off the sides of the wooden crate, pulling out the nails to make it easier to pry. I'd finished one crate and discovered that the chickens were frozen in a solid block. I was prying one out with the crowbar, covered in sweat, when the head of the kitchen came by and gave me quite the look.

He shouted, "What are you doing, Foley?[10]"

I answered, "Preparing the chicken like you said, Sir!"

He retorted, "No! You're wasting time!"

Can you guess what he did?

---

[9]Kitchen Patrol, i.e., cooking.

[10]Slightly paraphrased from the original naval method of speaking.

He grabbed a fire ax from the wall and began swinging with great speed and force on one of the wooden crates. He kept at it until the crate was broken into large chunks. Then he used a shovel to dump the chunks into the giant pot and handed the ax to me. I asked, "But Sir, how will that make soup?" His reply was simple and to the point: "Wood floats and nails sink. We'll scoop 'em out later"

And that is how you made chicken soup in the Navy.

? Scaling up food

Imagine you have been hired by a company to break the Guinness Book of World Records for a food item such as pizza. How would you modify the traditional recipe for that item so that it can break the current world record? Consider that the finished product should be both food-safe and edible.

One must not forget the heat transfer aspect of cooking in an oven: the outside temperature of a cut of meat will be much higher than the target temperature unless special care is taken to remove the meat from the oven before it reaches the target temperature for "carry-over" cooking.

To further reduce the chances of failure, we can take a lesson from the current food movement of Sous-vide water baths similar to the Paté cooking described by McGee (2007), p. 171:

- $FR_1 =$ Heat breast meat to a maximum 68 °C;
- $FR_2 =$ Heat thigh meat to a minimum 72 °C.

- $DP_1 =$ Immerse plastic-sealed breast meat chunks in 68 °C water until equilibriated;
- $DP_2 =$ Immerse plastic-sealed breast meat chunks in 72 °C water until equilibriated.

It would seem that we have found the perfect turkey cooking method, and in fact, this is similar to what is done to cook turkey meat in restaurants when it is used as a component or covered in sauces. Unfortunately, we have not considered our customer's needs carefully enough as in Vossebeld et al. (2018), and Girgenti et al. (2016). The customers want the food to be presented in a particular way, not just be at the correct temperature.

- $CN_1 =$ Put a cooked whole bird on the table so it looks pretty;
- $CN_2 =$ The skin must be crispy.

We need some way to cook certain parts of the bird selectively to address these needs without going back into our coupled state and without mechanically separating them.

? Super crispy

How do you make food crispy? Is it about the temperature? Is it about the cooking process? How would you keep food crispy if it needs to be stored for at least a week?

15.3.3   How Do People Really Cook a Turkey?

Several innovative solutions have arisen to address these challenges to varying degrees. With minimal effort, one can find videos and equipment for deep fat-frying a turkey to speed up the process, obvious even in 1962 (McGee 2007; Goodwin et al. 1962). While faster, this greatly increases the chances of injury as the ice crystals (or just moisture) may cause the hot oil to splatter and atomize, occasionally turning the cooker into a fireball of epic proportions (Butler 2015; Osias 2006). The issue is a large enough concern that there is a patent on a deep fryer that claims to make this process safer (Osias 2006).

? Fire in the hole!

Working with hot oil near an open flame is dangerous. How would you design an oil-based cooking process that is less likely to destroy your kitchen? Consider the axioms for guidance.

Defrosting the turkey ahead of time also can assist, if planning permits. This does not address the problem of the differing composition of dark and white meat resulting in certain parts cooked while the others are not. Again, necessity has bred innovation in the form of placing aluminum foil as a radiant heat shield over the white meat areas. One suggestion was to place ice packs over the white meat to cook them selectively. As well as some of these approaches work, they still require significant effort and quite a bit of skill to apply for repeatable success. This makes it clear that cooking the turkey is a "complex system" in the Suh sense.

The concept of brining a turkey was the initial issue of Cooks Illustrated in 1993 since updated in 2004 (Hays 2004). Very recently, Lan Lam, Senior Editor of "Cook's Illustrated" re-examined the turkey process to see if the process could be further streamlined in Lam (2016). Brining a turkey allows us to remove the contradiction inherent in our two incompatible target temperatures by changing the meat chemistry in a way that it can accept a larger variety of temperatures and maintain a high level of moisture. This wider range of acceptable temperatures could be considered "softening the spring" in Suh's terminology. Lam's improved recipe replaces the short brining with a long refrigerated salting step, which accomplishes the same goal and reduces the moisture to improve the skin's crispiness. Doing this with a small amount of sugar also caused the skin to brown nicely, effectively caramelizing the skin.

The previous recipe suggested starting the turkey upside down so that the majority of the heat focused on the dark meat (on the bottom of the bird). Lam wanted to find an easier way to apply more heat to the bottom without the extra effort and found it in the current method of making pizza at home: a pizza stone. This large stone, when preheated correctly, stored enough heat that the turkey could simply be placed in the roasting V-rack and not have to be manipulated. This innovation caused the dark and light meat to finish cooking at the same time.

- FR_1 = Keep white meat tender at 72 °C and higher;
- FR_2 = Crisp skin of turkey;
- FR_3 = Heat meat to 72 °C.

- DP_1 = Salt to change the protein structure of meat to retain water;
- DP_2 = Sugar solution;
- DP_3 = Preheated pizza-stone, heated enclosure at 180 °C, and thermometer probe in meat.

In effect, the new procedure is effectively uncoupled as shown in Eq. 15.5. Each of the FRs is only affected by its DP.

$$\begin{Bmatrix} FR_1 \\ FR_2 \\ FR_2 \end{Bmatrix} = \begin{bmatrix} X & 0 & 0 \\ 0 & X & 0 \\ 0 & 0 & X \end{bmatrix} \begin{Bmatrix} DP_1 \\ DP_2 \\ DP_3 \end{Bmatrix} \tag{15.5}$$

As can be easily seen, the continuing innovation in cooking a challenging roast such as a turkey involves understanding the coupling and information content inherent in each of the process choices made for having it arrive on the Thanksgiving table.

15.4 Baking an Apple Pie

A famous simile often used in the United States is "As American as Apple Pie." This references the idolized atomic family period of the 1950s where the working spouse would arrive home to the smell of a freshly baked apple pie (Fig. 15.4).

? Think Global, Act Local

In the North East of the United States in 1980–1990s, it was popular to go to a "pick your own" apple orchard to get apples for making apple pies (see Sect. 15.4) and other dishes. These orchards had significant financial troubles due to an interesting change: China has flooded the market with cheap applesauce. Why does this matter? It turns out that after the apple picking season is done, most orchards take the remaining apples, turn them into applesauce, and sell them to packaged food producers as a healthy way to add flavor and sweetness to food. China and cheap shipping have

Fig. 15.4 A classic apple
pie. (Reproduced with
permisssion from America's
Test Kitchen (1997),
©America's Test Kitchen)

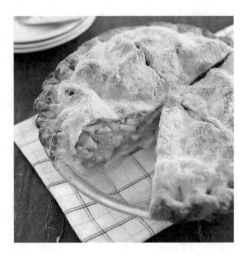

suddenly caused this to often not be worth the effort to compete: the US producers
cannot make up the costs in labor for producing the sauce.

It turns out that the successful orchards have noticed that this is an issue and
have examined their CNs to realize that people come to an orchard not only for the
apples but for the experience. This has caused smart orchard owners to expand their
operations into baked products and amusement rides to bring people in to make back
that lost profit. What happens to the leftover apples now?

Consider a local business in your area that is having trouble competing with a
global competitor. Are there CNs and FRs that the local business have missed to
maintain their business or even grow? Propose a design of how this concept might
turn into a business venture.

The concept of a pie and apples themselves did not originate in the US (Eschner
2017). In fact, the association seems to have come about due to WW2 involvement
by the US (Kohatsu 2017). One of the author's own experiences in baking pies
allowed him to immediately identify what makes them challenging when following
the traditional approach:

- CN_1 = Top and bottom crusts should be flaky;
- CN_2 = Crust should hold the fruit in but not be thick like pizza.

- FR_1 = Separate many small blobs of fat and wheat flour;
- FR_2 = Roll crust to consistent thickness of $3\,\text{mm} \pm 1\,\text{mm}$.

- DP_1 = Butter cut into flour at a cold temperature until pea-sized lumps form, then
  made into a ball and rolled out;
- DP_2 = Water added until it can be manipulated with a rolling pin.

The problem becomes clear when examining the design matrix in Eq. 15.6:

$$\begin{Bmatrix} FR_1 \\ FR_2 \end{Bmatrix} = \begin{bmatrix} X & X \\ X & X \end{bmatrix} \begin{Bmatrix} DP_1 \\ DP_2 \end{Bmatrix} \tag{15.6}$$

This concept is coupled because the water affects the layers of the starch and fat. If you do not add enough water, the dough is hard to work with: it does not stay together, crumbles, and is very fragile. If you add too much water, the dough is no longer flaky when baked. The more you manipulate the mixture, the more gluten forms and it gets leathery in texture.

In addition, unless the cook can work in a refrigerator, the butter will begin to melt as it is worked. This creates a time dependence and reduces the chances of success. Depending upon your dietary preferences or desired tastes, you can use hydrogenated vegetable shortening, coconut oil, or even traditional lard (Lopez-alt 2007). Many of these fats fix the melting problem but does not have much taste, so some butter needs to be added back in.

What we need is a different fluid that does not interact with starch and fat to eliminate coupling. The choices of liquid in the standard kitchen are limited to mostly water-based hydrolysates and oils. Pastry already has a fat, so additional oil will affect the butter-starch interaction. Julia Childs comes to the rescue in the form of the only other commonly available liquid: alcohol (Lopez-alt 2007). Alcohol acts similar to water at room temperature but disappears at oven baking temperatures. Also, alcohol inhibits the gluten-forming process, ensuring that flakiness is preserved as you work the dough into shape as shown in Fig. 15.5.

These changes affect our DPs:

- DP_1 = High-melting temperature fat with low moisture content cut into flour at a cold temperature until pea-sized lumps form then made into a ball and rolled out;
- DP_2 = Vodka added until it can be manipulated with a rolling pin.

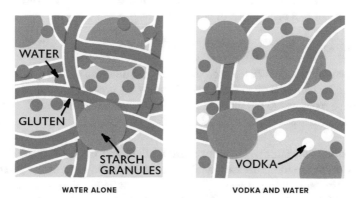

Fig. 15.5 Effect of alcohol on pie dough. (Reproduced with permisssion from Lopez-alt (2007), ©America's Test Kitchen)

$$\begin{Bmatrix} FR_1 \\ FR_2 \end{Bmatrix} = \begin{bmatrix} X & 0 \\ 0 & X \end{bmatrix} \begin{Bmatrix} DP_1 \\ DP_2 \end{Bmatrix} \qquad (15.7)$$

As shown in the Design Matrix in Eq. 15.7, these two small changes have reduced complexity by removing coupling between the various elements, increasing the chances that we will meet our requirements.

15.5   The Complexity of Reverse Engineering a Recipe

The complexity of cooking becomes painfully clear when a recipe needs to be reversed engineered. Typical examples of this are found in a cooking show produced by Endemol, "Herman Against the Others" (inspired by the German show "Kitchen Impossible") in which top chef Herman den Blijker challenges known and award-winning chefs to reproduce a foreign regional signature dish. A third foreign award-winning chef prepares the pretty complicated signature dish, typically a regional specialty, and challenges Herman and his opponent to reproduce it. The chefs have no or little experience in preparing it, as it is a regional dish that does not meet their expertise. By tasting the food and observing its structure and characteristics, they have to find out what the exact ingredients are and determine the right procedure for preparation. They can taste the dish, take pictures, ask employees in stores, and/or ask people in the streets. Obviously, time is limited so they have to apply readily available knowledge for reproduction. The competing chefs both present their dish to a qualified local jury consisting of 6–8 local experts that will taste the dish, assess, and rate it. As the cooking show presents a battle between top chefs, complexity is desired to make the show interesting for its viewers. This is not unique as there are situations where complexity is desirable (Foley et al. 2016). However, complexity should be reduced by the acquisition of knowledge at the end of the show (Puik and Ceglarek 2014a, 2015). A few typical situations are described and analyzed from a perspective of complexity in AD.

? Taste Testing

How well could you identify the ingredients the last time you ate out or ate food that was created by someone else? Could you identify the process used to cook it? Can you estimate measures to tell when the food is finished being prepared?

The Axiomatic Maturity Diagram (AMD) (Puik and Ceglarek 2014b) will be applied to visualize the processes, analyze the scores, and explain the complexity of the reverse engineering process. The AMD, as applied in Figs. 15.7, 15.8, 15.9, 15.10 and 15.11 plots the status of the Axioms through the development process (in time). The actual position of design activity in the AMD is determined by the extent to which the Axioms are satisfied. The Independence Axiom is plotted on the horizontal axis of the AMD and it describes the organization of a product design or in this case the understanding of the cooking process. The vertical axis plots the Information Axiom which is a measure for the robustness of a product's design and in this case, it plots how well the cooking process is executed. The goal of the design process is the top-right dot in the AMD; both axioms are fully satisfied and the design may be considered a "Good Design" (Suh 1990).

In this chapter, the process of cooking is considered to be a design process and the process of reconstructing the dish after reverse engineering is plotted in the AMD. In the cooking show, the chefs' performances are rated with a grade on a scale of 1–10. To visualize this, the AMD is expanded with scores around the dot at the top right side. The grades of the jury members (6–8 people) are averaged into a single score. The open dot at the end of the development path represents the average and final score per dish of the jury (one extra decimal for accuracy on a scale of 0–100). The lines represent the development path that the chefs followed during their quest to reconstruct the dish.

15.5.1 Reproduction of Braised Lamb Ribs

Michelin Guide "Bib Gourmand" awarded Icelandic chef Gísli Matt prepares Lamb Ribs in a sweet and sour sauce (Fig. 15.6). While reverse engineering, the competing chefs are both quite successful in determining the ingredients of this dish. Even the way of preparing the dish is chosen well, both chefs infer that the meat is braised. Unfortunately, the also Michelin Guide "Bib Gourmand" awarded chef Alain Caron, who was born in France and moved to the Netherlands at the age of 26, is mistaken about the exact cut of meat to choose. He chooses a lamb loin instead of the lower ribs. Because of this, his cooking result is not satisfactory. The lamb loin does not have enough fat to make the meat soft during the braising process. His perfect reconstruction of the sweet and sour sauce cannot prevent that his dish is assessed disappointingly by the jury. Alain has made a structural error by selecting a wrong DP (loin instead of ribs). Figure 15.7 shows the AMD.

The process of reconstructing the dish starts at the lower left of the AMD, where ingredients and preparation methods are still unknown. The analysis of the Icelandic dish leads to the organization of the recipe, coupling FRs and DPs, and as such

Fig. 15.6 Example of braised lamb shanks. (Reproduced with permission from Gough (2019))

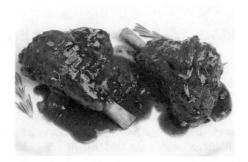

Fig. 15.7 Analysis of chef
Alain's mistake. There is a
structural error in the design
of his recipe. Though the
cooking process is executed
well, he cannot recover from
the mistake, but he
minimalizes damage as
much as possible.
(Reproduced from Foley
et al. (2019), originally
published open access under
a CC BY 4.0 license: https://
doi.org/10.1051/matecconf/
201930100007)

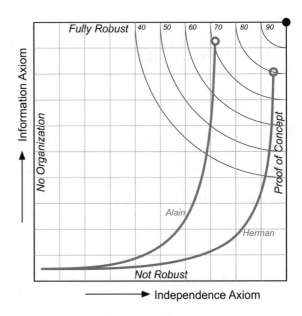

satisfying the Independence Axiom. Unfortunately for chef Alain, the FR "delivering soft but rich mouth feeling" cannot be addressed by the DP "braised lamb loin" because the muscles in the loin are too rigid and will not become soft enough within the available time. In his recipe, the Independence Axiom is not fully satisfied and the curve in the AMD does not reach the right side of the AMD. His perfectly executed sweet and sour sauce brings him quite high in the AMD (correct ingredients that are perfectly treated). His final score is a mere 71 points, while Herman's dish scores 80 points while not being executed to perfection.

> **? Morbitity and Mortality**
>
> Have you ever had a sense that your recipe was going to turn out well or not? What was instinct telling you at the time? How did you feel at that moment? Did you do a post-mortem of a failed recipe to determine what was wrong?

15.5.2 Reproduction of Scottish Haggis

The second example is about replication of the Scottish Haggis (Fig. 15.8). Haggis is a savory pudding consisting of sheep's pluck (liver, lungs, heart). It is prepared by Haggis champion and butcher Fraser MacGregor. Herman's opponent is Maaike Dogan, a specialist in merging western and middle eastern food. In this battle, Herman has a substantial advantage; he is familiar with Haggis, recognizes the dish, knows about the ingredients, and instantly has ideas to reproduce it. Maaike is not familiar

Fig. 15.8 Example of Scottish Haggis. (Reproduced with permission from Stockcreations (2019))

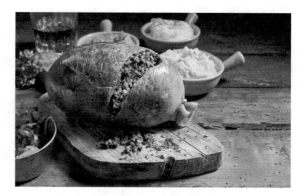

Fig. 15.9 Herman starts off perfectly well, however, though all his ingredients and procedures are perfectly chosen, he is not capable of matching the right flavors and loses the battle. (Reproduced from Foley et al. (2019), originally published open access under a CC BY 4.0 license: https://doi.org/10.1051/matecconf/201930100007)

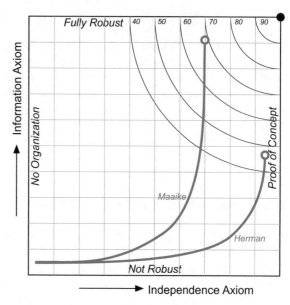

with the dish at all, and she is not able to determine the right ingredients. In fact, she is far off. Instead of using lamb's pluck, she is using minced beef and beef liver. Halfway through the cooking process, it seems that her last chances of a good result are gone when she almost burns her ingredients. This, however, is where the odds turn. Though her ingredients are not the right ones, she shows her excellent cooking skills and qualities in tasting. Due to her middle eastern origin, her skills of seasoning with herbs and spices appear decisive in replicating the right flavor. Where Herman had a big lead, he loses due to Maaike's excellence in reproducing the right taste. The AMD is shown in Fig. 15.9.

Though Herman's potential is considerably better than Maaike's, Herman gets lower grades due to the incorrect flavor of his dish (68 vs 47 points).

Fig. 15.10 Example of
Bavarian Hay Soup (Swiss
Hay Soup image not
available). (Reproduced with
permission from DM-Media
(2019))

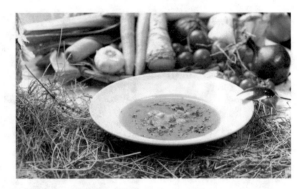

? **Death by Chocolate**

Imagine you are trying to make a chocolate cake with these ingredients: eggs, water, butter, wheat flour, cocoa, baker's chocolate. Without looking at an existing recipe, develop the FR–DP matrix and fill in the transfer coefficients to determine what you think are the correct ratios. Consider each ingredient and write down what you think will happen if you add too much or too little of the ingredient. Try baking your recipe and evaluate its result. How close were you in your first attempt? What would you change in the next attempt?

15.5.3   Reproduction of Swiss Hay Soup

The third and last example is the reconstruction of a Swiss "Hay Soup." It is a rare Alpine dish usually only served above 1000–2000 m altitude and made of dried alpine grass, flowers, and herbs. The dish is prepared by top chef Lukas Pfaff by infusing the local hay with water (like preparing hot tea). The hay extract is mixed with beef/veal and vegetable stock. It is served with a milk-foam and ashes from burnt hay. Herman's opponent is Jermain de Rozario, a young talented and fanatic chef who recently received his first Michelin star.

This is a very unusual recipe because hay is an unaccustomed ingredient for soup and the ashes of burnt hay on top of the milk-foam is a challenging attribute to recognize. Both competing chefs are completely unfamiliar with the concept and ingredients of hay soup and have knowledge making it difficult to properly reproduce it. At this stage, Jermain takes a lead; being a young and eager chef he is willing to learn. He has tasted the ashes of hay in the foam because he suspects that hay is used in that part of the soup. Further, he shows two valuable behavioral characteristics:

- He visits a farm to acquire hay and gathers knowledge by asking the farmer about the preparation of the soup. He does the same in the stores he visits. This is how he learns about the right ingredients and the preparation of the soup;

Fig. 15.11 Jermain applies an iterative approach in which he optimizes his recipe several times before he finalizes it. He reflects after every attempt and gathers an understanding of the dish leading to an excellent score. (Reproduced from Foley et al. (2019), originally published open access under a CC BY 4.0 license: https://doi.org/10.1051/matecconf/201930100007)

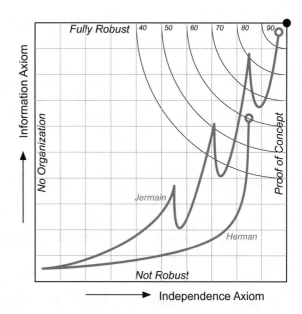

- While preparing the dish, he iterates the recipe of the soup. He tries something, evaluates the result very explicitly, and adjusts the recipe to approach the flavors of the soup as close as possible. This is how he improves his recipe several times and executes that step again and again. Herman, on the other hand, compiles the soup in a single procedure. Obviously, he tastes the result several times but he does not change his recipe, he continues with what he has cooked in the last step.

Again the AMD of these processes is derived (Fig. 15.11).

Jermain's performance is praised by the jury and they can hardly believe that this soup was made by a different chef since he is so close to the initial dish. His score is a total of 95 points in the AMD. Though Herman has used the right ingredients, his hay is not infused in the right way. The process of infusing took too long and made the soup bitter. His average grade does not go beyond 60 points.

? Delicacies

Iceland has several foods that are "delicacies" eaten at certain times of the year: fermented Greenland shark, fermented whale fat, and blowtorch-seared split sheep's head.[11] To many people, this food seems very strange (similar to the previously described hay soup). Determine why these foods became part of the Icelandic culture. Do you have similarly highly-regional foods that are not found outside of your region of the world? How did this happen?

---

[11] The eyeball is a particular delight to many.

15.6   Achieving Functional Requirements with Less Waste

With the move from family farm-centered food distribution to supermarkets, the need for food packaging has increased. In today's busy world, convenience is the name of the game. Disposable, single-serve food items have become a staple at the grocery, and even if you are preparing your meal at home, many of the ingredients come packaged in a variety of different materials. With an AD viewpoint, convenience is an FR that is customer need-driven, and the common DP is usually centered around easily disposable packaging.

> **? The Dangers of Too Much Coffee**
>
> Due to the high price and significant processing of coffee, it tends to be a crop that uses a lot of pesticides. Read about how coffee is produced and look for the coupling elements. Propose changes to eliminate that coupling such that the need for pesticides is lower while maintaining coffee quality.

More recently, sustainable/earth-friendly packaging is becoming an FR born out of the moral and ethical responsibilities felt by the actual consumer of the product. Although this customer need is being driven by the actual consumer of the product, could "The Environment" be the actual customer representing this need? The AD framework provides a way to express the environment as a customer and derive FRs based on the needs of the environment.

For choosing DPs to minimize the impact that a product or process has on the environment, we can use the Design For Environment (DFE) methodology. The DFE methodology provides the means for an organization to minimize the impact of its product and processes on the environment (Ulrich and Eppinger 2015) and could aid in choosing more earth-friendly DPs. To understand how adding FRs derived from environmental needs can affect the product design, the first axiom can be used to understand the resulting path dependency of the design.

One FR could be, "Ensure product packaging is sustainable." For example, there are many possible DPs that could achieve this requirement such as recyclable materials, biodegradable materials, or even returnable/reusable packaging. The question is what effect does the addition of an FR related to sustainable packaging have on the ability to achieve the other FRs?

Consider the "K-Cup" for a moment shown in Fig. 15.12. This invention has brought the ultimate convenience to brewing a cup of coffee in the morning, but at the expense of millions of single-use plastic cups hitting the landfill every day. A few companies have recognized this incredible amount of waste and have added an FR to "reduce packaging waste" to their product design to remedy the problem. Biodegradable K-Cups (Fig. 15.13) are now manufactured by those companies, and the customer experiences the same level of convenience as a normal K-Cup, but without the pollution waste from the plastic. The coffee may even taste better since it is not being brewed in plastic.

Fig. 15.12 Traditional K-Cup. (Reproduced from Foley et al. (2019), originally published open access under a CC BY 4.0 license: https://doi.org/10.1051/matecconf/201930100007)

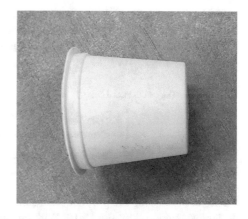

Fig. 15.13 Compostable K-Cup. (Reproduced from Foley et al. (2019), originally published open access under a CC BY 4.0 license: https://doi.org/10.1051/matecconf/201930100007)

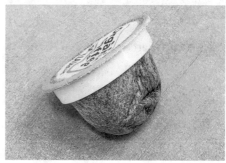

The effect of adding a DP for sustainable packaging can be seen in the comparison of the design matrices for Design A (generic plastic K-Cup, Eq. 15.8) and Design B (Biodegradable K-Cups, Eq. 15.9). Both designs are coupled. How can the marketplace accept and use product designs that are seemingly coupled?

Design A:

$$\begin{Bmatrix} \text{FR}_{\text{Convenient}} \\ \text{FR}_{\text{Low Cost}} \end{Bmatrix} = \begin{bmatrix} X & X \\ X & X \end{bmatrix} \begin{Bmatrix} \text{DP}_{\text{Convenient}} \\ \text{DP}_{\text{Low Cost}} \end{Bmatrix} \tag{15.8}$$

Design B:

$$\begin{Bmatrix} \text{FR}_{\text{Earth-Friendly}} \\ \text{FR}_{\text{Convenient}} \\ \text{FR}_{\text{Low Cost}} \end{Bmatrix} = \begin{bmatrix} X & X & X \\ X & X & X \\ X & X & X \end{bmatrix} \begin{Bmatrix} \text{DP}_{\text{Earth-Friendly}} \\ \text{DP}_{\text{Convenient}} \\ \text{DP}_{\text{Low Cost}} \end{Bmatrix} \tag{15.9}$$

With AD, the designer can achieve the design intention by choosing DPs that decouple a design (Suh 2001), but this decoupling can also result from customer perception and acceptance of a DP. For example, packaging coffee into single-serve plastic cups results in a higher cost per cup of coffee for the consumer, thus the choice of DP for convenience will affect the achievement of a low-cost cup of coffee, but the choice of DP for the low cost may also affect the achievement of convenience. Therefore, the design is coupled, but with the sales and widespread success of single-serve coffee makers, clearly, the consumer is willing to pay more for convenience. For the consumer, there may be no significance of the increased cost for added convenience. Therefore, there is little to no relationship between low cost and convenience as expressed by Eq. 15.10.

Customer-Perceived Design A:

$$
\begin{Bmatrix} FR_{\text{Low Cost}} \\ FR_{\text{Convenient}} \end{Bmatrix} = \begin{bmatrix} X & 0 \\ X & X \end{bmatrix} \begin{Bmatrix} DP_{\text{Low Cost}} \\ DP_{\text{Convenient}} \end{Bmatrix} \tag{15.10}
$$

Also, customer perception may affect the design matrix for Design B which considers the earth-friendly FR. For instance, a consumer looking to purchase a more earth-friendly K-cup may not perceive additional cost or less convenience to be a barrier to purchasing the product. Therefore, Design B becomes a partially coupled design as expressed by Eq. 15.10. Both customer-perceived designs become lower triangular.

Customer-Perceived Design B:

$$
\begin{Bmatrix} FR_{\text{Earth-Friendly}} \\ FR_{\text{Low Cost}} \\ FR_{\text{Convenient}} \end{Bmatrix} = \begin{bmatrix} X & 0 & 0 \\ X & X & 0 \\ X & X & X \end{bmatrix} \begin{Bmatrix} DP_{\text{Biodegradable}} \\ DP_{\text{Low Cost}} \\ DP_{\text{Convenient}} \end{Bmatrix} \tag{15.11}
$$

The thinking is that customer perception and the acceptance of innovations can decouple designs that were previously considered to be coupled. Design intention allows the designer the opportunity to recognize that if the customer accepts the addition of an FR, then a seemingly coupled design can become decoupled. In this way, a designer can rely on marketing to create the customer need that drives this additional FR.

15.7 Conclusion

In this chapter, we have considered several complex kitchen-related tasks and operations in the lens of AD. When cooking a turkey, it advises the cook to decouple the different incompatible cooking materials: dark meat and white meat. If dis-assembly was not acceptable, the cook needs to increase the design range by brining and changing the heat-transfer between the different compositions of meat.

For apple pie, the coupling appears in the choice of fat, moisture, and its interaction with gluten in making a pie crust. The traditional recipe is high-information content because it requires tightly controlled conditions to have a crust that is flaky but can be manipulated into the proper shape. AD again asks us to find ways to uncouple these three elements by finding a different working fluid, alcohol, which separates the workability from gluten formation.

Reverse engineering of food has many similarities with traditional reverse engineering of product and system designs and AD's complexity definition may be well used. As an analog to traditional engineering, knowledge acquisition is the central theme here. Knowledge and complexity have an inverse relationship; as relevant knowledge increases, complexity is reduced. Just like a product designer that is learning while designing, a chef reconstructing a dish needs knowledge and understanding of the recipe: structured analysis in (re)evaluation supports this process.

In addition to the recipe, food preparation requires the equipment and the food as the raw materials. Innovation in both equipment and packaging design was discussed from the customer viewpoint. AD was used to describe that customer acceptance of equipment and packaging innovations can decouple designs that are coupled. The K-Cup was used to illustrate these points and further illustrates the significance and consequence of design intention.

We hope these examples of complexity in the kitchen have inspired you to look for your own opportunities to create food the way you like it more easily and robustly.

Problems

1. Kolmogorov complexity measures complexity by considering how difficult it is to describe a sequence using a programming language. Is this an effective measure of complexity in a cooking recipe? If not, how would you adjust Kolmogorov's complexity to give an effective measure of complexity in a cooking recipe?
2. One of the big innovations in beer packaging was the incorporation of a small plastic ball in Guinness cans to ensure that the foamy "head" that was produced when pouring was similar to a draught from a tap. Consider another packaged food item that you found inferior to the product in another venue. Based upon these differences, build up a CN to FR to DP mapping and look for where the complexity is coming into your perception of the product. Propose a solution.
3. With the popularity of cooking game shows, it is challenging to come up with a new concept. The Desirable Complexity approach in Foley et al. (2016) states that for a "fun" game, you must use invert AD best practices to create appropriate challenges. Based upon violating Axioms 1 and 2, develop a cooking game show that would be at an appropriate level for amateur cooks.
4. You are developing new Meals Ready to Eat (MRE) for extreme adventurers going into remote locations. What are the CNs, FRs, and DPs you would choose to keep the adventurers fed when you are unsure of where they will be going? How would you deal with the constraints of someone with a nut allergy or a religious food restriction?
5. In US homes, a staple for sending food for children to school is the peanut-and-jelly sandwich.[12] Such food is not appropriate for feeding in homes for the elderly due to the high risk of inhalation and suffocation. Design a better portable and convenient food item for distribution to the elderly during outings.

---

[12]The lead author is not a fan of these due to his severe nut allergy.

6. Consider the task of feeding yourself (or your family). Apply the Complexity Theory method to this problem. Start with CNs, FRs, and develop DPs. Create a Design matrix, design decomposition, or Design Record Graph (Iino and Nakao 2016) to show the dependencies between the FRs. Finally, consider the complexity for the design of the meal: time-independent real complexity for meeting each of the goals outlined in the FRs (such as having food ready at a given time) and time-dependent combinatorial or periodic complexity as appropriate.

7. How to consider the level of recyclability in a product (such as a K-cup) is hard to incorporate into the design methodologies as described. Is it possible to use the "battery symbol" approach described in Iino and Nakao (2016) to tag elements that can be recycled easily? Discuss how you would modify AD to better incorporate sustainable elements such as this.

8. Consider a single-use food preparation item such as the K-cup. Develop the Design Matrix for it from the user's standpoint. Develop the Design Matrix for it from the product designer's standpoint. Why are they different? How would you adjust the design to include sustainability in the design intent?

References

America's Test Kitchen (1997) Recipe: Classic apple pie. https://www.cooksillustrated.com/recipes/1377-classic-apple-pie

Atshuller G (1994) And suddenly the inventor appeared. Technical Innovation Center, translated from Russan by Leev Shulyak

Bradford W (1981) Of Plymouth Plantation 1620–1647. Modern Library, New York, first printed in entirety 1856

Bramlett J (2018) The unconventional thinking of dominant companies. CreateSpace Independent Publishing Platform

Butler G (2015) 15 greatest deep-fried turkey disasters caught on video. https://www.oregonlive.com/cooking/2015/11/12_greatest_deep-fried_turkey.html

Chang HC, Carpenter JA, Toledo RT (1998) Modeling heat transfer during oven roasting of unstuffed turkeys. J Food Sci 63(2):257–261. https://doi.org/10.1111/j.1365-2621.1998.tb15721.x

Cochran DS, Foley JT, Bi Z (2016) Use of the Manufacturing System Design Decomposition for comparative analysis and effective design of production systems. Int J Prod Res 55:870–890

Davis K (2001) More than a meal. Lantern Books, New York, NY, USA

DM-Media (2019) Bavarian specialty, special soup, hay soup with bread and spices, vegetarian. Photo licensed from Shutterstock, ID: 667673017

Donovan M (2006) On food and cooking: the science and lore of the kitchen, 2nd edn. Gastronomica: The J Crit Food Stud 6(4):117–118. https://doi.org/10.1525/gfc.2006.6.4.117, http://gcfs.ucpress.edu/content/6/4/117, book Review

Eschner K (2017) Apple pie is not all that American. Smithsonian. https://www.smithsonianmag. com/smart-news/why-apple-pie-linked-america-180963157/

Foley JT (2017) Tutorial: Axiomatic Design for everyone. In: Slătineanu (2017), p 68

Foley JT, Harðardóttir S, (2016) Creative Axiomatic Design. 26th CIRP Design Conference. Procedia CIRP, Elsevier ScienceDirect, Stockholm, Sweden, pp 688–694

Foley JT, Puik E, Cochran DS (2016) Desirable Complexity. In: Liu (2016), pp 101–106. https:// doi.org/10.1016/j.procir.2016.05.023

Foley JT, Puik E, Cochran DS (2017) The faucet reloaded: improving Axiomatic Design by example. In: Slătineanu (2017), p 7. https://doi.org/10.1051/matecconf/201712701009

Foley JT, Puik E, Puik L, Smith J, Cochran DS (2019) Complexity in the kitchen. In: Liu A, Puik E, Foley JT (eds) 12th International Conference on Axiomatic Design (ICAD), MATEC web of conferences. Sydney, Australia, p 12. https://doi.org/10.1051/matecconf/201930100007

Girgenti A, Pacifici B, Ciappi A, Giorgetti A (2016) An Axiomatic Design approach for customer satisfaction through a lean start-up framework. In: Liu (2016), pp 151–157. https://doi.org/10. 1016/j.procir.2016.06.101

Goodwin TL, Mickelberry WC, Stadelman WJ (1962) The effect of freezing, method of cooking, and storage time on the tenderness of pre-cooked and raw turkey meat. Poultry Sci 41(4):1268–1271. https://doi.org/10.3382/ps.0411268, https://academic.oup.com/ps/article/41/4/1268/1614461

Gough J (2019) Roasted lamb shanks. Photo licensed from Shutterstock, ID: 55000708

Gualtieri L, Rauch E, Rojas R, Vidoni R, Matt DT (2018) In: Puik et al (2018) Application of Axiomatic Design for the design of a safe collaborative human-robot assembly workplace. p 01003. https://doi.org/10.1051/matecconf/201822301003

Hays R (2004) How to brine a turkey. Cook's Illustrated. https://www.cooksillustrated.com/articles/ 36-how-to-brine-a-turkey#print

Iino K, Nakao M (2016) Design Record Graph and Axiomatic Design for creative design education. In: Liu https://www.sciencedirect.com/science/article/pii/S2212827116307764

Iino K, Nakao M (2018) Human design parameters for safety of products and systems. In: Puik et al, p 01002. https://doi.org/10.1051/matecconf/201822301002

Kohatsu K (2017) Why are we 'as American as apple pie'? Huffington Post. https://www.huffpost. com/entry/why-are-we-as-american-as_n_6227462, originally published 2014

Kujawa K, Weber J, Puik E, Paetzold K (2018) Exploring and ADAPT!—extending the ADAPT! method to develop reconfigurable manufacturing systems. In: Puik et al (2018), p 01006. https:// doi.org/10.1051/matecconf/201822301006

Lam L (2016) Easier roast turkey and gravy. Cook's Illustrated. https://www.cooksillustrated.com/ articles/331-easier-roast-turkey-and-gravy

Liu A (ed) (2016) 10th International Conference on Axiomatic Design (ICAD), vol 53, Procedia CIRP, Elsevier ScienceDirect, Xi'an, Shaanxi, China

Lopez-alt JK (2007) Foolproof pie dough. Cook's Illustrated. https://www.cooksillustrated.com/ articles/37-foolproof-pie-dough

McGee H (2007) On food and cooking. Scribner, revised from 1984 version

McGee H, Mcinerney J, Harrus A (1999) The virtual cook: modeling heat transfer in the kitchen. Phys Today—PHYS TODAY 52:30–36. https://doi.org/10.1063/1.882728

Osias J (2006) Safe turkey deep fryer. US Patent 20060272633A1

Papasidero D, Pierucci S, Manenti F, Piazza L (2015) Heat and mass transfer in roast beef cooking. temperature and weight loss prediction. Chem Eng Trans 43:151–156. https://doi.org/10.3303/ CET1543026

Pétursson E, Karlsson IN, Garðarsson OG, Pálsson P, Saulius Genutis VO, Foley JT (2017) Axiomatic design of equipment for analysis of SMA spring degradation during electronic actuation. In: Complex systems engineering and development proceedings of the 27th CIRP design conference, Procedia CIRP, Elsevier ScienceDirect, Cranfield University, UK, pp 261–266. https://doi.org/10.1016/j.procir.2017.01.055

Puik E, Ceglarek D (2014a) A review on information in design. In: Thompson. https://axiomaticdesign.com/technology/icad/icad2014/9-Puik-et-al-paper.pdf

Puik E, Ceglarek D (2014b) A theory of maturity. In: Thompson. https://axiomaticdesign.com/technology/icad/icad2014/17-Puik-et-al-paper.pdf

Puik E, Ceglarek D (2015) The quality of a design will not exceed the knowledge of its designer; an analysis based on axiomatic information and the cynefin framework. In: Thompson et al. https://doi.org/10.1016/j.procir.2015.07.040

Puik E, Foley JT, Cochran D, Betasolo M (eds) (2018) 12th International Conference on Axiomatic Design (ICAD), MATEC web of conferences, Reykjavík, Iceland

Rolli F, Fradinho J, Giorgetti A, Citti P, Arcidiacono G (2018) Axiomatic decomposition of a zero-sum game: the penalty shoot-out case. In: Puik et al, p 01005. https://doi.org/10.1051/matecconf/201822301005

Schorger AW (1966) The wild turkey: its history and domestication. University of Oklahoma Press, Norman

Slocum AH (2008) FUNdaMENTALS of design. MIT precision engineering research group. http://pergatory.mit.edu/resources/FUNdaMENTALS.html

Slătineanu L (ed) (2017) 11th International Conference on Axiomatic Design (ICAD), MATEC web of conferences, Iasi, Romania

Smith JJ, Shah SA, Cochran DS (2018) Prevention, early detection, and reversal of type-2 diabetes using Collective System Design. In: Puik et al, p 01018. https://doi.org/10.1051/matecconf/201822301018

Stockcreations (2019) Cooked sliced open haggis and vegetables with mashed turnip, potato and fried onions on a rustic wood table with copy space. Photo licensed from Shutterstock, ID: 611174096

Suh NP (1990) The principles of design. Oxford University Press

Suh NP (2001) Axiomatic design—advances and applications. Oxford University Press

Suh NP (2005) Complexity. Oxford University Press

Suh NP (2015) Challenges in dealing with large systems. In: Thompson et al, pp 1–15, keynote

Thompson MK (ed) (2014) 8th International Conference on Axiomatic Design (ICAD 2014), vol 33. CIRP, Axiomatic Design Solutions Inc, Lisboa, Portugal

Thompson MK, Giorgetti A, Citti P, Matt D, Suh NP (eds) (2015) 9th International Conference on Axiomatic Design (ICAD), vol 34. Procedia CIRP, Elsevier ScienceDirect, Florence, Italy

Ulrich K, Eppinger S (2015) Product design and development, 6th edn. McGraw-Hill Education, New York, NY

United Stated Department of Agriculture (2015) Turkey basics: safe cooking. https://www.fsis.usda.gov/wps/portal/fsis/topics/food-safety-education/get-answers/food-safety-fact-sheets/poultry-preparation/turkey-basics-safe-cooking/CT_Index

Vossebeld DM, Foley JT, Puik E (2018) The complexity of mapping customer needs ... (and the myth of a unanimous customer). In: Puik et al, p 7. https://doi.org/10.1051/matecconf/201822301024

Weinersmith Z (2011) Saturday morning breakfast cereal comic: dinosaur to turkey. https://www.smbc-comics.com/comic/2011-11-08

Weinersmith Z (2018) Saturday morning breakfast cereal comic: GMO. https://www.smbc-comics.com/comic/gmo

Wettasinghe CM, Koh TH (2008) Axiomatic Design Theory for the analysis, comparison, and redesign of curriculum for special education. Disabil Rehabil Assist Technol 3(6):309–314. https://doi.org/10.1080/17483100802281012

Wright AH (1914) Early records of the wild turkey. The Auk: A Q J Ornithol 31(3):334–358

Design of Organizations

16

Nam Pyo Suh

Abstract

Sound well designed organizations are most important organizations should be design well for many different reasons, such as efficiency, reliability, rational decisions, and productivity, and most of all, in achieving the mission of the organization. Some of the significant failures of high-technology products and major corporations, as well as successful enterprises and products, may be attributed to organizational and personnel issues.

People design a variety of organizations that are fundamental units of human society to achieve specific goals such as those related to educational, manufacturing, financial, legal, and political purpose. An organizational unit could be a nation, industrial firm, university, army, hospital, and a non-profit organization. An organization may consist of several lower level organizations, forming a hierarchical structure among higher level and lower level units to fulfill the missions and objectives of the organization.

Organizations have missions or goals, i.e., *raison d' être*. They must operate within a set of external and internal constraints such as governing rules and legal regulations that may constrain the decisions and activities of the organization. Organizations need resources, i.e., operating funds, people, and infrastructure. Most of all, the organization must have a leader or a group of leaders to oversee the entire design, operation, execution, and administration of the organization to achieve its stated goals.

The first step in the design of an organization is the establishment of its goal and mission. The process of design begins with the identification of problems the organizations must overcome to achieve the established goal. The design of an organization follows the same transformational process as any other design. The goals and problems must be translated into functional requirements (FRs), which

N. P. Suh (✉)
M.I.T., Cambridge, MA, USA
e-mail: npsuh@mit.edu

© Springer Nature Switzerland AG 2021
N. P. Suh et al. (eds.), *Design Engineering and Science*,
https://doi.org/10.1007/978-3-030-49232-8_16

is then followed by the transformation of FRs into design parameters (DPs) and finally into process variables (PVs). One significant difference between organizational design and other designs is that in organizational design, DPs are people, whose future behavior and performance are not always predictable.

The design of the organization should be either uncoupled or decoupled for the organization to be effective. When the structure of the organization is a coupled design, the organization cannot function effectively. Then, the decisions made in one part of the organization may conflict with decisions made in another part of the organization, thus compromising the attainment of the overall goals. Organizations with coupled FRs are resource-intensive with uncertain outcomes.

Organizations—their missions and goals as well as personnel—may evolve or change over time. Many organizations are complex time-dependent systems with functional periodicity. Thus, a periodic re-initialization of the system should be required.

The role of the chief executive officer (CEO) is most important in any organization. Many CEOs play two roles: both the role of a composer of music and the conductor of a symphony that plays the music. A wise CEO creates an uncoupled organization. The CEO then can delegate each one of the highest level FRs to each one of the executives who report directly to the CEO. The role of the CEO is to achieve corporate goals by modulating and combining the outputs of all FRs. When the CEO designs a coupled system, the organization cannot effectively achieve its goals. The organization that couples FRs will be chaotic, undoing the actions of other parts of the organization.

In large organizations, many lower level FRs are the responsibility of lower level DPs. The organization must be sure that all the decisions made throughout the organization are consistent with the highest level goals. Before any decision is made, one should ask "Is this decision good for our organization?" If the answer is not affirmative, one should not implement the decision.

Complexity theory applies to organizational design. Time-dependent combinatorial complexity should be avoided, whereas time-dependent periodic complexity should be built into renew the goals of the organization periodically.

Finally, this chapter presents the idea of S-factor, S-Gap, and Delta (δ) to illustrate why it is difficult to change the relative standing of organizations and what the leader of the organization must do to put the organization on a different trajectory to make the organization to be outstanding and distinguished.

16.1 Why Design an Organization?

Beginning in prehistoric days, humans have instinctively designed and implemented organizations at all levels, probably to improve collective survivability[1]. They probably used trial-and-error processes to act in unison and survive in a

---

[1]This instinct for survivability seems to be possessed by all animals. The schools of deer that come around our yard also have a hierarchy; the mother deer always protects her young breeds. However, their organizational hierarchy seems to be shallow, being limited to one generation.

hostile environment and address everyday needs and common problems collectively. Today, we have a variety of organizations to deal with diverse human needs and societal goals, promote economic and technological advances, and ultimately achieve national and global aspirations for a better quality of life.

Organizations are the basic units of society, nations, and humanity. Each one of them has a purpose and objectives. They perform a variety of functions and achieve specific missions and goals. The size of the organization may vary, from a few people to millions of people. Within an ideally designed organization, people share common values and depend on each other for collective well-being. Without organizations, individuals may not be able to function, survive, and secure basic needs.

The goal of organizations is to achieve a set of missions that must be addressed to meet human, societal, national, and international needs. Different common laws and regulations of a nation may govern each one of these organizations, which were established for governance. Ultimately, the overarching legal basis for these organizations is the constitution of a nation or a royal decree, which may impose the ultimate limits of acceptable designs.

Many different kinds of organizations exist to serve a variety of different societal goals. Well-known organizations are schools, industrial firms, banks, governments, manufacturing organizations, religious organizations, military, charitable organizations, the World Bank, and many others. As human knowledge expands and the population increases, "super" organizations (e.g., the United Nations) have been created to deal with a common interest and to assure the collective survival and collaboration.

Many of the modern non-governmental organizations are chartered legal entities (e.g., schools, companies, law firms, schools, hospitals, churches), each with a mission or objectives. In the case of a university, the mission is to generate highly educated people for various fields of human endeavor, who can advance organizational or societal goals. For an industrial firm, the mission could be the manufacture of specific products by hiring people and gathering human and financial resources and generate profit for those who have invested in the firm.

Both the design and operation of all of these organizations must be done well to achieve their stated goals. From time to time, these organizations need to be re-designed (or re-initialized), often within the same legal framework, to be more productive or compatible with the changed external conditions and needs. To achieve this goal, many organizations change their internal structure from time to time to respond to the external changes through the re-initialization of the organizations.

In many countries, regionalism, race, sex, and religion still affect or influence the organizational structure as a means of protecting their diverse interests. In some countries, the tribes used to be the basic unit of societal organizations, i.e., people belong to tribes for security, jobs, marriage, the survival of posterity, and family life. In some countries, hiring and promotion of people in an organization are not done based on merits and potential contributions, but rather on some other criteria such as "whom one knows" and "what region one is from." In such a society, a real democracy based on individual merits cannot survive for long.

Organizations need resources—human and financial—to sustain the organizations. Therefore, securing these resources is the most critical responsibility of the chief executive and the management.

Industrial firms exist to generate wealth through their activities. There are two kinds of industrial firms: those privately owned by individuals or a group of individuals, and those publicly traded companies that derive their finance through the issuance of company stocks in the public market. Public companies are controlled by regulations and rules of the national and local governments. The board of directors (BoD) governs the public companies, whose primary function is looking after the interest of the shareholders of the company. The BoD appoints the chief executive officer (CEO) of the company, who holds the executive power for operation of the company. The CEO or the board nominates the board members, and the shareholders typically elect the board members at their annual meeting. For the CEO, the membership of the board is vital for two reasons, i.e., to get sound advice and support for the CEO's actions. Many CEO attempts to create a friendly board that backs the CEO's position and policies.

Relevant units of an organization typically include the following functions: chief executive, finance, information, marketing, sales, operations, human resource/personnel, physical facilities, and the board of directors. For non-profit organizations, similar functions are performed but often under some other names. The board of directors of a public company protects the interest of the public (i.e., shareholders) and also appoints the chief executive. The chief executive officer (CEO) is responsible for all operational aspects of the company. Having an outstanding CEO is a prerequisite for a successful public company. The CEO appoints all key personnel of the organization. The fortune of a company often depends on the ability of its CEO. There are many examples of renowned companies facing bankruptcy because the board chose an inept CEO. Unfortunately, it takes a few years to find out the actual ability of the CEO, sometimes too late to save the company.

The CEO must identify the problem(s) that the organization must address or solve. Depending on the selection of a specific nature of the problem(s) the organization must address, different FRs may be selected, and thus, the outcome can be substantially different. It is the responsibility of the CEO to determine FRs. Therefore, the selection of the CEO is the most important decision the board of directors makes. The CEO is also responsible for the operation of the organization. She/he must design the organization to achieve the goals of the company. The CEO then must select the right, able, and ethical people (i.e., design parameters (DPs)) who can perform their functions (i.e., FRs) effectively.

University presidents are also CEOs, although their role differs from profit-oriented organizations, and the issues and goals are different. However, many issues that must be handled by university presidents are similar to corporate CEOs.

Design Story 16.1: Important Roles of CEO in a Major Corporation

In many major public industrial corporations, the chief executive officer (CEO) is also either the president or the chairman of the company. The COE performs the most critical role in determining the future of a company. The CEO designs the organizational structure in consultation with the CEO's staff, including COO (Chief Operating Officer), vice presidents (VPs), CFO (chief financial officer), and legal counsel. CEOs develop policies and strategies, as well as implement them. CEOs can make or break the company.

The board of directors of a company determines the compensation package (i.e., salary, stock options, etc.) of CEOs and senior executives of companies based on their performance. Sometimes, they gather data on the compensation of other similar companies to justify their decisions to shareholders. Relative to the average salary of employees in the company, many CEOs of American companies are well compensated. In many high-tech companies in the United States, CEOs hold about 2% of the company stock as incentives for outstanding performance. If the company does well, the CEO of profitable companies can become quite wealthy.

Outstanding CEOs of companies deserve every penny they earn for their performance. Under a strong and capable CEO, the shareholders of these companies have seen their investment grow by leaps and bounds. In 2018, Amazon, Apple, Boeing, Facebook, Google, Broadcom, and Microsoft were such companies. Amazon is the largest and fastest growing e-commerce company in the United States. Apple, Inc. is known as the dominant American company in portable telephones worldwide and is one of the largest multi-technology, multi-national companies in the world. Broadcom is the leading manufacturer of critical semi-conductor devices that are used in making telecommunication, computation, and other applications. The gross revenue of these high-tech companies exceeds that of all the oil companies of the world combined, although they use less natural resources than many others for their business. One of the remarkable things about many of these high-technology companies is that the founder of the company is still a dominant business leader of their industries.

Inept CEOs can ruin a reputable company. One CEO has ruled a major and oldest public company in the United States with iron hands for 15 years. The company used to be one of the original companies listed on the New York Stock Exchange. Until early 2000, the company was one of the fast-growing multi-technology companies in the world. Today, the company is a much-diminished company with many questions about its future. Many of its shareholders lost their investment.

Notwithstanding the poor performance, the high-level executives of the company were well-compensated relative to their performance and the compensation of its employees. There may be many reasons for the demise of the company that outsiders can only speculate. However, some of the contributing factors might have been due to the poor design of the company strategy. From the AD perspective, the lingering questions are did the CEO understand the problem(s) the company had to address? Did the CEO define a correct set of FRs and select the right set of DPs? Did the design of the company couple FRs?

Why did this company fail to perform under the leadership of this new CEO? It is difficult to judge without access to the inner workings and the business strategy of the company. However, it appears that he was a manager, not a leader with a vision. He enjoyed the trappings of being the CEO of a large conglomerate but did not have a clear understanding of his FRs and DPs. He made promises that he could not deliver or would not deliver. The board of directors (BOD) is partially responsible for letting the CEO manage without a clear strategy for a highly diversified global company. It may be safe to assume that the FRs and DPs were not carefully designed, and the company was an organization with coupled design. The BOD should have replaced the CEO within five years rather than waiting for 15 years. Oriental folklore says that "even mountains move in 10 years!"

Functional Periodicity, discussed in Chap. 12 on complexity, is highly relevant in corporate management. Corporations should review their strategy and execution periodically, and re-initialize and execute the plan well!

Design Story 16.2: Organizing a Start-Up Industrial Firm

Researchers at a university developed a new technology to measure the moisture content in hygroscopic polymers such as nylon and PVC (polyvinyl chloride) in situ. These plastics tend to adsorb moisture because these polymers are made of polar molecules. When the moisture in the plastic pellets exceeds a certain minimum level, the long-chained molecule of the polymer breaks down (i.e., molecular cession) during processing in high temperatures in extruders and injection molding machines, degrading the physical properties of the polymer. Therefore, these polymers are typically dried before processing. It is desirable to measure the moisture content in situ before processing the polymer pellets. Under the sponsorship of industrial firms, students developed a means of measuring the moisture content of such polymers based on the measurement of the dielectric properties of the polymers.

The industrial firms that sponsored the research wanted to use the technology. The professor, who conceived the idea for the measurement technology, asked two of his graduate students who just finished their masters' degrees if they would be interested in starting a new venture firm to commercialize the monitoring technology. They were enthusiastic about the idea of starting a new high-tech company. The professor raised funds from his friends and relatives to commercialize the technology to dispense with the time and effort required to raise funds from venture capitalists.

Some of the investors and the professor hired a lawyer to incorporate a company, which is relatively simple in the United States. They formed a board of directors and appointed one of the newly graduated engineers as the president and CEO of the company. The CEO hired several of his friends to develop the technology further and commercialize it. Creating a new business was relatively easy. However, making the company profitable was not easy!

They thought that the most crucial part of the new company is technology. That was naiveté or a significant mistake. They did not fully appreciate the fundamentals of what it would take to commercialize a high-tech product successfully. Many things, such as the importance of the reliability of the instrument in the production environment, sales, marketing, manufacturing, and financing of a company, were not fully appreciated. Because they did not have sufficient background in the commercialization of new technology such as marketing and economical manufacture of the product, the company was not successful in becoming a viable commercial venture after they exhausted the capital raised. They did not appreciate how difficult it is to make reliable industrial equipment. They learned an expensive lesson, and the investors lost money.

They learned a few lessons from the failure. The market size for the new product was much smaller than they had assumed. Furthermore, the instrument had to be calibrated for every material at the operating temperature. The organizational design was also flawed because they did not correctly define the "problem." They also learned that it is not a good idea to have inexperienced people to take on the critical task of making business decisions. They should seek out highly qualified people to join the board of directors to benefit from their knowledge and experience.

The young engineers who operated the company learned a lot, perhaps more than they would have learned in a business school, at a great expense to the investors. The professor learned a lot, too, about the commercialization of new technology and how not to start a new venture firm. The key lesson learned was that a new venture firm must be designed correctly with the clear identification of FRs, DPs, and PVs. Perhaps an equally important lesson was that experience in starting a new business can eliminate apparent mistakes made by novices.

Design Story 16.3: Organizing an Industrial Firm—Story of Another Venture Firm

A bright young graduate, who studied business management at a leading technical university and inherited some money from his family, joined a successful industrial firm. He was soon fired because he raised too many questions about the way the company was operating as a young engineer/manager. Then he joined another company and was fired there also. After he was fired the third time, he joined a new start-up company established by a brilliant technologist who graduated from the same university a few years earlier. The only product made by the company was the testing equipment that measured the quality and functionality of semiconductor chips that were just manufactured through complicated fabrication processes. He became the second in command in charge of marketing the new product. The company did very well, especially after the CEO, the technologist who founded the company, left the company, leaving the helm of the company to him as the new CEO. The company grew rapidly as the semiconductor industry expanded at an unprecedented rate for the next three decades. They defined the problem well in the early phase of the semiconductor industry by identifying the need to measure the quality of each one of the semiconductor devices.

This new CEO knew the importance of the underlying technology and had expertise in and appreciation of the importance of finance, marketing, and human resources in newly launched high-technology companies. He was a brilliant designer of organizations and a superb leader of his employees. He hired outstanding technologists and treated them with respect. They continued to improve and innovate their products to be able to deal with ever more complicated semiconductor chips being produced by companies such as IBM and Intel. His CEO office was a small cubicle just like those of low-level engineers because he knew that the most valuable asset of his high-tech company, i.e., the creative and productive technologists, must be treated with respect and fairly. He used to say that the most valuable assets of his company went home every day at 5 p.m. Everyone in his company, regardless of their job title, traveled in the same class of the airplane when they were on business trips.

In these high-technology companies, the chief financial officer (CFO) is the second most important executive in the company, who oversees nearly all aspects of managing high-technology companies, including sales, manufacturing, marketing, engineering, and legal. Successful companies always need more capital to expand their business. They raised the capital by selling the stocks of their company in the public market. The CEO and CFO of this company worked together well for a few decades. They also had an active board made up of experienced business and technology leaders.

He became super-rich and funded many other new start-up companies. He became successful in his business because he was ethical and moral, in addition to his expertise in marketing, financing, and high-technology. He commanded the respect of those who worked with and for him in many different capacities. He became a philanthropist who funded many programs at universities, hospitals, and other worthy causes. People like him render hope and faith in continuing the advancement of humanity for the better. His name was Alex d'Arbeloff.

Government organizations are designed to achieve the goals established by the laws of the nation. For example, the U.S. Congress established the U.S. National Science Foundation (NSF) by enacting the NSF Act of 1950. It specified its mission of the agency (i.e., to promote the progress of science and engineering; to provide welfare, health, and prosperity to people; and to secure national defense), a broad outline of its organizational structure, including the appointment of the leaders of the organization, i.e., presidential appointees, (the director, deputy director, and a few assistant directors). It also specified how the agency is to be financed and the chain of command under the presidency of the United States (e.g., the NSF director reports directly to the President of the United States). Its budget plan is approved by the White House through the Office of Management and Budget (OMB) and submitted to the U.S. Congress for final approval. Unlike other government agencies, the NSF Act mandate that a board (i.e., the National Science Board) be appointed by the President to oversee the activities of NSF.

Design Story 16.4: Design of Government Organizations[2]

A professor, who was just sworn in as a new presidential appointee of a government agency of the United States, came into his office after waiting for 6 months for confirmation of his appointment by the U.S. Senate after receiving the clearances of the Federal Bureau of Investigation (FBI) and the Presidential Appointment Office of the White House. It was an unexpected turn of events in his career since going into government service was not part of his career plan! He took the job of serving in the government in a critical position, although his family had to suffer financially.

When he entered his large office, he was impressed by its cleanliness with a new carpet on the floor and a fresh coat of paint on the wall. It was apparent that the staff members, who were extremely dedicated and competent, worked hard to make the office as pleasant as possible for the new appointee. The bookshelves were empty, and the desktop was polished. Then, he noticed a piece of paper on his desk with a drawing similar to that shown below. The caption said, paraphrasing it "A political appointee comes to Washington, thinking that he/she can make a big difference in government. Then after two years, they return home not having achieved anything, mired in Washington bureaucracy with is tail between the hind legs like a scared dog." The cartoon was amusing but did not deter this new political appointee from his goal of changing how engineering research and education were funded to strengthen U.S. engineering education and research in the twenty-first century (Fig. 16.1).

He decided to re-design his directorate to make it more effective in fulfilling the duties and responsibilities outlined in the NSF act of 1950, as amended. He began this process of designing the new NSF Engineering Directorate by defining the problems that must be overcome, translating the issues identified into FRs. A new structure was created by specifying DPs (e.g., divisions). Division Directors designed the programs within the divisions in consultation with the Engineering AD. The appointment of the AD by the President of the United States gave him the authority to make these decisions.

NSF was created to achieve three tasks: to promote the progress of science and engineering; to provide welfare, prosperity, and health to people; and to secure the national defense. The newly introduced changes were to deal with these three tasks more effectively and make the United States more competitive in engineering in the twenty-first century. One result of this change was more support for younger researchers and new fields of science and technology. Also, it was to promote multidisciplinary research, in some cases with the support of and in collaboration with industry. The new design of the NSF Engineering was well received by many, including those in the U.S. Congress, the White House, universities (especially young professors), and industry, but there was strong opposition, too, from those who benefited under the old system. The new system was to support new and innovative research rather than refining the well-established ideas and technologies.

---

[2]This story is partially told in Sect. 3.6.1.

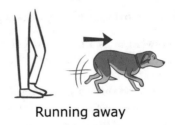

Running away

Fig. 16.1 A cartoon to make fun of presidential appointees running away from Washington after having failed to achieve anything meaningful during their tenure. (Copyright 2013, Center for Shelter Dogs, Cummings School of Veterinary Medicine at Tufts University. Illustrated by Lili Chin. Reproduced with permission)

The hostility of those who opposed the changes made at the NSF Engineering Directorate lingered. Their feeling was reasonable and understandable in the sense that they had been champions of their fields, many of whom had made significant contributions. However, the new direction and policy of the Engineering Directorate, which was to support more emerging technological fields and younger researchers who are entering the profession for the first time, resulted in the loss of easy access to research grants to established professors. This loss of easy access to government support changed the quality of life of these well-established professors, who used to get the NSF support easily working on more or less similar problems for decades. These changes instituted by this presidential appointed have had a lasting positive impact on the nation's research and education infrastructure, although some senior professors criticized him at the time.

In the new design of the NSF Engineering Directorate, there were seven FRs the new organization was designed to satisfy with seven DPs. Seven divisions were proposed, increasing the number of divisions from four to seven to assure the independence of FRs. Then, the chief financial officer (CFO) of NSF warned that Congress would reject the new organizational structure, because there would be too many divisions that had to be headed up by additional senior executives, increasing the top ranks of civil servants. As a result of the CFO's advice, he compromised by combining two proposed divisions into one. Therefore, two of the seven FRs had to be administered by one division director. The result was not satisfactory because one of the FRs of the two FRs in this division was not given the same priority as the other FR by the division director. He tended to favor the FR he was most familiar with and neglect the other FR. Therefore, after waiting for a year, this division was split into two, so each division can handle only one FR and its lower level FRs.

The Congressional Committee that had the oversight on NSF did not have any concerns about the number of divisions in the new organization. The new FRs of NSF Engineering changed the landscape of engineering research and education of many engineering schools in the United States. For the first time, NSF Engineering supported research in micro-technology, design, and newly emerging fields of technology. Also, NSF established the Engineering Research Centers (ERC) to promote multidisciplinary research in collaboration with industry. Many outstanding scholars from universities and industry joined the NSF Engineering Directorate to make their share of contributions toward newly emerging fields. The overall consensus was that the transformation resulted in the stronger engineering research community in the country.

When he decided to go back to his university after almost four years of government service, the U.S. Congressional Committee with oversight on NSF commanded the NSF Engineering AD for the job well done. NSF awarded him the Distinguished Service Award and a Gold Medal, notwithstanding the cartoon that was on his desk on the first day of his arrival in his office at NSF.

Finally, it should be noted that such significant changes in a government organization, programs, and policies are challenging. There are too many forces that try to maintain the status quo at any given instant in the institution's history. In institutions in any country, there are always those who benefit from the existing system, although it may no longer serve the interest of the people. One must be devoid of personal agenda if one wishes to make such a significant change. In fact, in the case of NSF *Engineering Directorate, about 1,600 engineers of "Concerned Engineers of America" sent a petition into the White House asking the President to fire the NSF AD, although the appeal was not heeded. Some eminent professors even "blackballed" him to prevent his election to a particular academy. Unless one is willing to swallow some of these abuses, one should not assume the position. Also holding the government job was extremely expensive for the professor with a large family.*

Notwithstanding the cartoon of the dog, many leave their government positions after two years of service for financial reasons. However, the most important reason to accept such an assignment is because of the unique opportunity to serve one's nation with a critical mission. For him, it was an honor to get a telephone call from the White House.

16.2 How Should We Design an Organization?

The CEO of an organization has a great deal of latitude in designing his/her organization. CEO typically decides on a set of FRs the organization must achieve during her/his tenure as the CEO. The CEO gets the approval of the board of directors for the plan. In the case of universities, the governing body is often called the Board of Trustees, which plays a similar role as the board of directors of companies.

To achieve the highest level FRs, the CEO must decide on a strategy of satisfying the FRs by coming up with a plan (i.e., DPs). The CEO has to find the right person to be in charge of each set of FR/DP/PV. In general, it is not a good idea to have one person to be in charge of more than one FR, since the person may make "coupled" decisions, which forces the upper management to check double all the decisions made by his/her subordinates, leading to micro-management. As we decompose the design of the organization, the person in charge should design the organization by decomposing the highest level FR and DP and appointing the right people to be in charge of the next-level FRs and DPs. One of the most successful CEOs, who have received the highest compensation based on his performance among all CEOs in the United States, gives his key division managers only one specific FR to achieve after he designs his company's strategy.

Many firms and organizations have tried to improve their operations by trying many different forms of organizational structure, including "matrix organization," "flat organization," "hierarchical organization," and others. However, the common mistake many CEOs have made was creating the organizational structure first before deciding on the goal of the organization and FRs. That is, the CEO must determine the overall goals and select specific FRs. After the FRs are chosen, the CEO can create an organizational structure and choose the right person to lead each pair of FR/DP. Then, the CEO can monitor the progress made toward achieving the overall goal of the company. The CEO should construct a master design matrix to quickly identify decisions that can lead to the coupling of the highest FRs of the company.

As the following example shows, a large organization designed based on Axiomatic Design (AD) is much easier to operate and achieve its goals. It also illustrates how difficult it is to change the existing design of an organization.

Design Story 16.5: Transformation of a Science and Technology University

Research universities are distinguished from other universities because they conduct significant research and have active graduate programs that emphasize research and original contributions to their fields. There are many excellent research universities throughout the world, which have contributed to the development of modern society and laid the foundation for human advancement. Some of the leading research universities have generated societal leaders, scholars, and researchers who have contributed to humanity through innovative ideas, scientific discoveries, and technological advances. For example, their research has played a significant role in the agricultural revolution, technological innovation, scientific discoveries, and medical advances. In the twentieth and twenty-first centuries alone, they played important roles in creating an electric power distribution system, automobile revolution, electronics, digital technologies, computers, software revolution, fission and fusion of atoms, scanning electron microscope, printing technologies, mobile telephones, and many others. Many of the older research universities, e.g., Harvard, Cambridge, MIT, and Oxford, have evolved and advanced over a long period. However, there are some outstanding young research universities, which are less than 50 years old. Initially, many of these younger institutions tried to emulate older research universities. They were partly successful, but many of them are still not competitive relative to the best research universities in the world. The main reason is that universities with more resources and reputation advance faster than those without them and tend to receive more financial support from both public and private. For younger universities to become a great university, they must make their unique contributions to humanity with visionary goals and programs, in addition to emulating the excellent features of leading older universities.

Background:

An Science & Technology university was established in an Asian country about 50 years ago in 1972 when the nation was in the early stages of industrialization. It was founded as a government-funded, but independent graduate school in science and technology. It had its board of trustees as the governing entity, unlike national universities that are run by the government. The goal was to generate human resources in science and technology to support the ambitious industrialization plan of the country.

To attract the best talents to this university, the government gave particular support to this then-new university, its students, and faculty. For example, once admitted, students were waived from military service. To attract best faculty members from abroad in its early days, the university offered the professors salaries comparable to those paid in the United States, about three times higher than the current salaries of national universities. They built a new campus in 1986 away from the highly congested capital city. At the same time, it also absorbed a nearby undergraduate school of science and technology, making it a university with about 3,200 undergraduates and 6,000 graduate students. In 2006, there were about 400 professors. It became one of the most selective universities in the country. Many of its students were top graduates of "science high schools," an exclusive high school for gifted students. Students were adequately supported, i.e., no tuition, free room, and board. Professors were as well compensated as those at comparable leading universities in the United States. It was a good university but was not rated as being one of the best in the world. Its ranking was about 200th in the world in 2006.

Problem Statement in the Customer Domain:

The university elected a new president from overseas because the board of trustees and the government were interested in improving its quality, global status, and competitiveness. The customers, i.e., the government and the public, were not satisfied with the rate of progress being made at the university. Their aspiration for this university was to see it become one of the leading universities in the world. What should this new president do?

His first task upon assuming the job was to define the "problem" the university is facing before he could design a solution. Before assuming the position, he collected information about the university by talking with young alumni/ae of the university, asking for written inputs of the department heads, and talking to the board of trustees. He also spoke to outside people such as journalists, government officials, and politicians—all to identify and understand the problems faced by the university. He accepted the invitation to be the president of this university because he realized that this university had the potential of becoming a world-class university under the right circumstance. The university had built-in advantages such as generous government support, a special admissions policy that enabled it to attract the best students, and public support for education.

As explained in Chaps. 1 and 2, the first thing we have to do in designing a university is to define the problem that must be solved to transform this university to achieve its goal of becoming one of the best universities in the world. The new president, in consultation with members of its faculty and staff, surmised that the following are the problems that must be addressed to move forward:

- The University has not progressed in recent decades because of the use of a seniority system rather than having a merit-based system.
- Professors were not pursuing new intellectual challenges in their research and education, because the number of publications rather than the impact made by the researchers measured their performance. Many professors published papers by letting bright graduate students research a topic the professor is already familiar with rather than pursuing intellectually challenging new issues that are important in the future development of science and technology.
- The senior professors who joined the faculty when they were young in the early days of the University continued to dominate the university culture for decades, depriving young faculty members do their challenging work and creating a crony system.
- The University depended on the government for funding, personnel, and operation of the University. The government bureaucrats controlled the University through its budgetary process. As a result, the median age of the faculty was 55 years, with almost no faculty members in the thirties and some in the forties.
- Because the students were fully supported and were waived from serving in the military, many of the students had delayed their graduation to improve their grade point average by retaking the same subject to improve the grades and replace the poor grades. Thus, the number of undergraduate students was higher than what the budget allowed by about 800, which strained the housing and other operating expenses.
- The University did not raise any funds by soliciting private gifts, and therefore, the University did not have any endowment.
- The infrastructure was not maintained since they were built in the 1980s. The buildings did not have adequate heating and cooling system. Therefore, they closed all research buildings at night during the winter season.
- Faculty members were appointed to key administrative positions for two years with extra compensation. Under this rotational system, inexperienced faculty members without managerial expertise often made significant mistakes.
- The number of female faculty, as well as non-native faculty members, was only about 10%.
- Because teaching and all the administrative functions were performed in the local language, its graduates were not prepared for jobs in major industrial firms, which sell their products overseas and thus, conduct their business in the English language.

The problem he identified was the "stagnation" of the university as if the forward motion of the university was frozen in place. The cause for the stagnation was the "intellectually lazy" culture that permeated throughout the university, i.e., many of the faculty members and students were happy with the then prevailing status quo, although they could achieve a lot more if they tried to distinguish themselves. They also depended too much on government bureaucrats' directives and did not attempt to be the leaders in their professional fields. They were satisfied with the status quo. The idea of becoming one of the leading universities in the world was beyond their imagination or dream, i.e., they thought that it could not be done! The university had gradually deteriorated over the previous 30 years since they moved into a brand new campus.

The most challenging part of becoming a professor or student at this university was "getting into the university." Once one becomes a professor at this university, the job was secure for life. Similarly, a student admitted to the university graduates from the university with a degree. Students also get free room and board for at least four years. Once one gets into this university, there were no incentives and reasons to perform. The prestige of the university guaranteed a good life for a lifetime for most graduates and faculty of the university. Professors' salaries increased each year regardless of the performance, too.

When the university was established some 50 years ago, it started with full of enthusiasm, because the government conferred special status to the university to nurture highly educated engineers and scientists. They worked hard to make the university to be one of the best in the country, but the notion that they could make their university to be the world's leading university was dismissed as being unrealistic. The university administration and the faculty blamed the government for all their shortcomings.

Having identified the "problem," i.e., the "stagnation," the following FRs were established to solve the problem and achieve the goal of making it one of the best universities in the world:

FR1 = Increase the faculty size from 400–700 to be competitive with the best universities in the world;
FR2 = Hire only the best scholars regardless of their field of specialty;
FR3 = Work on important problems of the twenty-*first century;*
FR4 = Increase government support for research;
FR5 = Change the language of instruction to English;
FR6 = Increase diversity;
FR7 = Increase the overhead rate to recover the indirect cost of sponsored research;
FR8 = Increase externally funded research;
FR9 = Improve the decision-*making process;*
FR10 = Raise gifts from donors;
FR11 = Require students to complete their degree requirements on time;
FR12 = Recruit and admit the best students;
FR13 = Strengthen interdisciplinary research;
FR14 = Improve and expand physical facilities;
FR15 = Replace the seniority-based compensation policy to a merit-based system.

Many of these FRs are what a typical research university would aim to achieve. However, there are a few that deserve further explanation regarding their issues:

FR1: A few universities would dare to commit to increasing the faculty size by 75% without a financial guarantee either from the state resources or a significant increase in the endowment. However, without such an increase in the faculty size, it was clear that this university will not be able to be as good as some of the world's leading universities. The government bureaucrats were extraordinarily skeptical and in some ways annoyed by such a daring plan when they had no intention of increasing its support of this university even by 10%.

FR2: Most universities have traditionally allocated a fixed number of faculty positions to different departments; for example, 50 faculty for physics, 20 for biology, 50 to mechanical engineering, and ten in civil engineering, etc. *In many cases, the number of faculty members was determined based on student enrollment and tradition. However, in some ways, they are entirely arbitrary. Students do not prefer specific departments because there are more professors in the department. The number of students in a given department tends to fluctuate over the years. Sometimes, the professors from other departments may have to help out if the enrollment suddenly jumps, but it rarely happens. At this university, it was decided that every department head should hire as many outstanding professors as they can find, provided that they have exceptional intellectual accomplishments and are incredibly gifted. Initially, there were many skeptics of the idea that each department could hire as many new professors as they could find, provided that they are truly outstanding people.*

FR3: Many professors are under pressure to publish. Some end up publishing papers that are neither good nor important to increase the number of publications. FR3 states that professors should work on significant problems rather than on frivolous or trivial issues.

FR4: The government allocates about 5% of the national budget for research support. Some of this fund is available to researchers on a competitive basis. Winning proposals can receive this grant under the competitive government program.

FR5: In science and technology, English is used globally. For example, seminal papers are written in English for a broader readership. Many international journals are in English. Many of the new scientific and technological keywords are in English. Also, this country depends on foreign trade for the economy. Young people are learning English at a very young age. For these reasons, the language of instruction should be in English.

FR6: Male professors with limited international representation dominated this university. The number of women students in science and technology is too small, being about 25%. The brainpower of both genders should be utilized to be active in the twenty-first-century economy.

FR7: The prevailing overhead rate was too low to recover the overhead cost of sponsored research. Thus it should be raised.

FR8: Competing for publically available research funds has many excellent benefits. It improves the quality of research and also focuses the attention of researchers on critical research issues.

FR9: Departments could not make any difficult decisions because the senior members of the faculty controlled the department by developing consensus, and the central administration controlled the real power by over-*riding department decisions.*

FR10: The university depended primarily on government largess. The new administration undertook significant fundraising activities.

FR11: The old system allowed students to stay at the university indefinitely, receiving free room and board without paying any tuition. This system enabled students to stay longer taking the same subject over and over again until they got a better grade, replacing the lower grade received in the past. Professors also liked this old system, since they were not paying for the student support, and therefore, they tended to keep their Ph.D. students longer, since they were more useful to the professor.

FR12: This university attracted the best students in the country because of its prestige, free education, military service deferment, better educational environment, and future career development. Many students came from "science high schools" that were extremely selective. Some bright and able students from regular high schools could not get admission to this university, except a few, for a variety of different reasons, often financial. Therefore, 15% of the admitted students to the university were selected from these high schools based on the recommendation of the school principal, who was asked to nominate one student. These students did as well as those who graduated from science high schools.

To satisfy the FRs, we may choose the following DPs:

DP1 = Increased faculty size to be competitive with MIT. Hiring criterion: Department heads to search for as many high-quality faculty members as they can find irrespective of their field of interest and department size;
DP2 = Quality as the sole selection criteria for new faculty;
DP3 = Emphasis on energy, environment, water, and sustainability;
DP4 = Active solicitation of government support for bold new research projects;
DP5 = Faculty support for the change of the language of instruction;
DP6 = Active recruitment of woman students and faculty;
DP7 = New rate with faculty and government;
DP8 = Active proposal submission;
DP9 = Department head system (rather than chairman system);
DP10 = Active fundraising;
DP11 = Time-Limit on financial support (i.e., 4 years only for undergraduate students, and 6 years only for Ph.D. students);
DP12 = Special admissions policy to supplement the regular admissions policy.

These DPs were chosen to satisfy the FRs. Some of these FRs and DPs had to be decomposed, which will not be presented here.

There was strong resistance to some of the DPs chosen, especially on DP5 (the language of instruction), DP9 (the department head system), and DP11 (new tuition system). There were many reasons for the resistance, some quite understandable.

Rationale for Making Design Decisions (i.e., Experience and Knowledge Matters!)

The person in charge of an organization cannot choose specific DPs without a plan of implementation in mind. For example, how would anyone dare to increase the faculty size from 400 to 700 without any guarantee of funding from the government funding agencies for the contemplated increase in the faculty size? Since there were no available funds and no outstanding commitment for future funding, the leader of the organization must have had a plan for implementation when one chooses a particular DP. Otherwise, one may quickly become a laughing stock by creating false hope and talking about a project without the ability for actual implementation. Based on his experience in his previous jobs, he had contingency plans in mind for implementing the plan. His rough thinking and strategy were as follows:

At a typical research-intensive university, the fraction of the salary fund that goes toward paying professors is approximately 16% of the total salary pool of the university. After a rough calculation, he affirmed that this ratio was also valid at this university, which he just joined as the new president. Although he let every department hire as many professors as they can find, it would be difficult for them to meet the highest criterion established for the quality of faculty. He also knew that it would be difficult to find more than 40 (i.e., $\sim 10\%$ of the existing faculty) highly qualified faculty candidates. If the government does not provide the additional funding needed to increase the faculty by 10%, he identified how he could generate 1.6% of the budget required to pay for the newly hired professors from the existing resources by eliminating unproductive activities.

He also realized that the university could raise a lot more research funds if the professors were more active in generating creative ideas for their research. Many professors had been attempting to increase the number of publications by refining what they had done before. Furthermore, at this university, professors did not have to seek external research support because the graduate students were paid from the central university budget. Therefore, the professors did not have to raise research funds to support their research students. This system created a culture where professors relied mostly on the university to support their research rather than seeking external funding. Thus, their competitiveness in research had not been tested. Also, a few professors, who brought in outside research funds, complained about the overhead charge, although it was only 10%, which would be the envy of all professors at research universities in the United States, where the overhead rate would be more than 50%. Such a low overhead rate meant that the university was, de facto, subsidizing the externally funded research from internal resources, because the real cost of supporting research was about 50%! Therefore, professors were encouraged to seek research funds from external sources to pay part of their research cost. The overhead rate was increased from 10% to 25% to reflect the actual research cost!

The president of the university also initiated activities to raise new external support from two external sources: (1) government funding for special education and research projects, (2) the generation of large gifts from private donors. Through active solicitation, both of these financial plans succeeded in a country that did not have the philanthropic culture. The university increased its faculty size to 650 from 400 by hiring 350 new faculty members in five years and built 17 new buildings to accommodate the increased faculty size and expanded research activities as well as new student dormitories to retire old dilapidated facilities.

The faculty hiring was done solely based on the qualification of the individual faculty candidate regardless of their field of research interest. By eliminating the departmental quotas for the faculty size, each department had to concentrate on the intellectual quality of the faculty candidate under the new faculty hiring policy.

Result:

The hiring of the best faculty, regardless of their disciplinary interest, strengthened its research and teaching activities, promoting interdisciplinary research. The central administration approved hiring most professors who appeared to be outstanding irrespective of their professional specialization. As a consequence, some departments grew faster than those that could not recruit exceptional people. The new policy accelerated the initiation of new research programs, especially interdisciplinary research, which has resulted in significant advances in science and technology. The faculty members were encouraged to conduct bold research or technology innovation, i.e., two ends of the research spectrum. Many pursued innovative research at both ends of the research spectrum. The quality of the work replaced the number of publications as the primary criterion for promotion and salary raise.

These highly capable professors brought in significant research funding, which also generated additional overhead income, strengthening the financial resources of the university. Teaching in English made both the students and faculty not only more proficient in collaborating with their colleagues in many countries but also made them more active and competitive, enriching both education and scholarly activities of the university. Physical facilities were expanded drastically to accommodate the increased number of professors and enhanced teaching and student activities by constructing 14 new buildings. A new teaching format was introduced, which eliminated formal lectures and introduced a discussion format for learning, aided by making formal lectures available through the Internet. In five years, the sponsored research volume and the overhead income increased by a factor of 2.7.

The number of publications and patents obtained increased, although qualitative measures replaced the quantitative measures of performance. Professors became active globally than ever before. For instance, the robotics team of this university won in an international robotic contest that carried $2 million prizes, competing against the leading universities in the world. The university also introduced the world's first wireless transportation technology (i.e., On-Line Electric Vehicle) and "mobile harbor" technology. The electric vehicle is commercially operating in five cities.

The international standing of this university rapidly advanced, becoming #6 among the top ten most innovative universities in the world, the only non-U.S. based university to be in the top ten.

It should be noted that such a rapid transformation of a university could not be done without the personal sacrifice of the leadership of the university and strong outside support of the government and the citizen of the country. Significant financial donations came in response to the new direction established for the university, which helped in building 16 new buildings and increasing the faculty size from about 400–630 by hiring 300 new faculty members based on their quality regardless of their specialization. The "faculty union" opposed many of the changes from the beginning, mainly because the old seniority-based system was replaced by the merit-based system, including compensation, i.e., younger professors could be paid more than senior professors, depending on their performance as a researcher, teacher, and scholar. They also opposed the change of the language of instruction to English from their native language. However, the majority of the faculty, especially the younger professors, supported the move. The support of the newspapers and the average citizen was instrumental in implementing the difficult changes. They helped the changes because they were well aware of the abuse of power by the senior faculty, which prevented the advancement of the university despite the generous resource allocation by the government.

Design Story 16.6: Designing a Competitive Industrial Firm through Merger and Consolidation

In the early twentieth Century, Henry Ford revolutionized the automobile industry. He did not invent the automobile but knew the "problem," i.e., the high cost of manufacturing automobiles due to the practice of assembling the entire car by a team of craftsmen. He introduced the concept of the moving assembly line to reduce the manufacturing cost of automobiles. In this new Ford production system, the car was assembled on a moving production line by a large team of workers, each of whom performed only a limited but highly specialized assembly task as the vehicle came to his/her station. When the car reached the end of the assembly line, the fully assembled vehicle was driven off the production line. Today, the production rate is about one car a minute.

Thanks to the Henry Ford idea for mass production, a large number of small industrial firms were created to manufacture machines and automotive components in Detroit, Michigan, U.S.A. The Detroit area was the center of technology innovation and wealth generation of the United States during the first half of the twentieth century. Many automobile companies were sprung up around the state of Michigan and nearby states. Besides Ford Motor Company, many automotive companies were established and competed. Ford dominated the automotive business for a long time. Many smaller companies did similar things to produce automotive components and automobiles. Many of them were not competitive. Finally, many of the automobile companies merged to form the General Motors Corporation (GM), which dominated the automobile business in the United States for decades until the mid-*twentieth century. Alfred P. Sloan was one of the founders of General Motors Corporation.*

A monopoly is harmful to the overall economy because it may lower the overall efficiency of capital utilization and innovation. At the same time, the scattering of resources by a large number of sub-critical enterprises that cannot withstand significant risks involved in technology innovation cannot be sustained. The optimum consolidation of a given industry yields substantial benefits through the better service of customers and enhanced innovation and innovation activities. GM became the wealthiest and most profitable automotive company by the mid-twentieth century. It became more prominent than the Ford Motor Company.

In the twenty-first century, one of the dominant industries is the semiconductor industry. They manufacture semiconductor devices that are used in computers, cameras, and all other instruments and equipment that used information technology. There were many competing companies in semiconductor fabrication and systems that use semiconductors. A brilliant and capable CEO of a semiconductor device manufacturing company designed a strategy for creating a dominant semiconductor company by acquiring or merging with companies in similar businesses (a la the old GM model) and established a dominant high-technology company in the semiconductor device industry. He eliminated redundant R&D and consolidated product lines. He also concentrated on critical technology products to become the most competitive firm in that space. His company has grown by leaps and bounds by being the most productive and efficient firm in the semiconductor industry.

His organization tends to be simple, although it has become a hundred billion-dollar company. Each product line is managed separately and independently, all reporting to the CEO directly without going through a COO (Chief Operating Officer). This organizational structure enabled the CEO to monitor each highest FR, which may be possible only when the CEO knows the technology associated with the FRs. In this type of organization, R&D groups are closely tied to product divisions. His goal is to produce the best products in each business area. One of the criticisms has been that he does not invest in long-term R&D, which cannot be substantiated unless one is more specific about the goals of long-term research that have been neglected. In a matter of about ten years, the company has become one of the leading semiconductor device manufacturers in the world, a major success story of the twenty-first century.

16.3   Operation of Organizations

The raison d'être of any organization is to achieve its missions by solving a set of challenging problems. For example, universities exist to educate the future leaders of society and to pursue scholarships for enlightening and improving the quality of life of people through the generation of knowledge. Nearly all universities do not have financial gains as their goal. Industrial firms exist to produce goods and services to improve the quality of life of people and to generate wealth for a higher standard of living, especially those who take risks investing their wealth for a better future. Most industrial firms must make financial gains to attract investment in their firms. Organizations must be administered well and efficiently to achieve these societal and institutional goals,

To accomplish the mission of the organization, they must be organized as it was discussed in the preceding section. Many organizations have a tree-like structure with the CEO at the top, leading and orchestrating the operation of the organization. Most of the legal entities have a board of directors or trustees to be sure that the organization does indeed abide by laws and protect the investors or stakeholders. CEOs of industrial organizations tend to have nearly absolute power since they drive the organization toward achieving their corporate goals. At most universities, the power is distributed between the administration and the faculty. Individual members of the faculty contribute to the financial and operational well-being of universities.

As a consequence, some universities deliberate even simple issues endlessly because of the broad participation in the decision-making process by both faculty, students, and the administration, whereas timely and efficient decision-making ability is essential for the well-being of an institution. There are pros and cons to these power structures. For a quick response to changing the external environment, the concentration of power at the top can be justified, since consensus-based decision-making can take much longer, and some decisions must be made on a timely basis. Furthermore, there is no guarantee that consensus-based choices are superior to the decisions made by professional administrators with appropriate prior experience and specific knowledge that applies to a particular situation.

One of the interesting things about the operation of an organization is that one's perspective changes drastically once one assumes the role of CEO. There may be many reasons for it. First, being a CEO is like being both the composer and the conductor of a symphony. The CEO must know where the organization should be headed and gather all the resources to generate the orchestrated music. CEO must make sure that the entire organization is moving in the direction to achieve its mission, which requires knowing the overall make-up of the organization and placing the right person in the right job. CEOs may not be the best violinist of the symphony orchestra but must know what kinds of musical sound should come out of the violin section of the symphony. The CEO has to identify and assign the best person for the critical position of the company. However, when a wrong person has the power of the CEO, he/she can run the company into the ground. There are well-known cases providing examples of how a CEO has ruined a great company because of the inept top management.

16.4   Design and Decision-Making in an Organization

Like other designs, once an organization is designed and finalized, the organization must perform as intended to achieve the FRs of the organization. To achieve this organizational goal, people at all levels of the organization must strive to make the right decisions consistent with the overall organizational goals. However, it is impossible to guarantee that everyone in the organization would make the right decisions. Therefore, one of the challenges in designing and implementing organization goals is how to ensure that people in the organization make the right decisions.

Thus, the critical question is "How should decisions be made at all levels?" If the CEO has to make all the decisions within an organization, the organization cannot function and move forward. Everyone in the organization has to make decisions that belong to the person's organizational purview. Furthermore, every decision cannot be monitored by someone else because there is not sufficient bandwidth and resources to do so. At the same time, we must make sure that everyone in the decision-making chain of command makes the right decisions.

One criterion for sound decision-making by everyone in the organization is "Is this decision right for my organization?" In the case of the university: "Is this decision good for the university?" In the case of people in a company, "is this decision right for my company?" In the case of a citizen, the question to ask is "Is this decision good for our country?" The decisions made cannot be alike, but we know that everyone has done their best to make the right decision. Having asked this question, they can later evaluate the quality of their decision and attempt to make improvements if their decision was a misguided one.

Finally, everyone at all levels must ask this simple question. "Is the decision made good for my organization and humanity?"

16.5   Typical Organizational Design

Question 16.1:

Which industrial/commercial firm between Amazon and Walmart has a better business model and a stronger corporate structure?

The main point of this book is that systems, including organizations, must be designed based on FRs that were created based on the problem(s) the organization must solve. If an organization is designed based on DPs (rather than FRs), it may become a personality-cult based organization rather than a goal-oriented company. By choosing FRs first and then identifying the right DPs (e.g., the most qualified persons) who can satisfy the FRs best, the organization can achieve the goals of the organization. If DPs are chosen first, one may end up having to teach FRs to stubborn old-timers. Sometimes, the conventional wisdom states that it is difficult to teach new tricks to old dogs—"old" meaning in terms of attitude rather than physical. In this transformational process of defining FRs to solve a problem identified, and then selecting DPs, followed by resource allocation (i.e., PVs), may create an organization that is efficient in terms of making the right decisions and implementing them. For example, Walmart may not be able to become Amazon, whereas Amazon can easily compete with companies like Walmart, because to an outsider, it appears that Amazon is a very functional organization, whereas Walmart is a mix of FR-based and DP-based organizational structure.

Re-construction of the FRs of an existing business is challenging. It is most likely that the reconstructed FRs may not be what they had in mind. However, to an outsider, the highest FRs of Amazon appears to be the following:

FR1 = Sell to customers electronically without the physical display of merchandise;
FR2 = Quick delivery of goods;
FR3 = Guarantee return policy;
FR4 = Centralize warehousing of some goods;
FR5 = Centralize the financial and administrative operation using computers;
FR6 = Integrate merchandise-delivery services with manufacturers;
FR7 = Electronic display of merchandise;
FR8 = Contract with manufacturers for guaranteed return policy;
FR9 = Collect payment as soon as a customer orders the merchandise.

Assuming that these nine FRs are indeed the correct ones, what should be the corresponding DPs? This question is given as a homework problem #4 presented at the end of this chapter.

16.6   When Should an Organization Be Re-designed?

Changing any organization involving a large number of people is not a trivial task. Typically, the rationale for not changing, or resisting changes, at some leading departments and universities are "we must be doing well to be so highly ranked. Why change?" They often forget that their reputation was based on what they did in the past. However, organizations are like living beings that must do well in the future in a continuously changing environment. The FRs change because society and business continually evolve, requiring re-examination or transformation of missions, goals, internal policies, the organizational structure, allocation of resources, and make-up of the personnel.

Many different symptoms or indicators suggest the need for reorganization. When it is not addressing the problem(s) identified or when it does not have an organizational structure that can implement FRs, sometimes organizations may not be performing their intended functions or have low productivity. In some cases, the organizations are merely repeating its traditional role that worked well in the past, although the FRs had changed and are no longer valid because the society surrounding the university is no longer the same as when the policies were enacted.

Implementing a new organizational design to replace the one that has existed for many years or a few decades is not a trivial matter. Depending on the organization, one may create committees to study the proposed new organization to make sure that enough people buy in the new organizational structure. It is particularly difficult at universities where the faculty and students are significant stakeholders as the following example shows.

Design Story 16.7: Re-organizing the Departmental Structure at a Leading Research University

Most engineering schools have chemical engineering departments. In the U.S. they were established in the 1920s in response to the need for petrochemical engineers as the automotive industry expanded, requiring more petroleum for automobiles. Later as the nuclear power industry developed beginning in the 1950s, some of the chemical engineering departments merged with nuclear engineering. Later some universities made nuclear engineering as an independent department. The latest trend has been to transform the chemical engineering department into the bio-chemical engineering department. Now some schools made bio-engineering into a separate department. All these permutations of the chemical engineering department are somewhat meaningless unless the FRs are identified and stated.

At a leading university, there once was a department of food technology. The department had significant problems of not attracting undergraduate students to major in their discipline. Even their graduate program had a problem in enticing outstanding graduate students to their programs. People consume vast amounts of food, but the discipline of food technology was not the most challenging or attractive to prospective students. Finally, they changed their department name to "Department of Applied Biology." However, the mission of the department was ambiguous because the university had a separate department of biology. In other words, they could not state their FRs succinctly. Having had years of unsatisfactory performance of the department, the administration of the university decided to eliminate the Department of Applied Biology. Then, some of the faculty members of the universities start condemning the university administration, arguing that the administration took administrative action without due consultation with the faculty. The university delayed making this tough decision for several decades, probably because some of the administrators did not deal with the vocal group of faculty. Indeed the provost of the university who made the decision has been hounded for decades. When another university was considering him for the presidency of their university, his detractors campaigned to deny him the opportunity. Sometimes, administrators at universities do not make the decision they need to make, for this reason, leading to bloating administrative structure and the number of committees, increasing the cost of running a university. At many universities, the number of students and faculty has not changed, but their cost and administrators increased the significantly untenable situation.

Since they did not wish to dismiss tenured faculty, the university provided three different options: join the Department of Biology (if invited), or the Department of Chemical Engineering (if invited). Professors who were not welcomed by either biology or chemical engineering departments belonged to the Provost office and continue their research work without any teaching duties. This reorganization was a suitable arrangement because it strengthened both the biology department and the chemical engineering department. A few who could not join these two departments continued to research the umbrella of the Provost Office.

Under an ideal scenario, each academic department should transform itself periodically based on the changes that have occurred in their field or to respond to socio-economic changes that have occurred. It takes a leader who is willing to face fair criticisms and still do what is right. The design is the required first step in improving an organization, but the subsequent difficulties that accompany changes are an integral part of the transformation of institutions.

Design Story 16.8: Periodic Re-initialization of Organization at a Medium-Sized Producer of Consumer Goods

Starting from the previously outlined AD based complexity theory, a long-term study performed in a medium-sized industrial company investigated the effects of economic periodicity as a trigger for a regular organizational reset on the agility and performance of the corporate system.

The company was founded in the early 80 s and literally started in a garage. For almost two decades, the founder himself managed the entire value chain with only a few employees: from product design to procurement, materials management and production to sales and marketing. However, the person-centered approach of the company structure set a strong growth limit. Finally, due to growing market demand and the associated need to overcome organizational constraints, a new organization was designed and implemented in 2000 that allowed the company to take a major step forward in growth in just a few years. However, a market-driven explosion of product variants quickly pushed the organizational system to its limits. In the first 5-year interval, a gradual deterioration in organizational efficiency was observed, which finally led to quality problems and efficiency losses until 2005. The decision was made to carry out a further reorganization, this time with a focus on assembly, materials management, and product development. Assembly was restructured and a new hierarchical level of assembly team leaders was introduced. Purchasing was separated from Materials Management and the Materials Management position was assigned to a new young manager. In product development, a new profile of an innovation project manager was introduced. Continuous performance monitoring showed that the organization had again lost performance between 2006 and 2011. This time, the focus of the organizational changes had to be on sales and marketing. Due to further growth, the organization of the company was completely revised again in 2017. This time it was done to consider the development of a new strategy and its impact on management processes.

The long-term study showed that the company had "intuitively" established an organizational "rhythm" (i.e., periodicity) to overcome time-dependent complexity. In order to continue with the good experiences made in the past, now a regular 5-year reorganization rhythm was introduced in order to prevent future organizational performance losses.

The previous example in Design Story 16.8 shows that an organization needs to change periodically: a maximum performance can be achieved only if an organizational structure matches the rate of change in its environment. The organizational structure and the underlying design principles are, therefore, key factors for a company's successful and sustainable development within a turbulent environment.

The logic behind can be explained with the life cycle model of the Systems Engineering concept (Matt 2011), which roughly divides the life span of a distinct artificial system into design, realization, utilization, and disposal stages. For organizational design, this model might be adapted.

The first stage is the system's design initialization. It follows the general principles of AD: identify customer attributes, derive FRs, and finally assign suitable DPs so that the final result of the organizational design ideally satisfies the two design axioms. T_0 represents the start of the very first design of a completely new system. Within an ideally very short time frame (t_0-t_{01}), the system is set up for the first time, and the introduction of the new organization starts at t_1. However, as we know from experience, any organizational model "deteriorates" after a certain period due to internal (e.g., fluctuation of personnel, new strategy, new products) and/or external changes (e.g., market changes, environmental requirements, new competitors) and thus needs to be updated. It is necessary to find a viable way to make necessary adjustments to internal and external events on the one hand, but on the other hand not to have to re-design the organization with every single change event fundamentally. For this time-dependent need for change in an organizational model the AD-based complexity theory delivers a helpful approach. The complexity of any dynamic system is determined by the uncertainty in achieving the system's FRs and is caused by two factors: by a time-independent poor design that causes a system-inherent low efficiency (system design), and by a time-dependent reduction in system performance owing to system deterioration or to market or technology changes (system dynamics).

There are two types of time-dependent complexity: the so-called periodic complexity exists only in a finite time period, resulting from a limited number of probable combinations. These probable combinations may be partially predicted based on existing experiences with the system or with a very systematic research of possible failure sources. The second type of time-dependent complexity is called combinatorial complexity. It increases as a function of time proportionally to the time-dependent increasing number of possible combinations of the system's FRs. Leaving the pre-defined flexibility tolerance of a system design, it may lead to a chaotic state or even to a system failure. The critical issue with combinatorial complexity is that it is completely unpredictable.

To control combinatorial complexity, a functional periodicity must be introduced. First, a set of FRs that repeats cyclically must be identified. Among these, those FRs and their related DPs must be identified that may be the subject of a combinatorial process. To introduce functional periodicity, the selected set of FRs must be re-initialized at a defined (periodically turning) point in time t_2.

16.7 Institutional Development: The S-Curve, S-Gap, and Vector Delta (δ)[3]

Many organizations aspire to be one of the best in their fields. However, history shows that only a few surpass the leading organizations in terms of the institutional reputation, accomplishment, and development. Most stay where they are over many decades relative to other institutions in the same field. Sometimes, it appears that the leading organizations do not have to try very hard to remain as the leading institutions. There may be many different reasons for this comparative standing. First, human and financial resources tend to go to the leading institutions rather than to those that are in dire need. There may be many reasons for this situation. Is it possible to change this situation? It is the question every leader is striving to answer with varied conclusions. In this section, one way that has successfully transformed three major institutions is discussed.

The strategy for transforming an institution for the better was designed based on AD. It was implemented at three major institutions—a government agency and two top universities. These institutions were significantly improved through transformational changes, thanks to the re-design. The strategy used in these three institutions is outlined in this section. The central idea is encapsulated in the S-Curve, S-Gap, and Vector Delta (Δ).

If we define the "S-Factor" as the integrated total measure of the quality of a university, the development of the institution over as a function of time may be depicted as shown in Fig. 16.2. This figure assumes a linear upward change of both A and B, which would be the case when each institution works hard to improve productivity, quality of education, and increase its financial resources. These curves are a simplified depiction of the progress made, although the improvement of an institution may be highly non-linear.

The development of an institution appears to be similar to the change in the wealth of two individuals. As shown in Fig. 16.3, one with much more wealth than the other. T. Piketty, a French economist, demonstrated that the rate of capital return in developed countries is persistently higher than the rate of economic growth of poorer nations and that this will cause increasing wealth inequality in the future. Based on the historical data in France, he showed that wealth produces more wealth faster than the wealth that can be generated through productivity increases and hard work when the rate of return on capital is higher than the rate of economic growth over the long term. Consequently, rich people (or rich nations) tend to get richer faster because of the wealth that they already possess, i.e., wealth breeds more wealth than just harder work or more productivity increase. This finding is schematically shown in Fig. 16.3. Similar phenomena may be present in the development of research universities (Picketty 2014).

---

[3]Based on the paper: Nam P. Suh, Presented at the Univer-Cities conference, Newcastle, Australia, November 14, 2016

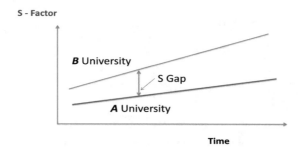

Divergence of University Development: the S-Curve

Fig. 16.2 The development of two universities is shown as a function of time. It shows that university B is developing faster than university A, but both universities are improving linearly as a function of time. The gap between these two universities is denoted as the S-Gap. This change of S-Factor may not be a realistic depiction of what happens

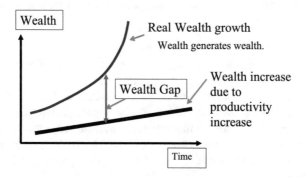

Fig. 16.3 The Picketty curve of wealth growth. The curve on the top shows that the wealthier person gets richer at a much faster rate than the person who tries to accumulate wealth by working harder

A similar phenomenon seems to occur with institutions such as universities. The leading universities in all of their chosen fields have a much higher probability of growing even stronger, because of the intellectual, human, and financial resources that they already have. If we designate the aggregation of all the elements that make a university strong, the "S-Factor," the growth may be depicted as shown in Fig. 16.4. The figure is a composite strength of a university, represented as the S-Factor, as a function of time. The top curve is for a stronger university, and the lower curve represents a less well-known university. The stronger university tends to attract better faculty, students, and significant financial gifts. Thus, the gap between the two, the "S-Gap," grows as a function of time. The S-Factor is a composite measure made of many elements that make a university great, such as the

Development of Universities
(Hypothesis on "Strength" of a university)

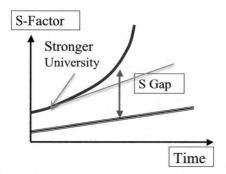

Fig. 16.4 The S-Factor of a university is a composite index of what constitutes the reputation of a university. The lower curve represents a university with a lower S-Factor, which develops more or less linearly with time through hard work, etc. The S-Gap between the wealthier institution with a higher reputation grows by a combination of linear growth and the compound rate due to the leading status. The S-Gap between these two universities continues to increase unless some drastic actions are taken

quality of faculty, students, and staff; the size of the endowment and financial resources; its current reputation; past academic and scholarly achievements; and prospects. Stronger universities with more "intellectual and financial assets" will grow faster than universities with a low S- factor. Therefore, the gap between them, the "S-Gap" shown in Fig. 16.4 will grow larger with time. For this reason, stronger universities attract more resources and people, which accelerate their growth.

The much faster growth (or advance) of the university with a higher S-Factor is due to many factors. The principle ones may be the following:

- more competitive students and faculty go to universities with better reputations and resources;
- resources (financial gifts, funds, etc.) tend to concentrate at richer universities or better known universities;
- faster growth of the S-Factor (e.g., outstanding faculty, students, facilities, reputation, etc.) at stronger universities may be due to the existing advantages;
- safety factor—for students and faculty members considering their choice of a university, joining a successful enterprise may be deemed safer;
- quality of life may be better at wealthier institutions;
- more opportunities may exist at a university with a higher S-Factor.

Universities that have a low S-Factor at a given instant in time (indicated by the lower curve) should not stay on their current trajectory if their long-term goal is to become one of the best universities in the world. They must transition to a higher

Fig. 16.5 For the university represented by the lower curve to be better than the university represented by the upper curve, it has to adopt non-linear changes indicated by vector δ

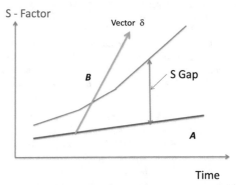

Ways of becoming one of the best universities: Leap frogging from *A* to *B*

Vector δ: Actions that may change the trajectory of a university.

trajectory as indicated by taking actions to go from the lower curve to the upper curve employing Vector δ as shown in Fig. 16.5, by adopting significant changes. The changes may take many different forms depending on specific institutional conditions. For example, the necessary actions may include the following: adding a large number of outstanding faculty members, attracting the most competitive students, generating significant financial resources, making major scientific discoveries, and innovating new technologies.

Case Studies at Two Different Universities

University A: This university, University A, had been rated as one of the top three universities in the United States for decades. Among the more than 20 (twenty) academic departments, this department had been rated to be the best in the country ever since various organizations ranked universities. Because the department was so far ahead of other similar departments in the United States, the department personnel, especially the professors, were very proud of their achievements. In some ways, they became complacent. However, young professors in the department were concerned about the stagnant nature of their department. It had not changed much during their days in the department as students and later as faculty members. They became restless.

When an opportunity came along to look for a new department head, they advocated the idea of finding who can take the department to new heights. They recommended one of the senior professors, who has transformed some other institutions as well as creating new research paradigms in the past, which had become a national model throughout the country. After thinking about two options he was presented with at the same time, he agreed to stay on, although compensation, etc., were less attractive than other offers. One big reason was that his family loved where they had been living for many years, and he loved the institution where he also attended as a student.

Among all its peer departments in the country and the world, the department was on a steeper slope, making other universities to catch up, similar to the wealth gap between the rich and poor. The well-known professors in the department were so satisfied and proud of their achievements, and they did not see any reason to change the department or their research and teaching activities. However, the new department head did not agree with their views on the future direction of their department.

The department had become the leading department of its kind in the world by excelling in more traditional engineering science and technology. The professors in the department were leading scholars in fields that were fundamental in developing the industrial base in the first half of the twentieth century. Because they were so good, they wanted to replicate what they had built by hiring their former students who were also good in the same disciplines. Most other leading departments of its kind in the world followed their footsteps in programmatic undertakings and their disciplinary research. This happy situation has persisted for decades. Yet young professors knew that the world outside was changing rapidly, passing their department by, although their senior professors could not be happier with the status quo.

The new department head decided to transform the department to be ready for the twenty-first century. One of the significant issues was the disciplinary mix of the faculty. Then, the existing faculty members were the best in classical disciplines that were important in the first half of the twentieth century. The best strategy was to bring in new faculty members who had backgrounds in fields that could change the direction of the academic field of the department. The department had been active in disciplines of classical physics, but now it needed to build expertise in the fields that would be important in the twenty-first century, such as communications, biology, optics, nanotechnology, quantum mechanics, and the like. The department started hiring new professors whose doctoral degrees were outside of the traditional disciplines of the department. These changes constituted the big delta shown in Fig. 16.5.

These significant changes in the direction of the department did not sit well with the famous senior professors of the department. They said "we must have done something right to create this department of international repute. Why change?" They try to disrupt the new direction of the department by forcing the department head to step down. But the department head prevailed. Now two decades of the transformation, the department has become a model for other departments of the same university as well as departments at other universities.

***University B:** Another well-known university hired a new president because the internal candidates chosen from their current faculty have not satisfied the expectation of the public. The taxpayers had supported this university by granting them special privileges and generous financial support since its founding about 40 years ago. Right after its establishment, the university had developed rapidly. However, its development soon reached a plateau, because privileges given to the university by taxpayers had the opposite consequences. The faculty members were researching familiar topics they been doing research in for the sake of publishing more papers. The life was too comfortable to search for challenging issues, with full funding of their graduate students and selection of highly qualified undergraduate students under special provisions given to the university by the government as a means of generating human resources with advanced education.*

Because of the several privileges given to this unique institution, it gradually lost its competitiveness. The professors had repeated similar research over and over to publish more papers that were used as a metric for academic achievements, and teaching was neglected. They hired faculty members they were comfortable with rather than searching for the best. All of this nurtured the seniority-based culture rather than merit-based competitive culture. They were also content with the budget the government provided yearly with inflation-adjusted increases. No attempt was made to undertake innovative research as an institution.

This university needed the vector δ to become a leading research university by coming out of the comfortable nest they had built for themselves. The new president of the university had to institute several significant changes, which were opposed by the senior faculty. He recruited and hired new faculty members in massive numbers purely based on their intellectual and scholarly quality. The specific expertise and contributions of their research were given the highest priority in selecting new faculty members rather than their field of study. He abolished the headcounts for each department; a merit-based system replaced the seniority-based system for compensation and promotion; and innovative research was emphasized by eliminating the policy that emphasized the number of papers published, etc. New faculty members were hired to double the faculty size by raising external financial support. New faculty members were given two years of research support to allow them to explore new research topics rather than merely continuing what they had done before. Facilities and equipment were modernized and expanded by building new physical buildings. In short order, the global ranking of this university. At one point, this university was recognized as the most improved university in the world.

16.8   Concluding Remarks

Organizations constitute basic units of society, a nation, and a group of nations. They are designed to achieve specific goals and missions. Unlike other design tasks, organizational design often deals with or affects the immediate well-being of people or organizations or nations and, ultimately, the world. Therefore, it must be dealt with thoughtfully and carefully. Many societal and organizational problems are caused by and the people in and around them. Consequently, we must design organizations right, following a rational and wise implementation of the goals of the organization.

The design of organizations must be done rationally by identifying the problem that must be solved through the creation of a viable set of FRs that are consistent with the goals. The designers should go through the design process objectively and rationally to come up with the best sets of DPs and PVs. DPs are typical organizational entities (such as universities, divisions of a company, government agencies), and PVs are human and financial resources needed to enable DPs to fulfill the FRs.

Some designers, engineers, and technologists are less interested in non-technical societal issues. However, it should not be the case. Ultimately, most engineers and technologists function in organizational settings, and as they assume more responsibility in their organization, people and organizational issues become increasingly more important. They must face the people-related problems to be good technologists as well as outstanding leaders. Everyone ultimately influences the decisions being made by various groups in companies, universities, and governments. More often than commonly acknowledged, engineers and scientists neglect personal and humane aspects of organizational life at their peril.

Organizations perform certain functions relevant to their fields of specialization. Almost all organizations are subject to functional periodicity, which requires re-initialization from time to time to make them viable in fulfilling their missions.

This re-initialization is hard to do in organizations because organizations are made up of people since, invariably, some of them would oppose any changes. The most challenging organizations to change are the organizations that provide guarantees to those in the organizations, because changes may disturb a set comfortable life of those in the organization. However, periodic re-initialization will benefit everyone associated with organizations.

Problems

1. Is a matrix organization better than a straight hierarchical organization? From the AD point of view, is this matrix organization better than a vertical line organization, which is responsible for certain products, including design, development, and manufacture? How would you design the organization if you were the VP in charge of the R&D group? Is the matrix organization a coupled design?

2. A major automotive company just appointed a new VP for research and development. He received his Master of Business Administration (MBA) from one of the leading business schools. Before enrolling for his MBA, he worked as an engineer in another large corporation after receiving his bachelor's degree in engineering. As the first order of business, he decided to re-organize his R&D group, which consisted of 450 people in a matrix structure. The vertical line of the matrix organization was to be the line organization that consisted of several divisions headed by a Project Director (PD). The horizontal line of the organization was for professional expertise led by an Engineering Director (ED), i.e., ED for hydraulics, air-conditioning, materials, etc., who oversees the continuing development and advancement in these fields. The Project Director could draw in experts from various engineering groups as needed with the concurrence of the EDs. Engineers would typically be in the group headed by an ED, but the PD may hire them for a specific project. In this type of matrix organization, people with similar skills are pooled for work assignments, reporting to two bosses, i.e., the vertical line PD and the horizontal ED. Is this matrix organization a coupled design? How would you make this organization function as an uncoupled or decoupled system?

3. Is the design of the university presented in the main text (i.e., Design Story 16.7: Re-organizing the Departmental Structure at a Leading Research University) an uncoupled or decoupled design? Construct a design matrix for the department strategic plan.

4. The following nine FRs were presented as a possible set of FRs that Amazon might be satisfying:

   FR1 = Sell to customers electronically without the physical display of merchandise;
   FR2 = Quick delivery of goods;
   FR3 = Guarantee return policy;
   FR4 = Centralize warehousing of some goods;
   FR5 = Centralize the financial and administrative operation using computers;

FR6 = Integrate merchandise-delivery operations with manufacturers;
FR7 = Electronic display of merchandise;
FR8 = Contract with manufacturers for guaranteed return policy;
FR9 = Collect payment as soon as a customer orders the merchandise.

Develop nine DPs for these FRs that will satisfy the Independence Axiom. Construct the design matrix for your design. Then, for your design, establish the design range and the system range for your design. Show how the information content can be minimized.

5. Managing a hospital is a complicated task with so many patients with a variety of illnesses and managing outpatients as well as those admitted to hospital for extended in-house care. It has to manage its finances to be sure that it can sustain its operations without having to incur financial losses. Suppose that you are just appointed as the president of a mid-size general hospital with 300 beds and daily visits to the outpatient flow of 500 patients. What would be the FRs that you have to consider and design a management system for the hospital?

6. One of the leading engineering departments of the world has many giants (i.e., well-known professors) who have contributed to the development of twentieth-century technology. Consequently, the department has enjoyed a stellar reputation worldwide because of these leading scholars. They continued to hire their former students and new professors from other universities, who have done similar work. The problem faced by the new department head is that these well-known professors want to continue to expand their kind of research that was important some 30–50 years ago. However, the world is moving into new technologies based on telecommunications, digital technologies, biotechnologies, quantum computing, and quantum computers. Help the new department head in choosing a new set of FRs. How would you overcome the resistance of the influential professors in the department?

Reference

Piketty T (2014) Capital in the twenty-first century. Belknap Press of Harvard University Press, Cambridge, Massachusetts, USA, translated by Arthur Goldhammer from French

Further Reading

Belanger DO (1997) Enabling American innovation: engineering and the National Science Foundation (History of Technology). Purdue University Press

Matt DT (2007) Reducing the structural complexity of growing organizational systems by means of axiomatic designed networks of core competence cells. J Manuf Syst 26(3–4):178–187

Matt DT (2011) Application of axiomatic design principles to control complexity dynamics in a mixed-model assembly system: a case analysis. Int J Prod Res 50(7):1850–1861

Suh NP (1990) The principles of design. Oxford University Press

Suh NP (2001) Axiomatic design—advances and applications. Oxford University Press

Suh NP (2005) Complexity. Oxford University Press

Suh NP (2016) On strategy for developing an innovative university: S-factor, s-gap, and vector delta. In: Univer-Cities Conference, University of New Castle, Australia. https://www.newcastle.edu.au/community-and-alumni/-alumni-archived/univer-cities-conference-2016/program, session 3: strategic and evolving implications of the single key node Eco-system of globalizing Universities

Züst R, Schregenberger JW (2003) System Engineering: A Methodology for Designing Sustainable Solutions in the Field of Engineering and Management. Verlag Eco Performance, Zurich. https://www.swissinstitute.ch/publikationen/buecherjournal.html, distributed by Swiss Institute for Systems Engineering

Application of Axiomatic Design for the Design of Flexible and Agile Manufacturing Systems

17

Dominik T. Matt and Erwin Rauch

Abstract

In the previous chapters, we learned the basics of Axiomatic Design (AD) as Design theory. We learned that users very often express their wishes as customer needs (CNs). These wishes must then be examined by the designer in order to define functional requirements (FRs). Based on the FRs and the two axioms in AD, design solutions are finally derived, so-called Design Parameters (DPs).

AD can be applied in many different areas such as product development, healthcare, software development but also manufacturing system design. Manufacturing systems are complex entities which can be broken down into their functional elements or requirements by the application of AD and for which suitable DPs can be found.

AD has been used for many years for the design of manufacturing systems. The chapter also shows that the number of uses of AD in manufacturing has increased continuously. While in the past, there were many topics related to specific manufacturing processes and systems as well as lean manufacturing, the focus has changed somewhat in recent decades. Today AD is often used in manufacturing to derive design characteristics for the intelligent and sustainable manufacturing of tomorrow.

In this chapter, several case studies from the field of production management and manufacturing system design are shown. By means of these practical case studies, the students will understand in which cases AD can be applied in industrial practice.

D. T. Matt (✉) · E. Rauch
Faculty of Science and Technology, Free University of Bozen-Bolzano, Universotätsplatz 1, Bolzano, Italy
e-mail: dominik.matt@unibz.it

D. T. Matt
Fraunhofer Research Italia s.c.a.r.l., Via A.-Volta 13a, 39100 Bolzano, Italy

© Springer Nature Switzerland AG 2021
N. P. Suh et al. (eds.), *Design Engineering and Science*,
https://doi.org/10.1007/978-3-030-49232-8_17

The first case study deals with the derivation of design guidelines for flexible as well as changeable manufacturing systems. The second case study describes the digitization in shopfloor management by developing a tool for a systematic acquisition, analysis, and evaluation of production data. In the third case study, AD is used to design an assembly station in which robots and humans work together and collaborate safely. The fourth case study shows how AD can also be used to derive design guidelines for Industry 4.0 learning factories. Finally, the fifth and final case study deals with the re-design of a demonstrator for cyber-physical production systems.

At the end of all case studies there are short exercises, which students should work on. The exercises encourage students to reflect on what they have learnt, to think on it independently and to apply AD in practical case studies.

17.1 Introduction

Axiomatic Design (AD) is applied not only in mechanical engineering, but also in many other applications. Through the systematic approach and the consideration of Independence Axiom and Information Axiom, even highly complex projects can be mastered reducing the complexity in the design task. In addition to product design, system design, software design and many other fields, AD is, therefore, also used in the design of manufacturing systems.

The design of manufacturing systems has a major influence on the sustainability of manufacturing companies. On the one hand, an efficiently designed manufacturing system generates a higher profit for the company, which in terms of economic sustainability contributes to securing the existence and growth of a company and thus also to the prosperity of its employees. With regard to ecological sustainability, the reduction of energy consumption or the reduction of emissions during production can make a contribution to the preservation of our environment and our earth. Last but not least, a manufacturing system should also focus on the employee, and therefore contribute to social sustainability. This is reflected in the design of the work systems and in the organization of the working environment.

Manufacturing systems can also be subdivided fundamentally into three different design areas: (1) system, (2) organization, and (3) people. A functioning manufacturing system can only be achieved through a symbiotic design of all these three areas. Machines must be correctly selected and arranged and an organizational set of rules must ensure that people work in a structured manner in this production environment.

Engineers in the industrial sector have been working on the design of manufacturing systems for many decades. While in the past 20 to 30 years mainly organizational innovations with the concept of Lean Management have been introduced, the trend today, with the introduction of Industry 4.0 and Internet of Things, rather goes in the direction of technological innovations. This inevitably leads to the fact that the design of manufacturing systems has become a very complex task. Designers of manufacturing systems should, therefore, make use of methods and instruments to design manufacturing systems as efficiently as possible. AD is one such tool that allows manufacturing system designers to solve problems in a structured way, break them down into their functions and derive the right solutions and implementation measures.

Therefore, this chapter first gives an overview of the extent to which AD has been applied in manufacturing system design to date. In the following sections, various case studies are presented on how AD has been applied in practice.

Design Story 17.1: Changing Needs in the Design of Manufacturing Systems

A young graduate engineer started his career in a production company as a project manager in the department of process optimization. He was very much looking forward to his new job in a large company and was already excited about his area of responsibility. One of the first projects he was working on was the planning and design of a new production line for a new product line.

Although the task was very exciting, it was also very challenging. He knew neither the current processes nor the previous products, which made it difficult for him to get into the subject. He, therefore, tried to learn from proven methods and first looked at the old production facilities. They produced standardized product components for the automotive industry in large quantities. The young graduate thus began to use an old plan of a production line as a basis and adapted it to the new product line. The head of the department observed him in his work and let him work out an initial concept. The young engineer proudly presented his concept draft to the round and showed the advantages resulting from the application of best-practice design guidelines of the old production lines. At a certain point, the head of the department stopped the young engineer and asked him if he had considered what requirements the new product line would have in comparison to the previous products? The young engineer was not prepared to answer the question and was only able to make inadequate explanations. The manager replied that his approach would be very good in itself, but that the new product line contains a large number of variants that would continue to increase over the next few years. In addition, the product life cycle of the new product would probably be much shorter than that of the old products. The production system would, therefore, have to be much more flexible and changeable than the previous rigid mono-product lines.

So, the young engineer was tempted to reapply what had been tried and tested without pursuing new and creative approaches, even though he did not have the "operational blindness" that many long-standing engineers have. Besides, he has not dealt enough with the special needs arising from the new product design and the resulting FRs for the manufacturing system. The young engineer learned this and revised his concept, developing a much more flexible and adaptable design for the production line, which helped the company to save much money for otherwise necessary investments in dedicated machinery for new variants.

The story of the young engineer was told to emphasize the importance of initiating a design with a clear and unbiased view keeping the focus on the needs and FRs and using this information then for deriving the right design solutions for the design of the manufacturing system.

17.2 Use of Axiomatic Design in Manufacturing System Design

AD is a systematic approach for design by the top-down decomposition of "What we want to achieve," to "How we can satisfy the requirements." The theory of AD is applicable to many different kinds of complex systems. A manufacturing system can be defined as a dynamic and complex system, because it is subject to temporal variation and must be reconfigurable and adaptable. In such cases AD shows a suitable and helpful method to reduce complexity in the manufacturing systems design (Matt and Rauch 2011). As learned in the previous chapters, AD is based on four domains to transform the so-called customer needs or customer attributes (CA) into FRs, DPs, and process variables (PVs) (Suh 2001).

Through its top-down approach, AD is a very systematic and structured design methodology. Starting from a main goal, a hierarchically structured catalog of FRs with proposed design solutions is developed. By breaking down (decomposition) of the top goals and design proposals specific DPs can be identified at a lower operational level. This is helpful for manufacturing system designers, which start very often with an overall objective and need to develop the manufacturing system accordingly in all its details on an operational Shopfloor level.

The number of studies using AD principles is gradually increasing as AD's superiorities create important advantages for decision-makers in solving multi-criteria decision-making problems (Kulak et al. 2010). Investigating the scientific literature regarding works on AD in manufacturing using the keywords "Axiomatic Design" and "manufacturing system" there can be identified a trend toward an increasing use of AD in manufacturing. In the following a brief overview is given to summarize the most important use of AD in manufacturing system design over the last 20 years and to give students the opportunity to deepen their knowledge by looking up relevant literature:

> Cochran developed an approach for the design of manufacturing systems, which is based on the principles of AD (Cochran et al. 2001). Cochran's methodology "Manufacturing System Design De-composition" (MSDD) visualizes the derivative FR–DP tree in a very clear manner and is easy to understand. AlGeddawy and ElMaraghy (2009) describe AD as a very suitable and frequently used method to derive the target system as well as the requirements and evaluate the interactions of the identified requirements in a systematic way. Bergmann applies the MSDD-methodology and thus the AD approach for the derivation of requirements for a sustainability-oriented holistic manufacturing system (Bergmann 2010). The work of Bergman proves once again, that the application of the AD methodology is suitable for a systematic and structured derivation of requirements and DPs. Authors like Vinodh and Aravindraj (2012) apply AD for the development of lean manufacturing systems. Durmusoglu and Satoglu (2010), Matt et al. (2016) and Rauch et al. (2019b) use AD for the development of design guidelines to make manufacturing systems more flexible and agile. Cochran et al. (2016) extended later his Manufacturing System Design Decomposition approach to implement manufacturing systems that are sustainable. Puik et al. (2017) developed an assessment of reconfiguration schemes for reconfigurable manufacturing systems based on resources and lead time. The trend toward Industry 4.0 and Internet of Things had also an effect on AD. Farid (2017) used AD to design intelligent manufacturing systems and Cochran et al. (2017) to model human–

machine interaction in manufacturing cells. Also Delaram and Fatahi Valilai (2018) used AD to develop an architecture for an intelligent use of computer-integrated manufacturing in modern production systems.

In most of this research works the Independence Axiom is mainly applied and discussed by application of the decomposition of FRs and DPs. Contrary to this there are not so many research works dealing and investigating the Information Axiom in manufacturing systems design. This could encourage practitioners and scientists to discuss in the future also the quality of alternative solutions by the use of the Information Axiom. At the domain level, the decomposition between FR and DP are treated in most of the works. The discussion about CAs and PVs played up to now only a subordinate role. Due to the fact that CAs are important to define the right first-level FRs and DPs they should be considered more in future works. In the literature, AD is mainly used as a method for practical applications and case studies of manufacturing system design. The analysis of previous and actual specific topics of AD applications shows further, that it is increasingly used also for new challenges in manufacturing like sustainability in manufacturing, smart and cloud manufacturing or agile/changeable manufacturing systems (Rauch et al. 2016).

In the following, 5 case studies show how AD can be applied in different design tasks in manufacturing.

17.3 Case Study 1: Design of Flexible and Changeable Manufacturing Systems

In the first case study (see also Holzner, 2015), we want to design a flexible and changeable manufacturing system for a small industrial manufacturer. The firm in our case study is a small-sized company in the North of Italy with 25 persons employed, which started in 1995 as a small crafts enterprise processing solid surface material for bathroom furnishings, kitchens, and modern interior design. Over time, the firm focused its activity on the production of exclusive bathroom furnishings in solid surfaces. The company produces different types of furnishings for bathrooms: (a) washbasins, (b) shower trays, and c) bathtubs. The production of bathtubs is a highly specialized production process, while the production of shower trays and washbasins—even if they are entirely different products—need similar manufacturing and assembly steps. Today shower trays and washbasins are produced on different assembly workstations and go from milling/gluing to a next workstation for grinding. The aim of the application of AD in this case study was to develop a new concept for a more flexible and changeable manufacturing and assembly system for different types and dimensions of shower trays and washbasins.

The main difference between flexibility and changeability is that flexibility in manufacturing only permits a system change in a specific corridor. Changeability, however, describes the responsiveness over the existing flexibility corridor and usually requires a longer time for reaction (Zäh et al. 2005). In this sense, flexibility describes the ability of production to change a manufacturing system very quickly, with little effort, and therefore with low costs. By flexibility, it is possible, within a defined flexibility corridor, to adjust the manufacturing system. Further flexible manufacturing systems allow the adaptation of the manufacturing systems for the production also of new products, but only if those are very similar and of the same product family. We distinguish in literature different types of flexibility:

1. Variant flexibility: Ability of manufacturing / assembling multiple versions of a product.
2. Volume flexibility: Ability of adaptation of production systems to fluctuating sales volumes.
3. Internal flexibility: Ability to change the system without modifications (example change of internal numerical code program).
4. Staff flexibility: Ability to work with a variable number of employees and different worker skills.

Changeability, however, is the ability to switch from one product family to another and making the appropriate changes in the production capacity of a company or manufacturing system. A change can have a significant impact on the production and logistics systems. It also impacts on the equipment structure as well as on the organizational or operational structure. Such a change requires a longer lead time for planning and takes place relatively quickly. Wiendahl et al. (2007) define changeability as characteristics to accomplish early and foresighted adjustments of the factory's structures and processes on all levels to change impulses economically. To reach changeability in companies and manufacturing systems, five enablers (see Fig. 17.1) can be found in the literature.

Especially for small- and medium-sized enterprises (SMEs), costs and flexibility in a production system are very important issues because the products are generally produced in small batches. In addition to a high percentage of manual production, these kinds of enterprises use mainly universal machines to guarantee certain flexibility. SMEs that have a high degree of automation and manufacture in large batches have to address their production more flexible and changeable to react quickly to market changes and consumers' preferences. SMEs with a robust and highly flexible manufacturing system have usually a greater market share, a better financial condition, and a better sustainable technology.

As learned in the previous chapters, the AD-based approach starts with the identification of customer needs. In our case study, the company was asked about future challenges and changes in their business environment. Principal CAs for the future manufacturing system were defined as follows:

CA1 = Handle an increased variety of individual products (*Increasing variety and Individualization*);
CA2 = Being competitive in price and costs (*price competition in the market*);
CA3 = Handle increasing quality requirements (*increasing quality requirements*);
CA4 = Deliver products in shortest time (*increasing demand on delivery*).

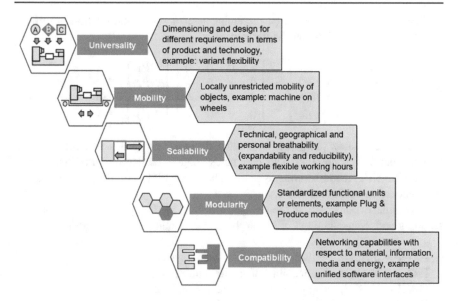

Fig. 17.1 Enablers of changeability in manufacturing systems. (Reproduced with permission from (Spena et al. 2016) (Reprinted from Procedia CIRP, 41, Pasquale Russo Spena, Philipp Holzner, Erwin Rauch, Renato Vidoni, Dominik T. Matt, "Requirements for the Design of Flexibleand Changeable Manufacturing and Assembly Systems: A SME-survey", 207–212, Copyright (2016), with permission from Elsevier.). Figure based on (Wiendahl et al. 2007) (Reprinted from CIRP Annals — Manufacturing Technology, 56, H.-P. Wien-dahl, H.A. ElMaraghy, P. Nyhuis, M.F. Zäh, H.-H. Wiendahl, N. Duffie, and M.Brieke, "Changeable manufacturing-classification, design and operation", 783–809, Copyright (2007), with permission from Elsevier).)

In the next step, these CAs were translated into FRs and DPs for manufacturing system design. The identified CAs were translated into further first-level FRs showing the technical and practical requests for manufacturing system design.

FR1 = Increase flexibility and changeability;
FR2 = Produce at lowest costs;
FR3 = Improve quality;
FR4 = Reduce lead time.

Corresponding DPs to meet these FRs were defined as follows:

DP1 = Flexible and changeable manufacturing/assembly system;
DP2 = Low-cost manufacturing systems;
DP3 = Zero defects and TQM in production;
DP4 = Pull principle and "0" WIP.

The design matrix on the first hierarchical level shows the relationship of the identified solutions (DPs) on the derived FRs:

$$
\begin{Bmatrix} FR1 \\ FR2 \\ FR3 \\ FR4 \end{Bmatrix} = \begin{bmatrix} X & 0 & 0 & 0 \\ 0 & X & 0 & 0 \\ 0 & 0 & X & 0 \\ 0 & 0 & 0 & X \end{bmatrix} \begin{Bmatrix} DP1 \\ DP2 \\ DP3 \\ DP4 \end{Bmatrix} \tag{17.1}
$$

The design matrix shows an uncoupled design. This means that FRs are distinguishable from each other. This case study focuses on the design of flexible and changeable SME manufacturing systems. Therefore, FR1 and DP1 are now further decomposed in additional AD levels.

Then, the decomposition process on the next hierarchy level continues with mapping and "Zig-Zagging". FR1 can be deduced into further two general FRs:

FR1.1 = Increase flexibility of manufacturing system;
FR1.2 = Increase changeability of manufacturing system;
DP1.1 = Flexible manufacturing systems guidelines;
DP1.2 = Changeable manufacturing systems guidelines.

The design matrix shows a decoupled matrix. Changeable manufacturing systems are usually flexible at the same time, while a flexible manufacturing system does not have to be changeable.

$$
\begin{Bmatrix} FR1.1 \\ FR1.2 \end{Bmatrix} = \begin{bmatrix} X & X \\ 0 & X \end{bmatrix} \begin{Bmatrix} DP1.1 \\ DP1.2 \end{Bmatrix} \tag{17.2}
$$

DP1.1 and DP1.2 are very general and abstract design solutions. Therefore, they need to be further decomposed in a next level to break down DP1.1 and DP1.2 into more tangible proposals for solutions according to the different types of flexibility in production:

FR1.1.1 = Produce different variants;
FR1.1.2 = Employ worker on different workstations;
FR1.1.3 = Increase or reduce quantity based on demand;
FR1.1.4 = Minimize time for changeover between different variants;
DP1.1.1 = Fixation positions for shower tray variants *(variant flexibility)*;
DP1.1.2 = Qualified personnel who know all variants and can work at flexible times *(staff flexibility)*;
DP1.1.3 = (De)Activation of assembly tables depending on demand *(volume flexibility)*;
DP1.1.4 = Memorized fixation positions changing with barcode scanning *(internal flexibility)*.

The revised design matrix of FR–DP shows a decoupled matrix.

$$\begin{Bmatrix} FR1.1.1 \\ FR1.1.2 \\ FR1.1.3 \\ FR1.1.4 \end{Bmatrix} = \begin{bmatrix} X & 0 & 0 & 0 \\ 0 & X & 0 & 0 \\ 0 & 0 & X & 0 \\ X & X & 0 & X \end{bmatrix} \begin{Bmatrix} DP1.1.5 \\ DP1.1.2 \\ DP1.1.3 \\ DP1.1.4 \end{Bmatrix} \tag{17.3}$$

After the decomposition of FR1.1 also FR1.2 needs to be further decomposed:

FR1.2.1 = Produce different products and product families;
FR1.2.2 = Extend the manufacturing system stepwise;
FR1.2.3 = Provide modular functional plug and produce units for working;
FR1.2.4 = Move machinery easily when changing product;
FR1.2.5 = Standardize connection of the manufacturing system;
DP1.2.1 = Universal assembly tables for shower trays and washbasins
            (*universality*);
DP1.2.2 = Scalable manufacturing layout (*scalability*);
DP1.2.3 = Selection of necessary tools on the table (*modularity*);
DP1.2.4 = Mobile arrangement of tools (mobility);
DP1.2.5 = Quick-connector for vacuum and power supply for quick start-up
            (*compatibility*).

$$\begin{Bmatrix} FR1.2.1 \\ FR1.2.2 \\ FR1.2.3 \\ FR1.2.4 \\ FR1.2.5 \end{Bmatrix} = \begin{bmatrix} X & 0 & 0 & 0 & 0 \\ X & X & 0 & 0 & 0 \\ X & 0 & X & X & X \\ 0 & 0 & X & X & X \\ 0 & 0 & X & X & X \end{bmatrix} \begin{Bmatrix} DP1.2.1 \\ DP1.2.2 \\ DP1.2.3 \\ DP1.2.4 \\ DP1.2.5 \end{Bmatrix} \tag{17.4}$$

Figure 17.2 illustrates the result of the conceptual design, based on the AD decomposition. The figure shows a proposal for a new universal assembly table. Instead of a process-oriented assembly it was developed as an object-oriented assembly bringing together the processes and technologies for gluing the different components, for milling and for surface finishing by grinding. The system allows a flexible positioning and fixation of different products (shower trays and washbasins) —therefore every assembly table is able to produce variants from both product families.

Exercise 17.1: Development of a Smart Assembly System for the Case Study Company

You are engaged by the case study company to develop a more intelligent assembly system as the one shown in Fig. 17.2. For this, you should use the concepts of Industry 4.0 and Internet of Things. Main objective of the re-design is to increase reactivity of the assembly system when a changeover to another product becomes necessary. What are your FRs? What are your corresponding DPs?

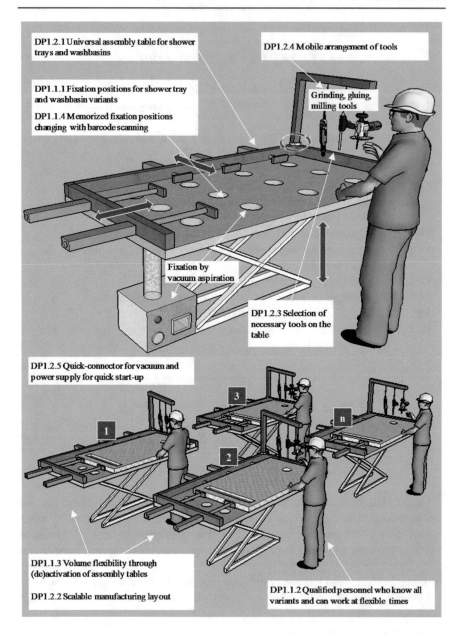

Fig. 17.2 Case study results—design of a universal assembly table. (Reproduced with permission from Holzner (2015) (Reprinted from Procedia CIRP, 34, Philipp Holzner, Erwin Rauch, PasqualeRusso Spena, and Dominik T. Matt, "Systematic Design of SME Manufacturingand Assembly Systems Based on Axiomatic Design", 81–86, Copyright (2015),with permission from Elsevier.).)

17.4 Case Study 2: Design of a Smart Shopfloor Management System

Traditional shopfloor management concepts are changing to new and digitally supported approaches for the coordination and management of production at the shop floor level. With Industry 4.0 and the Internet of Things production data will be provided in a completely new quality and with real-time information about production processes. This will be possible by the comprehensive equipping of production with sensors for data acquisition and the consistent integration of intelligent machines (so-called cyber-physical systems) and products. The future representation of the data models in real time makes production transparent and thus easier to control. In the future, such a production control system can also cope with short-term changes in demand and capacity utilization. The digitization and collection of production data promises also a better use of the data for shopfloor management to increase efficiency and sustainability. In this second case study, we report about the design of digital ad smart shopfloor management systems (see also Rauch et al. 2018).

In traditional lean management, shopfloor management has often taken place in the so-called lean war room (Japanese obeya) with the support of analog visualization and communication tools. The digitization of shopfloor management requires the introduction of specific software systems for production monitoring and management. Such mobile- and web-based software applications are suitable instruments for combining human decision capacities, methods, relevant production data, and innovative technologies in a smart shopfloor management.

The software company Solunio GmbH recognized the trend of the time and dealt relatively early with the development of a software to collect data from the production, to structure this data and to visualize it as relevant information for managers, shift leaders, and workers in production. Based on existing expertise in industrial companies the company developed the commercial software "Visual Shop Floor" for smart shopfloor management with three layers (see Fig. 17.3).

At layer 1 (*Data Collection*), data are collected by connecting the application with various systems and equipment in the company. Such systems can be the internal ERP (enterprise resource planning), a MES (manufacturing execution system) or MDA/PDA (machine or production data acquisition), as well as specific systems such as CRM (customer relationship management), APS (advanced planning system), QMS (quality management system), or intelligent sensors installed on machines.

At layer 2 (*Data Management*), all data collected is then aggregated and structured by filtering relevant data and transferring it into structured data models. The initially large data flood ("Big Data") is thus transformed into smart and relevant data ("smart data"). The data are then grouped into (i) order data, (ii) machine data, and (iii) worker data.

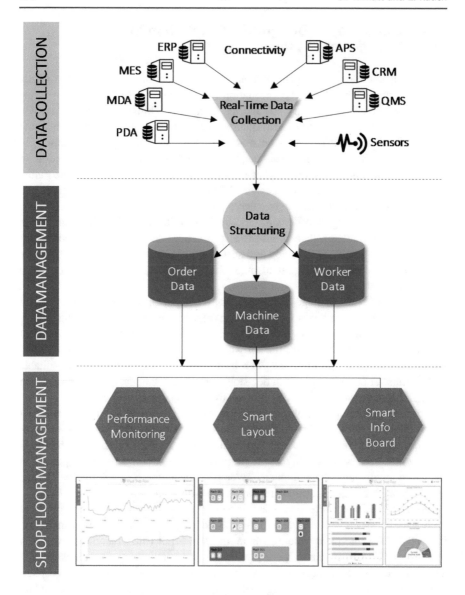

Fig. 17.3 Existing functionalities of the commercial software Visual Shop Floor. (Reproduced with permission from Solunio GmbH)

Layer 3 (*Shopfloor Management*) uses the data for shopfloor management by means of various functions. The "Performance Monitoring" module makes it possible to display key performance indicators (KPIs) or statistics in real time avoiding complex updating of reports. The "Smart Info Board" module enables general information to be displayed to all or specific monitors in production at the touch of a button, eliminating the need for time-consuming manual update of paper. The "Smart Layout" module enables the user to visualize the current situation in production by means of a dynamic graphical layout representation. If the user zooms in or out, more details such as machine status or job data appear.

However, the company, which is mainly run by software developers and not production experts, found it difficult to understand the comprehensive needs of the users for developing a new release of the software with additional functionalities/modules. In order to analyze the FRs in a systematic way and to define appropriate modules in the software, the company decided to use AD together with experts. As a first step, several workshops were held with production managers and staff to better understand the customer needs (see Fig. 17.4).

The highest level of FRs and DPs can be expressed as follows:

FR0   Manage the production shopfloor in a smart way.
DP0   Smart shopfloor management software.

DATA COLLECTION	DATA ANALYSIS	DATA ACCESS
• real time data • machine data • inventory data • energy consumption • staff information • process information	• data analytics algorithms • event-based warning and early warning systems • automatic maintenance detection	• reduction of routes for information procurement • terminals for employees • access with mobile devices
MONITORING	VISUALIZATION	CONNECTIVITY
• cockpit per management level • production status • machine status • performance/efficiency • alarm in case of deviation	• work instructions, quality checklists, inspection plans, order data, tool data • paperless production	• standardized interfaces • uninterrupted data flow • consistency of data in different systems
EMPLOYEES	USER-FRIENDLINESS	DECISION MAKING
• acceptance of employees • allocation of jobs according to age and competence • new competencies in data management required	• intuitive user guidance • recognition of the role of the employee (e.g. shift manager, worker) • image and media support	• rapid decision making and transmission • localization of a necessary decision • prioritization of decisions

Fig. 17.4 Customer needs collected in workshops with production leaders and workers. (Reproduced from Rauch et al. (2018), originally published open access under a CC BY 4.0 license: https://doi.org/10.1051/matecconf/20182230101)

Based on the results of the initial workshops the following high-level FRs and related DPs were defined:

FR1 = Collect real time data of machines, processes, resources, and energy;
FR2 = Avoid inconsistency of data;
FR3 = Visualize needed and related data everywhere for individual roles in production without using paper;
FR4 = Monitoring of performance (input–output) in production;
FR5 = Allow individual and production related data analysis;
FR6 = Avoid problems and increase reactivity in decision-making if problems arise;
FR7 = Facilitate acceptance of employees;
DP1 = Data collection module with interfaces and smart sensors;
DP2 = Data structuring module;
DP3 = Digital visualization technologies;
DP4 = Monitoring tools;
DP5 = Tools for production data analysis;
DP6 = Problem prevention and problem-solving tools;
DP7 = Dedicated training of employees and tutorials.

The design matrix on the first level is decoupled and shows the dependencies between the solutions (DPs) and the FRs:

$$
\begin{Bmatrix} FR1 \\ FR2 \\ FR3 \\ FR4 \\ FR5 \\ FR6 \\ FR7 \end{Bmatrix} = \begin{bmatrix} X & O & O & O & O & O & O \\ O & X & O & O & O & O & O \\ O & O & X & O & O & O & O \\ O & O & O & X & O & O & O \\ O & O & O & O & X & O & O \\ O & O & O & X & X & X & O \\ O & O & X & X & X & X & X \end{bmatrix} \begin{Bmatrix} DP1 \\ DP2 \\ DP3 \\ DP4 \\ DP5 \\ DP6 \\ DP7 \end{Bmatrix} \qquad (17.5)
$$

DP1 (data collection) does not need a further decomposition as this module is already realized in the existing commercial software and works well for the planned software re-design. Same as above occurs also for DP2 (data structuring). The data structuring method has already been realized and is not part of the re-design.

DP3 (digital visualization technologies) is supporting to visualize specific contents to operators or other users in production. Mobile apps help to visualize data everywhere, while an own function is visualizing only data relevant for the own position (shift-leader, operator, etc.) while an Info Board contains general information. Problems are visualized graphically in the layout as problem map.

FR3.1 = Visualize data everywhere;
FR3.2 = Visualize relevant data for the own role;
FR3.3 = Visualize general information;
FR3.4 = Visualize problems transparently;

DP3.1 = Mobile App module;
DP3.2 = MyRole View module;
DP3.3 = Info Board module;
DP3.4 = Problem Map module.

The design matrix shows a decoupled design. The Mobile App module consists of an app containing a mobile version of the software. Thus, it has a dependency to other FRs. The Info Board module is also able to visualize problems transparently.

$$
\begin{Bmatrix} FR3.1 \\ FR3.2 \\ FR3.3 \\ FR3.4 \end{Bmatrix} = \begin{bmatrix} X & O & O & O \\ X & X & O & O \\ X & O & X & O \\ X & O & X & X \end{bmatrix} \begin{Bmatrix} DP3.1 \\ DP3.2 \\ DP3.3 \\ DP3.4 \end{Bmatrix}
\qquad (17.6)
$$

DP4 (monitoring tools) needs to be further decomposed. Production performance indicators are monitored in a performance monitoring function, while energy consumption is monitored in an energy cockpit. The smart layout function shows changes in the layout.

FR4.1 = Monitoring of production performance;
FR4.1 = Monitoring of energy performance;
FR4.1 = Monitoring of changes in the layout;
DP4.1 = Performance Monitoring;
DP4.2 = Energy Cockpit;
DP4.3 = Smart Layout.

The design matrix shows an uncoupled design:

$$
\begin{Bmatrix} FR4.1 \\ FR4.2 \\ FR4.3 \end{Bmatrix} = \begin{bmatrix} X & O & O \\ O & X & O \\ O & O & X \end{bmatrix} \begin{Bmatrix} DP4.1 \\ DP4.2 \\ DP4.3 \end{Bmatrix}
\qquad (17.7)
$$

Also DP5 (tools for production data analysis) needs a decomposition. The software should not only allow to see general monitoring dashboards but also to do more detailed data analysis using the data stored in the software. Thus, the software should provide a digital value stream mapping function in order to compare different situations and to identify potentials for optimization. Further individual data analytics should also be possible.

FR5.1 = Allow lean production data analysis;
FR5.2 = Enable individual data analysis;
DP5.1 = Digital Value Stream Map;
DP5.2 = Data Analytics.

The design matrix shows an uncoupled design:

$$\begin{Bmatrix} FR5.1 \\ FR5.2 \end{Bmatrix} = \begin{bmatrix} X & O \\ O & X \end{bmatrix} \begin{Bmatrix} DP5.1 \\ DP5.2 \end{Bmatrix} \tag{17.8}$$

DP6 (problem prevention and problem-solving tools) needs a further decomposition. Problems due to machine stops should be avoided in future through early warning systems or predictive maintenance. A digital problem issue tracking function should also reduce the duration of the procedure to solve a problem. The introduction of a location-based decision-making can further improve also the reactivity for problem-solving. This means that, e.g., the nearest shift-leader will be informed if the production system identifies a problem where a certain decision is needed.

FR6.1 = Prevent stops of production machines;
FR6.2 = Reduce duration of problem-solving;
FR6.3 = Increase reactivity in problem-solving;
DP6.1 = Predictive maintenance module;
DP6.2 = Issue tracking;
DP6.3 = Location-based decision.

The design matrix shows a decoupled design. Predictive maintenance as well as issue tracking increases the reactivity for problem-solving showed in the matrix by the dependencies of the DPs with the last FR.

$$\begin{Bmatrix} FR6.1 \\ FR6.2 \\ FR6.3 \end{Bmatrix} = \begin{bmatrix} X & O & O \\ O & X & O \\ X & X & X \end{bmatrix} \begin{Bmatrix} DP6.1 \\ DP6.2 \\ DP6.3 \end{Bmatrix} \tag{17.9}$$

Also DP7 (dedicated training of employees and tutorials) needs a decomposition. It is crucial for the implementation of such a shopfloor management system that all user are accepting the software. Thus the design foresees two further lower level FR–DP pairs.

FR7.1 = Support users if problems arise;
FR7.2 = Increase skills of users in data management;
DP7.1 = Online Tutorial;
DP7.2 = Dedicated trainings in the shopfloor management software.

The design matrix shows a decoupled design. There is a dependency as the regular use of online tutorials is also helping to train people working with the software.

$$\begin{Bmatrix} FR7.1 \\ FR7.2 \end{Bmatrix} = \begin{bmatrix} X & O \\ X & X \end{bmatrix} \begin{Bmatrix} DP7.1 \\ DP7.2 \end{Bmatrix} \tag{17.10}$$

Figure 17.5 shows the final concept and structure of modules/functionalities of the software. The module "Data Analytics" enables the user to create individual data analyses in an intuitive way without any specific knowledge, thus using existing data effectively and efficiently. The "Mobile App" module enables the user to access the software system from mobile devices. In order to keep distances short and reaction speed fast, the module "Location-based Decision" supports calling the closest decision authority to the place of the immediate decision. The "myRole View" module enables the user to switch between a standard view and a role-specific view in order to display only that information that is important and useful for their role (e.g., worker, shift-leader). The "Smart Layout" module enables the user to visualize the current situation in production by means of a dynamic graphical layout representation. If the user zooms in or out, more details such as machine status or job data appear. The "Performance Monitoring" module makes it possible to display KPIs or statistics in real time avoiding complex updating of reports. The "Smart Info Board" module enables general information to be displayed to all or specific monitors in production at the touch of a button, eliminating the need for time-consuming manual update of paper. Based on internal data algorithms the "Predictive Maintenance" module determines automatically, when the next maintenance intervals are to be carried out. The "Problem Map" module graphically shows where quality problems arise in the company, and therefore enables intuitive and quick detection of problem areas or machines. The "Issue

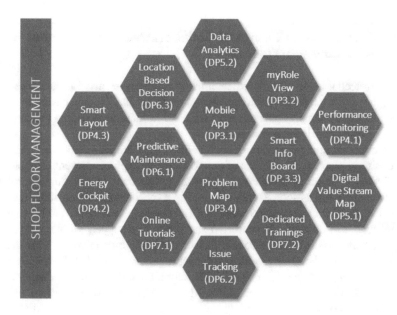

Fig. 17.5 Future modules of the Shopfloor management software. (Reproduced from Rauch et al. (2018), originally published open access under a CC BY 4.0 license: https://doi.org/10.1051/matecconf/20182230101)

Tracking" module digitally tracks the systematic processing of occurring problems in production by allowing the status of open problems to be continuously and in real time updated by the parties involved. The "Energy Cockpit" module shows the current energy consumption in the company and warns the user as soon as the consumption exceeds a defined warning limit or follows a negative or positive trend. The "Digital Value Stream Map" module is the digital image of a traditional value stream map, which is updated continuously and in real time and thus avoids time-consuming manual data collection. The "Dedicated Trainings" module offers access to training documents or video material directly at the workplace in order to facilitate the training phase of new employees at the workplace or during the start-up of new products. The last module "Online Tutorial" enables decentralized access to tutorials for problem-solving and for frequently asked questions (Rauch et al. 2018).

Currently, the company has already implemented the modules DP3.1, DP3.3, DP4.1, DP4.3, DP5.2, DP6.2 in a new software release. The other modules form the basis for further developments and will be implemented in subsequent releases.

Exercise 17.2: Detailed Design of a Shopfloor Management Software Module

Imagine you are in charge of implementing the remaining modules and planning their implementation. Pick a module that has not yet been implemented and try to design it with AD using a similar approach to the one in this case study.

17.5 Case Study 3: Design of Collaborative Human–Robot Assembly Workplaces

With new technologies and more intelligent control systems for machines and robots, the collaboration between human and machines has become easier. In smart manufacturing systems, robots are working hand in hand with people and support them, when their assistance is needed.

However, the implementation of such collaborative human–robot workplaces is not so easy in practice. The design of collaborative workplaces presents completely new challenges in terms of safety of the worker. Commercial collaborative robots are safe as such, but as soon as they are used in a specific application situation, this often changes. For example, the robot can enter or stop in a safety mode when in contact with the operator. However, if the robot is equipped with a dangerous gripper (sharp, pointed), the potential danger can change or increase. This means that the use of collaborative robotics no longer makes sense or that the robot can in turn be used only with a safe enclosure. Therefore, possible sources of danger must be identified and eliminated or minimized by appropriate design solutions of collaborative workspaces.

There are several international standards for the safety of workstations with robots. The various standards regulate different cases and situations and are often difficult to understand due to their complexity and scope. In particular, there is a lack of an overview of which standards can be applied and for which situations. Manufacturing system designers, therefore, often have difficulties in applying these standards in the right way (Gualtieri et al. 2018).

Such a complex problem requires a systematic and structured approach for concept design, in order to avoid loops in the design stage or even worse during implementation and to identify the relevant international standards for safety.

In this third case study, AD is used to examine how FRs can describe sources of danger and classify them according to the applicable standards (see also Gualtieri et al. 2018). This provides practitioners with a clearer overview of the most relevant safety standards to keep in mind when designing a collaborative workplace. In Fig. 17.6, we can see the main standards available for the design of the safety system in collaborative robotic cells.

Title	Code
Robots and robotic devices -- Safety requirements for industrial robots -- Part 1: Robots	**ISO 10218-1 : 2011**
Safety requirements for industrial robot -- Part 2: Robot systems and integration	**ISO 10218-2 : 2011**
Safety of machinery -- General principles for design -- Risk assessment and risk reduction	**ISO 12100 : 2010**
Safety of machinery — Safety-related parts of control systems — Part 1: General principles for design	**ISO 13849-1 : 2015**
Safety of machinery -- Minimum gaps to avoid crushing of parts of the human body	**ISO 13854 : 2017**
Safety of machinery -- Positioning of safeguards with respect to the approach speeds of parts of the human body	**ISO 13855 : 2010**
Safety of machinery -- Safety distances to prevent hazard zones being reached by upper and lower limbs	**ISO 13857 : 2008**
Safety of machinery -- Prevention of unexpected start-up	**ISO 14118 : 2017**
Safety of machinery -- Guards -- General requirements for the design and construction of fixed and movable guards	**ISO 14120 : 2015**
Robots and robotic devices -- Collaborative robots	**ISO TS 15066 : 2016**
Safety of machinery - Application of protective equipment to detect the presence of persons	**IEC 62046 : 2018**

Fig. 17.6 Collaborative robotic cell: main standards for the safety systems design. (Reproduced from Gualtieri et al. (2018), originally published open access under a CC BY 4.0 license: https://doi.org/10.1051/matecconf/201822301003)

The highest level of FRs and DPs are

FR0 = Reduce the mechanical risks that could arise from not intentional human–robot physical interaction;
DP0 = ISO 12100:2010 and ISO 10218-2:2011 (safe collaborative workstation by reducing as far as possible the risk probability and gravity).

The top-level FRs and relative DPs were defined as follows:

FR1 = Prevent unexpected human–robot contacts;
FR2 = Reduce the intensity of unexpected human–robot contacts;
FR3 = Avoid the access to the dangerous zone physically;

DP1 = Contact prevention measures according to ISO 13849-1:2015;
DP2 = Power and force limitation according to ISO 10218-1:2011 and ISO TS 15066:2016 (Sect. 5.5.5);
DP3 = Physical barriers/limitations according to ISO 14120:2015.

$$\begin{Bmatrix} FR1 \\ FR2 \\ FR3 \end{Bmatrix} = \begin{bmatrix} X & O & O \\ X & X & O \\ 0 & 0 & X \end{bmatrix} \begin{Bmatrix} DP1 \\ DP2 \\ DP3 \end{Bmatrix} \qquad (17.11)$$

FR1 (Prevent unexpected human–robot contacts) and DP1 (contact prevention measures) need a further decomposition on a lower level. The design of the safety systems that aims to actively prevent human–robot unexpected contacts can be satisfied using different complementary approaches. Depending on the final application, it is possible to apply one or more combined solutions. Starting from FR1, further FRs and DPs of the successive hierarchical level can be defined as follows:

FR1.1 = Determine the minimum distances to a hazard zone with respect to approach speeds of parts of the human body;
FR1.2 = Monitor when a person enters the safeguarded space;
FR1.3 = Timely sensing of a possible collision;
FR1.4 = Reduce speed if a robot comes nearby people;
FR1.5 = Prevent unexpected machine start-ups;
DP1.1 = Position safeguards with respect to the human body part speed according to ISO 13855:2010;
DP1.2 = Safety rated monitored stops according to ISO TS 15066:2016 (Sect. 5.5.2);
DP1.3 = Sensitive protection according to IEC 62046:2018;
DP1.4 = Monitoring of speed and separation according to ISO TS 15066:2016 (Sect. 5.5.4);
DP1.5 = Measures for prevention of unexpected machine start-up according to ISO 14,118:2017.

The design matrix shows a decoupled design:

$$
\begin{Bmatrix} FR1.1 \\ FR1.2 \\ FR1.3 \\ FR1.4 \\ FR1.5 \end{Bmatrix} = \begin{bmatrix} X & 0 & 0 & 0 & 0 \\ X & X & 0 & 0 & 0 \\ X & 0 & X & 0 & 0 \\ X & 0 & X & X & 0 \\ 0 & 0 & 0 & 0 & X \end{bmatrix} \begin{Bmatrix} DP1.1 \\ DP1.2 \\ DP1.3 \\ DP1.4 \\ DP1.5 \end{Bmatrix} \qquad (17.12)
$$

For FR2 (reduce the intensity of unexpected human–robot contacts) and DP2 (power and force limitation) there is no need for a further decomposition. The design of the safety systems that safeguard the operator during unexpected but allowed human–robot contacts can be achieved by reducing the energy exchange according to the "power and force limiting" approach. For the implementation of this DP, the guidelines explained in ISO 10218-1:2011 and ISO TS 15066:2016 Sect. 5.5.5 can be applied.

FR3 (avoid the access to the dangerous zone physically) and DP3 (physical barriers/limitations) need a further decomposition on a lower level. The design of the safety systems that aims safeguard the operator by avoiding human–robot contacts using physical limitations can be satisfied through the preventive design of the components of the robotic cell as well as the design of safeguards.

Starting from FR3, further FRs and DPs of the successive hierarchical level can be defined as follows:

FR3.1 = Prevent hazard zones being reached by operator during manual work activities;
FR3.2 = Avoid crushing of parts of the human body;
DP3.1 = Protective structures according to ISO 13857:2008;
DP3.2 = Minimum gaps relative to parts of the human body according to ISO 13854:2017.

The design matrix shows a decoupled design:

$$
\begin{Bmatrix} FR3.1 \\ FR3.2 \end{Bmatrix} = \begin{bmatrix} X & O \\ X & X \end{bmatrix} \begin{Bmatrix} DP3.1 \\ DP3.2 \end{Bmatrix} \qquad (17.13)
$$

Figure 17.7 explains a preliminary concept layout of the new collaborative workstation, including the main safety systems and their related standards. As shown, there will be a collaborative space, where human and robot will share the workspace in order to perform a common production task, and a not-collaborative space, where operators are not allowed and the robot can work, performing more.

Of course, different limited spaces involves different safety requirements and systems, which are regulated by different standards.

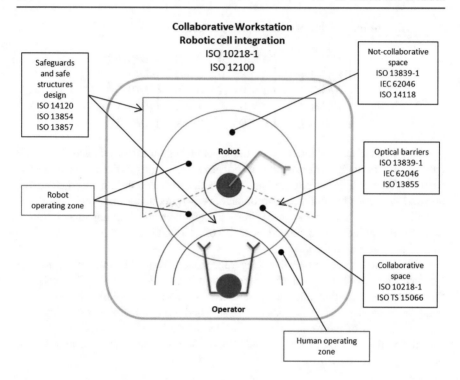

Fig. 17.7 Exemplary design of a collaborative assembly workplace. (Reproduced from Gualtieri et al. (2018), originally published open access under a CC BY 4.0 license: https://doi.org/10.1051/matecconf/201822301003)

Exercise 17.3: Design a Learning Factory Lab at Your University

Imagine you have to design a collaborative workplace for a previously purely manual assembly. Discuss in small groups, which possibilities exist in detail for the implementation of DP1.1 to DP1.5. If possible/available, use the relevant standards as an aid and then present your proposals to the group.

17.6 Case Study 4: Design of a Learning Factory for Industry 4.0

Learning factories are an idealized representation of real production environments. In the last decades numerous learning factories have been built in industry and academia. The first example of a learning factory was established in the United States at Penn State University in 1994. Later in the 1980s, one of the first learning factories in Europe was established with the "Lernfabrik" for computer-integrated manufacturing (CIM) at the research center Fraunhofer IAO in Stuttgart. Since the last decade more and more learning factories appeared like the Process Learning Factory at TU Darmstadt, Pilotfabrik at TU Vienna, ifactory at the University of Windsor or the Laboratory for Manufacturing Systems and Automation at University of Patras. The specific objectives of learning factory concepts in an academic environment are mainly to offer a practice-based engineering curriculum, balancing analytical and theoretical knowledge with manufacturing skills as well as hands-on experience in the design of manufacturing systems and product realization. While the majority of learning factories have mainly worked on concepts of lean management, today the trend is going toward learning factories for Industry 4.0 (I4.0). Modern learning factories are, therefore, acting as application centers for Industry 4.0 in order to familiarize with new technologies, to test them in practice and to learn how to use them in the industrial environment.

When setting up such I4.0 learning factories, it is important to define the extent to which the learning factory is to act. Here, the requirements of students and stakeholders, i.e., companies, must be taken into account. This case study attempts to explain the use of AD to derive design guidelines for I4.0 learning factories. The case study is based on the development of an I4.0 learning factory at the Free University of Bolzano named Smart Mini Factory showing the single steps how the design guidelines were implemented in practice (Rauch et al. 2019a).

According to the collective system design approach of Cochran and Kim (2010), it is important to include all members of a design (user and stakeholder) in the design process in order to achieve a collective agreement on the requirements of the system. Based on a literature review and workshops with user and stakeholders, their needs in engineering education were identified (see Table 17.1). The "X" in Table 17.1 means that the identified need can be assigned to one or more stakeholders. University students, high school students, researchers, teachers, and experienced people from industry were identified as main users, while universities, high schools, and industrial companies are the main stakeholders.

After the collection of CNs in Table 17.1, the next step in the design approach was to define top-level FRs to start with the development of an FR–DP decomposition. For the purpose of this work, the following top-level FRs–DPs were defined:

FR0 = Increase the qualification level of engineers and technicians in Industry 4.0 technologies;

DP0 = I4.0 Learning Factory for practically oriented engineering education.

According to AD, this vague and very abstract design solution in DP0 needs to be further decomposed until DPs are detailed enough to work with them. Based on FR0–DP0, the following first-level FRs and DPs as well as design fields (DF) were defined. For this first-level DPs, so-called design fields (DF) were defined, where a DF is a main field of responsibility. In case of the identified DFs, the approach suggests one responsible for each.

FR1 = Transfer newest insights from research in Industry 4.0;

FR2 = Teach industry 4.0 technologies and methods in a practically oriented way;

Table 17.1 Collectively identified customer needs (CNs) of users and stakeholders. (Reproduced with permission from Rauch et al. (2019a).)

CN	Customer Need (CN)	University	High School	Industry
CN1	Real-world practical experience (Cochran and Smith 2018)	X	X	X
CN2	Safe and comfortable environment to ask questions (Cochran and Smith 2018)	X	X	X
CN3	Interesting contents (Cochran and Smith 2018)	X	X	X
CN4	One-to-one interaction with instructor (Cochran and Smith 2018)	X	X	X
CN5	Application of theories (Cochran and Smith 2018)	X	X	X
CN6	Chance for trial and error without negative consequences (Cochran and Smith 2018)	X	X	X
CN7	Getting in contact with new and emerging (I4.0) technologies	X	X	X
CN8	Understanding if an engineering study could be the right choice		X	
CN9	Training the own teachers and instructors in new technologies		X	
CN10	Training the own skilled workers or engineers already hired			X
CN11	Test new technologies before investing and implementing them		X	X
CN12	Use equipment to perform experiments or for research purpose	X		X

Reprinted from Procedia Manufacturing, 31, Erwin Rauch, Florian Morandell, and Dominik T. Matt, "AD Design Guidelines for Implementing I4.0 Learning Factories", 239–244, Copyright(2019), with permission from Elsevier

FR3 = Exploit the resources and competences developed in the lab;
FR4 = Provide the resources to sustainably establish and run a learning factory;
DP1 = Research projects and collaborations *(DF1: Research)*;
DP2 = Education program in the learning factory *(DF2: Teaching)*;
DP3 = Collaboration models with local industry *(DF3: Industry)*;
DP4 = Funding for setting up a learning factory and business model *(DF4: Management)*.

Based on the top-level FR–DP pair and the first-level decomposition, the following lower level FR–DP pairs could get derived (see Fig. 17.8). On the left side, we can see "what" should be achieved (FR) and on the right side "how" it could be satisfied (DP). The sum of the lowest level DPs of every branch (highlighted in blue) builds the final list of a total of 20 design guidelines (DG) for I4.0 learning factories for practically oriented engineering education in universities.

The Smart Mini Factory Laboratory at the Free University of Bozen-Bolzano has been successfully set up using the previously shown design guidelines to convert the learning factory from a lean oriented lab to an I4.0 learning factory. Table 17.2 summarizes the DG and the activities implemented in the Smart Mini Factory:

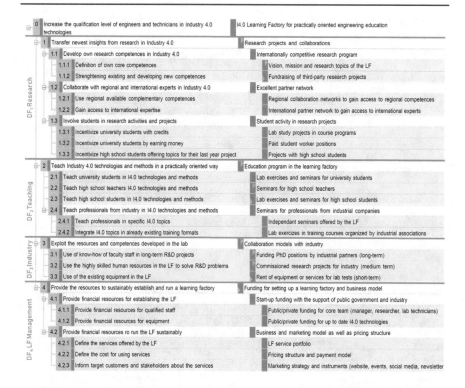

Fig. 17.8 Axiomatic Design mapping and decomposition of FR0–DP0. FRs on the left side and corresponding DPs on the right side, the in blue highlighted DPs represent the derived design guidelines for learning factories (LF) (screenshot created with AD software Acclaro DFSS). (Reproduced with permission from Rauch et al. (2019) (Reprinted from Procedia Manufacturing, 31, Erwin Rauch, Florian Morandell, and Dominik T. Matt, "AD Design Guidelines for Implementing I4.0 Learning Factories", 239–244, Copyright (2019), with permission from Elsevier.)

Exercise 17.4: Design a Learning Factory Lab at Your University

As a student, you are one of the main users of learning factories alongside other possible target groups (such as companies). As a student, consider the requirements you place on a possible learning factory laboratory at your university. Then define the FRs, derive possible design proposals (DPs) and check your design in each step by using a design matrix. Discuss your design with your professor. He will be grateful for your valuable input from a student's perspective.

Table 17.2 Collectively identified customer needs (CNs) of users and stakeholders. (Reproduced with permission from Rauch et al. (2019a).)

DG_i	DP_i	Exemplary application in the Smart Mini Factory (SMF) lab
DG_1 – Vision and mission	$DP_{1.1.1}$	A new vision and mission statement as well as I4.0 oriented research topics were defined for the SMF (see also the following link: www.smartminifactory.it)
DG_2 – Fundraising	$DP_{1.1.2}$	To strengthen existing and to develop new I4.0 competences, fundraising was started acquiring 1.25 mio Euro from 2017–2018 for research projects on Industry 4.0 related topics
DG_3 – Regional collaboration network	$DP_{1.2.1}$	SMF is member of a trans-regional network of partners from Italy and Austria working on innovative education and training models (ongoing research project "Engineering Education 4.0")
DG_4 – International partner network	$DP_{1.2.2}$	An international network of I4.0 and learning factory experts could be developed through an international researcher exchange project on Industry 4.0 funded by the EC H2020 MSCA RISE program as well as through the participation at the Conference on Learning Factories
DG_5 – Study projects	$DP_{1.3.1}$	Students from university were involved in research projects through thesis projects for undergraduate and graduate students as well as mandatory study projects for graduate students
DG_6 – Student assistant positions	$DP_{1.3.2}$	Students were involved financing "120 h student jobs" where students assist research teams in the conduction and preparation of research activities on Industry 4.0
DG_7 – Projects with high schools	$DP_{1.3.3}$	High school students were involved in research projects serving as test persons for lab experiments or by outsourcing parts and tasks of research projects
DG_8 – Exercises and seminars for university students	$DP_{2.1}$	The learning factory is used in ten lectures in the undergraduate and graduate program for practical lab exercises and case study trainings. Further, students can participate to Industry 4.0 seminars for industry
DG_9 – Seminars for high school teacher	$DP_{2.2}$	The learning factory offers two Industry 4.0 seminars to high school teacher from technical or scientific high schools to enforce the knowledge transfer to the high school level
DG_{10} – Exercises and seminars for high school students	$DP_{2.3}$	The learning factory is used for practical lab exercises and case study trainings with high school classes. The goal is first to promote engineering study courses and secondly to

(continued)

Table 17.2 (continued)

DG_i	DP_i	Exemplary application in the Smart Mini Factory (SMF) lab
		increase the qualification level of technicians with high school degree
DG_{11} – Specific I4.0 seminars for industry	$DP_{2.4.1}$	The SMF offers nine specific Industry 4.0 seminars for professionals in industry in order to increase the qualification level of existing workforce in industrial companies
DG_{12} – I4.0 exercises in executive training courses	$DP_{2.4.2}$	The SMF offers practical training sessions integrated in training programs organized by other associations and the local Chamber of Commerce
DG_{13} – Funding of PhD positions	$DP_{3.1}$	Through the funding of PhD positions with a duration of 3–5 years, industrial companies can outsource long-term research projects to SMF and often take over the doctoral candidate afterwards
DG_{14} - Commissioned industry projects	$DP_{3.2}$	For medium-term research projects, industrial companies engage single researchers or individual teams in the SMF to work on a specific research problem
DG_{15} – Rent of equipment or lab tests	$DP_{3.3}$	In case of short-term necessity of equipment of the SMF as well as the conduction of tests, industry companies can engage the SMF (equipment is, therefore, well described on the website of the SMF)
DG_{16} – Start-up funding for core team	$DP_{4.1.1}$	The SMF received public funding of 2.3 mio Euro for financing a core team consisting of a lab manager, post-doc researcher, and lab technicians
DG_{17} – Start-up funding for I4.0 equipment	$DP_{4.1.2}$	0.5 mio Euro of the total funding of 2.3 mio Euro from public is addressed to finance up to date equipment and technologies related to industry 4.0
DG_{18} – Service portfolio	$DP_{4.2.1}$	According to the results of the conducted AD decomposition, the SMF offers services in the following fields: (i) Research, (ii) Teaching, and (iii) Industry
DG_{19} – Pricing and payment	$DP_{4.2.2}$	In case of the SMF, the definition of the pricing structure and the payment model was supported by a market analysis of common prices for training courses as well as by discussions with local providers of training courses for professionals. This was necessary to avoid that SMF owned by the university is in competition and in conflict with private provider of training courses
DG_{20} – Marketing strategy	$DP_{4.2.3}$	Creation of a professional and responsive website for the SMF lab. Further marketing instruments were posting of regular news on the website, brochures for high schools and brochures for industrial companies, the organization of regular

(continued)

Table 17.2 (continued)

DG$_i$	DP$_i$	Exemplary application in the Smart Mini Factory (SMF) lab
		events or workshops with companies and the organization of lab visits for target groups (high school students and industrial companies). In a next step also the activation of social media channels will be started in order to reach companies (LinkedIn), students (facebook) and scholars (ResearchGate)

Reprinted from Procedia Manufacturing, 31, Erwin Rauch, Florian Morandell, and Dominik T. Matt, "AD Design Guidelines for Implementing I4.0 Learning Factories", 239–244, Copyright (2019), with permission from Elsevier

17.7 Case Study 5: Design of a Demonstrator for a Flexible and Decentralized Cyber-Physical Production System (CPPS)

Cyber-physical production systems (CPPS) are equipped with intelligent units, so-called cyber-physical systems (CPS), and enable new possibilities in the factory of the future through the connectivity between the digital world and the physical production system. Many enterprises are still quite skeptical regarding the vision of Industry 4.0. The term CPS stands for the continuously increasing presence of computing and communication capabilities in physical objects in the real world. The decision-making process of such systems in production may be supported or handled autonomously by computational intelligence.

It has been so far difficult to transfer such advantages and concepts in a clear and practical-oriented manner. It is not always possible to train and show these emerging concepts directly in a real factory environment. Therefore, demonstration models are a popular alternative and complementary solution, where the concepts and technologies can be demonstrated and explained in a miniaturized way to employees as well as to students. Therefore, Fraunhofer Italia Research built a demonstration model for a flexible and decentralized CPPS system for showcase purposes (Egger et al. 2017). The demonstration model created by Fraunhofer Italia is intended to facilitate the knowledge transfer of Industry 4.0 concepts and CPPS to project partners, industrial firms as well as students from schools and universities.

The case study shows an AD based re-design of the realized demonstration model of a flexible and decentralized CPPS. The previous demonstration model was built by a team of Fraunhofer Italia researchers and students to demonstrate the potentials of a CPPS in the factory of the future. Mainly the model aims to demonstrate the following concepts of typical and modern factory of the future concepts to students and companies (see also Fig. 17.9):

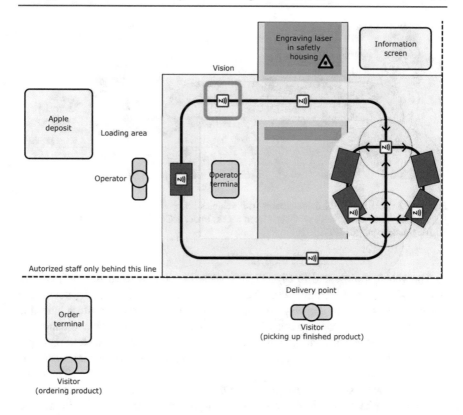

Fig. 17.9 Previous architecture of the CPPS demonstrator at Fraunhofer Italia Research. (Reproduced from Egger et al. (2017), originally published open access under a CC BY 4.0 license: https://doi.org/10.1051/matecconf/201712701016)

- flexible Transport System;
- intelligent Work-piece Carrier;
- decentralized Control;
- digital Interconnection;
- efficient Human–Machine Interface.

Figures 17.9 and 17.10 illustrate the system architecture and the realized demonstration model consisting of:

- laser engraving head;
- safety housing (custom design);
- fume extraction unit;
- air compressor;
- NFC (near field communication) pads;
- vehicles for product transport.

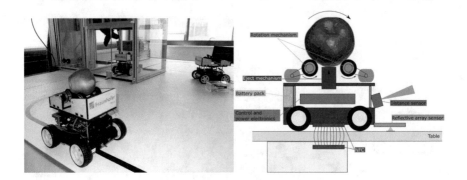

Fig. 17.10 Realized CPPS demonstrator with vehicles for product transport. (Reproduced from Egger et al. (2017), originally published open access under a CC BY 4.0 license: https://doi.org/10.1051/matecconf/201712701016)

The vehicles presented in Fig. 17.10 consist of a commercial robotic platform with 4 DC motors, an Arduino-compatible controller board, an internally developed apple-spin mechanism (apple symmetry axis aligns to spin axis), a custom built line sensor with eight analog sensors, an IR distance sensor for collision avoidance, an apple-eject mechanism, and a control algorithm (line follower) with routing capability and the ability to detect and take crossings. In addition, a user interface was developed to get orders from a computer terminal. Visitors may enter their name and a personal message to be engraved on the apple. When ready, a screen informs the visitor to pick up his apple. Visitors need to present their RFID card in order to start the delivery of the apple.

The research team collected the main requirements and needs for the re-design of the CPPS demonstrator and categorized them as shown in Table 17.3. The table shows also if the needs were fully or only partly fulfilled (improvable) in the previous demonstration model or if they are new.

The highest level of FRs and DPs are

FR0 = Demonstrate Industry 4.0 concepts for CPPS in a practical way;
DP0 = Demonstration Model for a flexible and decentralized CPPS.

Based on the outcome of the initial workshop, the following Cs for the (re) design were defined:

C1 = Maximum total budget of 20,000 Euro for new investments;
C2 = Maximum space of 6 square meters;
C3 = Modular structure with standard components;
C4 = Mobility of the demo model for flexible use.

Table 17.3 Collectively identified customer needs (CNs) of users and stakeholders. (Reproduced from Egger et al. (2017), originally published open access under a CC BY 4.0 license: https://doi. org/10.1051/matecconf/201712701016)

CN	Customer Needs	C, FR, n-FR	Existing
CN1	Demonstrate intelligent and decentralized control of individualized production (lot size 1)	FR_4	Yes
CN2	Permit rapid scaling of the capacity up and down automatically	FR_2	In part
CN3	The product should have a local link	$n\text{-}FR_1$	Yes
CN4	The model should be realized with students for training purpose	$n\text{-}FR_2$	Yes
CN5	The demonstration model should show a complete production process	$n\text{-}FR_3$	In part
CN6	The maximal budget for realization are 20,000 Euro	C_1	Yes
CN7	Modularity in order to reuse the single components also in other educational or research settings	C_3	Yes
CN8	Maximum space for the demonstration model is 6 m^2	C_2	Yes
CN9	The demonstration model needs to be movable to use it in different events and facilities	C_4	In part
CN10	Safety for user and visitors has to be guaranteed	FR_3	Yes
CN11	Allow interaction between visitor and the CPPS demo model	FR_3	Yes
CN12	Traceability of orders	FR_4	In part
CN13	Quality check of the order before delivery	FR_3	In part
CN14	Delocalization of order entry (e.g., on mobile devices)	FR_3	Yes
CN15	Demonstration of advanced industrial robotics in the CPPS	FR_1	No
CN16	Experience the production from the point of view of the product	FR_5	No

Further, the following FRs were defined:

n-FR1 = Products should have a local link;
n-FR2 = The model should be realized and run with the support of students for training purpose;
n-FR3 = The demonstration model should show a complete production process.

Finally the remaining CAs were associated to top-level FRs deriving DPs:

FR1 = Apply advanced industrial robotics in the CPPS;
FR2 = Allow automatic scaling of capacity up and down;
FR3 = Ensure safety during operation of personnel, visitors, and equipment;
FR4 = Event-based dynamic control and monitoring of a production line for mass customized products;

FR5 = Visualize the production from the point of view of the product;

DP1 = Lightweight robot and vision system for bin picking at the loading station;

DP2 = Buffer for waiting vehicles and automatic call;

DP3 = Safe user interface between user/visitor and the cyber-physical system;

DP4 = Intelligent and autonomous vehicles driven by a decentralized control architecture;

DP5 = Camera system on the work-piece carrier.

The design matrix on the first level is decoupled and shows the dependencies between the solutions (DPs) and the FRs:

$$
\begin{Bmatrix} FR1.1 \\ FR1.2 \\ FR1.3 \\ FR1.4 \\ FR1.5 \end{Bmatrix} = \begin{bmatrix} X & 0 & 0 & 0 & 0 \\ X & X & 0 & 0 & 0 \\ 0 & 0 & X & 0 & 0 \\ X & 0 & X & X & 0 \\ 0 & 0 & 0 & X & X \end{bmatrix} \begin{Bmatrix} DP1.1 \\ DP1.2 \\ DP1.3 \\ DP1.4 \\ DP1.5 \end{Bmatrix} \qquad (17.14)
$$

Regarding FR1–DP1, industrial robotics can be integrated using a lightweight robot for picking apples from the container and loading them on the vehicles. Starting from FR1, further FRs and DPs of the successive hierarchical level can be defined as follows:

FR1.1 = Localize and identify apple for flexible feeding;

FR1.2 = Grasp sensitive products;

DP1.1 = Lightweight robot combined with vision system for bin picking of the apple;

DP1.2 = Flexible gripper for complex and sensitive products.

The design matrix shows an uncoupled design:

$$
\begin{Bmatrix} FR1.1 \\ FR1.2 \end{Bmatrix} = \begin{bmatrix} X & 0 \\ 0 & X \end{bmatrix} \begin{Bmatrix} DP1.1 \\ DP1.2 \end{Bmatrix} \qquad (17.15)
$$

For flexible feeding, the research team used existing equipment. A mobile station with a mounted UR3 lightweight robot combined with a camera system allows flexible feeding without additional investments. For grasping the apples, a flexible and sensitive gripper is required to avoid damages to the product.

Scalability (FR2-DP2) is a major requirement of modern production systems. While in the current demonstration model the number of vehicles is fixed, a buffer should be created in the re-designed demonstration model. All other stations (laser engraving and robotized loading station) are sufficiently rapidly scalable in their performance. Vehicles not needed in periods with low demand can be parked in the buffer to reduce energy consumption in the system, while they are called automatically, when demand is rising. FR2 can be decomposed further as follows:

FR2.1 = Provide function for rapid scaling down;

FR2.2 = Provide function for rapid scaling up to guarantee capacity for higher demand;

DP2.1 = Crossing points with NFC pads to detect vehicle direction for ejection of the vehicles in a buffer line;

DP2.2 = Buffer line with sufficient length to guarantee the needed capacity.

The design matrix shows an uncoupled design:

$$\left\{ \begin{array}{c} FR2.1 \\ FR2.2 \end{array} \right\} = \begin{bmatrix} X & O \\ 0 & X \end{bmatrix} \left\{ \begin{array}{c} DP2.1 \\ DP2.2 \end{array} \right\} \tag{17.16}$$

To realize the buffer line some more NFC pads had been integrated in the demonstration model. In addition, the dimensions (length) of the buffer line were defined according to the maximum number of vehicles, in order to guarantee the expected performance of the model during visitor presentations.

For FR3–DP3 (safe user interface) the model should allow interaction between the visitor/user and the CPPS. In the previous demonstration model, visitors may create an individual order for writing an individual text on an apple by using a desktop station or their smartphone. Any order requires approval by a supervisor. To avoid injuries and malfunctions of the production equipment, the visitor cannot touch the vehicles or any other stations, and the finished apple ejects to a withdrawal tray, where the visitor may grasp it without interfering with the vehicle itself. In the previous system, a quality check was missing for the simulation of a complete production process. Further, in addition to the visualization on a screen, the result of the quality check as well as the availability of the apple at the delivery station should be sent to the visitor via app. Thus, this new functions had to be integrated in the re-designed demonstration model. FR3 could be decomposed in the following lower level FRs and DPs:

FR3.1 = Prevent direct intervention by the user in unsafe areas;

FR3.2 = Create individual order in situ or remotely;

FR3.3 = Check compliance of incoming orders;

FR3.4 = Check the quality after processing;

FR3.5 = Inform user/visitor about the order progress;

DP3.1 = Separation of unsafe areas (e.g., through acrylic glass screen);

DP3.2 = Order creation (individual text on the apple) at the order terminal or via smartphone (app);

DP3.3 = Approval by supervisor on a monitor screen;

DP3.4 = Camera system at laser engraving station to compare the result with the text in the order;

DP3.5 = Notification to the visitor after laser engraving station and at delivery station.

The design matrix shows a decoupled design:

$$
\begin{Bmatrix} FR3.1 \\ FR3.2 \\ FR3.3 \\ FR3.4 \\ FR3.5 \end{Bmatrix} = \begin{bmatrix} X & 0 & 0 & 0 & 0 \\ 0 & X & 0 & 0 & 0 \\ 0 & X & X & 0 & 0 \\ 0 & 0 & 0 & X & 0 \\ 0 & 0 & 0 & X & X \end{bmatrix} \begin{Bmatrix} DP3.1 \\ DP3.2 \\ DP3.3 \\ DP3.4 \\ DP3.5 \end{Bmatrix} \tag{17.17}
$$

While DP3.1 to DP3.3 were already part of the original model, the other two DPs were implemented in the re-designed demonstration model.

The decentralized control (FR4–DP4) as well as the traceability of mass customized products in the demonstration model was previously solved by the use of intelligent (NFC technology) and autonomous vehicles. FR4 can be decomposed in the following lower level FRs and DPs:

FR4.1 = Vehicles shall be aware of their position and communicate with the CPPS;
FR4.2 = Bring mass customized products decentralized to their next processing station;
DP4.1 = NFC technology for both communication and location awareness;
DP4.2 = Autonomously navigating vehicles with their own drive, routing capability, and controller for every work-piece carrier.

The design matrix shows an uncoupled design:

$$
\begin{Bmatrix} FR4.1 \\ FR4.2 \end{Bmatrix} = \begin{bmatrix} X & O \\ 0 & X \end{bmatrix} \begin{Bmatrix} DP4.1 \\ DP4.2 \end{Bmatrix} \tag{17.18}
$$

The choice for NFC is motivated by the fact that it provides superior robustness against electromagnetic disturbances typical for an industrial production environment and the well-defined range of operation, which allows its use not only for communication purposes but also for unambiguous position detection. Same also for the modular vehicles built with standard components, and hence there were no design changes in this FR–DP pair.

Regarding FR5–DP5 (user experience), the demonstration model should allow the visitor to follow the steps in the production process from the point of view of the product. In the previous demonstration model this function was not integrated. There is no need to decompose this FR–DP pair any further, as DP5 can be implemented through a standard camera mounted on the vehicle. The livestream of the camera was realized by transmission to the information screen and allows now the visitors following the production process from loading the apple, rotating the apple in the right position, laser engraving, and ejection in the delivery station.

Most of the improvements are reflected in the layout of the demonstrator illustrated in Fig. 17.11. In the re-designed demonstration model there is a clear distinction between active waiting for jobs (green), active waiting for delivery (purple), and standby in the buffer line (blue) vehicles. The loading mechanism not

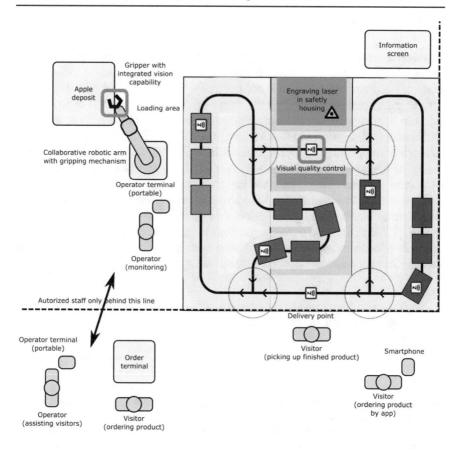

Fig. 17.11 System architecture of the re-designed CPPS demonstrator. (Reproduced from Egger et al. (2017), originally published open access under a CC BY 4.0 license: https://doi.org/10.1051/matecconf/201712701016)

only grips the apples and places them on the vehicles, but also aligns them so that the rotation mechanism of the vehicles becomes obsolete. Hence, the vison process is now part of the loading. The operator is relieved from repetitive loading and may assist visitors. In addition, visitor may place orders remotely.

Exercise 17.5: Re-design of the Demonstrator Considering Artificial Intelligence

Artificial intelligence (AI) is the next trend that will strongly influence production in the coming years. The task is to demonstrate the possibilities of AI based on the current demonstration model. Discuss this in a small group and define the CNs resulting from this brainstorming. Derive then the top-level FRs from them and perform a decomposition to obtain possible DPs for a combination of an AI and CPPS demonstrator.

17.8 Conclusions

As this chapter has shown, AD is a highly suitable design theory that can be applied to the design of complex tasks in manufacturing systems design. The various examples and case studies also show the many possible uses of AD. Thus, both very technical problems regarding the design of individual machines or production cells can be addressed as well as more extensive projects for the design of the entire production system with additional organizational or strategic aspects. With the increasing introduction of topics such as Industry 4.0, Digitization and AI, the design of manufacturing systems will very often be expanded to include topics relating to software instruments for the acquisition, analysis, and evaluation of production data. The case studies have also shown that AD provides very valuable input here. Students should get an insight through the different case studies how AD can be applied in the most different questions in production and how an AD project can be handled in its approach. The different exercises at the end of each case study should also encourage the students to think along.

Problems

Students should choose two of the exercise problems given in the main text of this chapter and work on them.

References

AlGeddawy TN, ElMaraghy HA (2009) Changeability effect on manufacturing systems design, Springer, Chap 15. Series in Advanced Manufacturing

Bergmann L (2010) Nachhaltigkeit in Ganzheitlichen Produktionssystemen. Vlukan, Essen (in German)

Cochran DS, Kim YS (2010) Collective system design in systems engineering education. American Society for Engineering Education

Cochran DS, Arinez JF, Duda JW, Linck J (2001) A decomposition approach for manufacturing system design. J Manufact Syst 20(6):371–389

Cochran DS, Arinez JF, Collins MT, Bi Z (2017) Modelling of humanmachine interaction in equipment design of manufacturing cells. Enterp Inf Sys 11(7):969–987

Cochran JJ, Smith (2018) A Systematic Design Approach to Manufacturing Education. Procedia Manufacturing, 26:1369–1377

Delaram J, Valilai OF (2018) An architectural view to computer integrated manufacturing systems based on axiomatic design theory. Comput Ind 100:96–114

Durmusoglu MB, Satoglu SI (2011) Axiomatic design of hybrid manufacturing systems in erratic demand conditions. Int J Prod Res 49(17):5231–5261

Egger G, Rauch E, Matt DT, Brown CA (2017) (re-)design of a demonstration model for a flexible and decentralized cyber-physical production system (cpps). In: Slătineanu L (ed) 11th International Conference on Axiomatic Design (ICAD), MATEC Web of Conferences, Iasi, Romania, p 01016

Farid AM (2017) Measures of reconfigurability and its key characteristics in intelligent manufac-turing systems. J Intell Manuf 28(2):353–369

Gualtieri L, Rauch E, Rojas R, Vidoni R, Matt DT (2018) Application of axiomatic design for the design of a safe collaborative human-robot assembly workplace. In: Puik E, Foley JT, Cochran D, Betasolo M (eds) 12th International Conference on Axiomatic Design (ICAD),

MATEC Web of Conferences, Reykjavík, Iceland, vol 223, p 01003, doi: https://doi.org/10.1051/matecconf/201822301003

Holzner P, Rauch E, Spena PR, Matt DT (2015) Systematic design of sme manufacturing and assembly systems based on axiomatic design. Procedia CIRP, Elsevier 34:81–86

Kulak O, Cebi S, Kahraman C (2010) Applications of axiomatic design principles: a literature review. Expert Syst Appl 37(9):6705–6717

Matt DT, Rauch E (2011) Continuous improvement of manufacturing systems with the concept of functional periodicity. Key Eng Mater 473:783–790

Matt DT, Rauch E (2016) Design and implementation approach for distributed manufacturing networks using axiomatic design. In: Farid AM, Suh NP (eds) Axiomatic design in large systems, Springer, Cham, chap 9, pp 225–250

Puik E, Telgen D, van Moergestel L, Ceglarek D (2017) Assessment of reconfiguration schemes for reconfigurable manufacturing systems based on resources and lead time. Robot Comput-Integ Manufact 43:30–38

Rauch E, Matt DT, Dallasega P (2016) Application of axiomatic design in manufacturing system design: a literature review. In: Liu A (ed) 10th International Conference on Axiomatic Design (ICAD), Procedia CIRP, Elsevier ScienceDirect, Xi'an, Shaanxi, China, vol 53, pp 1–7

Rauch E, Morandell F, Matt DT (2019) AD design guidelines for implementing I4.0 learning factories. Proc Manufact 31:239–244

Rauch E, Spena PR, Matt DT (2019) Axiomatic design guidelines for the design of flexible and agile manufacturing and assembly systems for smes. Int J Interact Des Manufact (IJIDeM) 13 (1):1–22

Suh NP (2001) Axiomatic design—advances and applications. Oxford University Press

Vinodh S, Aravindraj S (2012) Axiomatic modeling of lean manufacturing system. J Eng Des Technol 10(2):199–216

Wiendahl HP, ElMaraghy HA, Nyhuis P, Zäh MF, Wiendahl HH, Duffie N, Brieke M (2007) Changeable manufacturing-classification, design and operation. CIRP Ann 56(2):783–809

Zäh MF, Mäller N, Vogl W (2005) Symbiosis of changeable and virtual production the emperor's new clothes or key factor for future success. In: Proceedings (CD) of the international conference on changeable, agile, reconfigurable and virtual production, Munich, Germany

Design of the Assembly Systems for Airplane Structures

18

Mustafa Yurdakul, Yusuf Tansel İç, and Osman Emre Celek

Abstract

This chapter deals with the design of automated assembly systems of airplanes. Axiomatic Design (AD) methodology is used to develop a general design hierarchical tree for the assembly of an airplane fuselage panel. Introduction of new and advanced machinery and assembly equipment in material handling, measurement, robotics, plant modeling and simulation, manufacturing processes require the usage of systematic methodologies for the design of assembly systems. In this chapter, multiple alternative design solutions are demonstrated from the general hierarchical tree, which are compared for their acceptability in satisfying various factory objectives. In two case studies presented in this chapter, design solutions are obtained and described in detail. The first assembly system alternative consists of the following: (1) an automated laser tracking measurement system, (2) reconfigurable fixtures for fixing the panels, (3) frame clip riveters in frame assembly cells, (4) 3D projection devices to control the position of the fastener on the panels, (5) autonomous mobile robots for material handling, and (6) automatic riveting machines for the final fuselage panel assembly. The second assembly system alternative includes the following:

M. Yurdakul
Faculty of Engineering, Department of Mechanical Engineering, Gazi University, Eti Mah. Yükselis Sokak, No: 5, 06570 Maltepe/Ankara, Turkey
e-mail: yurdakul@gazi.edu.tr

Y. T. İç (✉)
Faculty of Engineering, Department of Industrial Engineering, Baskent University, Bağlıca Kampüsü, Fatih Sultan Mahallesi, Eskisehir Yolu 18.km, 06790 Etimesgut/Ankara, Turkey
e-mail: yustanic@baskent.edu.tr

O. E. Celek
Turkish Aerospace Headquarter, Havacılık Bulvarı No: 17, 06980 Fethiye Mahallesi, Kahramankazan Ankara, Turkey
e-mail: oecelek@tai.com.tr

(1) robotic measurement systems, (2) robotic stringer placement robots for stringer positioning, (3) reconfigurable fixtures for holding the panels, (4) frame clip robots to assemble clips to frames, (5) 3D projection devices for fastener position controls on the panels, (6) modular crane for material handling, and (7) mobile automated drilling and fastening robots for final fuselage panel assembly. These two alternative designs are compared, and results are made available for system designers to assess the capabilities of each alternative. The application of the proposed design methodology provides a reference guide for system designers to apply in designing assembly systems in an aerospace assembly factory.

After studying this chapter, the reader should know the following:
(1) How we can design airplane fuselage panel assembly systems. (2) How to develop a general assembly system design hierarchy tree. (2) The clear understanding of functional requirements (FRs) and design parameters (DPs) at each level of the assembly system design hierarchy tree. (4) How to obtain various alternative solutions from design hierarchy tree of the assembly system. (5) Using simulation to compare alternative design solutions.

One of the Most Important Questions to Think About throughout This Chapter:
This chapter presents multiple alternative solutions instead of a single solution. Although with multiple solutions the general decision tree is larger and more widespread, it lets the system designers to see all solutions. The system designer can make a more thorough comparison among the solutions and then make recommendations for final selection.

18.1 Introduction

Aerospace manufacturers are bursting at the seams with a backlog of orders. To remain competitive, aerospace manufacturers must reduce time-to-market on new airplane variants, improve capability, increase flexibility and shorten lead time to reduce backlog on current orders (Groover 2007). One viable solution is to automate their factories. The industry is investing heavily in systems that reduce cost, improve quality, and boost productivity. Systems include lightweight fixtures, reconfigurable tools, automated part positioning, automated scanning, countersink control, automatic riveting, and robotic measurement. Furthermore, investments are made in state-of-the-art robots for drilling, riveting, sealing, coating, and painting applications, in addition to material handling, carbon fiber layup, and advanced machining operations.

Airlines will need 38,050 new airplanes valued at more than $5.6 trillion in the near future. Asia Pacific region (China, Northern Asia, South Asia, Southeast Asia, and Oceania) is expected to have the largest expected deliveries in total as shown in Fig. 18.1.

Fig. 18.1 New airplane deliveries by region (2015–2034)

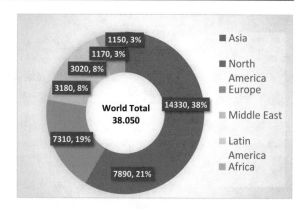

Based on the growth trends in air travel demand, airplane production volumes have been increasing over the years, as shown in Fig. 18.2 especially for single-aisle airplanes such as A320 or B737. Boeing increased the production of its popular narrow-body single-aisle 737 jets from 42 airplanes to 52 in 2018. The company plans to ramp up production volume on the more technically complex B787 to 14 airplanes per month by 2020. The aerospace giant currently has more than 5,700 airplane on order, valued at more than $450 billion. Boeing's archrival, Airbus, also plans to boost output of its most popular airplane, the A320. Airbus expects to ramp up production rates from 42 planes a month to 50 units. Airbus plans to crank up A320 production to 60 planes a month at its factories in China, France, Germany, and the United States. That kind of production volume would be unprecedented in the commercial aerospace industry (Weber 2015).

Assembly lines at major suppliers, such as GE Aviation, Honeywell, Rockwell Collins, Spirit Aero Systems, and UTC Aerospace Systems increased production rate. Pratt & Whitney invested $1 billion worldwide to prepare its factories for jet engine production increases. The facility featured an overhead horizontal moving assembly line in order to produce the Pure Power PW1100G-JM engine for the Airbus A320neo (Weber 2015).

Automation in assembly lines of aerospace companies is necessary for minimizing hand assembly operations in order to increase the efficiency. Benefits of automation include lower manufacturing costs, increased quality levels, consistent and higher throughput rates, and fewer repetitive motion injuries. When all the benefits are added, automation is continually replacing human workers not only in the final assembly line but also in the sub assembly lines.

The assembly centers within airplane factories are the focal points for collecting all the varied pieces of an airplane and bringing them together to be joined into an airframe. The airframe is approximately 75% of the cost of the airplane; assembly is approximately 65% of the cost of the airframe; and drilling and fastening is approximately 65% of the labor cost of assembly. The greatest opportunity to reduce costs is based on unchanged processes and activities related to the assembly line of the airframe (Bullen 2013).

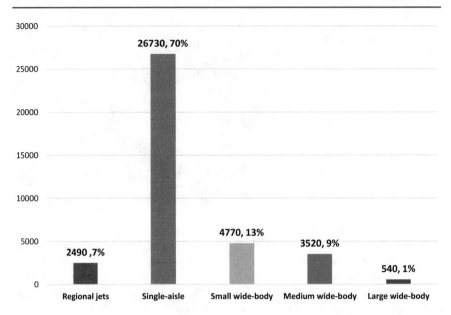

Fig. 18.2 Airplane Deliveries: 38.050 (2015–2034)

The fuselage is the main structure or body of the airframe of an airplane. It provides space for cargo, controls, accessories, passengers, and other equipment. In single-engine airplane, the fuselage houses the power plant. In a multiengine airplane, the engines may be either in the fuselage, attached to the fuselage, or suspended from the wing structure. Wings, tail cone, vertical fin, and engine are attached to the fuselage in an airplane. In some airplane designs, the engines and landing gear are also attached directly to the fuselage structure. In modern airplanes, as shown in Fig. 18.3, the fuselage takes the form of a tube, which houses the flight deck, passenger cabin, freight holds, and the majority of the equipment required to operate the airplane. For passenger airplanes that fly above 10,000 ft. the fuselage also forms a pressure hull so that a cabin altitude of 8,000 ft. can be maintained throughout a normal flight (Federal Aviation Administration 2018). The airplane fuselage consists of six different panels, namely, lower, lower left, lower right, upper, upper left, and upper right.

A typical airplane fuselage panel is mainly composed of skin, stringer, clips, frame, and other support parts. Main components of a fuselage panel assembly are presented in Fig. 18.4. Skins carry the major stresses and functions as the main part of the airframe. Stringers are the main lengthwise members of the fuselage panel structure. Stringers work in combination with the skin to create a strong beam. Stringers prevent tension and compression from bending the fuselage. They have some rigidity but are chiefly used to give the fuselage shape and attach the skin.

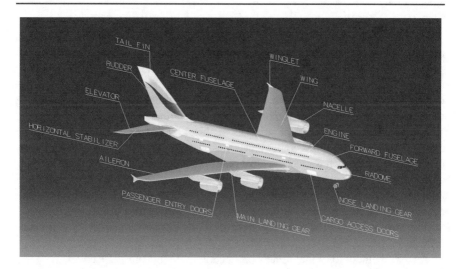

Fig. 18.3 Airplane structural components

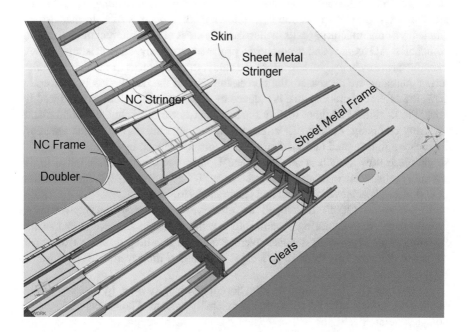

Fig. 18.4 Main components of a fuselage panel assembly

Frames on the other hand serve a dual purpose, they give cross-sectional shape to the fuselages, and also they add rigidity and strength to the structure. The shape and size of these members vary considerably depending on their function and position in the fuselage. They have multiple functions and break up skin panels so that they behave as panels supported on all four edges. They distribute applied loads created by doors and fairings and maintain the cylindrical shape of the skin. Frame assemblies are the most numerous and important members of the fuselage. Clips are structural elements that connect stringers to skins. Also, frames are attached to the stringers with stringer clips. Sometimes frames attach directly to the skin by means of shear ties (Jeppesen Sanderson, Inc. and Atlantic Flight Training, Ltd. 2007).

All these members are delivered to fuselage panel assembly center and are joined together to form fuselage panel assemblies. In this study, AD principles are applied to develop alternative assembly systems for a fuselage panel assembly.

The most relevant studies to the content of this chapter are briefly discussed as follows:

An AD methodology that relates production system design objectives to operational DPs was developed at Massachusetts Institute of Technology by Reynal and Cochran. The methodology also focuses on the design of production operations by eliminating non-value-added operations. Internal and external customer requirements are also taken into consideration with this methodology. It is used to increase the efficiency of manufacturing cells in the assembly areas of two different manufacturing companies. AD axioms and decomposed processes are analyzed in existing and new manufacturing systems. As a result of the study, the part stocks in the first manufacturing company are decreased, the processing time of the detail parts is reduced by 50%, the assembly process time is reduced by 60%, and production area reduced by 40%. Production of a higher quality final product is provided. In the second manufacturing company, bottlenecks in manufacturing area are solved. Some assembly fixtures are re-designed and loading process time is reduced by 30 s per piece. The single-piece flow system is integrated and U shape arrangement is applied in the assembly cells. Work in process time reduced by 80%. The objective for the production of 400 pieces is achieved (Reynal and Cochran 1996).

Kulak et al. (2005) developed an effective methodology of converting a process-based manufacturing system into a cellular one in a conventional manufacturing firm. Their study reduces average material handling distance from 67 to 31 m and delivery time from 18 to 7 days. The biggest improvement is observed in 80% reduction of overtime.

Jefferson et al. (2016) addressed the design complexity issue by creating design methodology for a novel reconfigurable assembly system. Their methodology is a holistic, hierarchical approach to system design which integrates reconfigurability principles, AD, and design structure matrices. A wing assembly case study is used to illustrate how the methodology translates reconfigurability requirements into a system that is scalable and flexible from the outset. The resultant reconfigurable cell design assembles the wing's spars and ribs with ramp up capability from 40 to 100 airplane per month.

18.2   Case Study: Airplane Fuselage Panel Assembly with Axiomatic Design Principles

This section presents a case study of the assembly of the fuselage panel to develop a cost-effective assembly system to ramp up to future production rates based on the AD methodology.

Figure 18.5 shows typical airplane fuselage sections. Airbus and Turkish Aerospace have signed the contract related with the manufacturing of Single-Aisle (A319/320/321) Airplane Section 19. Turkish Aerospace started manufacturing of Section 19 shells under the first phase of the program and started deliveries of these shells to Premium Aerotech Augsburg facilities. At the second phase, in addition to the shells, Turkish Aerospace will also manufacture Section 19 barrels and deliver these barrels to RUAG Oberpfaffenhofen facilities (Turkish Aerospace 2020).

Based on the contracts signed by the Turkish Aerospace, the customer needs and input constraints for the assembly of airplane fuselage structures are as follows:

- rate 5–20 airplane fuselages per month for the first ramp up;
- use certified processes and materials;
- meet all Airbus regulations and certifications;
- limited assembly area.

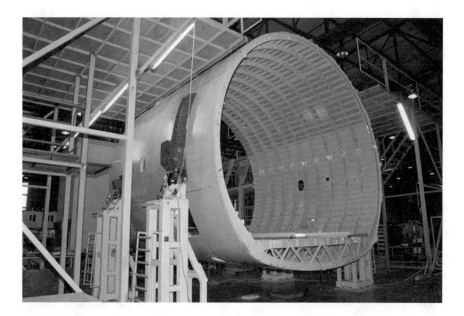

Fig. 18.5 Airplane fuselage section

Customer needs and input constraints convert FRs into (DPs) and process variables (PVs) to determine design properties of the assembly system. The decomposition process is designed to create a discrete system in order to make the system parameters independent of each other. They are consistent with constraints and needs. The first-level FRs and DPs for fuselage panel assembly is specified as follows:

FR1 = Assemble Airplane Fuselage Panels at Required Rate;
DP1 = Flexible and Scalable Assembly System.

At this stage, DPs and FRs are decomposed to their next levels, which are presented in Table 18.1. Focusing on the DPs, the methodology provides a solution for reconfigurability characteristics. Customization and scalability are embedded in the DPs. For second-level FRs and DPs to be consistent with the first-level and requirements are specified. The second-level FRs and DPs are specified as follows:
As an example, Consider FR13 and DP13 shown in Table 18.1, FR13 is needed to be satisfied by DP13 which is an automated drilling and fastening system. The systems are generally capable of carrying out drilling, countersinking, and fastening operations automatically by using computer-controlled numerical codes. They are originally designed to drill and to fasten airplane parts like panels, stringers, frames, and sections.

Table 18.1 Second-level FRs and DPs for fuselage panel assembly system

FRs-1	DPs-1
FR11: Position and locate beam component to fixture	**DP11**: Fixture system
FR12: Position and locate skin-stringer-clip components to the beam with tack rivets	**DP12**: Fixture system
FR13: Drill all components	**DP13**: Automated drilling and fastening systems
FR14: Remove components from the fixture deburr and clean	**DP14**: Scalable manual deburr and clean
FR15: Apply promoter, sealant relocate all components to the fixture	**DP15**: Scalable manual promoter, sealant application and relocation
FR16: Complete manual operations before final fastening	**DP16**: Scalable semi-automatic riveting system
FR17: Final fasten and assemble all components	**DP17**: Automatic riveting machine systems
FR18: Complete manual operations after final fastening	**DP18**: Scalable manual after machining operations
FR19: Apply paint, sealant, and varnish	**DP19**: Scalable robotic painting, sealant and varnish application

Also at this stage, the design equation is written to check if the system is coupled, decoupled, or uncoupled. Since the design matrix is diagonal, the system is an uncoupled design. The design matrix is constructed with the DPs where the FRs are met for this level as follows:

$$\begin{vmatrix} FR_{11} \\ FR_{12} \\ FR_{13} \\ FR_{14} \\ FR_{15} \\ FR_{16} \\ FR_{17} \\ FR_{18} \\ FR_{19} \end{vmatrix} = \begin{vmatrix} 1 & 0 & 0 & 0 & 0 & 0 & 0 & 0 & 0 \\ 0 & 1 & 0 & 0 & 0 & 0 & 0 & 0 & 0 \\ 0 & 0 & 1 & 0 & 0 & 0 & 0 & 0 & 0 \\ 0 & 0 & 0 & 1 & 0 & 0 & 0 & 0 & 0 \\ 0 & 0 & 0 & 0 & 1 & 0 & 0 & 0 & 0 \\ 0 & 0 & 0 & 0 & 0 & 1 & 0 & 0 & 0 \\ 0 & 0 & 0 & 0 & 0 & 0 & 1 & 0 & 0 \\ 0 & 0 & 0 & 0 & 0 & 0 & 0 & 1 & 0 \\ 0 & 0 & 0 & 0 & 0 & 0 & 0 & 0 & 1 \end{vmatrix} \begin{vmatrix} DP_{11} \\ DP_{12} \\ DP_{13} \\ DP_{14} \\ DP_{15} \\ DP_{16} \\ DP_{17} \\ DP_{18} \\ DP_{19} \end{vmatrix} \qquad (18.1)$$

Design decomposition is divided into subgroups by the zigzagging method, in which the design is expressed in more detail. It is aimed to obtain a physical and reasonable solution. The decomposition of the parameters continues until an existing solution becomes concrete and further decomposition is not physically possible. For the third level, the FRs and DPs are created as follows in Table 18.2.

The Following FRs and DPs in Table 18.2, FR132 is needed to be satisfied by DP132 which is frame assembly cell. In order to transfer holes to frame and fasten clips to frame, a more specific frame assembly cell is required. Frame assembly cell is capable of carrying out drilling, countersinking, and fastening clips to frame in airplane fuselage components either by using robots or advanced drilling and fastening machines.

Design decomposition proceeds with the same method and FRs and DPs are created for the fourth level as in Table 18.3.

DPs and FRs are specified at the next level, they are decomposed to be detailed more. *The Following FRs and DPs in* Table 18.3, FR1322 is needed to be satisfied by DP1322 which is frame clip robot. Frame clip robots that can be used as an alternative to frame clip riveters are designed for assembly of frames to clips in different types of airplane fuselage panels. The robot moves on rail systems which is robot's seventh axis movement. The accuracy of the robot is ±0.3 mm, repeatability is ±0.05 mm. The precision is achieved by calibration, pressure, and temperature compensation. Clamping force is 3000 daN, drill speed is 80 daN and

Table 18.2 Third-level FRs and DPs for fuselage panel assembly system

FRs-13	DPs-13
FR131: Constrain and positions clips	**DP131**: Manual operator
FR132: Transfer holes to frame and fasten clips to frame	**DP132**: Frame assembly cell
FR133: Increase drill rate for ramp up	**DP133**: Scalable architecture
FR134: Fasten components temporarily with tack rivets	**DP134**: Tack riveting module

Table 18.3 Fourth-level FRs and DPs for fuselage panel assembly system

FRs-132	DPs-132
FR1321: Fasten with riveting machine	**DP1321**: Frame riveter assembly cell
FR1322: Fasten with riveting robot	**DP1322**: Frame clip robot

drill spindle speed 500–6000 rpm with a peck-drilling functions. The robots are capable of clamping, drilling, countersinking, 5/32″, 6/32″, 7/32″, 8/32″, fastener insertion and squeezing processes up to 7 mm thickness of components. Figure 18.6. shows drilling and fastening robot similar to the frame clip robot.

FRs and DPs are created for the fifth level as in Table 18.4.

The Following FRs and DPs in Table 18.4, FR13222 is needed to be satisfied by DP13222 which is an all-electric riveting head. The all-electric riveting head includes drill feed unit, rivet inserter, rivet injector, tool changer, drill spindle, resynch camera, distance and normality sensors, rivet length measurement sensor, drill lubricator, pressure foot, and sealant applicator.

FRs and DPs at the lowest level correspond to a specific part feature, mechanism, or system. Finally, design hierarchy decomposition is illustrated as an example up to level 6. FRs and DPs are created for the sixth and last level as shown in Table 18.5.

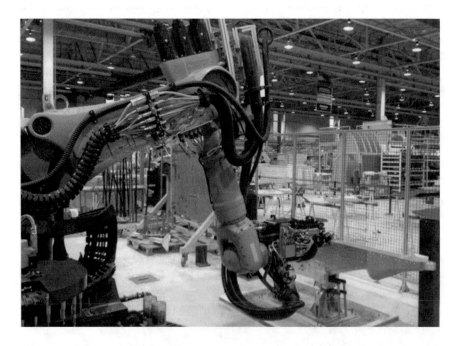

Fig. 18.6 Drilling and fastening robots

Table 18.4 Fifth-level FRs and DPs for fuselage panel assembly system

FRs-1322	DPs-1322
FR13221: Move the robot for appropriate position	**DP13221**: Rail platform
FR13222: Fasten clips to frame	**DP13222**: All electric riveting head

Table 18.5 Sixth-level FRs and DPs for fuselage panel assembly system

FRs-13212	DPs-13212
FR132121: Position the fuselage panel	**DP132121**: Position sensors
FR132122: Select appropriate drill bit and drill the component	**DP132122**: Drilling unit
FR132123: Insert rivet	**DP132123**: Rivet inserter
FR132124: Squeeze rivet	**DP132124**: Upper pressure foot and lower anvil

General assembly system design hierarchy tree (Fig. 18.7) is obtained using FR and DP information which is explained in detail above. Different alternative systems can be obtained by using the general assembly system design hierarchy tree. Figures 18.8 and 18.9 present an alternative assembly system. This system includes primarily an automatic riveting machine and autonomous mobile robots. On the other hand, a second alternative which includes riveting robots and modular crane for panel handling purposes is presented in Figs. 18.10 and 18.11.

18.3   Assembly System Design Alternatives Simulation Results

The first assembly system design alternative includes fully automated laser tracker for measurement systems, reconfigurable fixtures for fixing the panels, frame clip robots in frame assembly cells for the clip to frame assembly, 3D projection devices for fasteners position controls on the panels, autonomous mobile robots for material handling, and automatic riveting machines for final fuselage panel assembly.

Second assembly system design alternative includes robotic measurement systems for measurement, robotic stringer placement robots for stringer positioning, reconfigurable fixtures for fixing the panels, frame clip robots for clip to frame assembly, 3D projection devices for fasteners position controls on the panels, modular crane for material handling and mobile automated drilling and fastening robots for final fuselage panel assembly.

After completion of simulations, results show that the second alternative is better than the first alternative by production rate.

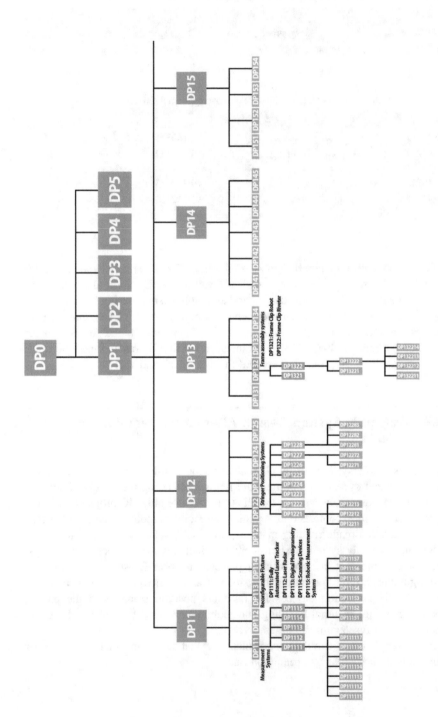

Fig. 18.7 General assembly system design hierarchy tree

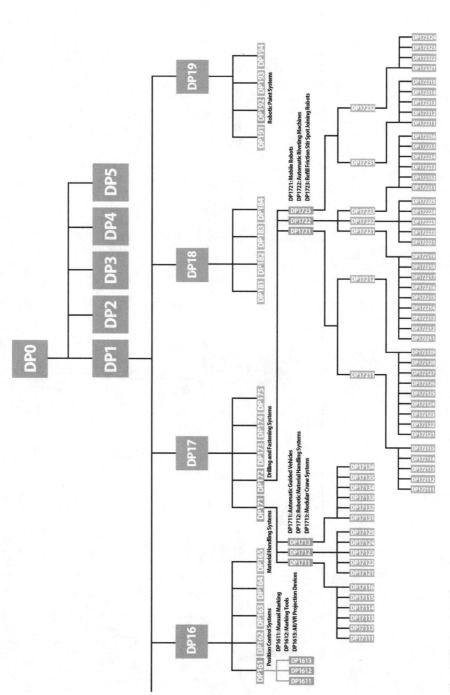

Fig. 18.7 (continued)

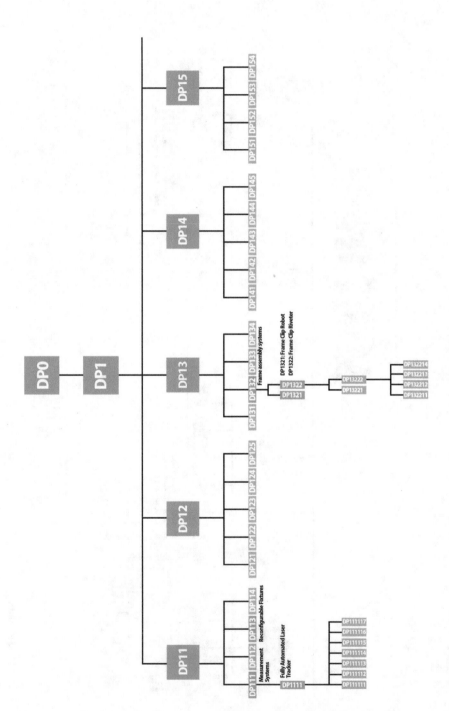

Fig. 18.8 Assembly system design alternative-1

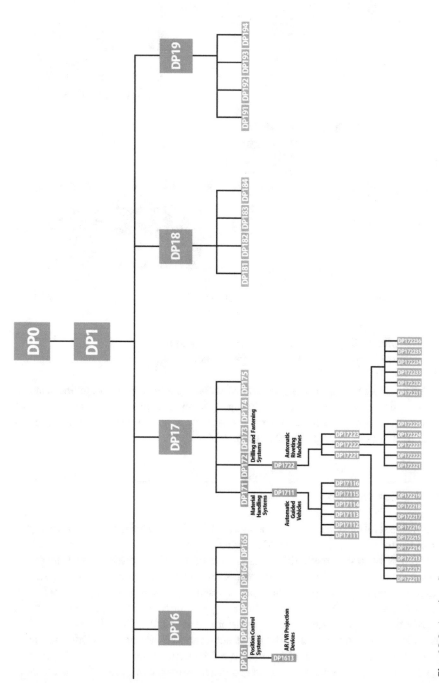

Fig. 18.8 (continued)

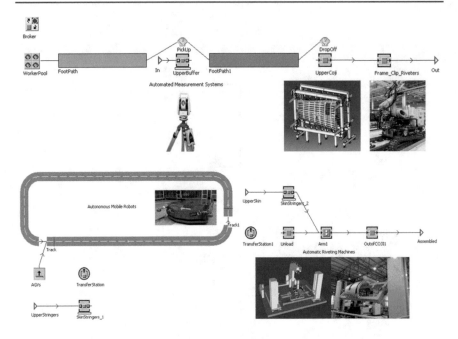

Fig. 18.9 Simulation of assembly system design alternative-1

- **First alternative:** 138 fuselage panels per month.
- **Second alternative:** 153 fuselage panels per month.

Koren and Shpitalni (2010) developed a comparison table for combine features of reconfigurable/flexible manufacturing systems (dedicated or random order). A new table is created for comparison results of assembly system design alternatives for airplane fuselage panels (Table 18.6).

18.4 Conclusion

A novel assembly system design methodology is developed by using AD principles in order to propose a solution to design airplane fuselage panel assembly. The framework of design methodology is developed based on system design methods, academic research, industry requirements, and industrial case studies. An Airbus A320 airplane Section 19 fuselage panel assembly case study is carried out for a better understanding of how the methodology is applied. Customer requirements are transformed into FRs, and FRs are transformed into DPs. The DPs are detailed in the design structure matrix and related sub-functions are created. Different alternative systems can be created by using the design hierarchy tree. Accordingly, two system alternatives for airplane fuselage panel assembly are presented to illustrate

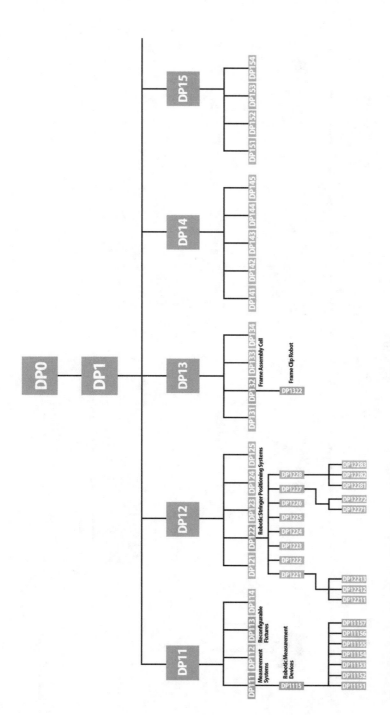

Fig. 18.10 Assembly System Design Alternative-2

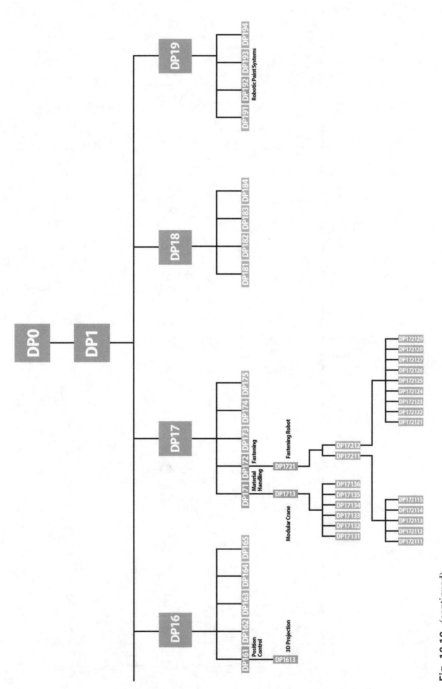

Fig. 18.10 (continued)

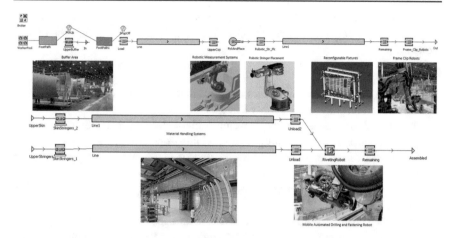

Fig. 18.11 Simulation of assembly system design alternative-2

Table 18.6 Comparison of the assembly system design alternatives

	Assembly system design for airplane structures	
	Alternative-1	Alternative-2
System structure	Fixed	Adjustable
Machine structure	Fixed	Adjustable
Customization[a]	Yes	Yes
Convertibility[b]	No	Yes
Scalability[c]	Yes	Yes
Modularity[d]	No	Yes
Integrability[e]	No	Yes
Diagnosability[f]	No	Yes
Reconfigurability	Customized	Customized
Throughput	High	Very high
Productivity	High	Very high
Lifetime cost	High	High
Configuration time	High	Medium
Time loss	Low	Very low

Customization[a]: flexibility limited to part family
Convertibility[b]: design for functionality changes
Scalability[c]: design for a capacity change
Modularity[d]: components are modular
Integrability[e]: interfaces for rapid integration
Diagnosability[f]: design for easy diagnostics

the application of AD methodology. This case study is aimed to be used as a reference guide for the design of similar assembly systems in the aerospace industry.

Problems

1. What can be the system-wide FRs and DPs that can be put at the first level of a design hierarchy for an assembly system?
2. Return back to the case study. Develop a hierarchy tree that provides a single system solution instead of multiple ones. Compare your result with the solutions obtained in the case study. Discuss whether it is better to limit your solution space in developing your decision hierarchy.
3. What advantages did the usage of AD methodology bring to the assembly system design?
4. Does the proposed approach always encourage usage of automated and advanced but more expensive technologies? Under which conditions more conventional technologies can be recommended for usage in assembly systems?
5. One of the authors stated that "Application of the AD Approach required a detailed and complete review of all technologies that are used/have potential to be used in a fuselage panel assembly system." The authors spent more time and effort in this review process than the development of the hierarchy tree. Test the correctness of the above statement by applying AD approach to a simple assembly system?
6. Are there any other design approaches available in the literature that can be used in development of alternative assembly system solutions? Try to apply those approaches to the same case study.

References

Bullen GN (2013) Automated/mechanized drilling and countersinking of airframes. SAE International, Warrendale, Pennsylvania, USA. https://www.sae.org/publications/books/content/r-416/, product code: R-416

Federal Aviation Administration (2018) Aviation Maintenance Technician Handbook—Air-frame, vol 1. US Department of Transportation. https://www.faa.gov/regulations_policies/handbooks_manuals/aircraft/media/amt_airframe_hb_vol_1.pdf, document FAA-H-8083-31

Groover MP (2007) Automation, production systems, and computer-integrated manufacturing, 3rd edn. Prentice Hall, Upper Saddle River, NJ, USA

Jefferson TG, Benardos P, Ratchev S (2016) Reconfigurable assembly system design methodology: a wing assembly case study. SAE Int J Mater Manufact 9(1):31–48. https://doi.org/10.4271/2015-01-2594

Jeppesen Sanderson, Inc, Atlantic Flight Training, Ltd (2007) Airframes and systems: JAA ATPL training, 2nd edn. No. 4 in ATPL series, Jeppesen Sanderson, Inc., Neu-Isenburg, Germany

Koren Y, Shpitalni M (2010) Design of reconfigurable manufacturing systems. J Manufact Syst 29(4):130–141. https://doi.org/10.1016/j.jmsy.2011.01.001

Kulak O, Durmuşoğlu B, Tufekci S (2005) A complete cellular manufacturing system design methodology based on axiomatic design principles. Comput Indus Eng 48(4):765–787. https://www.sciencedirect.com/science/article/pii/S0360835204001901

Reynal VA, Cochran DS (1996) Understanding lean manufacturing according to axiomatic design principles. The Lean Aircraft Intiative Report Series, URL https://axiomaticdesign.com/technology/papers/RP960728Cochran_Reynal.pdf, document RP96–07–28

Turkish Aerospace (2020) AIRBUS—PAG SA Section 19 Shells&Barrel Program. https://www.tai.com.tr/en/product/airbus-pag-sa-section-19-shellsbarrel-program

Weber A (2015) Assembly automation takes off in aerospace industry. Assembly Magazine. https://www.assemblymag.com/articles/92790-assembly-automation-takes-off-in-aerospace-industry

Healthcare System Design

19

Inas S. Khayal and Amro M. Farid

Abstract

This book includes several design applications in several fields: energy, large systems, manufacturing, and many more. In this chapter, we turn our focus to the design of healthcare systems. But first, we ask what exactly do we mean by healthcare systems? This chapter will describe the large scale and scope of what is meant by the phrase "healthcare systems." A broad definition of Healthcare System Design consequently leads to the recognition of the large number of stakeholders affected by such designs. The need for appropriate, effective, timely, sustainable, and cost-effective healthcare services has been recognized globally, and has led to an increasingly growing healthcare sector. As the healthcare sector continues to expand, there are several unique challenges that have risen due to the many siloed designers acting on different parts of the healthcare system. The goal of this chapter is to orient the reader to the various scale and scope of healthcare systems and to present a structure that allows the reader to thoughtfully consider the design process relative to stakeholders, system boundary, system functions for functional requirement (FR) selection, system form for design parameter selection (DP), and consequently the process variables (PV).

I. S. Khayal (✉)
The Dartmouth Institue for Health Policy and Clinical Medicine and Biomedical Data Science, Geisel School of Medicine at Dartmouth, Lebanon, NH, USA
e-mail: ikhayal@berkeley.edu

I. S. Khayal · A. M. Farid
Department of Computer Science, Dartmouth College, Hanover, NH, USA

A. M. Farid
Thayer School of Engineering at Dartmouth, Hanover, NH, USA

A. M. Farid
MIT Mechanical Engineering, Cambridge, MA 02139, USA

© Springer Nature Switzerland AG 2021
N. P. Suh et al. (eds.), *Design Engineering and Science*,
https://doi.org/10.1007/978-3-030-49232-8_19

19.1   Introduction

19.1.1   Motivation

As a reader of this book, your career may include designing across multiple sectors or may focus on a single sector. This chapter will focus on healthcare. While it may seem like a niche service, healthcare is currently the largest employer in the United States, accounting for about 18% of the gross domestic product (GDP) or an expenditure of $11,000 per person in 2018. Why is that?

People are living longer today than in any time in human history. The aging population along with a continuous growth in medical spending has led to an increased rate of healthcare jobs in the United States and globally. Interestingly, although science and technology have allowed for significant advancements in health treatments, humanity is facing an unprecedented chronic disease burden. While we may live longer, most will struggle with many more long-duration chronic diseases—such as diabetes, heart disease, autoimmunity, and cancer. Such a significant disease burden has caused the healthcare sector to expand to address the many challenges that arise when treating or managing health conditions today. This sector is one of the most labor-intensive fields, requiring expensive medication and individualized services, and highly educated service personnel.

19.1.2   Chapter Outline

Section 19.2 starts with how to define the healthcare system. Healthcare design has many varying levels of scale and scope. Therefore, understanding and identifying the scale and scope is critical to a successful design [Sect. 19.2.1]. Then, Sect. 19.2.2 presents a framework for thinking about what the healthcare system does (*functions*) and who or what performs these functions (*resources*). While many engineered designs are for stock products, healthcare designs are in many cases customized and will vary by region, country, culture, or even individual patients. Understanding the variation in FRs and/or DPs in this broad context is discussed in Sect. 19.2.3.

Section 19.3 discusses the characteristic and often unique challenges found within healthcare systems. The discussion addresses the significant heterogeneity of function and form even within a specific country, region, or hospital [Sect. 19.3.1]. While many engineered systems are typically defined as technical systems, healthcare is fundamentally socio-technical. Unique implementation and outcome challenges emerge as a result [Sect. 19.3.2]. Despite the range in scale, scope, heterogeneity, complexity, and regional impact of healthcare services, there is a need to interconnect healthcare systems. Consequently, designing for interoperability is a critical consideration for success [Sect. 19.3.3]. Finally, healthcare is a legacy system. It is hard to change what has been already designed—be it technical in nature or social in nature. Therefore, understanding the existing system, which of its aspects are flexible, and why is a critical consideration to healthcare design [Sect. 19.3.4]. Finally, Sect. 19.4 summarizes the key takeaways and conclusions.

19.2   Defining a Healthcare System

Defining a healthcare system includes identifying the system boundary, the scale and scope of the problem, and a framework to organize the system. As described in previous chapters, with a dedicated chapter to the topic (Chap. 5: *Problem Definition*), *accurately identifying the problem* is absolutely critical. This section will stress the importance of *accurately identifying the problem* and consequently help the design reader to distinguish between "what is designed" and the remainder of the healthcare system.

Design Story 19.1: Pacemaker

In 1951, a Boston cardiologist is given credit for ushering in the modern era of clinical cardiac pacing, the fitting of a device—a pacemaker—to maintain a regular heart rhythm. Since then, cardiac pacemakers have advanced tremendously. One of the primary customer requirements for a permanent (internal to the body) pacemaker is its ability to function for a long period of time, to avoid further invasive surgeries to the patient. This customer requirement appears as a design constraint on two DPs: the size of the battery and the power consumption of the pulse generator.[1] Traditional biomedical engineering design devotes much effort to continuously improve on this customer requirement. Despite these efforts, the traditional pacemaker design neglects an important FRs, namely, to turn it off!

A classic "device-engineer" may wonder, "why would you ever need to do that?" In reality, the complex needs of today's diverse cardiac patients have made this FRs evermore critical to not just the patient, but also their entire healthcare team. Unfortunately, such a requirement did not arise from a sterile stakeholder requirement identification process but rather from design failure and emotional heart break.

Although people are living longer today, they are often doing so with chronic as-yet incurable diseases. For example, dementia is a progressive condition where the brain deteriorates, and the individual loses their ability to remember. Such a condition is emotionally, socially, and physically taxing on both the individual and their family. Many patients with dementia, typically in their 60s, 70s, or 80s, also tend to have deteriorating heart conditions. Many of them received a pacemaker prior to dementia or during its early onset. Some patients believe that as dementia

---

[1]Interestingly, this design constraint creates an inevitable coupled design between the battery and the pulse generator. Such a coupled design appears in many applications where "on-board" energy storage and the need for miniaturization create an energy budget and a constraining volume for the device as a whole.

comes to a late stage, it can cause so much suffering that they would prefer not to prolong their lives with artificial measures like cardiac devices. In the United States, patients at least have the right to refuse or discontinue treatment, including a pacemaker that keeps them alive. Physicians also have a right to refuse to turn it off. These two seemingly contradictory legal rights have raised a significant ethical question. Is it ethical to deactivate a pacemaker in patients with a chronic debilitating condition given that its use in such patients significantly extends their life, but at a questionable quality of life for both the patient and their family? Many engineers would consider this a "messy" ethical or legal issue. However, in reality, the identification of the "turn-off" FRs is a fundamental engineering design question that would have alleviated many stakeholder ramifications. From a design perspective, we can include an FR to "turn-off" the device with a corresponding DP. Where the issue becomes difficult is setting up a corresponding DP that addresses the various types of individuals that may turn-off the device (e.g., clinicians, family members, etc.) and a thorough protocol to do so that considers the ethical, moral, and religious questions of who makes the decision to "turn-off" the device. Therefore, the design of healthcare protocols and procedures that resolve these ethical questions is an integral part of healthcare organizational design.

19.2.1 Healthcare System Boundary, Scope, and Scale

The concept of the system implies and requires a boundary that distinguishes it from everything else. Such a boundary can be defined with varying scope. For example, one may be interested in reducing knee pain, which may be stated as an FR. A designer can create one or more systems defined with increasing scope: "a knee implant," "a knee replacement surgical suite," "a knee replacement service including the surgical suite and surgical team," "an orthopedic clinic with integrated physical therapy services," or "a hospital". Each of these scopes provide additional functions that ultimately serve to reduce knee pain. The logic here is that while a knee implant can reduce knee pain, it has limited efficacy without the technical facilities and human resources to conduct the knee replacement, the post-surgery follow-up care, and the integration with other healthcare services that may be required in the event of complications. A designer may be responsible for designing a healthcare system with any of these degrees of scope. Consequently, the choice of a widening system boundary may result in a design that could be described as a "product," "software," "both product and software," and "organizations" (see Chap. 16).

Unfortunately, the designer may not necessarily have control over the delineation or the clarity of the system boundary. Its specification may be set externally, by the design-client organization, by politics, or even healthcare regulation laws. While external specification of the system boundary alleviates this design choice from the designer's responsibility, it does not alleviate the burden of ensuring that the to-be-designed-system integrates well into the larger healthcare system and produces the expected health-outcome results. In short, and like many other large-scale systems, the designer is only *responsible* for the "system" but is actually *accountable* for its integration with a larger *"whole-system."*

The choice of the system boundary and scope also implies the scale of the system design. As the designer broadens the scope of their healthcare system, they are inevitably forced to view the system's function and form at a fairly high level of abstraction. Rather than focusing on the individual features of a given device, they must now consider entire healthcare system resources be they operating rooms, departments, or entire healthcare facilities. Once the designer has chosen such a scale, the system can then be decomposed iteratively into its component parts, starting from the highest FRs and DPs to a lower level FRs and DPs. Once the decomposition is done up to a point without introducing any coupling of FRs, the lower level FRs can be parceled out and given to different groups for further decomposition and implementation. This is how complicated systems such as airplanes (see Chap. 18) and wireless electric buses (i.e., On-Line Electric Vehicle (OLEV) (Suh and Cho 2017)) have been created. The important thing to implement in this process is the careful monitoring of the design tree and the creation of the Master Design Matrix discussed in Chap. 3 to quickly identify any coupling in the design that may be introduced by one of the participants in the design group.

It is generally accepted that after 1000 components have been identified, the system can no longer be practically designed by a single designer. In such a case, the designer must form a design team to address different part of the system which can be later integrated. At a scale of 10,000 components, the system can be referred to as a system-of-systems that inevitably requires multiple design teams. In such a situation, the coordination of the design effort becomes as significant as the design itself. The possibility of introducing coupling due to the decisions made by a designer who is working on other branches of decomposition exists, which can be prevented if the team under the system architect follows the entire process and constructs the master design matrix to identify any inadvertent coupling of FRs.

Design Story 19.2: Endovascular Aortic Aneurysm Repair Device

A company in California manufactures an internal implant called an endograft used in a procedure called an endovascular aortic aneurysm repair (EVR). EVR was developed almost three decades ago as a minimally invasive alternative to a surgical procedure to address abdominal aortic aneurysms (AAA)—a bulge in the wall of the main blood vessel leading away from the heart to the abdomen. They innovatively designed their endograft to have the main body stabilized by resting directly on the aortic bifurcation rather than using hooks for fixation with the fabric of the endograft affixed to the stent skeleton only at the top and bottom of the device. This design created a novel sealing concept that reduces the possibility of device migration and leakage (i.e., reducing the risk of what is considered a type 1 endoleak—flow around the proximal or distal seal zones of the endograft).

At the time of initial manufacturing, the graft was a stratra fabric. Upon introduction into the healthcare delivery system, it yielded increased reports of Type III endoleaks (i.e., those caused by defects in the endograft device) for patients with significant aortic remodeling. Endoleaks are a type of uncommon but nevertheless serious late stage complication that has a high risk of rupture and death. A study found that there was a 24% chance of Type III endoleaks due to fabric breakdown. The company consequently provided a safety notice to providers. The United States Food and Drug Administration (FDA) classified this notice as a Class I recall (i.e., the most serious). Since then, the company has updated their graft material to a new formulation.

This design story demonstrates how a new and unique biomedical product can be completely successful upon first use, but later have unintended life-threatening consequences as the human biology (in the form of aortic remodeling) adapts to the integration. Furthermore, the device's novelty created an endoskeleton design that may complicate guidewire and device entry on redo procedures. Such a design considers the biological integrity of an initial procedure, but neglects the very realistic potential for complications in this relatively minimally invasive EVR procedure.

The above discussion emphasizes the importance of the system boundary in healthcare system design. Not only does it affect the scope and scale of the design, but it also requires a deep appreciation of how the system will affect and be affected by its introduction into the healthcare delivery system. The chapter now provides a formal systems framework for the description of a healthcare system.

19.2.2 Healthcare System Function and System Form

In addition to the system boundary, a system is defined by *what* it does—its *system function*, and *how* these functions are performed—its *system form*. The system function is made up of a set of functions that fulfill the system's *FRs*. The system form (in large-scale systems) is made up of a set of resources that are described by *DPS*.

An understanding of system function and form is now particularly important as the designer begins to understand the state of the healthcare system today. Historically, the healthcare system has been organized based on form and *not* function. A typical hospital has a departmental structure that addresses specific body parts (e.g., Rheumatology [Joints], Neurology [Brain], Cardiology [Heart], Endocrinology [Hormones], etc.). Similarly, at a higher level of aggregation, healthcare systems are also defined by location. For example, a typical hospital has inpatient and outpatient wings to distinguish between patients that will or will not stay overnight.

Furthermore, within these wings and departments, healthcare is typically described by *who* provides the function, rather than the function itself. Simply speaking, when someone needs care, they go to see a general physician, surgeon, or psychiatrist. In other words, the hospital is organized by system resources rather than the system functions that they provide. While it seems intuitive to describe surgery-care by the resource performing the surgery (i.e., the surgeon), from a system design perspective, such a description omits the inclusion of the care-function itself! For example, surgery can be defined as "a procedure that involves *cutting* of a patient's tissues or closure of a previously sustained wound." Furthermore, the Merriam-Webster Medical Dictionary defines surgery as a noun and not a verb. To a lay patient audience, this system resource-based description of healthcare may be appropriate. However, it is pervasive and appears as an integral part of clinical models used in professional practice and academic research (e.g., behavioral health models, serious illness care models). Consequently, the very models used as a system-level description of clinical practice do not define the needed functions but instead describe the type of provider that should be performing these non-explicitly stated functions.

While healthcare is not perfect, it does seem to be functional. At first appearance, patients receive the care that they need. So, what is the problem with how the healthcare field describes and defines its system? The answer lies in the nature of the care itself. Conventional clinical practice utilizes a reductionist approach directed primarily toward acute conditions. In recent years, however, healthcare needs have significantly shifted from treating acute conditions to treating chronic conditions. 78% of total healthcare costs in the United States are now due to chronic disease. Consequently, clinical medicine needs to shift toward addressing the growing chronic disease epidemic. Unlike acute conditions, chronic conditions are particularly complex in that they tend to involve multiple factors with multiple interactions between them. The medical science literature has now established that combating chronic disease requires treating the patient holistically. Doing so will require systems thinking that entirely redesigns existing healthcare approaches rather simply "reworking" or "reapplying" of acute care models.

Despite the growing need posed by chronic conditions, the relative absence of systems-level engineering design descriptions of healthcare inhibit designers and non-medically trained individuals from understanding the field and its terminology. This linguistic and conceptual gap has isolated healthcare, leaving many engineering design efforts to contribute in a siloed fashion. For example, biomedical engineering focuses on developing devices that measure and deliver treatment. The growing efforts in health informatics develop software solutions that support clinical decision-making. Finally, the field of healthcare logistics optimizes the flow of the patients through the healthcare system. Nevertheless, it is less than clear how these disparate efforts actually improve patient outcomes. In contrast, the recent efforts in healthcare system design focus on redesigning the clinical patterns of practice with patient outcomes firmly in mind, drawing upon not just medical science but also the many types of engineering solutions mentioned above. Here, the designer(s) must intersect engineering, systems thinking, and formal design methods from a diversity of practitioners in different fields. The first step in doing so is getting everyone "to speak the same language." That is, the designer must gain an awareness of and reconcile the linguistic and conceptual discrepancies between these many fields.

In the past, designers remained within the technical realm; thus, avoiding much of these discrepancies. They could become experts in knees or hearts; addressing the acute injuries to these parts of the body. However, the chronic diseases of today are multifaceted and consequently require services from several healthcare departments in potentially different locations. In effect, the patient experience of a multifaceted chronic condition creates a significant need for integration. Therefore, designers must simultaneously understand how their technology, devices, and software affect the patient experience and integrate within the larger healthcare system. For example, at the outset, diabetes care involves an endocrinologist to regulate the insulin hormone. However, advanced diabetes patients can experience complications. Foot damage requires podiatry, eye damage requires ophthalmology, and kidney damage requires nephrology. These many types of medical specialists are not typically trained to coordinate care between each other. Consequently, Diabetes Centers have emerged as places where all of a diabetes patient's needs can be provided. Despite the presence of such facilities, and patients' preference for them, most patients still receive care in a typical, medically siloed, healthcare environment.

Healthcare systems are complex. Introducing technical artifacts that were designed using Axiomatic Design (AD) is one level of complexity. Using AD to design the healthcare system incorporating many technical and human resources is more complex. The following emergency department design story describes the importance of the need to understand the many aspects of a healthcare system.

Design Story 19.3: Emergency Department

Emergency departments (EDs) are considered the safety net within the United States healthcare system. Unlike typical healthcare departments, emergency departments are open 24 hours a day, 7 days a week. Emergency departments provide care to individuals with illnesses or conditions requiring immediate attention. They are also a safety net for uninsured individuals that only have emergency departments as care options.

Growing demand for emergency departments have *not* led to increases in ED capacity. On the contrary, ED numbers are decreasing. Consequently, challenges of ED overcrowding have led many medical professionals to turn to systems scientists and complex system designers in order to find robust solutions.

With the understanding that the ED is a complex system that is working toward specific goals, it is necessary to understand those goals clearly on all levels in order to properly analyze and re-design the system (Peck 2008). The design team developed a four-level emergency department design decomposition (ED^3). Initial analysis showed very high levels of coupling between the DPS and FRs, thus a clearly coupled system. This design example focuses on one area of the ED—triage to address and manage patient flow. The classic system of triage sorts patients based on urgency called the emergency severity index (ESI). When using the ESI system to facilitate patient flow, its original purpose may suffer due to a coupled design. The use of AD led to the creation of a new index based on how long a patient is likely to remain in the ED. By introducing a new index for patient flow, the design problem was then uncoupled. By doing so, patient wait times were significantly decreased ($\sim 50\%$) compared to typical operations.

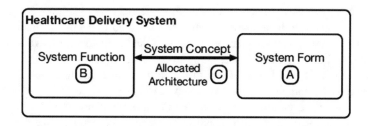

Fig. 19.1 Diagram showing system form, system function, and the allocation of the latter to the former called the system concept. (Reproduced from Khayal (2019), originally published open access under a CC BY 4.0 license: https://doi.org/10.3390/systems7010018).

The remainder of this section describes a system model architecture for personalized healthcare delivery (Khayal and Farid 2018). It formally defines the *system function* and *system form* for healthcare. A visual representation is shown in Fig. 19.1.

System Functions

The primary functions in healthcare are identified based on how clinical medicine is practiced: the diagnostic model. First, it examines the individual's concern or complaint. Second, it attempts to determine its cause. Third, it applies a treatment regimen to that cause. Using solution-neutral language, these functions sequentially are.

(1) measurement: understand, quantify, or classify individual health state;

(2) decision: determine what to do for the individual and when;

(3) transformation: perform treatment service(s) for the individual;

(4) transportation: move the individual between any of these processes, if needed.

Here, it is important to recognize the term "individual" as the primary operand of the healthcare system. It is used instead of the more common term "patient" to reflect that the current "healthcare" system is actually a reactive "sick-care" system that treats individuals only after they have become ill. In order to design a proactive "healthcare" system then the primary operand must be a healthy individual who uses the system to maintain or improve a healthy state, prevent its degradation, and only recover the health state if illness prevails.

Measurement is a cyber-physical process that converts a physical property of the operand (i.e., the individual) into a cyber, informatic property to ascertain their health state. Typical healthcare measurement processes include clinical evaluation, diagnostic tests (e.g., blood, urine, and stool) and diagnostic procedures (e.g., medical imaging, endoscopy, and electrocardiography).

Decision is a cyber-physical process occurring between a healthcare system resource and the operand-individual. In cooperation with the individual, the healthcare system resource generates a decision on how to proceed next with the healthcare system. Several types of decision processes exist. Planning is defined as the decision of which healthcare system functions need to occur for the individual in the form of a treatment plan or strategy. Scheduling includes two integrated decisions; a choice of who/what is going to perform the functions in the treatment plan, and a choice of when to do so in the form of an individual's booking. The distinction is important because, in many cases, exclusivity relationships may appear between the individual and the healthcare system resource, be it imposed externally as in the case of many healthcare insurance providers or freely chosen as rapport is developed between a medical professional and the individual. This chapter focuses on the atemporal aspects of planning and scheduling decisions; those that directly affect the choice of treatment and who/what is going to execute it. While many engineers may gravitate quickly toward the development of measurement and treatment technologies, human-centered design encourages us to step-back and understand how the clinician and the individual will together decide on using the measurement or treatment technology as part of a larger treatment plan. For example, the best way to see and address gastro-intestinal and colon cancers is through preventative colonoscopy. The procedure uses a device called a colonoscope. It is a long, flexible, tubular instrument used to image the lining of the colon and take biopsy samples. During the procedure, it is inserted through the rectum and advanced to the other end of the large intestine. Many individuals refuse this uncomfortable procedure and select a less-effective imaging-based procedure instead. Such a planning decision naturally draws upon further information such as cancer risk, family history, and reaction to drugs.

Transformation is a physical process that transforms the operand, specifically, the internal health state of the individual. Such processes include surgical procedures such as amputation, ablation, and laparoscopic surgery, and therapeutic procedures such as pharmacotherapy, chemotherapy, and physical therapy.

Transportation is a physical process that moves the individual between healthcare resources. It is included here for the sake of completeness because only incapacitated individuals need to be moved. For example, a nurse can move an individual from the emergency department's operating theatre to the recovery room.

System Form

As mentioned previously, the system form (in large-scale systems) is made up of a set of resources that are further described by DPs. Each of the resources defined below includes a set union of human and technical resources. In the healthcare field, a designer should expect that each newly designed technical resource requires a human resource to operate it. For example, the operation of a push wheel chair can be performed by any adult whereas the operation of a surgical robot system requires years of specialist clinical training. Again, the design of a technical resource must explicitly consider the system boundary and more specifically the often non-technical nature of the human operator. The consequent implementation and outcome challenges are discussed in Sect. 19.3.

A *Measurement resource* is a resource capable of measuring the operand; here, the health state of an individual. Human measurement resources include MRI technicians, sonographers, and phlebotomists. Technical measurement resources include magnetic resonance imaging scanners, ultrasound machines, and syringes.

A *Decision resource* is a resource capable of advising the operand-individual on how to proceed next with the healthcare delivery system. Human decision resources include oncologists and general practitioners. Technical decision resources include decision support systems and electronic medical record decision tools.

A *Treatment resource* is a resource capable of a transformative effect on its operand: the health state of an individual. Human transformation resources include surgeons, oncology infusion nurses, and physical therapists. Technical transformation resources include operating theatres, chemotherapy infusion rooms, and physical therapy rooms.

A *Transportation resource* is a resource capable of transporting the operand-individual. Human transportation resources include emergency medical technicians, clinical care coordinators, and transporters. Technical transportation resources include ambulances, gurneys, and wheelchairs.

19.2.3 Variations of Healthcare System Function and System Form Across Cultures and Regions

Engineering design is often viewed as the utilization of universal scientific first-principles to produce designs that can be used universally across cultures and regions. More recently, the field of manufacturing has recognized that many products must be "mass-customized" in order to serve the preferences of a wide variety of customers. In much the same way, and probably to an even greater extent, the healthcare system has many levels of design that are impacted by the biology and culture of people in different regions.

National-Financial Level

While the term healthcare elicits a focus on medicine, the financing of healthcare is a significant driver of how, where, when, and what healthcare services are available to a population. For example, Japan simultaneously faces a growing aging population and a shrinking young population. Consequently, the healthcare industry has focused on developing technical resources like social robots rather than human resources like home-nurses. Such a design decision delivers a healthcare system delivery model within the financial constraints of the country.

Social Level

The social level affects many aspects of healthcare services; most importantly its community-wide acceptability.

Healthcare systems are increasingly utilizing new community structures to deliver their services. For example, many healthcare systems are utilizing social media platforms to provide peer-patient-to-peer-patient support networks. Alcoholics Anonymous is one such successful network in the United States. Such peer networks create a strong emotional bond across individuals with a similar condition. In certain cultures, however, there remains significant social stigma towards certain diseases. For example, in some cultures women have significant difficulty marrying if they are identified as having certain diseases. Furthermore, some societies, cultures, and/or religions place restrictions on certain types of healthcare interventions like birth control and abortions.

Biological Level

In addition to national and social factors, healthcare system design must also consider variations in biological factors. The testing of healthcare treatments today requires that clinical trials specifically note the ethnicity of the studies' participants. Medical science has generally accepted that such variations as they stem from ethnicity and culture affect study efficacy.

Medical research today has also recognized that although new treatments are tested for a wide variety of ethnicities, the design of new treatments still follows a one-size-fits-all approach. The latest healthcare trend advocates for "personalized medicine" where therapies are tailored to specific individuals. Such an approach takes into account an individual's unique molecular and genetic profile to predict whether a given medical treatment will be safe and effective.

Design Story 19.4: Healthcare Labor Market Volatility Assessment

The quality and reliability of a nation's healthcare system is often driven by the number and diversity of its healthcare professionals. Unfortunately, many developing nations often suffer from very constrained segments in their highly skilled labor market and hence must "import" this human capital. Volatility in key healthcare professions can threaten reliable and sustainable healthcare delivery. In this design story, AD was used to develop a system to assess volatility of healthcare human resource in a country in the middle east. The FRs for the system were defined and aggregated as a set of healthcare professions: FR = {Healthcare Professions}. The functional domain is only addressed at this level of hierarchy as it is important to be able to distinguish between these individual healthcare functions throughout the analysis. In contrast, the physical domain can be analyzed at several levels of hierarchy. But one of the hierarchies would describe a decoupled system. Each individual healthcare professional is a distinct healthcare resource. Healthcare professionals can be aggregated by their professional licensing degree: DP = {Healthcare License Degree}. When designing based on resources, each individual can be aggregated based on where they practice: DP={Healthcare Facility} and in what region: DP = {Geographic Region}. For this example, the DP level is chosen such that this system is decoupled.

Example FRs include: and   Example DPs include:

FR#	Description
FR1	Nutrition
FR2	Pathology
FR3	Dermatology
FR4	Physiotherapy
FR5	Ophthalmology
FR6	Anesthesiology
FR7	Obstetrics and gynecology
FR8	Emergency medicine
FR9	Pediatrics
FR10	Radiology
FR11	Internal medicine
FR12	Midwifery
FR13	Surgery
FR14	Dentistry
FR15	Medical laboratory
FR16	Clinical support
FR17	Pharmacy
FR18	Nursing

DP#	Description
DP1	Nutritionist
DP2	Pathologist
DP3	Dermatologist
DP4	Physiotherapist
DP5	Ophthalmologist
DP6	Anesthesiologist
DP7	Obstetrics and gynecologist
DP8	Emergency medicine doctor
DP9	Pediatrician
DP10	Radiologist
DP11	Internal medicine doctor
DP12	Midwife
DP13	Surgeon
DP14	Dentist
DP15	Medical laboratory technician
DP16	Clinical support staff
DP17	Pharmacist
DP18	Nurse

19.3 Challenges Specific to the Design of Healthcare Systems

The previous section served to describe several systems thinking abstractions for a healthcare system: system boundary, scale, scope, function, and form. All of these are key aspects that need to be considered when designing a healthcare system. In doing so, Sect. 19.2 touched on several challenges specific to the healthcare field. This section enumerates four key challenges to consider when designing healthcare systems. They include healthcare as a socio-technical system (in Sect. 19.3.1), heterogeneity (in Sect. 19.3.2), complexity and interoperability (in Sect. 19.3.3), and understanding legacy systems (in Sect. 19.3.4).

19.3.1 Healthcare is a Socio-Technical System

Section 19.2 described that every designed technical resource requires a human resource to operate it. For many engineering designers, the defined system boundary may be a completely technical artifact (e.g., a knee implant). However, the success of this technical system is based on the success of the human user as a human resource. For example, the orthopedic surgeon must place the knee implant, and thereafter the physical therapist must rehabilitate the knee in order to achieve the highest likelihood for normal knee function with minimal pain. In many cases, it is not easy to distinguish whether an unsuccessful outcome is due to the human or technical resource. Years of clinical studies and reporting are often required to distinguish between these two factors. Returning to formal AD theory (and its Independence Axiom), the socio-technical nature of the healthcare solution means that the FRs of normal knee motion are achieved by two DPs in an inevitable coupled design.

The socio-technical nature of healthcare systems presents further design challenges. One may naively believe that an implantable device, such as a knee implant, will have hundreds or thousands of identical copies. In reality, the device itself is produced using materials and manufacturing methods that have quality tolerances that leave a level of variability in the final product. Similarly, the surgical team installing the implant provides several types of parallel and sequential services that also introduce a level of variability. The variability in the healthcare outcome can be further exacerbated by the orthopedic rehab center that provides inpatient and outpatient rehabilitation services, physical therapy services, and skilled nursing services. Only after all of these technical and human resources are combined can a health outcome be truly evaluated. Furthermore, in a clinical study, a sufficiently large sample of implants need to be placed by many different surgical teams and rehabilitated by many different orthopedic centers in order to truly assess the technical design. Consequently, the variability in the social aspects of the healthcare system must be controlled in order to maximize the likelihood of success of the designed technical resource. That said, the variability introduced by both the human and technical resource may need to accommodate the natural variations of the individual-patient. In short, the Information Axiom instructs the designer to achieve a successful healthcare outcome by minimizing the variability of both the human and the technical resources.

As medical advancements continue, especially in artificial intelligence (AI) and data analytics, some believe that we may, someday, minimize or eliminate human resources from healthcare solutions. Such a perspective, nevertheless, neglects the importance of the human-patient to human-doctor connection, be it conscious or subconscious, in providing care. Furthermore, their social connection, in terms of rapport and trust, shapes the patient and clinician's decision-making process, affects how patients proceed with healthcare options, and determines their degree of cooperation as they proceed with treatment. These many human aspects of healthcare are even more pronounced in services that require a high level of social connection like psychology, psychiatry, cancer, palliative care, and pediatric care.

19.3.2   Healthcare Delivery Heterogeneity

While the Information Axiom instructs the designer to minimize the variability in the human and technical resources of the healthcare system, there are practical limitations to doing so. Even as the technical resource is designed within very tight quality tolerances, it must also be designed to fit in a wide variety of heterogeneous healthcare delivery systems. This heterogeneity stems from its different human resources, in the implementation of the integrated design, and in the financial models under which the healthcare delivery system operates. Different doctors have different healthcare patterns and outcomes, different healthcare systems integrate technology in different ways, and the different financial models present hard constraints and soft influence on how healthcare services are chosen and delivered.

Heterogeneity in human resources

Beyond the heterogeneity in the different types of doctors (e.g., cardiologists, surgeons, psychiatrists), there exists variations in their number, training, expertise, and patterns of practice across a given region. These human factors affect the design of the technical resource. Even if the design is purely technical (e.g., social robots), the device's market uptake will depend on the number and nature of the doctors in that region. For example, rural areas are less likely to benefit from advanced healthcare technologies because they also suffer fewer doctors and specialists. Still other countries have shortages in certain types of doctors. Japan has a shrinking ratio of working individuals to aging individuals. In the United Arab Emirates, expatriates make up 85% of the healthcare workforce; and consequently, half the workforce is turned over every two years.

Heterogeneity in implementation into a healthcare delivery system

In addition to the heterogeneity in the DP of the healthcare system's human and technical resources, the healthcare system also introduces heterogeneity through the implementation of its PVs. One common problem is that the PV hierarchy is not decomposed to the same degree as FR and DP hierarchies. In other words, the PV are described at a high level with no specifics as to how the implementation is carried out in detail. For this reason, many medical advancements are never implemented and the typical implementation lag time is 17 years. To address this problem, a new medical field called "implementation science" was developed to study how to implement medical discoveries and interventions once they are known. It recognizes that the lack of detail of how a scientific discovery or intervention was tested in a clinical trial can lead to widely different outcomes. For example, in some cases the implementation of the electronic medical record (EMR) into the healthcare system has improved patient health outcomes and doctor productivity, while in other cases it degraded them. Similarly, some implementations of behavioral health and opioid recovery programs have improved patient health outcomes and lowered costs, while in others there has been little or no improvemen.

Heterogeneity in healthcare delivery system financial models

The operation of a healthcare system depends significantly on how it is financed. Many different payment strategies and stakeholders have been implemented, and each has its own set of stakeholders. For example, individuals can pay out of pocket, employers or individuals can purchase private healthcare insurance from private companies, or a country or region can provide public healthcare through the government. Furthermore, a healthcare system's financial model can and usually does vary over time.

Many countries are currently revising the financial models of their healthcare systems. The conventional model today is "fee-for-service"; a specific fee payment for every time a service is rendered. Much research suggests that such a payment model incentivizes the provision of large quantities of healthcare service with less attention to quality in terms of patient health outcomes. In contrast, a new concept called "value-based care" provides reimbursements for demonstrated value, and improved health outcomes at reasonable cost. Many countries are iteratively experimenting with reimbursement schemes for value-based care. As the associated financial incentives change, the efficacy of healthcare interventions has also been found to change as well.

19.3.3   Complexity and Interoperability

As mentioned earlier in the chapter, the current healthcare system developed organically to meet "one-off" acute illnesses and injuries. This same system is facing an unprecedented chronic disease burden. These conditions, unlike acute conditions, are particularly complex in that they are ongoing and tend to involve multiple factors with multiple interactions between them. Consequently, many patients require many different services and resources in their treatment of the chronic condition. A great deal of healthcare system complexity arises when a single patient utilizes many different types of services offered by different human and technical resources. For example, a cancer patient may meet with an oncologist in a clinic, receive chemotherapy from an infusion nurse at an oncology infusion-center, and receive imaging at an imaging center.

From the perspective of the patient, the complexity appears as the burden of moving between many human and technical resources. Meanwhile, from the perspective of the healthcare system, the complexity creates the need for coordination and communication of care between these resources. Such resources are accustomed to providing services without coordination despite the potential for adverse outcomes of varying severity: missed appointments, drug reactions, ineffective, delayed or inaccurate care plans, and other safety issues.

Greater healthcare system interoperability may alleviate some complexity. Here, it is equally important to improve the interface both within and between different healthcare systems. For example, an electronic medical record (EMR) system from a single vendor may enhance interoperability across healthcare systems. However, given the relative absence of EMR standards, data sharing across EMR systems from different vendors remains elusive. That said, it is not uncommon to find different EMR systems in different departments within the same healthcare system.

The lack of interoperability appears at multiple scales and scope. While interoperability concerns can occur between different healthcare systems, they can also be found within a single healthcare system (e.g., hospital), a single department (e.g., surgery), or a single resource location (e.g., operating room). For example, a given operating room utilizes a vast array of medical devices. They should ideally gather data from all available source sensors so that they can be processed (automatically) into actionable data for the surgical team. Instead, this device data is often uploaded into the EMR system and monitored manually. In this regard, interoperability presents a viable opportunity to improve patient safety.

Efforts to improve healthcare interoperability can have several drivers. From a regulatory perspective, the connection between patient safety and interoperability is likely to cause regulatory reform proactively or via the judicial system. Alternatively, when there is a pressing industry-wide need, industrial consortia will often form to write relevant standards. Finally, in some cases, EMR system vendors may recognize that proprietary but transparent interoperability standards is conducive to a "platform-economics" business model. For example, the DOC, XLS, PPT, and PDF file formats are all proprietary de-facto interoperability standards. There also exists the DICOM imaging file format in healthcare, a standard that revolutionized the ability to share images across boundaries.

19.3.4 Healthcare as a Legacy System

Finally, it is important to recognize that the healthcare system functions as a large flexible engineering system. Not only is it a "soft infrastructure system" composed of social elements like rules, regulations, policies, and institutions, but it is a veritable "hard infrastructure system" in terms of the billions of dollars worth of capital assets that constitute its technical resources. The sheer scale of the existing healthcare system means that a designer is obliged to recognize its legacy nature. Neither can its existing capital stock of technical resources be immediately replaced with a new set of new technologies, nor can its stock of human resources be fired and replaced with newly trained medical professionals. Doing so is not only cost-prohibitive but also entirely unsafe given that new technical and human resources often require significant time before they are properly integrated in the remainder of the system.

This distinction between large flexible engineering systems and new product design requires a fundamental change in the engineer's design methodology. As described earlier in this book, the forward-engineering "zig-zagging" method is no longer entirely appropriate. The designer cannot simply determine a high-level FRs, allocate it to a DPs, and then decompose the FRs into a set of lower level FRs, etc. Such an approach maximizes creativity, free of design constraints, and is most appropriate for new products. It is not appropriate for a large flexible engineering system design because it does not take into account legacy nature of existing technical and human resources.

Instead, in an engineering systems context, the functional and physical hierarchies must first be "reverse engineered." The designer must observe the physical hierarchy—particularly at a relatively detailed level, infer the associated FRs, then aggregate the DPs into their associated human and technical resources, and then repeat. Once the existing legacy structure of the healthcare system has been modeled in terms of its functional and physical hierarchies it can serve as the designer's "initial condition." From there, the designer can "evolve" the system to a more advance stage of development recognizing the design priorities that appear in a modified set of stakeholder needs and FRs. Furthermore, in developing the new design, it is often unnecessary to "reinvent the wheel." Well-known functions have tried-and-true physical solutions which may be re-implemented successfully. More specifically, the design of technical resources in a healthcare system often relies on an existing and extensive body of *validated* medical science and biomedical engineering research which can be leveraged as a rich repository from which to draw. Such a design approach recognizes and emphasizes the need for validation by clinical trial prior to system-level design. Similarly, the design of human resources in a healthcare system requires the designer to select appropriately qualified personnel given that the time and money required for training is practically limited. In short, the legacy nature of the healthcare system places practical constraints on methodology and outcome of any design effort.

19.4 Key Takeaways and Conclusion

In summary, this chapter has described some of the key considerations that a designer must make as they approach a healthcare system design project. It has discussed several systems abstractions in the context of healthcare systems: system boundary, scale, scope, function, and form. These abstractions were described in terms of practical limitations and requirements that are often imposed from outside of the system boundary. This chapter also described a system framework for designing healthcare systems that is consonant with Axiomatic Design's FRs, DPs, and process variable domains. The chapter concluded with four key healthcare design challenges that the designers must consider as they design healthcare systems at various scales and scope.

Problems

1. From Design Story 19.1, design a "turn-off" system for a pacemaker that addresses the ethical and policy issues of two types of turn-off functions. One of the turn-off functions is to be performed by a physician and the other is a more advanced turn-off system that can be performed by the user or family member, but that ensures it is performed with authorization and not by mistake or malice.

2. From Design Story 19.2, it was identified that the designed system makes for a complicated re-entry. What FRs would you add to the system to ensure that future surgical routing to fix any issues would be uncomplicated? How would you setup your FRs and DPs for this analysis?

3. You are hired to lead the design for a pacemaker. If the following high-level FRs are designated, design a set of DPs for an uncoupled system.
   FRs:

   1. produces rhythmic electrical signals;
   2. does not negatively affect the host body;
   3. produces safe signals regardless of external environment;
   4. eliminate surgical maintenance or expiration (does not need to be replaced).

4. You consult for a baby company that wants you to develop a baby monitoring system. Below are comments from parents. Convert each comment into a FRs.

   a. "I live in a rural area in a high-energy performance home (i.e., 12-inch thick walls) on a large lot."
   b. I work outside and I need a baby monitoring system that can provide a secure private connection that guarantees zero interference, clear sound, with range up to 1,000 feet.
   c. I need to know when my unit is out of range of the baby unit.
   d. I need to be able to respond to my baby so I can comfort them with my voice and face.
   e. I need the parent unit to function outside in wet or dry conditions, and under extreme hot and cold temperatures.

5. You are a design engineer traveling abroad to Africa for vacation. You notice a tired pregnant passenger on a local bus trying to get to a pre-natal visit at a local hospital (65 miles away). You converse with the passenger who tells you the following FRs for her ideal pre-natal care. Identify the DPs to develop a decoupled system solution.

   a. send me a reminder when I need to connect for a pre-natal visit;
   b. perform most visits virtually;
   c. communicate efficiently and with speed (within 30 min) between patient and clinician;
   d. allow for anonymous patient-to-patient communication that is monitored for clinical accuracy (so I can ask private questions that I don't want my doctor to know about me).

References

Khayal IS, Farid AM (2018) Architecting a system model for personalized healthcare delivery and managed individual health outcomes. Complexity 2018:24. https://doi.org/10.1155/2018/8457231

Peck JS (2008) Securing the safety net: applying manufacturing systems methods towards understanding and redesigning a hospital emergency department. S.m. thesis, Massachusetts Institute of Technology, Engineering Systems Division, Technology and Policy Program, 77 Massachusetts Ave., Cambridge MA 02,139, USA. https://dspace.mit.edu/handle/1721.1/42934

Suh NP, Cho DH (eds) (2017) The on-line electric vehicle: wireless electric ground transportation systems. Springer International Publishing

Further Reading

Crawley E, Cameron B, Selva D (2015) System architecture: strategy and product development for complex systems, 1st edn. Pearson

Farid AM (2016) An engineering systems introduction to axiomatic design. In: Farid AM, Suh NP (eds) Axiomatic design in large systems: complex products, buildings and manufacturing systems. Springer, Cham, Switzerland, Chap 1, pp 3–47

Khayal IS (2019) A systems thinking approach to designing clinical models and healthcare services. Systems 7(18):26. https://doi.org/10.3390/systems7010018

Khayal IS, Farid AM (2016) The need for systems tools in the practice of clinical medicine. Syst Eng 20(1):3–20. https://doi.org/10.1002/sys.21374

Functional Periodicity, "Function Clock," and "Solar Time Clock" in Design

20

Nam Pyo Suh

Abstract

Some systems are designed to perform the same set of functions cyclically and repeatedly. These systems have "functional periodicity." The best-known system with "functional periodicity" is a biological cell. A cell divides into two identical cells through mitosis, which involves five sequential phase transitions: interphase, prophase, metaphase, anaphase, and telophase. These transitions occur when the cell is ready for phase change rather than after a fixed time delay. Similarly, in engineered systems such as the "track machine" used in manufacturing semiconductor chips, functional periodicity can be introduced to the system to improve the reliability of the manufacturing system and overcome inevitable variations of processing times. The time duration of the functional period may vary from cycle to cycle for a variety of reasons.

There are other engineered systems that can benefit from functional periodicity, e.g., the assembly line of automobiles, the flight schedule of airlines, and operation of universities. We may incorporate "functional periodicity" in these design systems to maximize productivity or to improve system reliability. In each functional period, these systems perform an identical set of functions. Before initiating a new functional period, the system should be re-initialized for optimum operation of the system for next cycle. A designed system can extend its useful life when its functions at the beginning of each functional period are re-initialized.

In engineered systems, we use two different kinds of periodicity: time-based and function-based. The time-based systems use the conventional solar time clock to control the system. The function-based system uses the completion of the same set of "functions" before it initiates the next cycle. These systems with functional periodicity can be re-initialized at the beginning of each new cycle to

N. P. Suh (✉)
M.I.T., Cambridge, MA, USA
e-mail: npsuh@mit.edu

© Springer Nature Switzerland AG 2021
N. P. Suh et al. (eds.), *Design Engineering and Science*,
https://doi.org/10.1007/978-3-030-49232-8_20

get the best performance. The inclusion of the functional periodicity in designed systems generally improves their operations. An example of functional periodicity that is both time-based and function-based is the election of political leaders.

Application of functional periodicity in designed systems should lengthen the life of products, improve the efficiency of systems, reduce the downtime, increase the effectiveness of transportation systems, and minimize deterioration of political and socio-economic systems. For best results, the "re-initialization" of the system should be done at the beginning of each functional period.

In this chapter, two ideas are introduced and discussed: the application of "functional periodicity" in system design and the utilization of the concept of "function clock."

20.1   Introduction to Functional Periodicity and Re-initialization

A system must fulfill its functional requirements (FRs), at all times without failure, to be useful throughout its life. If the system is a production machine, its reliability, performance, and productivity are of utmost importance. A large, complicated system must run more or less continuously throughout its life, producing quality goods reliably, with occasional maintenance. On the other hand, if the system is a research university, it must perform its functions well. It must continuously improve and enhance its programs, contents, quality of human resources, and finances to provide the best education to students and create knowledge for humanity. If the system is a government agency, it must renew itself to be sure that it is fulfilling the original legislative mandate for establishing the agency. Many of these complicated systems must satisfy a set of FRs over a pre-determined period, as discussed in previous chapters.

The primary goal in design is to create a system that satisfies the FRs. An even more ambitious goal is to design a system that will renew itself periodically for an indefinite period to fulfill its original FRs. To achieve this goal, we introduced two concepts: "functional periodicity" and "re-initialization" to show how a system that renews its FRs and DPs periodically can be designed. One of the most well known among such systems is the democratic political system. Political leaders (e.g., president, members of Congress, etc.) serve a fixed term in office, and a new election is held. Academic programs re-initialize at least once a year to achieve this goal. These systems have time-fixed periods for renewal, i.e., each cycle ends at a fixed time.

Educational Institutions and Functional Periodicity and Re-initialization

Nearly all educational entities from primary school to colleges and universities have used functional periodicity and re-initialization, at least once or twice a year. Students change each year, but the educational programs are typically organized on a semester or yearly basis. In the United States, schools begin a new academic year and semester in the fall of each year. After four months of intensive study, students and teachers have breaks. Then the schools repeat the same process for different students.

Some systems have periods that end when their functions are finished rather than stopping at the pre-determined time. A well-known example is the Supreme Court of the United States. The Supreme Court justices do not have a term limit that occurs at the end of a fixed time. Similarly, some manufacturing operations do not end at the end of a set time but instead ends when its manufacturing task (i.e., a function) is finished. A biological cell undergoes five sequential phase transformations during mitosis to split into two identical cells when it is functionally ready rather than at a fixed time interval.

Actual Story: Is it a monopoly or an effective use of functional periodicity and re-initialization for an industrial firm?

New England of the United States consists of the six northeastern states of the United States, i.e., Maine, Massachusetts, Rhode Island, New Hampshire, Vermont, and Connecticut. The region is not only rich in history but also the center of higher education and the birthplace of many advanced technologies of the Americas. It is also one of the most scenic sections of the United States. Many of these states are culturally and politically liberal states vis-a-vis the conservative southeastern states of the United States. Economically, technically, and politically, these states have continued to evolve and transform. Many well-known universities have their roots in New England.

Until about 1950, New England was the home for many shoe-related businesses. There were many shoe factories and leather tanneries in Massachusetts and New Hampshire. The world's largest shoe machinery manufacturer, USM Corporation, was located in Beverly, Massachusetts, about 35 miles northeast of Boston. They dominated the machinery business worldwide. It was incredibly generous to its employees. It created wealth and many high-paying jobs in the Commonwealth of Massachusetts and the United States!

USM's business model was unique. Instead of selling their machines, they only leased them to shoe manufacturers. If someone wanted to go into the shoe manufacturing business, the company would set up a factory and install its machines on lease. Then, they would collect lease-fees each time one of their machines was used to manufacture shoes. They conducted active research and development to invent new machines, new materials, and processes. The main goal of their research and development was to innovate new technologies and secure patents to protect its market share. They had a warehouse full of modern machines they invented, but they did not sell them. They only leased some of their patented machines. The patents and their leasing policies protected them from their potential competitors.

Therefore, they had a de facto monopoly in the shoe machinery business worldwide. Once in a while, they would introduce new machines, but their business was based on leasing the same machines for many years, servicing them regularly, replacing bearings, etc., periodically. Anyone who wanted to get into shoe business could do so if they could meet the lease terms of USM Corporation.

They practiced functional periodicity to make their customers happy. After their machines had been used to manufacture a fixed number of shoes, they would periodically service them in the shoe factory. They replaced worn parts and bearings, etc., to make the machines function as if they were new. Since their machines were rugged to last for a long time, once the worn components were replaced, they worked like new machines again. Their business practiced "functional periodicity" and "re-initialization"—through the re-initialization of their leased machines, although they did not use those terms. The company had a gold mine because it was difficult for other companies to penetrate the shoe machinery business. They took care of their employees generously. Many stayed with the company throughout their lifetime until they retired.

Sometimes, good things cannot last forever! The U.S. government sued USM for monopoly and anti-trust practices, and the government won. The U.S. Federal Court ordered USM to sell their machines rather than only leasing them. When all those leased machines had to be sold to the shoe manufacturers all at once, USM became temporarily cash-rich. Unfortunately, USM invested their cash in the wrong businesses and could not compete in highly competitive companies; they did not have expertise and deep roots. USM, a great company, is no longer in business. In hindsight, the top management of USM chose a wrong set of FRs when they re-initialized the corporate strategy under the government mandate.

The lesson we should learn from the sad saga of USM Corporation is that the functional periodicity and re-initialization in business are effective strategies. However, the business model should quickly adapt to changing external conditions, such as changing Federal laws and regulations. That is one of the reasons why so many companies hire "lobbyists" to protect their back by influencing the process of enacting government regulations and laws.

Actual Story: Functional Periodicity and Re-initialization as a Design Tool

A couple of decades later after the demise of USM Corporation, the idea for incorporating functional periodicity and re-initializing FRs into a designed system was advanced to solve a problem encountered by a semiconductor equipment company.

Functional Periodicity and Re-initialization: Background Story

An executive of a company and a professor were waiting at the Armonk airport, a small airport, outside of New York City, near the headquarters of IBM (International Business Machines) Corporation, for their flight to Rochester, New York. They were on their way to visit the optics research laboratory at the University in Rochester. The executive and the professor knew each other well, having collaborated on many projects in the past. The professor was a board member of the company and recommended hiring the executive a few years earlier. While waiting for their flight, the executive described a problem the company had had with their "Track Machine." He stated that he had tried to hire a specialist in the field of operations research (OR) as a consultant to solve the problem. However, he said that he had decided against it. The OR specialist did not know the solution to their problem. Instead, he proposed a major research contract to the company. However, the problem needed an immediate answer because the track machines were being used in many semiconductor fabrication facilities (commonly known as FAB), causing production problems.

In FABs, silicon wafers are made into semiconductor devices (sometimes, called "chips"). One of the machines used is the so-called "track machine" (note: the old name "track" stuck, although modern tools do not use tracks anymore). "Track machine" performs many functions in conjunction with the lithography machine. It takes in wafers at a regular interval and clean the surface of semiconductors, etch the surface, spin-coat the surface of wafers with photoresist, and transport the photoresist-coated wafer to the lithography machine for exposure to UV light through photomasks to create electric circuits (line-width as small as 20 nm) on the surface coated with photoresist. After exposure in the lithography machine, the wafers are brought back to the track machine for removal of unexposed photoresist and cross-linking of the photoresist.

The process in the track machine begins when a silicon wafer is loaded at its loading station by a wafer-handling robot. There are many robots and many stations within the track machine for simultaneous transport and processing of many wafers. These robots carry the wafers from station to station for various operations done in the track machine. The operations include cleaning of the wafer surface, spreading photoresist, curing photoresist after exposure to UV light in lithography machine, etching, etc. After each operation, the wafer is moved to the next station in the track machine to complete another manufacturing operation. This process continues until the wafer has been subjected to all manufacturing processes, which follow a pre-determined sequence of operations. Since a large number of wafers must be processed, there are multiple stations for each one of the manufacturing operations. The processing time for each operation is different. Therefore, the robot must be instructed to transport a given wafer from its current station to the next station to complete the required manufacturing operations. The company used an artificial intelligence (AI) technique to program the transportation sequence of the robot based on "If ..., then do ..." type of AI algorithm. After the completion of each assigned manufacturing operation, the robot transports the wafer to the next station for the subsequent fabrication process.

The track machine made by this company normally functioned well, but then once in a while, the device would stop working, because the old AI-based algorithm—(if ..., then do) —would not know what to do next, i.e., the machine got "confused" after many hours of operation due to accumulated errors. When the machine stops, many wafers in the track machine at various stages of processing might become unusable. To continue the manufacturing operation, they have to re-boot machine, which is very disruptive and costly.

The executive thought that a better software program should be developed based on a better process model, perhaps using an optimization method developed in operations research (OR). They both agreed that the problem might have stemmed from the fact that there are slight variations at each station from the assumed processing times, temperature, etc. When the errors accumulate, the algorithm based on the "if, then" logic might fail to function correctly.

The professor made a different suggestion. "Why not introduce functional periodicity and automatically "re-initialize the machine" after one (or more) complete cycle measured from when a finished wafer leaves the track machine. The re-initialization is done by assessing the status of every wafer currently in the machine. For example, it determined how many more minutes a specific wafer has to be kept in Module A, which modules are empty and waiting for a new wafer to process. Then, decide on where each wafer has to go for the next operation, i.e., re-initialize the system for the next cycle. This idea became the basis for "functional periodicity" and "re-initialization." It turns out that Nature has been practicing "functional periodicity" and re-initialization to maintain life on Earth, which may be responsible for the incredibly healthy life of living beings!

The idea for functional periodicity and re-initialization was initially developed to solve a problem associated with the track machine used for semiconductor processing. However, the principles are equally applicable to other technical and non-technical systems. For example, companies that sell expensive automobiles provide regular "free" maintenance. During the maintenance, they replace parts that may imminently fail to enhance the image of the quality of their cars.

Nature, including all living beings, uses functional periodicity every day, which is known, in biology, as the circadian cycle. We sleep at night and study or work during the daytime, more or less, regularly. Our biological cells go through different phases in our body and divide into two "identical" cells once approximately every 24 h. When our biological systems lose functional periodicity and the ability to re-initialize, the system becomes chaotic and does not survive for too long.

Many human-designed systems have incorporated periodic changes to harmonize several actions taking place in engineered systems. Transportation systems are good examples. For instance, airlines schedule thousands of flights every day, covering vast geographic areas. The flight schedules repeat regularly, typically daily. When airlines must reschedule their flights because of the unexpected weather change, they can recover quickly because of the periodic nature of airline schedules. For instance, suppose that a hurricane hit the Atlanta airport in the State of Georgia. Therefore, they had to close one of the busiest airports for a day—this closing of the Atlanta airport forces airlines to divert the aircraft headed to Atlanta to other airports. The effect of closing the Atlanta airport will propagate to other airports. Some of the flights from Boston to other cities must be canceled because the aircraft from Atlanta to Boston has been canceled. A chaotic situation will arise not only in Atlanta but also in Boston and elsewhere, which may last hours. Passengers stranded in the Boston Logan Airport may have to sleep on chairs and floors at the airport. This weather in Atlanta may create chaos in scheduling problems that propagate throughout the country and even to other countries. However, if the weather finally clears up after so many hours or days, the airlines can re-initialize their system. They can dispatch the airplanes to various airports and gradually resume their flights on schedule. Airlines can resume their regular flights rather quickly because airline flights typically repeat on a 24-h cyclic basis. Most airline flight schedules have functional periodicity.

Many human-made systems have functional periodicity. Just like the airline schedule, we can build in functional periodicity in engineered systems. These systems with functional periodicity can be re-initialized to continue the operation without disruption. For instance, every morning, the availability and locations of airplanes should be determined to determine if the aircraft should be relocated or dispatched to different airports to meet flight schedules. When functional periodicity and re-initialization are designed into a system at the design stage, the system will be more robust and easy to maintain as well as lasting a long time.

The purpose of this chapter is to introduce the concept of "Functional Periodicity" and "Re-Initialization" of systems. The goal is to design a system with functional periodicity and re-initialize it periodically. A system that re-initializes periodically can continue its operation for an extended period without a chaotic breakdown of the system operation. Many large systems designed in the past have encountered problems both during the development stage and also in operation, because they had made design mistakes, introducing coupling of FRs. Had they introduced the functional periodicity and the means of re-initializing itself, they might have operated more robustly and survived longer.

20.2 "Function Clock" Versus "Time Clock"

Most people perform various tasks based on the time clock, i.e., 24 hours a day, 60 minutes per hour, and 60 seconds per minute. The time clock is used as the standard reference for most events that occur in our daily life. In the operation of design systems, we set almost everything based on the time elapsed instead the function accomplished. The time referred to is the "time clock," which is set to the rotation of Earth about its axis. However, in some cases, it is more appropriate to use the completion of "functions" as the reference frame, because some functions may take longer or shorter to complete. For example, suppose we create a school system based on the "function clock"[1] rather the "time clock" that is prevalent today. How would that school be different from the school that operates based on "time clock"?

Definition of "Function Clock"

A function clock is defined as the clock that tracks when a specific function of a system is completed. When there is a set of functions that must be satisfied to complete the task repeatedly, the function clock tracks the completion of each function. When a new cycle of functions begins, the function clock begins to tick again and monitors when all the functions are completed. There is no correlation between the time clock and the function clock.

Many things in Nature operate based on "function clock." For instance, in biological systems, the cell division, i.e., "mitosis," goes through four sequential phases before they split into two identical cells. However, the duration of each phase change does not occur at precisely the same time. The phase transition occurs after the functions of each phase are completed, which take different durations in terms of time. Similar variations occur in some manufacturing operations. For instance, consider the task of maximizing the productivity of the "track machine," which process semiconductor wafers by subjecting them to various manufacturing processes using many modules. In this machine, the wafers are moved from module

---

[1]The term "Function-Clock" is not a commonly used term. It is introduced in this book for the first time, because in some design applications, the concept of "Functional-Clock" may be useful.

to module using a robot after a given operation is completed. The wafer can be transferred to the next station of the track machine only after the current procedure is completed. The completion of each activity cannot be timed precisely because of variations in processes. The wafers can be removed from each processing station of the track machine only after the specific processing function is completed. The traditional way is to pre-program the robot motion to transport the wafer from a given station to the next module.

The difference between "function clock" and "time clock" may be illustrated using how the education of students can change under these two different systems.

Example 20.1 Difference between "Function Clock" and "Time Clock"

In nearly all countries, schools operate based on a fixed schedule. Schools in the United States typically starts new school year right after labor day, around September 4 and ends in the middle of June. They have a couple of weeks of a short break between December and January as winter vacation. The school year is divided into two semesters, each lasting about four months. Every student is taught various subjects during the semester. Most of these schools operate based on a "time clock." All students are evaluated for their understanding of the subjects taught by giving them "grades" after each semester. We can rationalize this system, but the system is unfair to slow learners who could do well given more time, even better than those who get good grades. It is also unjust to quick learners, because they may be wasting their time once they complete what they are programmed to learn. The school that operates based on the "time clock" justify their system by giving the students "grades" such as "A, B, C, D, and F" at the end of each semester, which is called the semester.

If schools operated based on a "function clock," each student will be asked to learn a given set of materials without any fixed time limit. Whenever the student masters the subject matter, she/he can move onto the next level of learning after demonstrating that they learned the subject matter. Some students may learn the subject matter in 45 days, whereas another student may take 120 days to learn the same subject matter. The students move up to the next level as soon as they master the subject matter. Under this system, the student follows the "function clock," which measures the progress made by each student in the understanding of the subject matter. Under this system of education, every student may achieve a complete understanding and comprehension of a given subject matter. Some students may "graduate" in one calendar year, whereas some others in ten years. Some countries in Asia had this system of individualized education before the twentieth century.

Example 20.2 Difference between Teaching and Learning in Terms of "Function Clock" and "Time Clock"

All the teachers were once students, too. As a student, she/he needed to satisfy the requirements and get passing grades. When someone becomes a teacher and teaches other people for the first time, the new teacher realizes that as a teacher, he/she must fully comprehend the subject matter. In other words, students operate based on "time clock," whereas the teacher must perform based on "function clock." The intensity of effort needed to operate under the "function clock" can be either higher or less than that required to operate under the "time clock," depending on one's knowledge base.

For some of the machines used in semiconductor manufacturing such as the "track machine" (shown in Fig. 20.1), it is essential that the machine continuously runs. The consequence of the machine stopping in the middle of its operation can be quite costly. To achieve the goal, some companies used the "if … then …" logic to

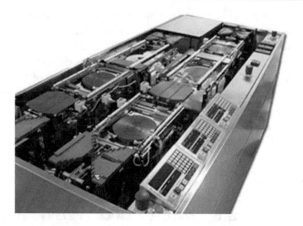

Fig. 20.1 SVG Track Machine, that cleans, coats with photoresist, and cures silicon wafer. A track machine is typically linked to a lithography machine. The number of stations of some track machines can be much larger than the one shown

schedule the wafer-handling robot in a track machine. Usually, such a system works well in production, but once in a while, the system would stop because the accumulated error is so significant that the system that uses "if ... then ..." logic to operate the machine breaks down. Then, the machine has to be re-booted at a great expense.

One way of overcoming this problem is to assess the state of the track machine when a finished wafer leaves the machine. That is, determine where the remaining wafers are located, what additional processing steps must be undertaken for each wafer. Based on the information, transfer and process the wafers until the next functional period, when the next wafer is ready to be removed from the track machine. Then, again re-assess the state of each wafer in the machine and decide for the next processing step. This "re-initialization" process should continue after each "functional period." This re-initialization should be done utilizing the information stored in the computer and quick sensing of the state of each wafer. This re-initialization process each time a finished wafer leaves the machine avoids the need to pre-determine the entire operation of the track machine by creating the "if ... then ..." rules a priori and eliminates the problem associated with accumulated errors related to "if ... then ..." rules.

Unlike the "time clock," the "function clock" starts ticking at the beginning of each new functional period of the designed system. For example, in the track machine used in semiconductor wafer processing, a new functional cycle of the system begins when a finished wafer leaves the track machine. In manufacturing airplanes, a new period starts when a finished aircraft leaves the assembly plant. Schools re-initialize twice a year. In all of these systems, the FRs of the system are "re-initialized" when a finished product leaves the system. Re-initialization is done using the latest information available on the status of each unfinished work-piece in the machine at the time of re-initialization. For example, when a finished wafer is taken off the track machine, another wafer in the track machine must be moved into the final module. The track machine is re-initialized after determining the status of each wafer in each module of the machine. The data are used to determine the best placement of the wafers for the next cycle. Based on the data of the initial state of each piece at the beginning of a new period, the best operational sequence for the new cycle can be determined. The "function clock" begins to "tick" at the beginning of each functional period. The function clock is not synchronized with the circadian clock. This process repeats as long as the system has to produce or operate.

20.3 Pros and Cons of "Function Clock" Versus "Time Clock"

Most of the societal functions are based on the "Time Clock" rather than the "Function Clock." In fact, the term "Function Clock" has not been used before and is not a commonly used term. However, there are many reasons for using Time Clock in many societal roles. The most important reason is that humans behave based on the circadian cycle. It is the least resource-intensive to plan group activities based on the Time Clock. Unlike controlling machine functions, the cost of operating a system that involves people based on the Function Clock can be high. Some people may not finish their tasks within an allocated time, slowing down the operation of the entire system. On the other hand, a highly efficient person may suffer in the system that uses "Time Clock" waiting for the less efficient person to finish their task. Although there is no definite proof or evidence, the overall efficiency of society and any organization with diverse activities and people with different levels of competency would be much higher under a system that use the "Time Clock."

"Function clock" is expected to be more efficient in a system that repeats a set of similar operations but with slight variations from cycle to cycle.

20.4 Periodicity and Re-initialization of Airline Scheduling

A major goal of airlines is to maximize their profit, just like most commercial firms. To achieve this goal, they attempt to transport as many passengers as possible in the shortest possible time. In the U.S., after airlines were de-regulated, airlines lowered the airfare of the economy class, eliminated many in-flight services (i.e., meals), and reduced the number of flight attendants. They also use smaller airplanes such as Boeing 737 and fill these planes to its full capacity with almost no empty seats. They often overbook, assuming that some customers will not show up. They also increased the number of seats by reducing the legroom between the rows of seats.

Some of the airlines adopted these and other extreme measures to reduce the cost of operation. Airline profits are affected by the cost of fuel, personnel, and equipment (i.e., airplanes). When the oil price is low, airlines make healthy profits and suffer when the fuel price is high. They tend to hedge against high oil prices.

Airlines provide direct, non-stop flight services between major hubs with sufficient passenger loads such as the New York–San Francisco leg. However, they eliminated many direct, non-stop flights between smaller cities because of the limited passenger loads. Therefore, they use regional hubs to collect passengers from diverse cities and then to transport them to their final destinations, using smaller aircraft. To achieve this goal, the airline synchronizes their flights by letting airplanes land and take off from a given airport nearly at the same time. Therefore, airports are busy at certain times of the day. Many flights of a given airline arrive and take off within a couple of hours of each other to allow passengers to transfer and reach their destination without long layovers. For example, airplanes from Europe typically arrive in Boston in the afternoon and flights from Boston to European destinations leave early in the evening, which is around mid-night in Europe due to the time difference. These airplanes then arrive in European cities early in the morning, after the airports officially open. (Airplanes are not allowed to land at the Frankfurt International Airport, Germany, before 6 a.m., probably for noise reduction.) Therefore, airlines have introduced certain functional periodicity to harmonize flights between various cities.

When severe weather forces airports to close, flights are either canceled or diverted to other airports. If the bad weather persists for an extended period, the airlines cancel their flights. However, when the weather clears, the airlines "re-initialize" their systems by relocating their aircraft to the right airports. The fact that at night the number of flights is small helps to relocate airplanes. Therefore, they can dispatch aircraft to the correct airports during the night to resume regular flights starting in the morning.

The important message of this example is that when a system is in operation for a long time, it is inevitable that errors accumulate, eventually resulting in system failures. These errors can be removed by re-initialing the system at the beginning of each functional period. Nature has evolved through the solar system that has yearly and daily periodicity. The periodic nature of biological systems has created functional periodicity and re-initialization through the long history of natural evolution.

Exercise 20.1: Travel to "Solar System II" in Distant Universe in Year 2520

Assume that by the thirtieth century, human beings finally developed spacecraft that can take people to another universe and found a solar system similar to ours. However, when they got there, they found two significant differences from our solar system of Earth in the twenty-first century. The planet revolves around its "sun" once every three months (rather than once a year) and rotates about its axis every 12 h, i.e., twice the rotational speed of Earth. The "people" on this newly discovered planet are very much like the people living on Earth but with some differences. What would be the difference? How would the difference in functional periodicity affect people? Perhaps the information given in the next section may help in thinking about this question.

20.5 Periodicity and Re-initialization of Biological Systems: Cell Division and Mitosis of Cells

Cells are the basic building blocks of all living beings. Cells in our body divide into two daughter cells, roughly once every 24 h. The phenomenon of cell division has been known since 1835 when Hugo von Mohl, a botanist, discovered the cell division in green algae in 1835.

Biological cells have functional periodicity, re-initializing after each cycle, i.e., cells replicate themselves periodically, following a sequence shown in Fig. 20.2. After the cells split into two identical cells, each cell goes through three different phases (in biology, it is called the "interphase"): the G1 phase, S-phase, and the G2 phase, before creating two identical cells through mitosis. The regular interval for the cell division is equivalent to the functional periodicity of biological systems. Another interesting fact is that the cell goes through re-initialization. The cell division process may halt for a while by going into the G0 phase until it is ready to resume the cell division process. This is equivalent to the "re-initialization" process. Biology textbooks provide the details of this process.

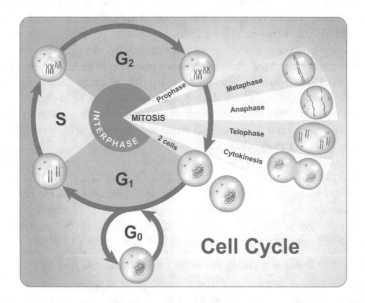

Fig. 20.2 Cell cycle. A cell goes through the interphase consisting of G_1, S, and G_2 phases. Through mitosis, one cell generates two daughter cells. Some cells go into G_0 phase, where the cell cycle is stopped until it is ready to repeat the cell division process by going through the cell interphase and mitosis. (Reproduced with permission from DAntes Design (2019))

20.6 Periodicity and Re-initialization in Manufacturing System Design

There are many different kinds of manufacturing systems, depending on the nature of the product, the production rate, and the total number of products to be manufactured. In "old" days, a large number of identical parts were made by machining and stacked up on a cart until the cart is fully loaded. Then, the cart was then taken to the next machining station for additional machining or to an assembly station to be joined with other parts. This type of manufacturing system is, in general, inefficient, because the inventory of parts is extensive. They may also need a large warehouse to keep the machined parts until they are required. Modern manufacturing factories may use a manufacturing cell, where a group of machines does various operations to a part until it is finished. In this type of manufacturing cell, a part is subjected to a series of manufacturing processes (e.g., cutting, milling, etc.). Similarly, if the manufacturing operation is an assembly operation, a number of assembly stations are placed in series to assemble the product in a continuously moving platform.

Henry Ford's Transformed Manufacturing System

One of the biggest revolutions in manufacturing is the mass-production system. The first such system was the manufacturing assembly line introduced by Henry Ford in the early twentieth century. He manufactured automobiles by assembling them on a continuous moving platform. Workers assembled automobile parts on a moving "conveyer" system, which substantially increased productivity and reduced the manufacturing cost of automobiles. Parts were brought to the assembly stations, which were assembled in a specific sequence as the platform moved along carrying the partially assembled cars. The assembly process was synchronized with the motion of the assembly line. When there is a problem at any station, the entire assembly line is stopped until the problem is fixed. Modern assembly plants roll out a new car one a minute.

20.6.1 Functional Periodicity in Design of a Simple Manufacturing Operation

Consider a simple manufacturing system with four machines, a, b, c, and d. The geometric shape of the part is so designed that it must be machined in all four stations in the sequence given, i.e., a, b, c, and d. The problem to be solved is the following: we want to maximize productivity and minimize the manufacturing cost. The operational time for machining and loading/unloading for each machine is different, the operational time at station b being the longest. The machining time at stations c and d are the same. There are several different ways of setting up the manufacturing system. One scheme is to run each machine as fast as the machine can be operated. Since it takes the longest at station b, parts that have gone through machining at the station a will pile up in front of station b. Station c will starve for lack of parts since Station b is slower than Station c.

Table 20.1 Design matrix
for machining parts at four
machining stations

	PVa	PVb	PVc	PVd
DPa	X	0	0	0
DPb	X	X	0	0
DPc	X	X	X	0
DPd	X	X	X	X

The best manufacturing sequence in terms of manufacturing cost and productivity is to adopt a functional periodicity based on the speed of machine b. When
machine b is to begin a new machining cycle, other machines, i.e., a, c, and d,
should be started at the same time. Machines a, c, and d should be slowed down so
that they would finish their operation at about the same time as machine b. Slowing
down the cutting speed may prolong the tool life, reducing the manufacturing cost.

The relationship between DPs (i.e., the shape of the part) and PVs (i.e.,
machining operation) are given by the design matrix given in Table 20.1.

The design matrix shows that the manufacturing system is a decoupled design.
Machining operation on "a" affects the functions of machines "b", "c", and "d".
Even if each machine is operated at its fastest speed, the productivity will not
increase. The production rate of machine b controls the number of parts that can be
assembled. The slowest machine controls the overall production rate. Machine b
controls the functional periodicity of this manufacturing system. Therefore, the
productivity is highest, and the cost is the least if all stations produce parts at the
rate machine b process the parts.

20.6.2 Functional Periodicity in Job Shop Scheduling

One of the classical problems in manufacturing research has been the scheduling of
job shops. A job shop is a manufacturing system with various machines to produce
machined parts for multiple customers on demand. The machining orders coming
into the job shop are unpredictable in terms of timing, specific machining needed to
make the part, the number of pieces, etc. Typically, in a job shop, a part is subjected
to various machining operations, and when the part is done with the final machining
operation, it is shipped out to the customer.

Consider a job shop with 20 machines of various kinds. Some of the commonly
used machines may be identical. However, the job shop must have a sufficient
variety of different tools to service whatever parts the customer orders for
machining. Typically, when an order comes in for machining, the foreman of the
shop attempts to process it as soon as possible based on a rule such as
first-in/first-out (FIFO). Each part may be subjected to several different machining
operations. Since several different components are machined in the job shop at the
same time, this FIFO process may not be the most efficient way of utilizing the
machine shop. Some parts will take up too much time on some machines, thus

denying access to these machines for other jobs. A classical question related to the job shop that has not been answered thus far is "How should the job shop schedule their operation to maximize the productivity of the job shop?".

A Possible Solution for the Job Shop Scheduling Problem Based on Functional Periodicity and Re-initialization:

When the first machining order comes into an empty machine shop, the issue is simple. i.e., use the available machines to manufacture the part. However, once the machine shop is 'fully loaded' with lots of orders, scheduling the sequence of machining different parts becomes a critical issue for maximizing the productivity of the job shop. The scheduling task is complicated because the job shop does not know the future incoming orders. How should we schedule the operation of the job shop? The answer to this question has eluded many researchers and scholars in production engineering.

Consider the manufacture of a part that requires the following machining sequence: milling on a milling machine, followed by machining on a lathe, grinding on a surface grinder, and electric-discharge machining (EDM). The last operation before the part leaves the job shop is the EDM process. We can set the functional period to be whenever the finished piece leaves the job shop. That is, for this particular part, when the EDM is done with the part, it will be the end of the functional period. We then re-initialize the parts still being processed to determine the next operation. The next part that is finished and leaves the job shop will be the end of another functional period, and the beginning of a new functional period and the time to re-initialize.

In job shops, the incoming orders are random and unpredictable in terms of specific machining tasks and the number of parts to be machined. The problem is to enable the job shop to schedule which part should be machined by what machine and in what sequence. It has been a difficult problem to solve, although many attempts have been made in the past. We will apply the functional periodicity and re-initialization to solve this job shop scheduling problem.

For this job shop problem, we will assume the following:

1. A new functional period to begin at that instant the latest finished part leaves the job shop, creating an empty machine, i.e., machine not occupied by a machining operation.
2. At that instant, a machine becomes available for another new workpiece.
3. At the beginning of this new cycle, re-initialize the entire system. The data include the status of each part, the status of each machine, and how long it would take to finish the piece.
4. Move partially finished parts to machines where subsequent machining should be performed.
5. Load a new piece to an unoccupied machine after moving the parts that have been machined at another station for following machining operations. This process can continue as long as there is a new stock to be machined.
6. There will be a buffer station to accommodate parts that cannot be moved to the next machining station right away, although it is done with a given operation.

After one functional period, i.e., when a completed part leaves the job shop, we assess the status of all the parts that are currently being processed. Then decide the best way of handling the remaining operations, i.e., which machining operation should be done next for part A, etc. To achieve this goal, we should make sure that functional independence is always maintained. Because we determine the quickest sequence of processing the parts in the job shop at the end of each functional period, this solution should maximize the productivity of the job shop. The prediction of which part will be the next that will be leaving the job can also be determined at the time of re-initialization. However, the uncertainty increases, because the next part that will be coming into the job shop is not known a priori. If we develop an algorithm, then we can do this more or less instantly in a computer to determine the next sequence of machining operations for the parts in the job shop at that instant.

Considering the forgoing discussion on the job shop scheduling problem, the FRs of a job shop may be stated as follows:

FR1 = Fulfill machining orders as quickly as possible.

FR1 may be decomposed as follows:

FR11 = Maximize the flow rate of completed job orders through the job shop;
FR12 = Minimize the number of idle machines;
DP11 = Scheduling algorithm;
DP12 = Load a part when a machine becomes available.

FR11 and DP11 may be decomposed as follows:

FR111 = Introduce functional periodicity to the job shop operation;
FR112 = Re-initialize the system when a completed part leaves the job shop, determining the remaining time on the current machine;
DP111 = Completion of a part for delivery;
DP112 = Assess the status of each part in the job shop, i.e., remaining machining time and subsequent machining operation to complete the part.

FR12 and DP12 may be decomposed as follows:

FR121 = Calculate the remaining machining time;
FR122 = Load empty machines at the time of re-initialization;
FR123 = Provide buffers for partially finished parts awaiting the next operation;
DP121 = Algorithm for calculating remaining machining time for all parts currently being worked on by various machines;
DP122 = Bring in a new part to the job shop;
DP123 = Buffer table.

Exercise 20.2: Job Scheduling

A job shop has two horizontal milling machines, two lathes, three drill presses, and a grinding machine. The job shop has received orders for the two parts: Part a and Part b. They have to make 50 pieces of each. For Part a, it must be milled for 15 min; turned on a lathe for 23 min; drilled to make two holes for 5 min each, and ground in the grinding machine for 35 min. For Part b, it must be machined in the machining center for 10 min, drilled for five holes which will take 7 min each, and ground by the grinding machine for 12 min. The loading time and unloading time of the parts on each machine are 6 min and 3 min, respectively. Develop the best schedule for the job shop.

Exercise 20.3: Scheduling for Construction Site

The engineer-to-order industry is under constant pressure to optimize production and deliver the right components at the right time. For instance, in the building industry, they have to install their parts at the construction site. Synchronization between fabrication and on-site installation is difficult to realize. Outline a plan of real-time-capable production planning and control in engineer-to-order companies by minimizing time-dependent combinatorial complexity in the value chain.

Exercise 20.4: Throughput Rate in Emergency Room (ER) of Hospitals

Emergency rooms (ER) of hospitals are one of the most demanding departments of hospitals to operate. Patients with many kinds of different illnesses come in for treatments without any prior appointments. Some with the urgent need for care, such as those who were in automobile accidents and gunshot wounds, need quick attention when they show up. Some patients with chronic illness come in because they feel worse than usual. The goal is to take care of ER patients well as efficiently as possible. The FRs of ER may be assumed to be the following three:

> *FR1 = Prioritize ER patients based on the urgency of the illness of the patients;*
> *FR2 = Separate patients who need to be admitted to the inpatient unit;*
> *FR3 = Estimate the duration of treatment;*
> *FR4 = Fast track (FT) patients who can be discharged after quick treatment.*

Design a system that will maximize the patient flow rate through the emergency room of a city hospital.

20.7   Periodicity and Re-initialization of Political Systems

Conceptually, it may be easier to understand the significance of periodicity and re-initialization in the design of systems by considering the political system. Many different political systems exist. (For example, the dictatorship a la North Korea; presidential system, a la the United States; parliamentary system, a la the United Kingdom, and a political system that is an amalgam of these systems.) Here, we will compare the three: the presidential system, the parliamentary system, and dictatorship. The key characteristics of these two systems are as follows:

1. Key features of a Presidential System:

- *president is elected by direct vote of voters or by electors elected by popular vote;*
- *fixed length of the term in power (periodicity and re-initialization applies)*;
- *checks and balance: Power sharing with legislative body, and judiciary*;
- *annual budgetary approval.*

2. Key feature of a Parliamentary System:

- *the prime minister is elected by majority party in legislature;*
- *no fixed length of the term in power, election has to be called once in a fixed period;*
- *checks and balance: Power sharing with legislative body, and judiciary;*
- *annual budgetary approval.*

3. Key feature of a dictatorship:

- *dictator controls power, often, until the dictator's death or forceful removal;*
- *no fixed length of the term in power;*
- *no checks and balance;*
- *personal enrichment.*

Under the presidential system, major new policies are advocated at the beginning of the president's term, which generally lasts four to six years. Then, the president has the rest of the term to implement the principal legislation, even if it is unpopular. Congress must pass new legislation that supports the new primary policy of the president if they are needed. The central power of Congress is the control of the budget. During the term of office, a presidential system allows the implementation of even unpopular changes because, during the term of office, the president cannot be removed except through impeachment. Functional periodicity exists in this kind of presidency. Re-initialization takes place at once every four years in the United States and every six years in France. This presidential appears to be superior to the parliamentary system because of a clear initiation point for re-initialization.

Under the parliamentary system, there has to be a general election at least every four or five years. As long as the party in power has a majority, they can re-elect prime minister as often as they like. If the majority party does not support the prime minister, the cabinet is dissolved, and a new election is held. The prime minister can set a new set of policies when the PM has the backing of the majority party when they take power. It is difficult to design new legislation on a long-term basis unless the party in control has a supermajority in the parliament and unified among themselves. The end of the term is not clear, although there is a period during which a new election does not have to be called. Some times the prime minister can call a snap election to prolong the control of power. In a parliamentary system, it is more challenging to create functional periodicity and re-initialize the system. Governments can be volatile, changing hands whenever difficult issues must be resolved.

In general, the worst political system is a dictatorship. In most cases, it does not have functional periodicity and re-initialization process, since there are no set terms for tenure. Often the consequence of losing their power is a significant upheaval. Some dictators seize control with good intentions, but they eventually lead the country into turmoil because of the absence of functional periodicity. The transition from dictatorship to a political system with functional periodicity is challenging. Many dictatorships fail, but the dictator tends to amass a significant fortune or leave the power with an unfortunate end. Ultimately, the country loses out when a dictator takes over a country.

When corruption in government is an over-riding issue, functional periodicity is even more critical. Unfortunately, in many of the countries where corruption of public officials is prevalent, it may be difficult to institute a functional periodicity. Under such a system, re-initialization may not be implemented peacefully.

The Miracle of South Korea and Dictatorship:

In 2018, most people in the world who visit Korea found it to be a modern and prosperous democratic nation built on an educated workforce and technology. Korea had gone through tumultuous periods since the beginning of the twentieth century to be where she is today. Korea is one of the few nations that transformed themselves through several re-initializations and the adoption of the political functional period that was part of the constitution.

Because of the political ineptitude and corruption of the ruling class, Korean people suffered for almost seven decades. Japan colonized Korea from 1909 until 1945. In 1945, Korea was split into two by the U.S. and Soviet Union, and then in 1950, communist North Korea invaded South Korea, which destroyed the country. Since 1953, the Koreas maintained armistice. In 1961, General Park Chung Hi took over South Korea through coup de ta. Then, Korea was an impoverished country with one of the lowest GDP in the world.

Many people give him credit for having created modern Korea. Modern Korea can trace back the beginning of many things that has made Korea a modern nation to him. He was not corrupt and was a visionary of what a modern country should be like. Most people would agree that he had built a modern nation in 50 years. During his presidency, Korea had a façade of democracy but was really under one-person control. He built from highway, world-class industrial firms, educational infrastructure that is highly competitive worldwide, but he was a dictator. In 1960, 'Korea's per capita income was than that of the Philippines and Egypt. Today 'Korea's economy is in the top ten in the world and has one of the most modern infrastructures. President Park had a vision, and he realized his vision. His economic plan set his government's functional periodicity. The ten-year period of the 1960s may be considered one period, where the emphasis was building on national infrastructure using low-cost labor. His second period of functional periodicity was in the 1970s, during which he emphasized the heavy industries, shipbuilding, automobiles, consumer electronics, and high-speed rails. Unlike the 1960s, the 1970s were a difficult period because the return on investment was not immediate in these heavy industries. After his assassination in 1979, Korea finally reached its initial goal of creating the base for heavy industries, unlike labor-intensive apparel business.

Throughout the presidency of President Park, Korea maintained the appearance of the democratic form of government, although the president had ruled the country with absolute power. He extended his tenure for more than two terms thorough questionable political maneuvers. He was an absolute dictator. The question remains: would Korea be where it is today economically if President Park Chung Hi served only two four-year terms? Two of the presidents who succeeded President Park, who used to be army generals, ended up in jails after their presidencies were over because of their financial corruption while in power. President Park did not enrich himself while in office. Fortunately for Korea, the industries that were nurtured by President Park became highly successful industrial firms, several becoming world leaders in their respective fields.

After the demise of two generals who became presidents after the assassination of President Park, Korea has become a genuinely democratic nation. The civilian presidents, who succeeded the generals, brought in real democratic reform without harming industrial infrastructure and economic development. Today, Korea is a truly free democratic country. Such an open political environment nurtured its economic growth, the foundation of which were laid during the Park presidency has been no less than spectacular and stellar. Today, Korea is one of the top ten economies of the world. One of the significant factors for this economic and technological growth is the zeal of Korea people for education in general and higher education in particular. 70% of high school graduates go to college. And equally important is the willingness to make massive investments in new technologies by major companies in Korea.

With economic prosperity and democratization of the political system, Korea has become a genuinely democratic nation. It has strengthened the independence of the three branches of the government. The president of the country heads the executive branch. Its legislative body is active with the usual chaos. The Supreme Court heads the judiciary branch. The system is similar to those of the United States of America. When the Korea War ended in 1953, Korea was one of the poorest countries in the world without any industry, natural resources, electric power, and infrastructure.

Exercise 20.5:

Many leading industrial firms of the 1960s are no longer leading industrial firms in their country or the world in the early part of the twenty-first century. Identify one of the large industrial firms that fit this description and show how you might revive the firm through re-initialization.

Exercise 20.6:

Some of the countries in the world have not improved their economies during the past several decades. How would you re-design their economic and industrial policies to improve their economy and quality of life?

20.8 Functional Periodicity and Re-initialization of Educational Systems

20.8.1 Academic Calendar

The school calendar is periodic and cyclic. The school year is punctuated by winter vacation and summer vacation throughout the world. Time off from intensive learning in schools is necessary to give young people to grow intellectually, psychologically, and physically. During the summer vacation, some students worked on family farms and other jobs, which helped their families and their finances. During the long summer holidays, students also rest and re-charge to meet another year's challenges. After each academic year, students are promoted to the next grade or level. In some ways, it is similar to the cell cycle of physical systems.

20.8.2 Research Universities

Before the Second World War, most universities in the world did not do extensive research. They were primarily teaching institutions. However, during World War II, some of these universities in the United States, especially those with strong science and engineering schools, actively researched to help the war effort. As the war was coming to an end, the United States government, under the directives of President Frank Roosevelt, decided to continue the involvement of universities in national efforts. The goal was to strengthen economic competitiveness and national security by enhancing universities. In 1950, the U.S. National Science Foundation (the NSF Act of 1950 of the U.S.A.) was established to support university research to promote science and engineering. It has provided funding for basic research in science and engineering.

During the Cold War following the Second World War, some universities in the United States received substantial research support through various government agencies and minor assistance from industrial firms. Today, many of the top 20 universities in the world are the universities in the United States. They have conducted extensive research mostly with public funds, a significant portion of which was provided by defense-related departments and agencies of the United States government. It should be noted that in 2019, the United States spent more on defense than the next 19 nations combined, including Russia, Germany, Japan, the United Kingdom, France, Korea, and China.

In the United States, the universities researched the significant investment made by the U.S. government through its many agencies and departments. Major universities established specialized laboratories devoted to defense and space-related research such as the Jet Propulsion Laboratory of California Institute of Technology, the Lincoln Laboratory of MIT, and the Applied Research Laboratory of Johns Hopkins University. In addition to NSF, the U.S. Government invested in defense-related research through the Defense Advanced Research Projects Agency (DARPA), the Office of Naval Research (ONR), the Air Force Office of Scientific Research (AFOSR), and as part of the development of various defense technologies as part of the advanced weapon development. The U.S. government also funded five National Laboratories such as the Lawrence Livermore National Laboratory, Sandia National Laboratory, Oak Ridge National Laboratory, Argonne National Laboratory, and Los Alamos National Laboratory. The U. S. government also supported basic research in the field of biology and health sciences, which has created some of the most prominent universities in these fields.

The research conducted by universities has created a new culture in universities as well as in the business world of generating new business ventures funded by venture capital (VC). The well-known firms that were created as a result of this new culture entrepreneurship are such firms as Microsoft, Apple, Google, Facebook, Amazon, and many others. These firms were created based on "innovative design using software." It is noteworthy that the combined revenue of these firms is much larger than the income of all oil companies and automotive companies of the world combined.

20.9　Conclusions

This chapter examined the design of systems that have cyclic behaviors. Two kinds of systems were considered: (a) a system that satisfies the same set of FRs cyclically; and (b) a system that satisfies the same set of FRs, but requires re-initialization of the system at the beginning of each new cycle due to variations of DPs in the previous period. An example of the second kind of a system that requires re-initialization is a biological cell that undergoes mitosis. The latter system follows a "function clock." That is, at the beginning of each new functional period, the FRs of the system must be re-initialized to assure the optimum operation in the subsequent cycle.

Problems

Take any two of the Exercise problems given in the main text and provide solutions.

Reference

DAntes Design (2019) Division cycle of eukaryotic cell divided into four phases: G1, s, g2 and mitosis. Photo licensed from Shutterstock, ID: 1251867079

Further Reading

Alberts B, Bray D, Lewis J, Raff M, Roberts K, Watson JD (1994) Molecular biology of the cell, 3rd edn. Garland Science
Suh NP (2001) Axiomatic design—advances and applications. Oxford University Press
Suh NP (2005) Complexity. Oxford University Press

Artificial Intelligence in Design: A Look into the Future of Axiomatic Design

21

Erwin Rauch and Dominik T. Matt

Abstract

In the previous chapters, we learned all about Axiomatic Design (AD), where AD comes from, how it was developed, the axioms, complexity theory, and in-depth content for learning AD. This chapter looks at how AD will evolve in the future and introduces an approach based on Artificial Intelligence (AI). The approach presented is to be understood as a hypothesis to venture into the future together with the students analyzing how AI will change not only their daily lives, but also the work of a design engineer.

Many of the technological innovations related to Industry 4.0 pave the way for achieving a next level in engineering and especially in manufacturing. For the next decisive steps, we need the combination of disciplines such as engineering design and AI to create assistance systems for designers of highly complex systems, which support them step by step in the design process as well as for the re-design of systems affected by time-dependent complexity.

In the proposed AI-assisted design approach, we propose to combine AD as an established and proven theory for the design of complex systems with the latest methods of AI. For the design phase, AI offers an enormous potential to transform customer needs into functional requirements (FRs) and to support the designer in identifying and selecting the best design solution for a design problem based on existing data sets of previous successful or not successful designs.

E. Rauch (✉) · D. T. Matt
Faculty of Science and Technology, Free University of Bolzano-Bozen, Universitätsplatz 1, Bolzano, Italy
e-mail: erwin.rauch@unibz.it

D. T. Matt
Fraunhofer Research Italia s.c.a.r.l., Via A.-Volta 13a, 39100 Bolzano, Italy

© Springer Nature Switzerland AG 2021
N. P. Suh et al. (eds.), *Design Engineering and Science*,
https://doi.org/10.1007/978-3-030-49232-8_21

Similarly, the combination of modern technologies for data collection and AI also holds great potential to monitor complex systems determined by time-dependent complexity, like manufacturing systems. Based on improved technologies for data collection and processing as well as AI we can generate data-based predictive suggestions for system adaptation or even optimization, either with or without the interaction of the designer.

The presented AI-assisted design approach has potential to usher in the next era of engineering design, which will take us a huge step toward the vision of intelligent and self-optimizing systems.

21.1 Introduction

For many years, designers have dreamt about having an intelligent design machine that automatically generates designs or design concepts superior to those currently available. Already in 1990, Suh and Sekimoto (1990) presented the idea of the "Thinking Design Machine" (TDM) with the aim to provide designers a powerful and computer-aided design tool to improve the quality of the design and to reduce the time needed for creating a high-level design concept.

Since 1990, the world has changed rapidly and significantly. Computer-aided tools have been improved and further developed in order to take later stages of the design process on a new level. Especially recent developments in computer-aided design (CAD) and computer-aided engineering (CAE) facilitated the work of designers in geometrical modeling and drawing as well as in structural and dynamic engineering of parts and products. In the meantime all larger and most of the smaller enterprises are equipped with latest computer software for 3D CAD drawing, which allows a completely new level of visualization and a better platform for discussing designs together with other specialists in the product development and realization process (manufacturing specialists, material specialists, quality experts, …). Technologies like Virtual Reality (VR) give designers now the possibility to immerse in the virtual world and to inspect their design in a virtual but realistic and three-dimensional environment by using VR headsets for some hundreds of dollars of investment. Such powerful 3D CAD tools allow to creation of a Virtual Mock-Up (VMU). Instead of testing a product design via crash tests or fatigue tests in the laboratory using Physical Mock-Ups (PMU), most of the testing can be done nowadays on a virtual level. As a result, costs for engineering and time to market could be reduced significantly over the last 30 years. Examples of such tools in the engineering phase of product development are tools for Finite Element Analysis (FEA) or multibody dynamics simulation. The ongoing trend toward open-source software especially allows also smaller enterprises to get access to simulation software and modern CAE technologies. Further developments in computational engineering will lead also in the near future to a further increase of tools that assist designers in their daily work.

While the last 30 years show many innovations in the later stages of the design and engineering process, there is little to no computational aid system available today in the early and conceptual design stage. As the most critical decisions are usually taken in the conceptual design phase this implies in many cases that a design with a lot of potential for optimization is handed over to the colleagues in CAD and CAE and thus creating problems and costs in later stages of the design or even worse during manufacturing or assembly of the product. Thirty years ago designers using AD in the conceptual design phase had only Microsoft Excel spreadsheets with very limited space and no automation to document and visualize their design decompositions and matrixes in a digital way. Nearly 20 years ago, Acclaro DFSS has been launched providing the designer with a computational tool to support the AD process in the early design stage. Acclaro DFSS allows the designer to document the steps from one domain to another by encoding CNs, FRs, and DPs. During the mapping and decomposition process, Acclaro DFSS helps the designer significantly to analyze the design according to Axiom 1 (Independence Axiom) providing an automatic check if a design is coupled, decoupled, or uncoupled. Further, the software tool includes a function to rearrange a decoupled design matrix in such a way that the designer automatically gets the ideal sequence for implementation. In addition to the before-mentioned functionalities, Acclaro DFSS provides different forms for visualization like the design matrix, the FR–DP tree, or process flowcharts.

After this pioneering step forward in the automation of the design process and computational support of designer using AD, there has not been any further innovation over the last nearly 20 years. Compared to the developments in CAD and CAE as well as in manufacturing and assembly (e.g., rapid increase in flexible automation, robotics, advanced manufacturing technologies as well as smart and connected factories) the early stage of design is still working with "stone-age" design tools.

The actual design solution depends mostly on the individual experience and knowledge of the designer itself. Up to now, there is no tool available for archiving past (successful and not successful) designs and to support the designer in decision-making or in finding better design solutions outside of the individual experience and knowledge of the designer. At the same time, we can observe that since some years AI has become a trend and will become much more important in the next years. Due to the introduction of the concept of Industry 4.0 (mainly used in Europe and Asia) and Smart Manufacturing (used in the US) data has become a new status in engineering. Based on new sensor technologies, industrial Internet, and smart and connected factories the amount of available data increased exponentially. This leads currently to a stronger focus on computational methods for taking advantage of this new quantity and quality of data. According to many experts, "data will become the new gold" and those that are able to use advanced AI methods for analyzing data in an intelligent way will benefit from a competitive advantage on the global market. The race to become leader in AI has already started. United States, China, and Europe are already developing and implementing important initiatives to develop their competences in AI.

Therefore, the hypothesis for the future development of AD is to take advantage of recent developments in AI. The time has come to make use of computational power, Big Data technology, and new AI methods to fundamentally renew and automate the design process. After many years of insufficient computational aid, AI has the potential to introduce a new era of AD and to realize the dream of the Thinking Design Machine.

21.2 Artificial Intelligence—The Next Hype?

AI is currently on everyone's lips. There are many examples of AI in our lives. Apple's Siri is one such example. Another is Amazon's Alexa. Natural language processing technology, a form of AI, is used to translate languages in Google Translate. Indeed, up to $30B has been invested in AI in the past five years and 90% of it on research and development by companies such as Google and Microsoft (Bini 2018).

In the annual Gartner Hype Cycle Curve, new promising innovations are examined again and again and their status is presented on the so-called "hype cycle curve." The main aim is to show to what extent a certain technology is still in an initial "hype phase" or whether it has already reached the "plateau of productivity" and is thus ready for practical application. AI is currently at the zenith of the hype curve, which means that a great deal of future potential is currently seen in this technology, but the extent to which AI will really change our lives and work is still outstanding. Besides the general Gartner Hype Cycle Curve there is also an own hype cycle curve for AI technologies, which allows an even deeper view into the current development and the future technology leaps of AI (Goasduff 2019). The following can be read from this curve, for example:

- **Speech Recognition** has already reached the "plateau of productivity" and is already used in many daily applications.
- Text- or voice-based **Chatbots** are still on the top of the hype curve offering a high potential for increasing efficiency in customer service. For example, the car manufacturer KIA talks to 115,000 users per week, or Lidl's Winebot Margot provides guidance on which wine to buy and tips on food pairings. Chatbots are changing customer service from "the user learns the interface" to "the chatbot is learning what the user wants."
- **Machine Learning** already passed the top of the hype curve moving toward a more realistic use of this technology. ML uses mathematical models to extract knowledge and patterns from data. Adoption of ML is increasing as organizations encounter exponential growth of data volumes and advancements in computer infrastructure. For example, Volvo uses data to help predict when parts might fail or when vehicles need servicing, improving its vehicle safety.

- **Augmented Intelligence** is at the beginning of the hype curve with an expected time of 2–5 years to reach a practical use in daily business. Augmented intelligence is a human-centered partnership of people and AI working together to enhance cognitive performance. It focuses on AI's assistive role in advancing human capabilities. AI interacting with people and improving what they already know reduces mistakes and routine work. The goal of augmented intelligence is to be more efficient with automation, while complementing it with a human touch and common sense to manage the risks of decision automation.

In other words, AI will have a huge impact on both our daily lives and the world we work in, perhaps more than any other technological innovation in recent years. This also means that engineers and engineering students should be more involved with AI to be prepared for these technological changes. For this reason, this chapter pays special attention to this topic. However, before we get into the application of AI in engineering and then in engineering design, we first want to better understand what we mean with terms such as AI, machine learning (ML), or deep learning (DL). Basically, we can say that these three terms are different concepts of different levels. In general, deep learning is a subset of machine learning, and machine learning is a subset of AI (Garbade 2018; Nicholson 2019) (Fig. 21.1).

Artificial Intelligence can be seen as the science and engineering of making intelligent machines. AI is a branch of computer science dealing with the simulation of intelligent behaviors in computers. A goal of AI is to further develop the capability of a machine to imitate intelligent human behaviors. In AI, a computer system is able to perform tasks that normally require human intelligence, such as visual perception, speech recognition, decision-making, and translation between languages (Skymind 2019). The main objective of AI is to teach the machines to respond like humans do to flows of data. Although AI is a branch of computer

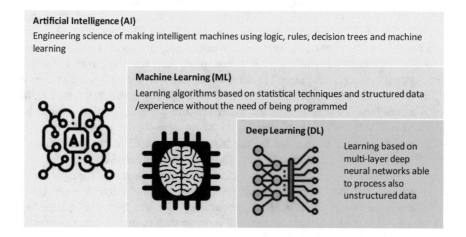

Fig. 21.1 Artificial intelligence, machine learning, and deep learning

science, there is hardly any field which is unaffected by this technology (Sadiku et al. 2019).

Machine learning is a subset of AI. That is, all ML counts as AI, but not all AI counts as ML. For example, rules engines, expert systems, and knowledge graphs—could all be described as AI, and none of them are machine learning. To give an example for rules engines: rules engines could be like an accountant system with knowledge of the tax code, which takes information you feed it, runs the information through a set of static rules, and gives you the amount of taxes you owe as a result. One aspect that separates machine learning from the knowledge graphs and expert systems is its ability to modify itself when exposed to more data; i.e., machine learning is dynamic and does not require human intervention to make certain changes. That makes it less brittle, and less reliant on human experts. As the name suggests, machine learning can be loosely interpreted to mean empowering computer systems with the ability to "learn." The intention of ML is to enable machines to learn by themselves using the provided data and make accurate predictions. In 1959, Arthur Samuel, one of the pioneers of machine learning, defined machine learning as a "field of study that gives computers the ability to learn without being explicitly programmed." The "learning" part of machine learning means that ML algorithms attempt to optimize along a certain dimension; i.e., they usually try to minimize error or maximize the likelihood of their predictions being true. This has three names: an error function, a loss function, or an objective function, because the algorithm has an objective. Here we need also "neural networks." They keep on measuring the error and modifying the parameters until they cannot achieve any less error (Garbade 2018; Skymind 2019).

Deep Learning is a subset of machine learning and also the next evolution of machine learning. DL algorithms are roughly inspired by the information processing patterns found in the human brain. Whenever we receive a new information, the brain tries to compare it to a known item before making sense of it, which is the same concept deep learning algorithms employ. Usually, when people use the term deep learning, they are referring to deep artificial neural networks, and somewhat less frequently to deep reinforcement learning. Deep artificial neural networks are a set of algorithms that have set new records in accuracy for many important problems, such as image recognition, sound recognition, recommender systems, natural language processing, etc. "Deep" is a technical term. It refers to the number of layers in a neural network making it able to process also unstructured data compared to machine learning techniques where features for classification need to be provided manually. Multiple hidden layers allow deep neural networks to learn features of the data in a so-called feature hierarchy, because simple features (e.g., two pixels) recombine from one layer to the next, to form more complex features (e.g., a line). Nets with many layers pass input data (features) through more mathematical operations than nets with few layers, and are therefore more computationally intensive to train. Requirements of DL are high-end computing machines and considerably big amounts of training data to deliver accurate results (Garbade 2018; Skymind 2019).

21.3 Examples of Artificial Intelligence Applications in Engineering

The literature contains various applications of Industrial AI in the fields of engineering and manufacturing. In the following, we want to give an overview of examples and applications of Industrial AI in engineering.

AI Technologies are already used also for **engineering design**. As an example, the generative design platform DesIA uses an object-oriented and open-source language to describe the specifications and the desired product/system. Afterwards, a rule based system combined with decision trees generates a number of admissible design concepts. In the next step, machine learning algorithms are used to choose the best design concept. In the last step, modern and advanced simulation and CAE tools help the designer to optimize the concept in its details (Masfaraud and Dumouchel 2019).

Kumar (2017) in his literature review describes a number of applications in **production planning**. AI technology has already been used in many computer-aided process planning (CAPP) applications in the past. Furthermore, AI is used in knowledge-based expert systems where AI technologies access the experience of experts (collected in databases) and give a designer or user suggestions for design solutions.

A further field of application of AI is **domestic or industrial robotics**. Today's AI-powered robots, or at least those machines deemed as such, possess no natural general intelligence, but they are capable of solving problems and "thinking" in a limited capacity. From working on assembly lines at Tesla to teaching Japanese students English, examples of AI in the field of robotics are plentiful. Home robots use AI to scan room size, identify obstacles and remember the most efficient routes for cleaning (Daley 2018). Fanuc, the robot manufacturer, uses AI-based tools to simplify to teach industrial robots to do their work. AI simplifies the training process, so the human operator just needs to look at a photo of parts jumbled in a bin on a screen and taps a few examples of what needs to be picked up, like showing a small child how to sort toys. This is significantly a less training than what typical vision-based sensors need and can also be used to train several robots at once (Shu 2019).

In **maintenance**, AI technologies are used for realizing predictive maintenance in the form of machine learning and artificial neural networks to formulate predictions regarding asset malfunction. Knowing that a certain component of a machine will fail with a defined probability on a certain day and at a certain time has an enormous influence on the way we organize maintenance work in the company in the future. AI in predictive maintenance allows for drastic reductions in costly unplanned downtime, as well as for extending the remaining useful life (RUL) of production machines and equipment. In cases where maintenance is unavoidable, technicians are briefed ahead of time on which components need inspection and which tools and methods to use, resulting in very focused repairs that are scheduled in advance (Kushmaro 2018).

Another potential field of application of AI in industry is **quality management and quality inspection**. Manufacturing units that make complicated items like microchips and circuit sheets are already making use of machine vision, which furnishes AI with amazingly high-goal cameras. Advanced vision systems combined with AI algorithms can pick even minute defects unmistakably, more reliably than the human eyes. Defects are identified immediately and a response is automatically configured, sent, and managed in order to reduce inefficiencies and waste of material due to non-quality. This helps to increase productivity and at the same time to improve, also, the ecological sustainability of modern manufacturing processes (Admin 2019).

The use of Industrial AI is not only increasing in manufacturing but also in **logistics and supply chain management (SCM)**. Supply chain planning is among the most important activities included in SCM strategy. Therefore, it is crucial to have reliable tools for developing efficient plans. Implementing AI or machine learning, the supply chain decision-making processes can be optimized significantly. The advantage in logistics and SCM is that we usually have a lot of data, which is a prerequisite for using AI or ML techniques. Analyzing huge data sets and applying intelligent algorithms, we can balance demand and supply, and at the same time optimize the delivery processes. In addition, human intervention is minimal. AI algorithms will do everything autonomously and save companies from making mistakes.

In addition to the above-mentioned examples of AI in engineering, a number of other examples for the application of AI could be listed (warehouse management, manufacturing system design, self-optimized machining, etc.). In summary, it can be said that AI is still in its infancy in the industrial environment and that not all potentials have been exhausted. In the future, the interdisciplinary combination of engineering competences and AI methods from computer science will enable us to take full advantage of AI in industry and engineering.

21.4 Axiomatic Design Knowledge Database as Basis for Artificial Intelligence in Axiomatic Design

As already mentioned in Suh and Sekimoto (1990), a computational aid system for AD requires a database. According to them, such a database needs to have at least enough knowledge to give the designer plausible design solutions. Such a database should also have the knowledge of many designers by providing a function to store past designs and to retrieve possible design solutions for a common set and subset of FRs. A FR–DP database may also be convenient to evaluate various functional aspects of a candidate DP, such as side effects not considered by the designer. According to Suh and Sekimoto (1990), DPs may be constructed and stored in different ways, such as (i) parts/components, (ii) systems and subsystems, (iii) materials, and (iv) physical phenomena/status. Since 1990, such a database has never been realized as the technical possibilities for storage of Big Data has been limited over the last years. Also Floss and Talavage (1990) already proposed in 1990 such a knowledge-based design assistant. Khan and Day (2002) developed a similar concept of a knowledge-based database some years later.

Due to poor scalability and low performance, many traditional computing technologies were inadequate for handling Big Data, which are characterized by the volume, velocity, variety, and veracity of the data (Cheng et al. 2018). The latest developments in the area of Big Data today also allow large amounts of data to be handled and processed. Big Data concern large-volume, complex, growing data sets with multiple, autonomous sources. With the fast development of networking, data storage, and the data collection capacity, Big Data are now rapidly expanding in all science and engineering domains (Wu et al. 2014). Research in the areas of computer graphics, database management systems, and AI along with the development of faster and more powerful hardware platforms accelerated and widened the use of computers for engineering problem-solving. Knowledge-based expert systems (KBESs) are one of the first realizations of research in the field of AI, in the form of a software technology. KBESs are computer programs designed to act as an expert to solve a problem in particular domain. The program uses the knowledge of the domain coded in it and a specified control strategy to arrive at solutions. Such systems consist of a knowledge base and an inference engine subdivided in one or more inference mechanisms (Krishnamoorthy and Rajeev 1996). The research findings of Quintana-Amate et al. (2015) provided by literature survey confirm the existence of a gap on knowledge sourcing in engineering, and more precisely they underlined the need for an extended knowledge-based engineering (KBE) development process which integrates AI tools and expert intervention to systematically manage the knowledge efficiently captured and modeled (employing AI algorithms and expert involvement). Therefore, there is a need for further research on the integration of KBE systems and AI implementations as a potential solution to achieve a next level of engineering design.

As seen before, with the recent progress in capability for data storage, handling, analysis as well as AI methods, such a database becomes much more realistic and opens completely new opportunities to take advantage for an optimized design. Such a database would be a complete novelty in the AD community as well as in the community for engineering design. Such a database means an immense concentration of knowledge, which would mature over years. As a side effect, this database would also play an important role for the practical application and teaching of AD, as examples can be taken from it for learning purposes. A big difficulty is surely the correct structuring of the database and the form in which the earlier designs are documented and archived, in order to be able to extract and use the data afterward in the best possible way. In the phase of building up such a database, first the ontology, architecture, and data representation of the database need to be defined as this is a fundamental basis that needs to be considered. As there is a great interest from the AD community to support the creation of such a database, there would be a high willingness of designers to fill the database with life. Another way of filling the databases is to use a reverse engineering approach (see also Girgenti et al. 2016; Vickery et al. 2018; Rauch and Vickery 2020). Such a reverse-mapping allows to decompose past designs easily into hierarchical FR–DP pairs. In a first step, such a database could be filled only with freely available designs or designs from Open Access papers. This means that people uploading their past designs give free access to this information. At a later stage, a model might be developed how designs can also be commercially exploited, e.g., by allowing the designer to access more than just the freely accessible data by paying a fee.

21.5 Vision of Combining Artificial Intelligence and Axiomatic Design

According to the sections before, we introduce the vision of an AI-assisted design and re-design of complex systems in engineering design. While a lot of research is currently focused on how to design products and systems according to the principles of the digital transformation in industry and Industry 4.0, the following hypothesis aims to innovate and automate the design process itself and thus to initiate a revolution in the field of engineering design.

Especially in the design of complex systems that are changing over time, e.g., manufacturing systems, the design process can be divided into a "new design" and adaptations ("re-design"). Adapting an existing system to changing environment or new requirements is a difficult mission. The world is becoming ever more short-lived, and product life cycles as well as system life cycles are becoming ever shorter. This also means that many products or systems have to be adapted at ever shorter intervals. Therefore, in the future, the design of products or systems must be as fast and agile as possible and be based on the principles of self-optimizing systems by using intelligent and smart technologies like AI.

Figure 21.2 shows the development of AD over the years focusing on the most important developments in AD theory, its field of applications, and tools to support the designer.

From the early phase of AD to the beginning of the twenty-first century, researchers focused more on the first axiom. In the following years, advances in complexity theory concentrated more on the second axiom and in the detailed analysis and procedure to define CNs in the customer domain and FRs in the functional domain. Regarding the application of AD in practice, it has been used in its beginnings mainly for the design of products and later for the design of complex systems (e.g., manufacturing systems, software design, and organizational design). In recent years, designers started also to use AD for the design of intelligent products and systems according to Industry 4.0 and Smart Manufacturing (Vickery et al. 2019). With the work of Kim et al. (2019), the first time researcher started also to use AI technologies for making a next important step in the development of AD in engineering design. As already mentioned in the introduction of this chapter there are only limited number of tools supporting the designer in using AD during the design process. From the 90s, the designer used Microsoft Excel spreadsheets for the application of AD with all its limitations in space as well as automation.

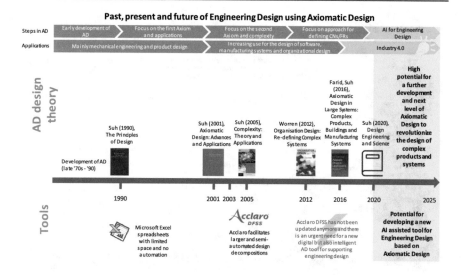

Fig. 21.2 Past, present, and future of complex system design using Axiomatic Design

Roughly ten years later, Acclaro DFSS has been launched facilitating larger design projects and offering functions for a semi-automated FR–DP decomposition. However, over the last nearly 20 years there were no more updates or launches of new aid tools for conceptual design based on AD, which is now (in an increasingly digital world) seriously limiting and affecting the use and dissemination of AD in design projects.

Therefore, the hypothesis is to realize in the future the vision of a Thinking Design Machine, as mentioned by Suh and Sekimoto (1990) by using recent AI methods or AI technologies to be developed in the near future creating the basis for a new platform of a computer-aided tool for conceptual design. In the following two sections, this hypothesis and vision of an AI-assisted design and re-design of complex systems will be described more in detail, thus giving an outlook on possible future developments in AD for engineering design.

21.6 Artificial Intelligence-Assisted Design of Complex Systems

Figure 21.3 shows the new proposed AI-assisted design approach (see Fig. 21.3). It starts with an automated clustering of customer feedbacks into meaningful CNs with the help of data mining and knowledge discovery methods. In previous approaches, this was usually done manually by collecting and looking over the customer feedback. The big challenge for users of AD in this phase is that large quantities of information in the customer domain can only be reduced with great effort to meaningful CNs in a manual way, whereby also a guarantee to consider all

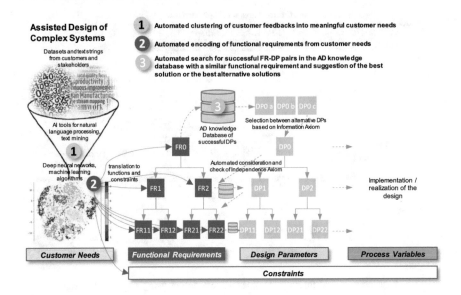

Fig. 21.3 Concept of AI-assisted design of complex systems

information as completely as possible is usually not given. Therefore, for the future, the development of assisted and intelligent methods is needed to simplify this and improve the quality of the data. Kim et al. (2019) are taking a first step in this direction showing in their work a first attempt/experiment based on available data of Airbnb (customer feedback) using Pytorch, an open-source deep learning platform, and MATLAB. By using a hierarchical clustering algorithm, customer feedback can be translated and clustered into key features, and therefore relevant customer needs. According to them a challenge will be to deal with different types and abstraction levels of customer feedback, which requires in future to find appropriate state-of-the-art algorithms for the automated identification, extraction, and clustering of CNs. Further research is still necessary, in particular, due to the need to transform unstructured and, sometimes, ill-defined user specifications into meaningful key CNs, which requires the research and application of state-of-the-art natural language processing techniques (Kulkarni et al. 2019; Kang et al. 2019a, b).

In the second step, these CNs will be encoded to FRs and to constraints. This describes the link from the customer domain to the functional domain, which should occur as automated as possible and without expensive involvement of the designer (except for logical checks). As also described in the work of Kim et al. (2019), one challenge lies in the automatic encoding and transition from natural language expression of customer needs to FRs that can be then further used in the AD design approach. First tested AI abstraction tools for natural language by Kim et al. (2019) have resulted to be not effective in extracting FRs. Word embedding tools are currently not directly capable of translating key CNs into functions of a system. It is also necessary to research, test, and validate possible AI solutions for this step in the AD design approach, or to determine whether fully automated solutions can be implemented or to what extent humans should intervene in a semi-automated solution. Using the proposed AD knowledge database, also a knowledge-based encoding of FRs could also be done, where based on earlier transitions from the customer domain to the functional domain, the designer is provided with suggestions for possible FRs for recurring or similar CNs.

In the third step, a semi-automated and AI-assisted FR–DP mapping and decomposition process takes place. During the mapping and decomposition, the proposed approach includes automated proof checking (Mantravadi et al. 2019) of the Independence Axiom (Axiom 1) to avoid a so-called coupled, and therefore complex design suggesting possibilities for a re-design or rearrangement of FR–DP pairs. The FR–DP mapping (finding a design solution for a certain FR) is semi-automated in the assisted design approach as the system will propose the designer automatically several alternative DPs for a certain FR. The selection of the best DP will be assisted by an automated check of the Information Axiom (Axiom 2), evaluating the complexity of a design solution. Similarly to this, such an AI-based approach is used also to propose possible decompositions of a higher level FR–DP pair into lower level ones based on similar decompositions found in the AD knowledge database. Prerequisite and crucial for this is a suitable ontology for the formal representation of such knowledge (Akmal and Batres 2013) and a central database in the background, which is fed with labeled successful and unsuccessful designs in order to be able to learn from past successes and failures through supervised AI techniques.

21.7 Artificial Intelligence-Assisted Re-design of Complex Systems

In Fig. 21.4, we can see the behavior of a system, e.g., a manufacturing system, over the time. Future events are very often unpredictable and might shift the system range away from the defined design range, and thus create time-dependent complexity. According to AD, the information content of a system with defined FRs is described by the joint probability that all FRs are fulfilled by the respective set of DPs and measured by the ratio of the common range between the design and the system range. As shown in Fig. 21.4, a system might deteriorate during its service life and its design range will move outside the required system range. According to AD, the first type of time-dependent complexity is periodic complexity, which can be managed through the analysis of previous typical time periods. Simple examples of periodic complexity are tools that wear out (Matt and Rauch 2011). If we are able to define the right periodic intervals for their change and re-design, this information helps to reduce complexity. The second type of time-dependent complexity,

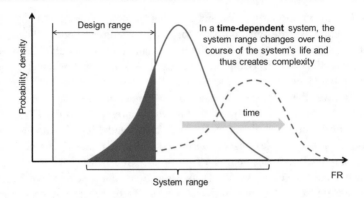

Fig. 21.4 Overlapping and shifting of design and system range

combinatorial complexity (Suh 2005), can be caused in case of a manufacturing system by the dynamics of unpredictable technological, socio-economic, or political influences. According to Suh (2005), this unpredictable combinatorial complexity can be managed by, transforming it into a periodic complexity. When the system does not renew itself by resetting and reinitializing, it becomes a reason for wasting resources. Manufacturing systems are especially characterized by such a combinatorial complexity and in order to be responsive to unforeseen changes. They must be reset in periodic intervals to avoid or minimize the effect of shifting outside of the design range. The time-dependent combinatorial complexity must be changed into a time-dependent periodic complexity by introducing functional periodicity. This allows trigger of the re-design of the system and to re-adjust to changing conditions. If this could be achieved, the system will be more agile and resilient than traditional ones.

In the proposed AD, approach for AI-assisted re-design the analysis of the system over time might show degrees of periodicity, which can be used to actively trigger the re-design of a company's manufacturing system or parts of it, before a too strong deviation of system range and design range force it to (see also Fig. 21.5). The analysis would imply searching for patterns in collected temporal

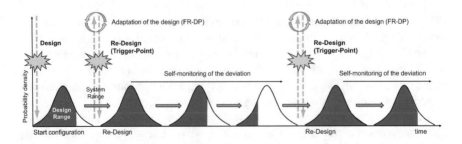

Fig. 21.5 Triggered re-design of manufacturing systems

series, like, for example, sensor measurements, evolution of performance measures, maintenance interventions (Pertselakis et al. 2019), and logging data for functional fault diagnosis (Ye et al. 2014).

Modern technologies of Industry 4.0, such as sensors and human–machine interfaces, enable the collection of large amount of data and thus the current status of systems like a manufacturing system to be called up in real time. A re-design should not be triggered only after an emergency alarm based on the self-monitoring, as this would mean a reactive re-design. Re-design must be based on the digest of the daily production measured over time (a trend over a longer period), not only in terms of the real-time data generated during the daily manufacturing process. Based on this fact also predictive suggestions need to be generated "it is worth to re-design before the end of the week/month/year" and only trigger alarms of the form "urgent re-design required" when the suggestions had been ignored and the "trigger point" had been reached without any measurable trend improvement. For self-monitoring, the tolerance bands of FRs and DPs are determined by metrics during the initial configuration or design of the system. Depending on whether the adaptation of the system can take place automatically (e.g., an adaptation of parameters of a manufacturing process) or whether human support is required, we speak of self-adaptation or assisted adaptation of the system. Due to technological or organizational changes, it may be that for certain FR–DP pairs, an earlier rejected DP alternative would achieve now a better result. To achieve this the "AI" must be able to doubt about its own beliefs. It is required that an "entity" able to simulate the use of "alternative" DPs to re-weight their influence on the overall performance. This topic is related to Reinforcement Learning (Lison 2012), a ML technique to find the best possible behavior or path in a specific situation. Similarly, new DPs may join the AD knowledge database (e.g., a new technology), which may replace an old DP due to better performance. In these cases, not only the previous status should be restored by self-adaptation, but the aim is to achieve a self-optimization of the manufacturing system. During this process, some DPs may save time and money by automatic adaptation, while other DPs may be of strategic relevance requiring a human-driven decision-making process.

21.8 Impact and Advantages of Artificial Intelligence in Axiomatic Design

In the current application of AD for the design of complex systems, there are and there have been certain limitations. Many experienced designers agree that AD helps them to cultivate insightful thinking. But many still find it difficult to apply AD principles to design practice since using AD effectively also requires designer's insights and experience in AD (Kim et al. 2019). Based on own experiences in research and industrial practice the following are currently detectable weaknesses of AD:

- need of experience in applying AD;
- difficulty in the holistic consideration of customer needs;
- designer very often struggle to define solution-neutral FRs;
- the identification of design solutions/parameters is based on their knowledge and experience;
- existing designs from other sources cannot be taken into account because there is no central data source;
- the process is very manual, and there is a very limited computer-aided support with current systems available;
- current approaches do not allow a real-time monitoring of whether the design parameters (DPs) still meet the FRs over time;
- not possible to automatically determine the time for a re-design of a system (trigger point);
- does not allow an AD-based self-optimization of the system.

However, the time may be now just right to take AD to a completely new and revolutionary level by taking advantage of modern technologies from Industry 4.0 (such as sensor technology, real-time data gathering, AI, deep learning, machine learning, or cloud computing) to eliminate the before-mentioned limitations. Planning can be carried out much faster, with less effort, with more accuracy, and an enormous planning quality through the presented AI-assisted and automated design concept. Table 21.1 shows the most important innovations due to the use of the proposed new AD design approach.

Table 21.1 Assisted (re)design of complex systems—traditional versus new proposed AI-assisted approach

Traditional AD design approach	New proposed AI-based AD design approach
Manual and subjective analysis of key customer needs through the designer or design team	Automated clustering of customer feedback into meaningful CNs
Manual and subjective translation of the CNs into FRs through the designer or design team	Semi-automated translation of CNs into FRs
Designer very often struggle to define solution-neutral FRs	System supports the correct syntax and formulation of solution-neutral FRs
Experience-based approach depending on the experience of the designer or design team	Knowledge-based approach depending on the quality and quantity of past designs in an AD knowledge database
No guarantee of a comprehensive consideration of all potential design solutions (DPs)	Due to an increasing filling level of an AD knowledge database over time, an immense compendium of potential DPs can be created.
Very manual process with only limited computer-aided support	Development of a highly automated computer-aided conceptual design (CACD) tool

(continued)

Table 21.1 (continued)

Traditional AD design approach	New proposed AI-based AD design approach
Difficult to apply for novices or people not experienced with AD	Many of the decisions and reviews (e.g., check of AD Axioms) are done automatically in the background, making it easy to use even for novice designers
No possibility for real-time monitoring of whether the DPs still meet the FRs over time	Integration of a self-monitoring with adjustable sensitivity limits and alarm if defined setting limits are exceeded
No possibility to automatically determine the time for a re-design of a system (trigger point)	Autonomous determination of the trigger point for a re-design of the system (or its parts) based on the self-monitoring
Does not allow a self-optimization of the system	Enables self-adaptation and self-optimization of a system

As mentioned above, such an AI-assisted design approach will have an important impact in the field of the design of complex systems. However going in this direction, there will be many related fields of action, where such an approach may help. A possible additional goal for the future is sustainability. The proposed approach could also provide information on the extent to which certain adjustments could also have positive or negative effects on the environment or sustainability in general in all their facets (economic, ecological, or social).

Problem

Students should concentrate on one domain (customer, functional, design domain) and discuss the potential of AI in the respective domain.

References

Admin (2019) 10 use cases of AI in Industry 4.0 revolution. GPUonCloud Website. https://gpuoncloud.com/10-use-cases-of-ai-in-industry-4-0-revolution/

Akmal S, Batres R (2013) A methodology for developing manufacturing process ontologies. J Jpn Ind Manag Assoc 64:303–316. https://doi.org/10.11221/jima.64.303

Bini SA (2018) Artificial intelligence, machine learning, deep learning, and cognitive computing: what do these terms mean and how will they impact health care? J Arthroplasty 33(8):2358–2361. https://doi.org/10.1016/j.arth.2018.02.067

Cheng B, Zhang J, Hancke GP, Karnouskos S, Colombo AW (2018) Industrial cyberphysical systems: realizing cloud-based big data infrastructures. IEEE Ind Electron Mag 12(1):25–35. https://ieeexplore.ieee.org/document/8322328

Daley S (2018) 19 examples of artificial intelligence shaking up business as usual. Builtin Website. Accessed 29 Oct 2019

Farid A, Suh NP (eds) (2016) Axiomatic design in large systems. Springer, Cham, Switzerland

Floss P, Talavage J (1990) A knowledge-based design assistant for intelligent manufacturing systems. J Manuf Syst 9(2):87–102. https://doi.org/10.1016/0278-6125(90)90024-C. http://www.sciencedirect.com/science/article/pii/027861259090024C

Garbade MJ (2018) Clearing the confusion: AI vs machine learning vs deep learning differences. Medium Magazine Website. https://towardsdatascience.com/clearing-the-confusion-ai-vs-machine-learning-vs-deep-learning-differences-fce69b21d5eb

Girgenti A, Pacifici B, Ciappi A, Giorgetti A (2016) An axiomatic design approach for customer satisfaction through a lean start-up framework. In: Liu A (ed) 10th international conference on axiomatic design (ICAD), Procedia CIRP, vol 53. Elsevier ScienceDirect, Xi'an, Shaanxi, China, pp 151–157. https://doi.org/10.1016/j.procir.2016.06.101

Goasduff L (2019) Top trends on the gartner hype cycle for artificial intelligence, 2019. Gartner Website. https://www.gartner.com/smarterwithgartner/top-trends-on-the-gartner-hype-cycle-for-artificial-intelligence-2019/

Kang S, Patil L, Rangarajan A, Moitra A, Jia T, Robinson D, Dutta D (2019a) Automated feedback generation for formal manufacturing rule extraction. Artif Intell Eng Des Anal Manuf 33(3):289–301. https://doi.org/10.1017/S0890060419000027

Kang S, Patil L, Rangarajan A, Moitra A, Robinson D, Jia T, Dutta D (2019b) Ontology-based ambiguity resolution of manufacturing text for formal rule extraction. J Comput Inf Sci Eng 19 (2):9. https://doi.org/10.1115/1.4042104

Khan A, Day AJ (2002) A knowledge based design methodology for manufacturing assembly lines. Comput Ind Eng 41(4):441–467. https://dl.acm.org/doi/10.1016/S0360-8352\%2801\%2900067-5#sec-ref

Kim SG, Yoon SM, Yang MC, Choi J, Akay H, Burnell E (2019) AI for design: virtual design assistant. CIRP Ann 68:141–144. https://doi.org/10.1016/j.cirp.2019.03.024

Krishnamoorthy CS, Rajeev S (1996) Artificial intelligence and expert systems for engineers, 1st edn. CRC Press, Boca Raton

Kulkarni S, Verma P, Mukundan R (2019) Assessing manufacturing strategy definitions utilising text-mining. Int J Prod Res 57(14):4519–4546. https://doi.org/10.1080/00207543.2018.1512764

Kumar SPL (2017) State of the art-intense review on artificial intelligence systems application in process planning and manufacturing. Eng Appl Artif Intell 65:294–329. https://doi.org/10.1016/j.engappai.2017.08.005. http://www.sciencedirect.com/science/article/pii/S0952197617301896

Kushmaro P (2018) 5 ways industrial AI is revolutionizing manufacturing. CIO Magazine Website. https://www.cio.com/article/3309058/5-ways-industrial-ai-is-revolutionizing-manufacturing.html

Lison P (2012) An introduction to machine learning. University of Oslo Website. https://heim.ifi.uio.no/plison/pdfs/talks/machinelearning.pdf, hiOA

Mantravadi S, Li C, Møller C (2019) Multi-agent manufacturing execution system (MES): concept, architecture and ML algorithm for a smart factory case. In: Proceedings of the 21st international conference on enterprise information systems (ICEIS), vol 1, pp 477–482. https://doi.org/10.5220/0007768904770482

Masfaraud S, Dumouchel PE (2019) DessIA—an engineering design software with artificial intelligence. Telecom Paris Website. https://www.telecom-paris.fr/wp-content-EvDsK19/uploads/2019/07/2-2b-JPE-TP-2019-KeynoteE_Dessia_Commercial_V6_short.pdf, keynote Paper Presentation

Matt DT, Rauch E (2011) Continuous improvement of manufacturing systems with the concept of functional periodicity. Key engineering materials, vol 473. Trans Tech Publications, Switzerland, pp 783–790

Nicholson C (2019) Artificial intelligence (AI) vs. machine learning vs. deep learning. A.I. Wiki on Pathmind Website. https://skymind.ai/wiki/ai-vs-machine-learning-vs-deep-learning. Accessed 28 Oct 2019

Pertselakis M, Lampathaki F, Petrali P (2019) Predictive maintenance in a digital factory shop-floor: data mining on historical and operational data coming from manufacturers' information systems. In: Proper HA, Stirna J (eds) Advanced information systems engineering workshops, CAiSE 2019. Lecture notes in business information processing, Rome, Italy, vol 349. Springer, Cham, pp 120–131, 3–7 June 2019

Quintana-Amate S, Bermell-Garcia P, Tiwari A (2015) Transforming expertise into Knowledge-Based Engineering tools: a survey of knowledge sourcing inthe context of engineering design. Knowl-Based Syst 84:89–97

Rauch E, Vickery AR (2020) Systematic analysis of needs and requirements for the design of smart manufacturing systems in SMEs. J Comput Des Eng. https://doi.org/10.1093/jcde/qwaa012

Sadiku MNO, Musa SM, Musa OM (2019) Artificial intelligence in the manufacturing industry. Int J Adv Sci Res Eng (IJASRE) 5(6):108–110

Shu C (2019) Industrial robotics giant Fanuc is using AI to make automation even more automated. Tech Crunch Magazine Website. https://techcrunch.com/2019/04/18/industrial-robotics-giant-fanuc-is-using-ai-to-make-automation-even-more-automated/?guccounter=1

Skymind (2019) Artificial Intelligence (AI) vs. Machine Learning vs. Deep Learning. https://skymind.ai/wiki/ai-vs-machine-learning-vs-deep-learning. Accessed 28 Oct 2019

Suh NP (1990) The principles of design. Oxford University Press

Suh NP (2001) Axiomatic design—advances and applications. Oxford University Press

Suh NP (2005) Complexity. Oxford University Press

Suh NP, Sekimoto S (1990) Design of thinking design machine. CIRP Ann 39(1):145–148. https://doi.org/10.1016/S0007-8506(07)61022-1

Suh NP, Cavique M, Foley JT (eds) (2021) Design engineering and science. Springer Nature

Vickery A, Rauch E, Brown CA (2018) Deriving functional requirements for industry 4.0 from industry's assessment of needs. In: Peruzzini M, Pellicciari M, Bil C, Stjepandić J, Wognum N (eds) Transdisciplinary engineering methods for social innovation of Industry 4.0: proceedings of the 25th ISPE Inc. international conference on transdisciplinary engineering. Advances in transdisciplinary engineering, vol 7. IOS Press, pp 23–32. https://doi.org/10.3233/978-1-61499-898-3-23

Vickery AR, Rauch E, Rojas RA, Brown CA (2019) Smart data analytics in SME manufacturing an axiomatic design based conceptual framework. In: Liu A, Puik E, Foley JT (eds) 12th international conference on axiomatic design (ICAD), MATEC web of conferences, Sydney, Australia

Wu X, Zhu X, Wu GQ, Ding W (2014) Data mining with big data. IEEE Trans Knowl Data Eng 26(1):97–107

Ye F, Zhang Z, Chakrabarty K, Gu X (2014) Knowledge discovery and knowledge transfer in board-level functional fault diagnosis. In: Purtell M, Mitra S (eds) 2014 international test conference (ITC), Washington, DC, USA, pp 1–10

Axiomatic Cloud Computing Architectural Design

22

John Thomas and Pam Mantri

Abstract

The design of modern cloud computing makes available a plethora of scalable cloud computing offerings. The cloud is increasingly becoming the backbone of the highly complex modern knowledge economy that includes social, mobile, IoT, Big Data, and AI. Knowledge-based products and services follow fat-tail distributions such as the power law that poses major opportunities and challenges for the designer. The Axiomatic Designer is uniquely positioned in designing for the de novo situations that the fat-tailed distributions expose. Also, the cloud frees up the architectural decision-making away from the legacy compatibility-burden, and toward various cloud-native (i.e., de novo/solution-neutral) as well as hybrid (on-prem/cloud and cloud/cloud) architectures. Furthermore, the competitive landscape around the cloud is not static; it is adaptive and evolving rapidly. Here again, Axiomatic Design (AD) is uniquely positioned in rising up to the various de novo challenges. This, however, requires contributions from frameworks such as knowledge as heterarchically hierarchical (KA|h|H), stigmergy, complex adaptive systems (CAS), Cynefin, Boyd's OODA loop theory of asymmetric fast transients, axiomatic maturity diagram (AMD), as well as Weick's loose-coupling approach to help unify and strengthen the axiomatic approach. This chapter unifies the above approaches in order to tackle the architectural challenges of cloud computing.

This chapter is an adaptation of the paper "Axiomatic Cloud Computing Architectural Design" presented by the same authors at ICAD 2019 in Sydney Australia (Thomas and Mantri 2019). This paper was published open access at https://doi.org/10.1051/matecconf/ 201930100024 under a CC BY 4.0 license.

J. Thomas (✉) · P. Mantri
New Rochelle, NY, USA
e-mail: johntom@cogtools.com

22.1 Introduction

The cloud is fundamentally disruptive. If its strategic import is properly understood, it has immense potential to help scale businesses in space (geographical space, product/service space, governance/regulation space, etc.) and time (start-up to IPO, industry business cycle, market seasonality, etc.).

With hindsight, it is understandable that the web would bankrupt a successful legacy business model such as the Borders bookstore that in the mid-90's mistakenly invested heavily on brick-and-mortar stores across the globe, failed to develop an e-reader, and outsourced its online sales (in 2001) over to Amazon. By the time (i.e., in 2008) Borders realized its online outsourcing error and retracted, it was too late. It filed for bankruptcy on February 16, 2011 (Wikipedia 2019a).

In hindsight, it is easy to see the strategic mistakes that the management at Borders bookstore had made. But from a mathematical perspective, what killed Borders was an inadequate appreciation of the power law (Wikipedia 2019b) that is operative in the modern knowledge-based, network economies. Human knowledge is a network of concepts which has been aggregating across millenniums. It has a certain shape, structure, and overall dynamic. But most significantly, it has a certain directionality in its growth patterns, as dictated by the power law which results from the phenomenon of preferential attachment (colloquially known as the Matthew effect or the Rich-Get-Richer effect). In other words, what is popular becomes even more popular by virtue of the fact that it is better known. Thus, a brick-and-mortar bookstore that tries to give equitable shelf space to the mega-successful Harry Potter books as well as the also-rans, simply cannot compete with an online store that only incurs remote-location storage cost that is comparatively cheap. Note that shipping costs are borne by the buyer who pays for it for the convenience of shopping from his/her home. Along with lower inventory costs, an astute vendor such as Amazon also gets to harvest critical insights about the knowledge growth patterns of the buyer (Siegel 2013). When this is aggregated across the population dimension that spans cities, states, and nations—it provides deep strategic insights about the meristematic growth patterns in the overall economy, and which may be gainfully tapped into. Note that it is not just the purchase of books that provide insights about the struggles and aspirations of a nation that is logging into browse and purchase. Each item that is being browsed and purchased has aspects of knowledge that went into its design and manufacture. The five-star rating that captures the *wisdom of the crowd* (Surowiecki 2005) is the engine that propels the preferential attachment and the resultant power law. These strategic insights help the company outsmart its competition.

The power-law distribution of knowledge-based products is fundamentally different from the familiar Gaussian-normal distribution. Power-law-based products exhibit fat tails that are often underestimated when mistakenly framed using the Gaussian distribution. Fat tails force the designer into the uncharted de novo space. And it is here that the AD approach has a unique role to play. Here, we trace the potential of AD in the context of de novo situations that fat-tailed distributions expose in the cloud.

Cloud computing provides various benefits, including agility, scalability, cost reduction, mobility, disaster recovery, etc. Also, the cloud ecosystem is fairly complex. Designing an adaptive architecture that can withstand the onslaught of change is fairly challenging. This chapter holistically unifies a smorgasbord of architectural concepts and frameworks that help unify and strengthen the AD approach for tackling cloud computing design.

Without the benefit of a holistic design framework, cloud architectures remain fragile. This is especially true in the context of cloud security. Unaddressed gaps in design become salient points of architectural weakness. Cloud offerings are increasingly vulnerable in this context, given the joint ownership model that the cloud operates within. The AD framework is rare in upholding the holism of design.

22.2 History of Cloud Computing

Cloud computing was born in the shadow of the Cuban missile crisis (1962) that almost precipitated a nuclear holocaust (Vleck 2019). During the crisis, the Pentagon discovered that its existing information infrastructure was practically unusable in a coordinated, large-scale, human–machine endeavor. Simultaneously, early prototypes of time-sharing systems were being developed in the early 1960s at MIT and BBN (Bolt, Beranek, and Newman) under the leadership of Prof. John McCarthy and Joseph C. R. Licklider (Lick). The missile crisis gave the necessary impetus to launch the time-sharing Project MAC (Multiple Access Computing) at MIT that spanned 1963–74. By 1969, Lick had expanded and democratized the time-sharing Project MAC vision to what he colorfully called the "*Intergalactic Computer Network* (Wikipedia 2019c)," which seeded the ARPANET—the historic precursor to the modern Internet and gateway to the cloud.

To help stabilize the infrastructure that was constantly being upgraded under Moore's law, the early 1960s also saw market-initiated (primarily IBM, GE, and Bell Labs) development of server virtualization (Wikipedia 2019d).

Cloud computing was born when these two seminal concepts (i.e., time-sharing and server virtualization) fused in the 1990s. The term itself was coined by Prof. Chellappa in a 1997 talk (Chellapp 1997):

> Cloud computing can be defined as a set of frameworks that provides **on demand**, **scalable**, **customized**, **quality services** in **Software**, **platform** and also provides **sharable infrastructure** through **internet** that are **accessible and available everywhere**. (Emphasis added.)

In 2011, NIST standardized the official definition of cloud computing (Mell and Grance 2011):

> Cloud computing is a model for enabling **ubiquitous**, **convenient**, **on-demand network access** to a **shared pool** of **configurable computing resources** (e.g., networks, servers,

storage, applications, and services) that can be **rapidly provisioned and released** with **minimal management effort** or **service provider interaction**. …Cloud systems automatically control and optimize resource use by leveraging a **metering capability** at some level of abstraction appropriate to the type of service (e.g., storage, processing, bandwidth, and active user accounts). (Emphasis added.)

Based on the NIST standard, cloud computing may be formally captured in the lower triangle, FR–DP configuration as shown in Fig. 22.1. The design leads off with two seminal concepts that historically define cloud architecture: virtualization and time-sharing. The virtualization design parameter (DP11) answers the Economies-of-Scope functional requirement (FR11) for abstracting away from the underlying hardware resources (compute, storage, networking) in order to set up highly customizable resources. Virtualization allows the user to break away from tight-coupling with any given hardware vendor (i.e., lock-in). It also allows the architect to mix-and-match technological offerings from various vendors that would have been impossible otherwise. Time-sharing (DP12) allows load-sharing-driven Economies-of-Scale of software/hardware resources for substantial cost reductions (FR12) across multiple users. The service is accessible (FR2) anywhere, anytime, for anyone, for any business, and from any of the client devices that can access the Internet (DP2). Given the virtualization functionality across time-shared resources, it is now possible to programmatically provide rapid elasticity (DP3) on an as-needed basis. Such rapid built-up and tear-down of an arbitrary set of resources from the resource pool would have been unthinkable in previous on-prem architectures. From an FR perspective, what this accomplishes is the agility to rapidly reconfigure and repurpose the strategic business thrust, and move on a dime (FR3). It is this agility that aligns closely with the Boydian strategy framework of asymmetric fast transients (see Sect. 22.9). FR4 demands that all of the above FR/DPs need to be managed and achieved on an automated (on the vendor side) and self-service (on the customer side) basis with minimal managerial overhead. Again, given the virtualization/time-sharing flexibilities, this requirement is also programmatically feasible (DP4). FR5 requires usage and billing transparency as provided by cloud telemetry (DP5) in order to honor the service contract as well as for providing usage feedback that the customer may use for adapting to changes in the demand curve.

With the above brief historical review of cloud computing along with the framing of the basic architecture using the AD, we may now review the rest of the 13 architectural concepts (Siegel 2013; Surowiecki 2005; Mell and Grance 2011; Vleck 2019; Wikipedia 2019c, d; Chellapp 1997; Grassé 1959; Parunak 2006; Fehling et al. 2014; Erl et al. 2017; Akhtar 2018).

22.3   Socio-Technical Stigmergy

Stigmergy (Grassé 1959) denotes call to work based on local signs or markings left by collaborating agents (α) at some time in the past and during the course of their work (either as a side effect of the said work or as something in addition to the

FR11		X							DP11
FR12		X	X						DP12
FR2	=	X	X	X					DP2
FR3		X	X	X	X				DP3
FR4		X	X	X	X	X			DP4
FR5		X	X	X	X	X	X		DP5

FR1: Configurable Resource Pooling for Economies-of-Scale and Scope → DP1: Customizable
   Resource (Storage,Compute, Memory, Location, Networking, etc.) Pooling

FR11: Provide Ability to Custom Configure Computing Resources for attaining Economies of
   Scope → DP11: Virtualization
FR12: Provide Ability to Share the underlying Infrastructure for attaining Economies of
   Scale→DP12: Time-Sharing
FR2: Provide Broad Network Access (Anytime, Anywhere, Any Device, Anyone, Any
   Business) to Compute Resources→DP2: Internet Access via heterogenous clients
FR3: Establish Business Agility by providing for Rapid Elasticity (scale-up/down/in/out) →
   DP3: Programmatic Rapid Built-up & Tear-Down of Pooled Resources
FR4: Minimize Managerial Overhead via Automatable, On-demand Self-Service →
   DP4: API's for Provisioning/Managing Pooled/Virtualized Resources, Access & Elasticity
FR5: Provide usage & billing transparency for Pay-per-Use→DP5: Measured Service
   Telemetry

Fig. 22.1 Cloud computing functional requirement–design parameter (FR–DP) map (using NIST definition (Mell and Grance 2011)). (Reproduced from Thomas and Mantri (2019), originally published open access under a CC BY 4.0 license: https://doi.org/10.1051/matecconf/201930100024)

work). These markings aggregate to provide organizational directives (β-logic) available at various levels, both within the environment and within and between agents. Thus, even though there is no one controlling the set of agents in a top-down sense, there is nevertheless system-wide control being established in a bottom-up sense. Case in point is the ant trail that emerges (see Fig. 22.2) from pheromone droppings by ant agents. The trail then helps organize the ant swarm in its various activities. Across multiple iterations, the stigmergic trail smoothens and tightens, thus indicating minimization of the embedded information content.

The concept of stigmergy was discovered while searching for governing organizational motifs among eusocial insects such as ants and termites. Research indicates that these same organizational motifs may be observed in various human activities. Parunak reports on a variety of such human-level socio-technical stigmergic processes, including forest trail formation, highway traffic flows, democratic elections, document editing, social media groupings, viral marketing, Google page ranks, peer-to-peer computing, Amazon-style recommender-systems, etc. (Parunak 2006) Stigmergic problem-solving occurs wherever the problem context is beyond the ken of any one agent. In other words, one should expect stigmergic solutions to dominate in regimes that would be considered as complex. Architecting solutions within the cloud computing/Big Data space clearly fall within this context. Indeed,

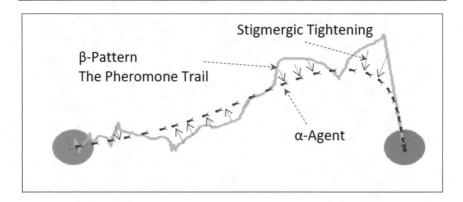

Fig. 22.2 Stigmergic trails by marching ants (created using NetLogo Wilensky (1997)). Note the tightening of the stigmergic trail. (Reproduced from Thomas and Mantri (2019), originally published open access under a CC BY 4.0 license: https://doi.org/10.1051/matecconf/201930100024)

the very essence of Big Data is in capturing and tracking stigmergic patterns of economically interesting behaviors across large population sets. This could be in the realm of finance, healthcare, threat modeling and cybersecurity, gaming, education, entertainment, etc. In architecting such systems, it is therefore important to track the stigmergic patterns that are forming across the vast cloud/Big Data ecosystem (Fehling et al. 2014; Erl et al. 2017; Akhtar 2018; Erl et al. 2016). Prior to the cloud, socio-technical stigmergic processes and patterns were either trapped in the confines of the enterprise or merely left as shallow traces across the lightweight Internet weblinks. The modern cloud has the potential to allow data flow patterns to aggregate without necessarily compromising privacy.

Stigmergic signals from the cloud include DP5: Telemetry-based transparency for usage-based billing (see Fig. 22.1). Organizations are perhaps unaware of the stigmergic significance of such accumulating data. Contractual agreements (Tollen 2016) with vendors need to be carefully negotiated, especially in the context of shape-shifting complex adaptive systems (see Sect. 22.4).

Example 22.1

Discuss stigmergic tightening from an AD framework.

Solution: Nature often starts with a coupled design. For example, to obtain the shortest path from point A to B, an ant trial starts with too many random detours away from a smooth ideal path. Each such detour that deviates from the ideal path may be accounted as a needless DP that over-complicates and adds needless information complexity to the travel path. Nevertheless, across multiple iterations, as the ants march back and forth across the jagged terrain, a number of these spurious, control-point DPs are eliminated, with the final result being a minimally complex information trail. Here, the design matrix begins with too many DPs, but over time, the design settles into a lightly decoupled (with necessary coupling between adjacent control points), lower triangular design.

22.4 Complex Adaptive System (CAS)

To fully understand the strategic import that design plays in the cloud, one has to appreciate the underlying adaptive dynamics propelling the cloud. As Urquhart suggests in Urquhart (2012):

> *Cloud as an adaptive system: The thing is, however, a certain class of complex systems, complex adaptive systems, have the additional trait that they can change their behavior in response to the success or failure of previous behaviors when a given event occurs—or when a certain series of events occurs. This ability to "learn" and adapt to the surrounding system environment creates amazing outcomes, including many of the most rich, enduring, and powerful systems in our universe.*

Shape-shifting adaptive dynamics makes the cloud ecosystem a complex adaptive system (CAS). As Prof. Holland describes it (Holland 2006), CASs *"are systems that have a large number of components, often called agents that interact and adapt or learn."* Holland then proposed a two-tiered system as shown in Fig. 22.3a.

The lower α-tier follows a fast dynamic and is engaged in the flow of resources between diverse agents, while the upper β-tier follows a slow dynamic that captures knowledge artifacts and aggregates from these which are then emitted system-wide as stigmergic signals that help the agents organize and scale.

Figure 22.3b is an iterative variation on the basic CAS. At each follow-on feedback-loop/iteration, the CAS trace bifurcates the target population into higher levels of organizational complexity. As evidence of the cloud bifurcation process, the Azure Resource Manager (Karthikeyan 2017) enables the organization and management of the cloud resource sprawl that used to exist in the classic model.

Example 22.2

Map the bipartite axiomatic FR/DP framework alongside the CAS α/β framework using Francis Bacon's dictum: *"Nature to be Commanded, must be Obeyed [Novum Organum]."*

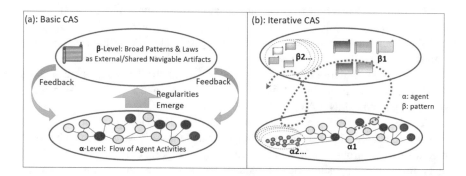

Fig. 22.3 Complex adaptive system. **a** Basic; **b** Iterative. (Reproduced from Thomas and Mantri (2019), originally published open access under a CC BY 4.0 license: https://doi.org/10.1051/matecconf/201930100024)

Solution: All designs involve working closely with base-level materials available in nature along with the laws that govern their behavior. It is in this sense that Bacon's dictum that nature to be commanded must be obeyed is relevant in design. To command nature (i.e., to design and compose with elements found in nature), it is wise to obey the laws that govern the basal elements as well as the adaptive, self-organizing structures and behaviors that they exhibit. Many complex natural as well as man-made systems (including biological, euso-cial, large-scale physical, as well as socio-technical systems such as the cloud) follow the iterative CAS processes that exhibit hierarchical as well as heterarchical patterns (see Sect. 22.5). In this context, the built-up of the bipartite β/α hierarchy (as shown in Fig. 22.3b) maps well with the bipartite FR/DP hierarchy. The fundamental difference between nature's CAS-driven hierarchy versus human-driven design hierarchy is that the former is often a long drawn-out, bottom-up zigzag process, while the latter is a relatively rapid, top-down zigzag process. But the elements of FRs and DPs may be discerned from carefully studying the elements available in the β and the α layers, respectively. In this sense, at all levels, design involves three distinct and strategic selections: the right FR elements from the β set, the right DP elements from the α set, and the proper mapping between the two.

22.5   Knowledge Hierarchy/Heterarchy

The following is a short review of the knowledge hierarchy framework (Thomas and Zaytseva 2016) which could aid in the mapping of various frameworks such as AD, Cynefin, OODA, agile, etc., into an integrated whole. Human knowledge is the engine that drives the knowledge economy. Given the abstract nature of human knowledge, it may be observed that domain knowledge is conical in shape; i.e., there are many more concretes than abstractions. The knowledge corpus captures the sum total of truths/facts gleaned from nature and painstakingly accumulated across time. Induction (depicted in Fig. 22.4a as the upward flowing arch) involves creating higher level generalizations. Note the similarity between induction and the upward flowing, regularity creating CAS emergence (Fig. 22.3a). In contrast, a deduction is the downward flowing arch involved in the application of the induced generalizations. The abductive cascade combines the inductive as well as the deductive flows into a long sequence of step-by-step problem-solving trace.

When multiple domains are mapped side by side along with their shared conceptual linkages, the various hierarchies map onto a heterarchical span that share and cross-pollinate across the domain barriers (Fig. 22.4b). Hierarchies are denoted as |H, heterarchies as |h, knowledge hierarchy as K|H, and knowledge as heterarchically hierarchical as KA|h|H.

Reverse salients are gaps that appear between knowledge hierarchies when mapped heterarchically, side by side. These create knowledge asymmetries between individuals and groups of individuals (including corporations and nations). Such units may hold opposing mental models based on the underlying knowledge asymmetries. For example, the management of Borders and Amazon was basing their corporate decisions on mental models that were at variance with each other. By the time gap closure had occurred, Borders as a corporation was bankrupted.

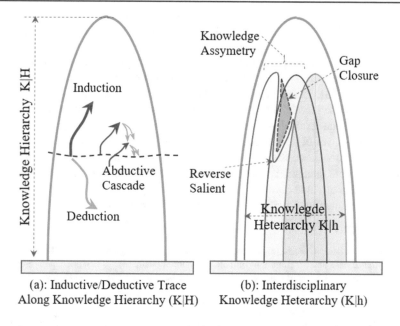

(a): Inductive/Deductive Trace
Along Knowledge Hierarchy (K|H)

(b): Interdisciplinary
Knowledge Heterarchy (K|h)

Fig. 22.4 Knowledge hierarchy/heterarchy. (Reproduced from Thomas and Mantri (2019), originally published open access under a CC BY 4.0 license: https://doi.org/10.1051/matecconf/201930100024)

Systems that display strong heterarchical engagements have very different growth patterns and architectural opportunities/vulnerabilities. For example, bacterial colonies exchange genetic material not just vertically (in a parent-to-child sense), but also laterally (Wikipedia 2019e) between cells that come into contact with each other. Vertical exchange is hierarchic and horizontal exchange is heterarchic. Evolutionary adaptation that uses the vertical exchange is slow as it has to work across organismal life spans. In contrast, an adaptation that uses lateral exchange is rapid as it is able to quickly share successful mutations across large populations. But when both mechanisms work in tandem, organisms can rapidly navigate large search spaces in order to solve species-wide existential threats. For example, this allows bacterial colonies to rapidly evolve and attain antibiotic resistance (Wikipedia 2019e).

The advent of social media, IoT (Internet of Things), Big Data, AI/machine learning, and mobile and cloud computing has accelerating such heterarchic linkages. Differences in heterarchic strengths and weaknesses could be complementary or noncomplementary. When pursued for competitive advantage, they result in asymmetric warfare (which is explored more fully in Sect. 22.9 under cloud OODA).

Heterarchic problems exist in the context of cloud data and cloud security. For example, the data modeling complexity involved in a Big Data/Data Lake context has to do with ironing out the inevitable ontological inconsistencies across multiple domains, each competing for abstraction dominance as well as in establishing a wider inductive base spanning structured, semi-structured, and unstructured data (Lee et al. 2018). Likewise, in the context of cloud cybersecurity, the current dominance of the hierarchical defense-in-depth (Igbe 2017) approach is vulnerable to heterarchic attacks. Defense-in-depth assumes that data/applications are secure in the innermost layer of its hierarchical and concentrically structured onion rings. But such an approach is vulnerable, especially in the increasingly IoTized technology landscape where data and applications are placed at the edge with both hierarchical and heterarchical vulnerabilities. Alongside defense-in-depth, what is therefore also needed is an integrated defense-in-breadth focus (Igbe 2017).

Example 22.3

Provide an example where large-scale/real-time heterarchic linkages between the customer experience base and the minute-by-minute operational business logs that are captured in the cloud could lead to rapid closure of the reverse-salient gaps between the two.

Solution: Stigmergic processes operates whenever and wherever problem contexts overwhelm the problem-solving capacity of the agents involved. The highly fractalized and heterarchic sprawl of modern business problems that clients and employees of a major cloud-based corporation faces often leads to reverse-salient gaps between the problem and the available solution base. By amassing and analyzing minute-by-minute operational logs being accumulated in the cloud, a business could quickly narrow down and pinpoint opportunities and business trends, their overall market potential as well as strategically generate valuable lead-customer (i.e., influencer)-driven design insights. In this sense, both problem abstraction and its rapid resolution are being done in a democratic, "*wisdom-of-the-crowd*" sense. Given the large-scale fractal sprawl of the cloud footprint, it would be valuable to incorporate principles of design into what is currently and predominantly an otherwise ad hoc process.

22.6 Power Law Versus Gaussian Distribution

Consider a variable which tracks a phenomenon that has multiple contributing factors, each of which obeys its own unique probability distribution. If these factors aggregate in an additive fashion, the resultant summing distribution that characterizes the phenomenon would be a bell curve. As per the central limit theorem, it would result in the Gaussian-normal distribution (Fig. 22.5a) if the contributing distributions were independent and identically distributed. The issue with the normal distribution shows up in the tail regions where the probabilities attenuate drastically. This gives rise to the problem of unreasonably thin tails. Seldom do natural phenomenon follow the Gaussian in the tail regions as it is attenuating too sharply by following the exponential of the negative square of the variable in question (Fig. 22.5a). Even so, many human-centric and natural phenomena approximately follow the Gaussian distribution. Examples include temperature distribution in a city at a given day of any year, height/weight distribution of a population, delays in the arrival of public transportation, size and weight of fruits and vegetables, experimental observational errors, etc.

In contrast, if these factors aggregate in a multiplicative fashion, the resultant multiplicative distribution that characterizes the phenomenon would be a power-law distribution which when plotted on a log–log plot shows up as a linear plot (see Fig. 22.5b). Note that from an empirical perspective, there could be many variations of the power law (Wikipedia 2019b), including the broken power law which consists of piecewise combinations of multiple power laws as well as smoothing of the power law with the exponential.

To illustrate the generative multiplicative process behind the power-law phenomenon, consider the following example of programmer productivity (Louridas et al. 2008; Ward 2016). To begin with, suppose that just a few software programmers are proficient in the software-creation tools at their disposal. Even small differences in better tool usage quickly aggregate to the advantage of the slightly exceptional individual. Each successful project completion builds confidence in the individual as well as in the eyes of the management that oversees the project. In time, with repeat deliveries and accrual of choice experiences, the end result is that these individuals are orders of magnitude more productive than the rest. Seeded by minor differences in the initial conditions (for example, here the slight difference in tool usage proficiency), the generative multiplicative process behind the power law has the potential to bifurcate target populations (in a CAS sense) into distinct groups and sub-groups. In time this could lead to deep-set social hierarchies between those who lead versus those who are led. Indeed, wherever human intellectual work is involved and made available to large populations in a free-market economy, the rich-get-richer style power-law distributions are also likely to show up. This is one of the reasons why the power law is increasingly relevant when considering a knowledge economy.

Other examples of the power law include earthquake intensities, city populations, best sellers sold, the number of citations received, etc. In (Barabási and Albert 1999), Barabási and Albert highlight the generative process behind the power-law distribution of the vertex degree in a network of webpage links:

> Because of the preferential attachment, a vertex that acquires more connections than another one will increase its connectivity at a higher rate; thus, an initial difference in the connectivity between two vertices will increase further as the network grows.

From a symmetry perspective, the above argument could also be extended to include preferential *detachment* for nodes that fall out of comparative favor. In time, this creates significant bifurcations between the haves and the have-nots. Given the foundational level wherein the generative multiplicative process behind the power law is operating from, no egalitarian legislative action could effectively overcome these biases without concomitantly also damaging the knowledge economy. Instead, the proper solution to the above politico-economic problem (in a knowledge economy) is to leverage the neglected heterarchy generation potential of the very same hierarchy generating power-law-driven, iterative CAS. Over and above

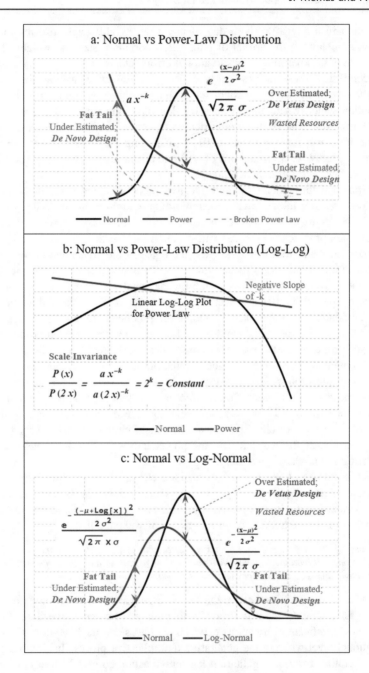

Fig. 22.5 Normal vs log-normal vs power-law distribution. (Reproduced from Thomas and Mantri (2019), originally published open access under a CC BY 4.0 license: https://doi.org/10. 1051/matecconf/201930100024)

the hierarchy generation potential, an iterative CAS module (if and when assisted by favorable factors such as the cloud) also has the ability to generate *heterarchic* hierarchies which (as explained below) is the fundamental solution to the above egalitarian conundrum. While knowledge hierarchies fragment and bifurcate a given domain (and therefore the social groups that cultivate it) into smaller and finer grains, knowledge heterarchies create bridging artifacts that allow concepts and propositions to disperse across the overall knowledge fabric. This is similar to the lateral transfer of genes in a bacterial population.

Mindless specialization (into ever-deepening hierarchies) is the bane of modern life. Fortunately, countervailing forces are at play that promises to link the hierarchies via heterarchic bridge artifacts. For example, AD (Suh 1990; Suh 2001) is fundamentally a hierarchy-bridging heterarchic artifact that considers all creative designerly activities under a common breadth-seeking rubric. It is breadth-seeking because the very same two principles of design (i.e., Axiom I and II) apply regardless of the domain of interest. In other words, regardless of whether the design pertains to engineering, software, education, organizations, medicine, etc., the same two design principles apply (Suh 1990).

By balancing the depth-seeking hierarchic drivers against the breadth-seeking heterarchic drivers, iterative CAS has the potential to coordinate and disperse knowledge agents across the totality of the knowledge economy, instead of crowding around just a few clusters. Thus, instead of egalitarially spreading the wealth (i.e., the product of human creativity) around, the heterarchy-generating iterative CAS is capable of spreading the wealth-generating engine of human creativity around. In colloquial terms, it is about *"teaching how to fish instead of giving fish"* (Wiktionary 2019).

Iterative CAS has the potential to flatten deep hierarchies in favor of a network economy that bridges isolated hierarchies using a multitude of lateral linkages. Furthermore, these heterarchic linkages allow the search space along all stages of the design process to be vastly improved. We may, therefore, be more confident that the search imperative embedded in Axiom II (i.e., minimize information content) is indeed delivering a true minimum. This is similar to how bacterial populations are able to rapidly navigate large search spaces in order to solve species-wide existential threats by utilizing both horizontal and vertical gene transfer mechanisms.

In a knowledge-driven political economy, the proper nurturing of the link between human creativity embedded in the act of design and finding meaning and fulfillment in life is of paramount importance. Note that in such an economy, the neglected art and science of design ought to be center stage. Also, in such an economy, the flattening of deep-set knowledge hierarchies in favor of heterarchic hierarchies allows for greater freedoms in human actualization. As an analogy, this is similar to the phenomenon of seed dispersal far removed from the parent, which allowed plants to colonize and spread itself across the globe. Dispersal of seeds opened up ecological pathways for the evolution of plants into rich, diverse forms that could successfully exploit the local micro-ecologies. However, the difference between seed dispersal and knowledge growth patterns is that while the available global surface area with sufficient sunlight for plant growth is limited, such is not the case for the highly fractalized heterarchically hierarchical knowledge architectures (Thomas and Zaytseva 2016). Indeed, such an abstract space is only limited by our imagination. In other words, there is sufficient *"surface area"* across the richly fractalized knowledge fabric for humans to flourish without having to dominate and extinguish the creative entelechy in each other in the narrow hierarchies of disjointed knowledge fragments. Such ought to be the proper solution to the Rich-Get-Richer power-law conundrum. And in this context, cloud computing is like the wind that is dispersing the seeds of human imagination into ever wider mash-ups of creative, uncharted territories.

While power laws go hand in hand with CAS-generated hierarchies, they do not necessarily vanish with CAS-generated heterarchic hierarchies. Both depth-driving hierarchies and breadth-seeking heterarchies are necessary for balanced growth, but need to exist in symbiosis. For example, the ancient redwood trees (symbolizing deep hierarchies) did not go extinct when grasslands (symbolizing wide heterarchies) started appearing 55 MYA. Instead, each continued to thrive separately within their respective niches while collaborating on the wider photosynthetic gas exchange cycles. Also, within its respective niche, each exhibits various power laws in its relevant allometric measurements (Anfodillo et al. 2013; Niklas 1994). In other words, it is not a single power law across the overall span. Instead, it is broken into separate segments, each governing a separate niche. This is what was referred to earlier as the broken power law (Fig. 22.5a).

In cloud computing, Loboz finds significant backing for the power law when he analyzed Microsoft's Azure Resource usage patterns (Loboz 2010):

> Analysis of daily resource usage by customer accounts on two Azure storage clusters had shown that the distribution of the resource usage on any given day is very heavy-tailed. We have found, for five different resource types that distributions are far from normal, exponential, or even log-normal—in fact they either are power-law or closer to power-law than any of the aforementioned distributions.

When jointly plotted against each other, the power-law distribution highlights key regions of over/underestimation of probabilities under the guidance of the bell-curve logic. As shown in Fig. 22.5a, the tails at the extremes are often underestimated, while the middle is overestimated. Underestimated tail regions are denoted as fat tails. For example, suppose that the T-shirt industry was to be designed under the guidance of the normal distribution but in fact exhibited power-law distribution. If that were to be the case, it would be as if ready-made clothes were being designed mostly for the middle region of the normal curve (i.e., small, medium, and large); but sizable populations continue to show up at the retail stores who are extremely large or extremely small. This, of course, does not happen in human body proportions which generally follows the Gaussian-normal curve. But if that were to be the case, huge sections of the market that pertained to the massive fat tail at the lower end (i.e., extra small) of the market would effectively be invisible to the designers. Likewise, some extremely large-bodied individuals would also not be serviced and therefore forced to obtain custom-tailored clothing. Also, in the middle regions (i.e., small, medium, and large), there would be a huge surplus and wastage. Clearly, misjudging the market would be a major problem for the designer.

Note that fat tails may also form under non-power-law situations such as shown in Fig. 22.5c which overlays the normal against the log-normal. Like the power law, log-normal is also multiplicative, but places restrictions such as stock prices never being allowed to fall below zero. Examples of log-normal distributions include the following:

- file size distribution on the Internet;
- the Internet traffic rate;
- how long users stay and peruse an online article.

As shown in Fig. 22.5b, the defining property of the power-law distribution is that it is scale-free. In other words, in transitioning from x to 2x (or any multiple), the ratio of the distribution is constant (i.e., invariant) no matter what that x is. In other words, it exhibits the fractal property of self-similarity (i.e., the whole has the same shape as the part). Under purely hierarchic dominance, the power-law structure that results would be the trivial and featureless straight line (Fig. 22.5b), but when mixed with heterarchic influences, the resultant broken power-law structure is far more interesting and realistic.

From an AD perspective, what is critically relevant about the power-law distribution is that the fat tails are often underestimated and fall outside the mainstream. This means that the design requirements need to be freshly induced, and the design itself needs to be attempted in a solution-neutral, de novo fashion. This is also probably the reason why the agile movement has resonated so well in our modern knowledge economy. If the requirements need to be freshly induced in order to cater for the fat tails, any top-down waterfall-type approach that caters to the middle regions of the bell-curve logic would incur major costs of wasted effort and misdirected resources. Power-law distribution is central to the modern knowledge economy. And fundamentally, given its structuring ability when dealing with solution-neutral/de novo problem contexts, AD is uniquely situated in rising up to the modern challenge of designerly misguidance under the normal curve.

Note that the two fat tails as shown in Fig. 22.5a are neither symmetric nor perhaps of equal significance. Given the relative probabilities between the two, occurrences of the fat tail at the short end at left are far more likely than that of the long end at right. In other words, there is far more statistics available for the short end as compared to the long end (for example, far more small earthquakes versus just a few really large ones). But from an impact perspective, events in the long end are probably far more consequential than that at the short end (for example, the energy released as well as damage from a very large earthquake). Also, tracing the causal linkages at the short end is far more hierarchical and Markovian (Wikipedia 2019f) (i.e., lacking in memory) than that at the long end. In contrast, the tracing of causal linkages in phenomenon that exhibit memory requires far more heterarchical thinking (which currently is more demanding and therefore in short supply).

Example 22.4

Compare and contrast the normal versus the power-law distribution from an AD perspective.

Solution: If the knowledge economy was to be erroneously considered as normally distributed, then the idea that the mass market is homogeneous and lumped in the central regions of the bell curve could have deleterious consequences in understanding the demand curve, including keeping major sections of the fractalized and non-homogeneous fat tails invisible to the designer who may be expecting the normal curve. It is effectively as if the designer is only aware of a single, homogeneous mass market FR from the central zone of the bell curve when, in fact, the power-law distribution exhibits at least three distinct FR regions:

   i. a mass market that is highly fractalized and located at the short end of the distribution;
   ii. a middle region that is thinner than the short end of the power-law distribution as well as the central zone of the bell curve; and
  iii. a high-impact fat tail at the far end that is thicker than the corresponding section of the bell curve.

From an axiomatic framework, such a problem-statement mismatch would be akin to designing for a single FR when the actual problem had at least three, if not more (especially in a broken power-law context). Given the cloud-driven acceleration of our knowledge economy, such broken power-law mismatches may be expected to increase if this problem is not properly understood and corrected.

22.7 Axiomatic Trace

Given the knowledge hierarchy framework, the AD trace may be depicted as shown in Fig. 22.6. Given that human knowledge is hierarchical, the design trace (Thomas 1995) that leverages this knowledge is likewise hierarchical. As explained in Sect. 22.6, fat tails expose designerly blind spots that need to be problem-abstracted afresh and designed in a solution-neutral, de novo fashion. De novo designs also occur in uncharted contexts (such as cloud-native architectures) that require the designer to freshly induce the highest level problem context that will govern the overall design. In contrast, on-prem designs that compete with the cloud have legacy commitments that need to be carefully re-engineered in the context of the cloud as they have substantial amounts of the designtrace locked up in long-shelf-life, cap-ex obligations. In all of these de novo, cloud-native/hybrid contexts, the axiomatic approach could provide critical insights as to how best to proceed.

As Prof. Suh indicates in (Suh 1990), design *"involves four distinct aspects of engineering and scientific endeavor"* as listed below:

- problem definition;
- creative leap;
- analytical process; and
- overall testing and validation.

Fig. 22.6 Axiomatic Design trace along K|H. (Reproduced from Thomas and Mantri (2019), originally published open access under a CC BY 4.0 license: https://doi.org/10.1051/matecconf/201930100024)

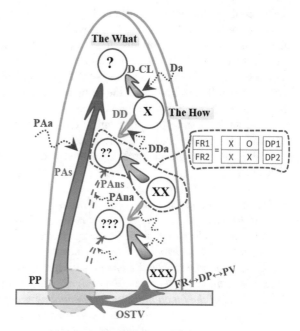

Abbreviations

PP: Problem Perception
PAs: Problem Abstraction-Synthesis
PAa: Problem Abstraction-Analysis
DCL: Design-Creative Leap
?: The What
X: The How
Da: Design Analysis
DD: Design Decomposition
DDa: Design Decomposition Analysis
PAns: Problem Abstraction (nested)-Synthesis
PAna: Problem Abstraction (nested) Analysis
FR: Functional Requirement
DP: Design Parameter
PV: Process Variable
OSTV: Overall System Testing & Validation

Problem definition involves problem perception (PP), problem abstraction-synthetic (PAs) as well as problem abstraction-analytic (PAa). PP is how we perceive the problem (e.g., patient perceiving pain in the chest and showing up at the doctors). PAs is the diagnosis of the problem at the right level of abstraction in an essentialized sense (e.g., the medical doctor having done sufficient tests on the patient decides that the patient has a life-threatening blockage in the coronary artery). When the patient takes the diagnosis and asks for a second opinion about the diagnosis that would be PAa: problem abstraction-analysis. If the presiding doctors were Sigwart and Puel (Wikipedia 2019g), the creative design leap

(DCL) could be the world's very first heart stent. Prior to the advent of the coronary stent, the medical profession has had close to two centuries of experience in stenting of vessels in other minor organs. All of this knowledge would be relevant as prior art and therefore inform the de novo design of the coronary heart stent. Ideally, it should be explicitly captured as part of the growing K|H. Along with the axiomatic tools and corollaries from AD, the prior art (whether implicitly or explicitly captured in the K|H) helps in the proper analysis of the design (i.e., in the Da: design analysis step). Despite the prior art, every de novo design probably has unique elements (that falls outside the current prior art) which requires rigorous testing.

Commenting on the hierarchical nature of design, Prof. Suh indicates in (Suh 1990) that

- *Everything we do in design has a hierarchical nature to it. That is, decisions must be made in order of importance by decomposing the problem into a hierarchy... When such a hierarchical nature of decision making is not utilized, the process of decision making becomes very complex.*
- *The designer must recognize and take advantage of the existence of the functional and physical hierarchies. A good designer can identify the most important FRs at each level of the functional tree by eliminating secondary factors from consideration. Less-able designers often try to consider all the FRs of every level simultaneously, rather than making use of the hierarchical nature of FRs and DP's.*

The above sentiment is the strongest indication that AD is closely aligned with K|H. The only distinction is that hierarchies are not just relevant in the top-down decompositional phase, but it is also of equal (if not more) relevance in the original problem abstraction phase too (i.e., PAs and PAa). The familiar set of design matrices (as shown in the red-dot-outlined offset in Fig. 22.6) also captures the hierarchical trace.

The step-by-step decomposition of the abstract design is aided by four auxiliary design processes:

- DD = Design decomposition;
- DDa = Design decomposition analysis;
- PAns = Problem abstraction (nested)-synthesis;
- PAna = Problem abstraction (nested)-analysis.

These steps are templated along the abductive cascade as shown in Fig. 22.4a.

The fourth major step in the design process, namely, overall system testing and validation (OSTV) makes sure that the original problem (in our above example, the pain in the chest) has been adequately addressed.

Tracing designs across the knowledge repository could be of value in at least six different ways:

- By tracing the design across a well-explicated heterarchic knowledge hierarchy, the design is also well documented. Documentation is apparently burdensome in modern agile practices on account of the effort involved. The design-trace approach could help to overcome this burden by leveraging and reusing that which is common.

- When the design trace is used for capturing evolving families of designs that are related by a common problem context, it creates a phylogeny which could be mined for stigmergic patterns which otherwise would be missed.
- The design trace would add a valuable pedagogic tool for teaching design.
- In the hierarchical composition/decomposition of the design, the trace could help assure that the conceptual order is being maintained. In other words, it would be out of place to witness higher level abstractions showing up at lower level designs. And vice versa, it would also violate the knowledge trace if lower level abstractions show up in the higher rungs.
- As per the *ironic process theory* (Wikipedia 2019h), attempts to suppress certain thoughts, unfortunately, make it all the more likely to happen. Colloquially this is called the *"don't think about the white bear"* problem which results in the subject trapped in the very same thought process that is taboo. Likewise, the requirement to think out of the box in a solution-neutral, de novo sense is much harder when a solution already exists. Such cognitive traps may be avoided if the mind could free-range and view the overall conceptual landscape with the current de vetus design being included rather than excluded.
- Given the nature of the intense specialization in modern knowledge economies (i.e., the problem of the dearth of generalists), problems and solutions are posed within the limited domain expertise of the designer. By tracing the design across the heterarchic knowledge hierarchy, such self-limiting parochialisms may be avoided.

These are some of the myriad ways that the tracing of design across the heterarchic knowledge hierarchy could benefit AD.

Example 22.5

Discuss the critical role that **PAns**: *problem abstraction (nested) synthesis* plays in the proper decomposition of a conceptual design.

Solution: Creative induction plays a significant role throughout the design process. This is especially true during the upward arching problem abstraction phase **PAs**: *problem abstraction-synthesis*. The inductive base for such an upward leap would involve amassing sufficient evidence from the forensic engineering of multiple cases that relate to the underlying problem. While it is clear that inductive synthesis plays a major role in the root problem-statement phase, it is less well known that induction is also involved in each of the decompositional phases of a conceptual design (i.e., **PAns**). Furthermore, higher up the conceptual hierarchy that the decompositional phase is situated, greater is the need for the nested **PAns**. Each of these **PAns** steps is creatively inductive, and therefore favoring the human touch. There is a fundamental difference between **PAs** and **PAns**: while **PAs** is open-ended and problem-focused, **PAns** is circumscribed by the conceptual design from above and is, therefore, solution-focused. Also, having a database of well-documented past designs could help rapidly triangulate and structure the otherwise error-prone inductive arch of **PAns**.

22.8   Cynefin

While earlier technologies had recognizable life-cycle trajectories that could be analyzed along simple, clear, well-structured, top-down frameworks such as SWOT matrices (Wikipedia 2019i), Porter's five competitive forces (Wikipedia 2019j), etc., the strategic- and business-oriented framing of cloud computing has been addressed in mostly a piecemeal fashion (as for example, frameworks for cloud security (Jansen and Grance 2011), governance (The Open Group 2019), migration (Passmore 2016), vendor selection (Cloud Industry Forum 2019), etc.). Snowden's Cynefin framework (Snowden and Boone 2007) is an integrated, inductive, bottom-up sensemaking framework that is complexity-aware and therefore of substantial relevance in the cloud context. It has, however, yet to be adapted for the cloud computing context (Wong 2011). Along with casting the Cynefin approach in the knowledge hierarchy framework, the following discussion highlights the cloud computing potential for Cynefin.

The Cynefin framework (Fig. 22.7) highlights both the opportunities and the challenges faced by architects embracing the complexity challenge (Snowden and Boone 2007):

> *In a complex context, however, right answers can't be ferreted out. It's like the difference between, say, a Ferrari and the Brazilian rainforest… Ferraris are complicated machines, but an expert mechanic can take one apart and reassemble it without changing a thing. The car is static, and the whole is the sum of its parts. The rainforest, on the other hand, is in constant flux—a species becomes extinct, weather patterns change, an agricultural project reroutes a water source—and the whole is far more than the sum of its parts. This is the realm of "unknown unknowns," and it is the domain to which much of contemporary business has shifted.*

Cynefin is unique in emphasizing distinct and discernable managerial realms and heuristics (Fig. 22.7) where either reductionism (i.e., the whole is the sum of its parts) or holism (i.e., the whole is more than the sum of its parts) is the dominant operative. Holism and reductionism have ancient Greek heritage. As shown in Fig. 22.8, cloud architects may present three distinct temperaments when considering holistic versus reductionistic tendencies. The ideal cloud architect (i.e., the architect engineer) is both a generalist (in a big-picture sense) and a specialist (from a fast-moving technology perspective). Such an architect is able to engage the α-β CAS structures seamlessly.

Such a skill-set profile could be characterized as the T-profile (i.e., broad as the head of the T as well as deep as the leg the T). The ideal cloud architect ought to be able to anticipate and envision technological shifts that might trigger business emergences as well as business shifts that might trigger technological emergences (in a CAS sense). Furthermore, the ideal architect ought to have the necessary people skills/soft skills to communicate, persuade, motivate, and navigate across complex corporate terrains in order to help bring about the requisite corporate realignments that the envisioned emergences entail. As mentioned in Sect. 22.6, given the fact that the AD framework is capable of both hierarchical and hierarchy-bridging heterarchic designs, it is uniquely positioned in training the

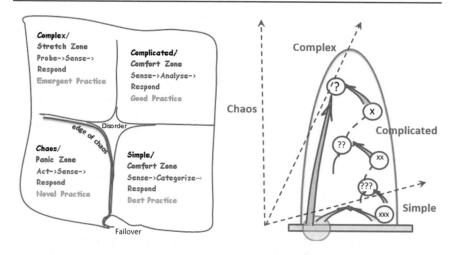

Fig. 22.7 Cynefin and knowledge hierarchy. (Reproduced from Thomas and Mantri (2019), originally published open access under a CC BY 4.0 license: https://doi.org/10.1051/matecconf/201930100024)

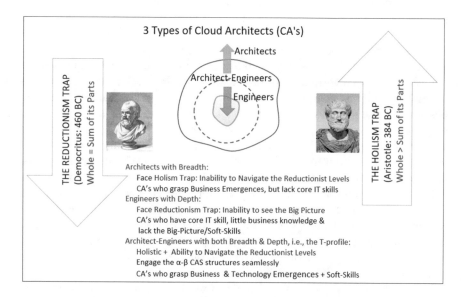

Fig. 22.8 Holism, reductionism, and cloud architects (Images from Wikipedia (Zapf 1801; Jastrow 2006)). (Reproduced from Thomas and Mantri (2019), originally published open access under a CC BY 4.0 license: https://doi.org/10.1051/matecconf/201930100024)

aforementioned architect engineer. Also, if the design trace is mapped against the knowledge hierarchy phylogeny, it could help anticipate potential emergences. Furthermore, given the fact that it is able to smoothly range across the abstraction spectrum, it is also able to assimilate both managerial and technical expertise into an integrated approach. Even the development of soft skills as a well-organized collection of building-block skill sets could be reduced to a problem of design (Sonmez 2014). Nevertheless, AD is not a panacea; it requires collaborative contributions from auxiliary frameworks (such as Cynefin) to help it in solving modern complex problems (such as cloud computing).

The vertical axis in Cynefin divides the ordered (on the right) versus the unordered (on the left). Of vital strategic essence is properly locating the problem in the proper regime. Here, the onus is to lead with bottom-up data in finding the right regime rather than applying any given framework in a top-down sense (i.e., let bottom-up induction have dominance).

By casting the Cynefin framework alongside the knowledge hierarchy framework (Fig. 22.7), it becomes clear that both the simple and the complicated are operating along well-structured knowledge hierarchies. In contrast, the necessary inductive base has yet to be established in both the complex and the chaotic regimes. The difference between the complex and the chaotic is that the former has at least partial conceptual order that overlaps with the conceptually known world. Furthermore, in the chaotic realm, higher values are under imminent threat (as in a medical emergency room situation) and require quick heuristic-based thinking and safety-enhancing actions. In the cloud context, chaos is when there is a major data breach with the host organization facing an existential crisis.

The knowledge hierarchy framework shows the continuum between the various regimes, i.e., reductionism and holism are not set against each other. Instead, each requires the other in order for knowledge to progress. Given that many of modern business problems manifest first in the complex realm, one should, therefore, expect that after analysis, some parts of the problem would be treated in a reductionist sense, while others in a holistic sense. Cynefin, however, warns about the danger of treating a complex problem as if it were simple or complicated. The warning is that this could lead to failover of the project into disorder (shown centrally as well as with a bottom swoosh in Fig. 22.7) where the managerial governance is itself lost. Problem-solving in the Cynefin world is to be contained within the separate regimes. Such a heightened sense of alarm would be short-sighted. As indicated above, the right approach would have been to partition and transition the reducible parts of the problem over to the simple/complicated regimes while dealing with the non-reducible parts in its own rights.

Consider, for example, some of the professional practices in software engineering. The top-down, deduction-biased, process-heavy, waterfall framework was perhaps adequately suited for an earlier era of simpler software development; it, however, fails in any of the other regimes where induction dominates, and the rigidity of the process becomes a bureaucratic ball-and-chain against agility and innovation. In contrast, the agile framework is better suited for the complicated regime. Also (with adequate care), it could iteratively move the complex into a more manageable "complicated" regime. This is similar to the transformation of time-dependent complexity in the Axiomatic Design/complexity theory (AD/CT) framework (Suh 2005) with the caveat that order and disorder are not merely temporal—it could also be geometric, chemical, informational, biological, etc.

The last line in the aforementioned quote (i.e., *...this is the realm of "unknown unknowns," and it is the domain to which much of contemporary business has shifted*) is relevant in the cloud context. The failure of design here is that while the majority of FR-DPs in a given problem context is situated in the well-established industry practices of the simple/complicated realms, a few top-level components of the problem are frequently situated in the complex realm. Failure also happens when engineering and management locate the totality of the problem in one or the other realms and therefore miss the combinatorial. These same blind spots probably existed even prior to the advent of cloud computing. But what has changed with the cloud is the rapidity with which novel, top-level problems with the potential for major impact shows up. The fundamental problem of cloud computing, therefore, involves expeditiously coming up with de novo designs for a few of the top-level, rapidly evolving FR–DP problem components even while much of the adjacent/lower level FR–DP components remain static and therefore re-targetable (with minimal change) from the existing legacy/de vetus play. The challenge, therefore, is in facing the rapidity with which the top layers need to be continuously shaped, reshaped, and reformulated. It is in these de novo, de vetus, and mixed cases that the sensemaking framework of Cynefin, along with the structuring that the AD framework provides, helps. In the presence of |h/|H, a judicious mixture of the various components (i.e., complex, complicated, and simple) would be more realistic.

Example 22.6

Cast the three types of cloud architects (CAs) in the axiomatic as well as the CAS α/β framework.

Solution: This is a case of two FRs and either one or two DPs. CAs need both breadth and depth. Satisfying just one of the job requirements would yield a coupled design. Architect-Engineers with both breadth and depth could satisfy both these requirements, thus yielding a decoupled design. This would have to be a lower triangle decoupled design as the breadth stricture sets the necessary context for the build-up of depth. Framing it now in a CAS framework, the scope and context for the breadth requirement form at the $\beta1$ level while that for depth forms at the $\beta2$ level. As a general rule, each new $\alpha \leftrightarrow \beta$ iteration increases the fractalization of the domain under purview.

22.9 Cloud OODA

We now turn to Boyd's OODA framework (Coram 2002) which is well placed in coming to terms with two of the most fundamental concepts in modern strategy, namely, asymmetric warfare and fast transients. Asymmetric warfare is related to heterarchies, while fast transients is related to hierarchies. Military strategist/systems architect (of the LWF: lightweight fighter program, which gave rise to the legendary F16 fighter plane) Colonel John Boyd highlighted the importance of fast transients in his OODA (observe–orient–decide–act) loop framework (see Fig. 22.9 as well as (Wikipedia 2019k)):

> *Idea of fast transients suggests that, in order to win, we should operate at a faster tempo or rhythm than our adversaries—or, better yet, get inside our adversary's Observation-Orientation-Decision-Action time cycle or loop.*

The four-stage OODA loop is depicted in Fig. 22.9a. In Fig. 22.9b, the four stages of the OODA loop (as well as that for OODA feedback) are traced across the knowledge hierarchy along with the trace for AD (i.e., key elements from Fig. 22.6) we had discussed in Sect. 22.7.

In (Richards 2004), Colonel Richards reviews the strategic value of the OODA framework:

> *What Boyd discovered was that the side with the quicker OODA loops began to exert a strange and terrifying effect on its opponent. Quicker OODA execution caused the slower side to begin falling farther and farther behind events, to begin to lose touch with the situation. Acting like the "asymmetric fast transients" experienced by fighter pilots, these mismatches with reality caused the more agile side to start becoming ambiguous in the mind of the less agile.*

The key phrase "*asymmetric fast transient*" needs to be carefully dissected and elaborated upon.

In both OODA and AD, the critical step is that of problem abstraction, which in OODA is denoted as the orientation stage. As Boyd writes (Wikipedia 2019k)

> *The second O, orientation—as the repository of our genetic heritage, cultural tradition, and previous experiences—is the most important part of the O-O-D-A loop since it shapes the way we observe, the way we decide, the way we act.*

Likewise, as Prof. Suh indicates in (Suh 1990):

> *It may be useful to state once more the importance of proper problem definition: the perceived needs must be reduced to an imaginative set of FRs as the first and most critical stage of the design process.*

Both approaches highlight the seminal value of problem abstraction. When placed in the K|H context, it becomes clear why the problem abstraction phase (i.e., orientation) has such strategic import. In comparison to every other step, it has the longest arc (i.e., PAs/PAa in Figs. 22.6 and 22.9b) along the K|H. Furthermore, being upward oriented, it is fundamentally inductive, which makes it more error-prone. The manner in which Boyd came up with the E-M (energy-maneuverability) theory (Coram 2002) that informs fighter-aircraft design illustrates the inductive challenge. The E-M theory resulted from synthesizing various contributing insights, including firsthand practical experience battling Mig-15 fighters in the Korean War, studies in strategic warfare, thermodynamics/aerodynamics as well as voluminous computer simulations designed to help create flight performance envelopes. From a design theory

Fig. 22.9 a The OODA loop; **b** OODA, K|H, and AD; **c** OODA strategies. (Reproduced from Thomas and Mantri (2019), originally published open access under a CC BY 4.0 license: https://doi.org/10.1051/matecconf/201930100024)

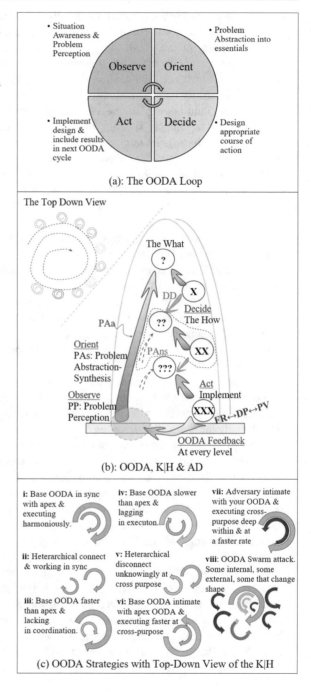

(a): The OODA Loop

(b): OODA, K|H & AD

(c) OODA Strategies with Top-Down View of the K|H

perspective, what was being induced was not the FR specifications for any specific fighter plane; instead, it was establishing the overall theoretical design envelope for all possible fighter planes. With the benefit of this framework, a fighter-aircraft designer could reasonably articulate a feasible set of FRs based on the perceived needs of the customer (i.e., the defense department).

But the E-M theory helps structure-only part of the OODA loop (i.e., PAa/PAs). Furthermore, it could not explain the 10:1 kill-ratio between the F-86 (predecessor to F-16) and the technically superior Mig-15 (higher ceiling, tighter turn radius, higher maximum speed). In fact, the Mig-15 was better positioned on the E-M profile. As Colonel Richards observed in (Richards 2004), the controversy was that the *"MiG's theoretically higher EM performance rarely led to wins in actual or even in practice air-to-air combat."* Puzzling over this ambiguity, Boyd noticed the following countervailing facts in favor of the F-86 (Richards 2004):

- The F-86's bubble canopy provided a simple, direct 360-degree field of vision that helped the pilot become better situationally aware (in visually detecting the enemy aircraft) as compared to the constraining view (i.e., the rear view was blocked) from the Mig-15 canopy. Engaging in a fast-transient dog fight requires better tools for situation awareness and problem perception (PP in Figs. 22.6 and 22.9b). This pertains to the observe phase of the OODA loop. Likewise, in the context of the cloud (with divided responsibility between the client and the cloud vendor), it is worthwhile creating automated monitoring algorithms based on the telemetric signals (i.e., DP5 in Fig. 22.1) along with simple dashboards to help the DevOps team be continuously situation-aware. Clutter, complexity worship and confusion need to be removed in favor of simplicity. This is in contrast to the Cynefin framework which cautions against moving from the complex realm into the simple for fear of falling into disorder. In other words, while Cynefin is valuable in becoming situationally aware as to where one begins with, it may not be the right choice in transitioning the problem (either whole or in part) from the complex into the more manageable complicated and simple regimes. Note that in pursuing the simple versus the complex/complicated, OODA agrees with AD's Axiom II which recommends the minimization of information content.
- The F-86 had fully hydraulic controls which allowed the pilot to command the aircraft with a single finger. In contrast, the Mig-15 pilot had to strenuously exert physical labor in controlling the aircraft that relied on mechanical linkages. The ability of the Mig-15 pilot to act in a consistent, coordinated fashion degraded under physical exhaustion. Note that this pertains to the act phase of the OODA loop. Poor actions in one loop feed every phase in the follow-on OODA loop, thereby creating vicious cycles. Here again, we see the importance of simplicity, but now in the realm of human action. The tactical end result of the hydraulic controls was that in comparison to the Mig-15 pilot, the F86 pilot could engage in faster transitions from one OODA maneuver to another.

Along with comparable EM credentials, the addition of a bubble canopy as well as hydraulic controls made the F-86 fighter plane strategically superior to the Mig-15 in an *"asymmetric fast-transient sense."* The asymmetry here is from the OODA-related strategic value of the bubble canopy as well as the hydraulic controls. And it is this asymmetry that is feeding the step-by-step degradation of the adversary, the process whereby the slower side begins *"falling farther and farther behind events"* and *"to lose touch with the situation* (Richards 2004).*"*

It is important to realize that cloud computing is strategic and needs to be considered in warfare terms. Critical assets deployed on the cloud are no longer business-as-usual; it, in fact, is being positioned on a winner-take-all basis. In this context (and as was illustrated in the fighter-plane example), every aspect of the OODA loop needs to be examined for its asymmetry potential. These insights, when abstracted and generalized using the KA|h|H framework along with AD, have the potential to scale.

It is true that as the top-level design is decomposed, there are many more nested abstractions (i.e., the steps denoted as PAns in Figs. 22.6 and 22.9b). Each of these is a baby step (compared to PAs) and closely triangulated with the aid of the downward arching deductive decompositions (i.e., the steps denoted as DD in Figs. 22.6 and 22.9b). These nested PAns are the orientation phases of the nested OODA loops which when viewed from the top create a fractal pattern of spirals (see top-left in Fig. 22.9b).

Consider once again the problem of problem abstraction (i.e., PAa/PAs). In a negative sense, if the problem is poorly stated, or worse if the wrong problem is being addressed, all downstream effort is wasted. In the medical context, this is called misdiagnosis. To put a human face on the cost of misdiagnosis, consider the following healthcare summary from a John Hopkins (Newman-Toker 2013) report:

- significant cases of permanent injury or death from misdiagnosis estimated to be 80 K to 160 K/year;
- diagnostic-error-related medical claims dominate in the total count (28.6%) and amount (35.2%);
- for new diagnosis, error may range up to 15%.

As we saw in Sect. 22.6 (where we discussed the problem of fat tails in the context of the power law), if we perceive the problem to be normally distributed when in fact it is operating under the power-law or log-normal distributions, it would force the designers to effectively *"bark up the wrong tree."* Referring back to the Borders bookstore case discussed in Sect. 22.1, the management failed to perceive the threat of the Internet as well as the demise of the brick-and-mortar, resulting in the bankruptcy of the firm in a short 10-year period.

In contrast, if designers could rapidly diagnose and orient (i.e., problem abstract in essentials) around real and pressing issues, it would make all the difference in orienting the design and execution teams in the right direction and solving the real problem.

Note that there are subtleties and nuances in the concept of asymmetric fast transients associated with the OODA loop. For example, in the above illustration of how hydraulic controls contributed to fast transitions from one OODA maneuver to another, speed is of the essence. But note that such an OODA loop is situated at the tactical level. In cloud computing, this would be similar to the roles and responsibilities of the DevOps team. In Fig. 22.9b, the tactical OODA has been demarcated within a red-dotted boundary in the middle. In contrast, in the case of the overall OODA loop which included the E-M theory, the issue is more strategic as it is not so much about physical speed; it is about swiftly tapping into accurate mental models (Coram 2002). In other words, the issue is not so much about how quickly the fighter pilot can tactically transition from one maneuver to another in order to get around and get behind the enemy aircraft for establishing air dominance in three-dimensional physical space; the issue is more about how quickly and efficiently the aircraft system architect could design, test, and transition from one configuration to another in the abstract conceptual space, as and when the requirements change.

Given the broad centrality and reach of cloud computing, the architectural design of the cloud is fundamentally strategic in nature. But given the speed at which cloud systems may be assembled and torn-down, everyone is operating under tactical time pressures. Change is relentless in the cloud, and time is of the essence. In other words, architects do not have the luxury of time in formulating their architectural designs. They have to deliver strategic designs under tactical time constraints.

In Cloudonomics (Weinman 2008), Weinman highlighted a similar theme in his 7/10 laws of Cloudonomics:

A real-time enterprise derives competitive advantage from responding to changing business conditions and opportunities faster than the competition.

It is in the fast-transient challenge that the cloud poses an "*existential threat*" to the legacy (e.g., banking) as well as an "*irresistible opportunity*" to the upstarts (e.g., FinTech).

As was the case with Boyd (who had hands-on experience flying sorties in the Korean war), the cloud architect needs to have hands-on experience in all facets of the cloud. And as indicated in Fig. 22.8, the cloud architect also needs to be able to span the strategic business/technological context in the widest possible abstract terms. In the context of cloud architecture, this means that in contrast to the tactically oriented DevOps role, the above strategically significant architectural role ought to be rightly designated as BizArch. Such combinations occur because the looping mechanism in OODA is a guided search that is looping across organizational levels and responsibilities in trying to solve the problem posed by the top-level FR–DP. Here OODA is genuinely heterarchical in creating and encouraging information flows across organizational/disciplinary spaces. In this process, OODA brings about creative mash-ups such as the aforementioned DevOps and BizArch. For example, ArchOps is a role being popularized by the Amazon Web Services (DevOps@Logicworks 2019; Hohpe 2019). In a similar vein, other such mash-ups may include GovArch and BizVend (with Gov for governance and Vend for vendor relations), etc.

While OODA is about decision-making in rapidly evolving strategic and tactical terrains, Boyd also highlighted the importance of exploiting strategic asymmetries between allies and combatants. Between two or more allies and/or adversaries, asymmetries may exist along various dimensions, including asymmetries in wealth, culture, manpower, mental models, technological prowess, physical skill sets, team cohesion, group dynamics, etc. For example, the bubble canopy as well as hydraulic controls pertain to technological asymmetries. But among all the above asymmetries, mental model asymmetries are unique in that they fall out of heterarchical knowledge asymmetries. And as indicated in Sect. 22.5, when corporations (such as Borders versus Amazon) lock horns across these asymmetries, they have the power to systematically and inexorably lay waste (in classic OODA style) the knowledge-gapped corporation or nation.

Figure 22.9c captures a few of the OODA patterns whereby asymmetric fast transients could make or break a corporation. The context is that of a far-flung, multi-national corporation that is hierarchically administered. The view is the top-down view as was described in the context of a similar view shown in the top-left of Fig. 22.9b. The various OODA strategies may be characterized as listed below:

i. Base OODA in sync with apex and executing harmoniously: This is the benchmark case where the apex and basal layers of the organization are working in close coordination (both in time-synchrony and in policy). In the cloud context, it means that the organization is well aware of the heightened cloud cadence and is fundamentally organized top to bottom with this in view.

ii. Heterarchical connect and working in sync: This is the more demanding benchmark that requires heterarchically hierarchical units of a far-flung multi-national corporation being able to work in close coordination. In the cloud context, it means that the corporation is deft and experienced in navigating the international regulatory strictures regarding data location, data privacy, and security.

iii. Base OODA faster than apex and lacking in coordination: This is where the apex and basal layers are asynchronous, with the basal layers evolving at a much faster rate. This situation is not uncommon, given that many corporations treat technology merely as an enabler, and not sufficiently strategic. In extreme cases, it could lead to counterproductive corporate pathologies such as insubordination and toxic workplace cultures. Such a situation might arise in the cloud context if the top management bought into the cloud-as-hype without properly understanding its strategic implications. In other words, there was no serious rethinking of the current architectural strategies in view of the cloud.

iv. Base OODA slower than apex and lagging in execution: This could happen when the founders of the firm who are technically and managerially astute are leading the firm, but under growth pressures they went on a hiring spree that failed to do due-diligence and quality check.

v. Heterarchical disconnect unknowingly at cross-purpose: This is the classic case of "*the left hand not knowing what the right hand does* (Wikipedia 2019l)." Given that there are no linking mechanisms between far-flung multi-national corporate units, the disconnect continues unabated for long durations. In the cloud context, such multi-national corporate dysfunctions could be disastrous given the fact that miscommunications and cultural insensitivities could escalate rapidly out of control (both within the firm and in the larger marketplace sense).

vi. Base OODA intimate with apex OODA and executing faster and at cross-purpose: This is clearly corporate sabotage. In a legacy corporation, there usually exists sufficient checks and balances to make sure that such intentional and highly coordinated actions and their actors do not find refuge. But in the cloud context, given the speed at which policies and personnel can change, it is not unlikely that highly coordinated sabotage teams could take residence, and no one is the wiser.

vii. Adversary intimate with your OODA and executing cross-purpose deep within and at a faster rate: This is the case of an external agent that is somehow privy to the internal corporate strategies and technological initiatives. Being intimate with the corporate agenda and capabilities, such an agent could competitively outsmart the corporation. This is the case of corporate espionage. In the cloud context, a single breach (at the firm, partner, or vendor boundaries) could drop unwanted listening assets within the vast sprawl of the firm's cloud belongings. Stigmergic listening (see Sect. 22.3) would fall in this category.

viii. OODA swarm attack—some internal, some external, and some that change shape: This is akin to the distributed denial-of-service (DDoS) attack. The classic DDoS swarm is synchronous and distributed but coordinated (in an algorithmic sense). It, however, lacks a clear center which could be targeted. Also, what it may lack in sophistication, it makes it up in the sheer number of resource exhausting attacks that are launched. A CAS swarm is similar, but it is shape-shifting and does not have to be synchronous. It could, therefore, play out in time, giving it more ambiguity and cover. An OODA-CAS swarm could be asynchronous, shape-shifting, and executing along asymmetric fast transients. If such sophistication exists on the cloud, it would probably be at the behest of a state sponsor.

Given the close alignment between OODA and AD, the question is what added value does OODA provide AD? Likewise, what added value does AD provide OODA? OODA was formulated for the purpose of establishing dominance in asymmetric warfare, i.e., how to exploit subtle differences (in mental models, technological prowess's, physical skill sets, and group dynamics between adverse and aligned participants) in order to obtain strategic (and often changing) objectives in fluid, fast-changing environments. In contrast, AD was formulated for the explicit purpose of establishing how design may be "*made into a science* (Suh 1990)." It is true that both OODA and AD track closely when mapped along K|H, but they are not dealing with the same issues. AD is more generic than OODA and could be used to enhance the design aspects of OODA. In other words, OODA could benefit from the logical tripartite mappings between FRs, DPs, and PVs. In a similar vein, AD could benefit from OODA in recognizing the strategic significance and asymmetric competitive value of certain key elements of a proposed design.

Example 22.7

How would you correct an organizational disconnect within a heterarchic multi-national such as shown in Fig. 22.9.c.v using the axiomatic approach?

Solution: The fundamental problem that organizations face is the rapidly increasing pace of business decisions that need to be synchronized across the global sprawl of far-flung multi-national units. In this context, the cloud computing initiative has only accelerated this pace. The differential rates in the OODA loop between two or more such organizational units often lead to a lack of coherence and synergy, both between individual units and in an overall sense. In the hierarchical case (i.e., Figures 22.9.c.iii, c.iv), the addition of an OODA-sensitive (vertical) synchronization control unit as an organizational DP would help coordinate the handling of the increasing pace of modern business decisions. The heterarchical disconnect as exhibited in Fig. 22.9.c.v would likewise require the addition of similar OODA-sensitive synchronization control units as organizational DPs to help smooth and coordinate the lateral disconnect. While organizational control units (i.e., the governance bodies) that synchronize business decisions (both vertically and horizontally) are not new, what is currently lacking is the awareness of the need for synchronizing the **rate of change** across the vast organizational sprawl.

22.10 Iterative Axiomatic Maturity Diagram (AMD) Ensembles

If failure could be de-stigmatized, it has potent stigmergic value in systematically learning and becoming familiar with the design landscape. Unfortunately, the various "Fail-X" phrases in use today have created needless confusion.

Failure as a worthwhile end goal does not make sense; it only has value in an interim sense when it is being harnessed for learning the topography of a complex design surface or improving a given design that is flawed. It is never the end goal. A company that prides itself on delivering nothing but failures will cease to exist before long.

Following are two Fail-X listings, the former which could lead to stigmergic learning, and the later which could very well thwart it. From a strategic OODA perspective, we would want our own teams (and those of our allies) to embrace the former while encouraging our adversaries to embrace the later:

Fail-X's that encourage stigmergic learning:

   i. Safe-Fail (Snowden 2006): Through deliberately engineered failures, designers learn the complex terrain being navigated.
  ii. Fail-Fast: To find if a system is ill-designed, best to quickly test it early on, rather than prolonging the discovery of the flaw.
 iii. Fail-Often: Setting up a sequence of small bite-size goalposts, which creates opportunities for many successes and failures.
 iv. Fail-Early: Provide greater latitude for failure, but only during the early phases of a project which could create the right attitude of seriousness toward successes and failures.
  v. Fail-Forward: In failure, take advantage of the lessons learned for the next iteration.
 vi. Fail-Small: Set up small, bite-size goalposts, which creates opportunities for small successes and failures.
 vii. Fail-Well: Compartmentalize and contain the failure from spreading. This agrees well with the uncoupled/decoupled design in AD.
viii. Fail-Safe: In production, if and when you fail, fail safely by not endangering life and property.

Fail-X's that discourage stigmergic learning:

   i. Fail-Backward: Lack of team resilience/ability to recover from failure, hence no learning.
  ii. Fail-Big: Fail colossally at something big. This is high risk for high rewards. It is not driven by incremental, iterative stigmergic learning.
 iii. Fail-Badly: When the system fails, it is catastrophic, and therefore no learning.
 iv. Fail-Silent: When failure happens, it is suppressed from public view with no indication of failure, and therefore no learning.
  v. Fail-Deadly: Mutually assured destruction (MAD) such as is the case for nuclear deterrence. Cloud development has yet to reach the stage of cloud wars where MAD may be relevant.

These are some of the colloquial ways to characterize candidate designs. In general, designs (as well as design processes) may be characterized and critiqued in at least six different ways:

   i. Viability of the select design in regard to the CRs/FRs. This includes the Independence Axiom.
  ii. Performance of the select design in functional comparison to a family of other valid designs. This includes the Information Axiom as a selection criterion.
 iii. Performance of the select design in cost comparison to a family of other valid designs.
 iv. Performance of the select design in view of the change dynamic that is evident in the phylogeny of the problem domain. In other words, what is the rate of

change in the FRs? And how does the candidate design cater to such a rate of change in the FRs?

v. Performance of the design process that created the design with respect to time-to-market? How quickly can such designs be designed and implemented?

vi. Performance of the design as part of a family of other designs that exist in the same enclave (for example, being hosted by the same cloud vendor).

vii. Performance of the design as well as the design process in catering to emergent FRs that may not be known a priori until the design/design process has matured sufficiently.

While the first two criteria from the above list do have axiomatic representation, the last five items do not have representation (except perhaps as rigid, a priori constraints). The agile methodology has made valuable contributions in addressing the last of the above cases, namely, how to go about designing in the complex realm (see Fig. 22.7) where FRs are emergent and unknown a priori, where statistics is rare, and where fat tails and power laws are common. AD could learn from the agile gambit and address this lacuna in a principled fashion without compromising its holistic strengths. Note that in a similar vein, items iii–vi above also remain unaddressed in AD.

As discussed earlier in Sect. 22.9, the problem abstraction phase (i.e., PAs in Fig. 22.9b) arches upward on the inductive design trace. But induction takes its own time; it does not have the same rapid cadence of deductive logic. In other words, it takes time to marshal the necessary holistic view that the axiomatic approach prefers.

Also, the inductive component is more error-prone. Misdiagnosis of the problem can be costly. Agile adopts various Fail-X approaches in order to mitigate this risk. For example, the safe-fail approach (Snowden 2006) accommodates FRs being emergent in a CAS sense. In other words, the FRs do not exist a priori. Referring back to the manner in which the β-layer forms in a CAS setup (Fig. 22.3a), agile seems to suggest that FRs are stigmergically emergent (using agile-style Post-It notes, etc.). They cannot be discerned a priori except through repeated trials and errors. They emerge along the design pathway that is engaged in solving a larger problem. In such a situation, a top-down linear approach such as the waterfall model that does not iterate back to the root FRs will misdiagnose the problem and therefore fail to address the emergent issues.

As would be the case in other approaches, true rapidity/agility in agile occurs in problem contexts that have been well plowed. And in problem contexts that are more bottom-up, inductive, and tentative in nature (such as Cynefin's complex regime), agile adopts an iterative approach of sprints and retrospectives which would necessarily take longer. If that is the case, where exactly is the agility in agile? In order to understand the agility aspect of agile, let us compare the waterfall approach to agile. If in waterfall-type approaches, spurious FRs are being addressed while relevant FRs (which happen to be emergent) are left unaddressed, it is obvious that such designs are never timely. As an analogy, if the train arrives at the wrong destination, it is indefinitely late for arrival at the right destination. The agility of agile is in solving the right problems, and not because it is inherently agile. In other words, it is fundamentally on the basis of the emergent FR problem (which is real and salient, especially in a knowledge economy) that agile has staked its claim on the totality of design.

However, such a broad claim on the totality of design needs to be challenged. For example, the differences between agile and a more formal/structured approach have been couched in the agile manifesto as "X over Y (Kern 2018)." Such a conflicted approach is unnecessary. For example, in the AD context (as shown in Fig. 22.10), it is more than likely that it is a case of "X because of Y." The industry is increasingly becoming aware of many of the agilist blind spots (Meyer 2014; Winters 2016; Brizard 2015).

Agile fails to master the problem of design in at least two significant ways:

- Design is holistic. Piecemeal designs seldom scale, especially in the complex regime. Given the significance of the emergent FR problem (especially in a knowledge economy), agile downplays the very concept of system-wide/holistic design. This can be a problem when considering cybersecurity which tends to expose unaddressed gaps in non-systemic, ad hoc designs. However, it would not be too difficult to bring in holism (especially during the final-stage sprints and retrospectives).

No	Agile (X over Y)	Axiomatic Design (X because of Y)
1	Individuals & Interactions over Processes and Tools	Individuals are able to creatively interact and engage vigorously because of the Processes and Tools that AD provides.
2	Working software over comprehensive documentation	Robust Products because of Principled, Comprehensive/Holisitic design which includes Succinct (FR=DMxDP) Documentation
3	Customer collaboration over contract negotiation	Customer Collaboration via Contractual Obligations as per CR: Customer Requirements which could be flexibly structured to support CR/FR emergences.
4	Responding to change over following a plan	Resilient to change because it is following a Plan (i.e., Design) which includes Design-for-Change.

Fig. 22.10 X over Y (Agile) versus X because of Y (AD). (Reproduced from Thomas and Mantri (2019), originally published open access under a CC BY 4.0 license: https://doi.org/10.1051/matecconf/201930100024)

- Without formal documentation, the stigmergic pattern-making process rarely takes root. In the current technological context where anything and everything is being dutifully noted and recorded (thanks to myriad IoTs and other instruments of constant vigil), it is unfortunate that seamless and effortless documentation is not de-jure in the design realm. The agile manifesto on documentation (i.e., "*working software over comprehensive documentation*") is therefore misguided. In the modern age, design documentation should be automated and effortless. The bias that agile has against documentation is quite anachronistic and self-defeating especially given the role that documentation plays in the formation of stigmergic patterns. Once again, it would not be too difficult to correct this problem.

From an AD perspective, there are valuable insights to be learned from agile. As mentioned earlier, the key distinction between agile and AD is in the context of emergent FRs. This is an area where AD could learn from agile. While keeping the holistic view, the axiomatic approach can strategically borrow agile's iterative stance (which incidentally agrees with the OODA loop). This is precisely what has been proposed in (Puik and Ceglarek 2018) wherein Puik and Ceglarek have advocated using the axiomatic maturity diagram (AMD) in an ingenious way for bringing synergy between the axiomatic and agile approaches. The following discussion extends the AMD approach by explicitly adding the stigmergic tightening of the AMD patterns along the time dimension (see Fig. 22.11).

As suggested in (Puik and Ceglarek 2018), the key is in understanding the competing thrusts of the main three drivers of the design process (Fig. 22.11a):

- **Do the right thing:** Find the right set of FRs, DPs, PVs that has total, holistic capture of the problem at hand and a design for it that satisfies the Independence Axiom (Fig. 22.11/X-axis).
- **Do things optimally:** Minimize the holistic, system-wide information content among candidate designs in order to find the right solution (Fig. 22.11/Z-axis)
- **Do things fast:** Navigate the design space in order to reach the target solution at a rapid pace, i.e., minimize θ, the temporal splay along Fig. 22.11/Y-axis.

Emphasizing any one of these drivers stand-alone or even two-by-two will only succeed up to a certain point. As suggested in (Puik and Ceglarek 2018), the axiomatic maturity diagram (AMD) could be modified ever so slightly to incorporate agile's iterative insight (Fig. 22.11b).

Normally, the AMD is a 2D plot that captures the path dominance between Independence and Information Axioms. For de novo designs, usually the Independence Axiom dominates the initial stages; it is only after the design trace has reached a certain level of maturity that the information axion is triggered. For de vetus cases, the Information Axiom may gainfully be put to use early on given the level of experience and history that is readily available. For the problematic case of emergent FRs (which by its nature is de novo), an iterative approach from the very beginning (i.e., as in Probe → Sense → Respond from the complex realm of

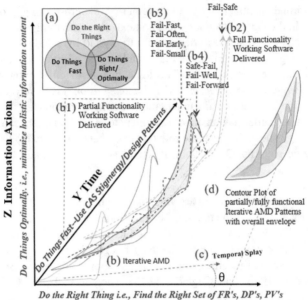

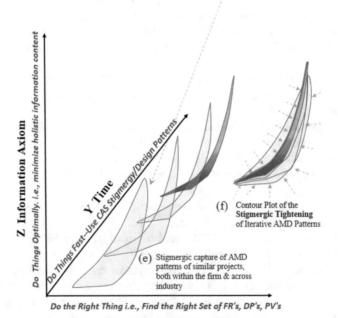

Fig. 22.11 Iterative axiomatic maturity diagram (AMD) ensembles (adapted from (Puik and Ceglarek 2018)). (Reproduced from Thomas and Mantri (2019), originally published open access under a CC BY 4.0 license: https://doi.org/10.1051/matecconf/201930100024)

Cynefin, Fig. 22.7) is probably the right way to proceed. Providing such early and repeated reality checks is one of the hallmarks of the agile approach. As suggested in (Puik and Ceglarek 2018), the dotted curves in Figs. 22.11b3 to b4 capture such agilest iterations that have been abstracted as the underlying wedge. The distinction between Fig. 22.11b3 and b4 is that the former (i.e., Fig. 22.11b3) has a slight bias toward the Information Axiom which should show up in colloquialisms such as Fail-Fast, Fail-Often, Fail-Early, and Fail-Small. In contrast, the latter (i.e., Fig. 22.11b4) is more conservative in its approach and might include colloquialisms such as Safe-Fail, Fail-Well, and Fail-Forward. These loose colloquialisms are merely suggestive and they are not categorical distinctions. The tan-colored wedge captures a variety of iterative/combinatorial possibilities that span between the boundaries of Figs. 22.11b3 and b4.

In each sprint (as Fig. 22.11b1 indicates), only a partial list of the required functionality is being delivered. There are four sprints that have been outlined, of which only the third is colored tan and bounded by Figs. 22.11b3 to b4. Figure 22.11b2 indicates the end of all sprints, with the full working functionality being delivered. Each of the sprints could have fresh additions (of emergent FRs). FRs may also be deleted from a previous partially working solution.

The slight temporal splay (θ) of the very first wedge captures the time taken in the underlying iteration (Fig. 22.11c). The agilest argument is that without an iterative approach, the splay would be much wider; the FRs often hastily and improperly induced; and the resultant design rigid, fragile, and even abandoned. These agilest arguments are completely valid. But there is nothing stopping the axiomatic approach from adopting an iterative stance as shown. And the comparative advantage of the axiomatic approach is that it never loses sight of the fact that the problem of design is holistic. With that ideal in mind, it is therefore motivated to reach for the holistic view.

The contour plot of the four sprints is depicted in Fig. 22.11d. It captures all four partial/fully functional iterative AMD patterns along with an overall containing envelope (in light green) that captures it in abstract. Just the abstract outline is repeated in the lower AMD figure in order to help capture the larger stigmergic patterns if proper documentation was to be enforced.

Figure 22.11e is the stigmergic capture of AMD patterns of similar projects (i.e., the phylogeny) which may exist both within the firm and across the industry. Figure 22.11f captures the contour plot of the **stigmergic tightening** of the various iterative AMD patterns as displayed in Fig. 22.11e. Such stigmergic tightening is feasible, given the fact that the axiomatics encourages holistic information minimization along with succinct, documentation-friendly, design matrix design capture. Thus, across multiple AMD wedge iterations (Fig. 22.11e, f), the axiomatic approach is capable of not just capturing the holistic demand, but it is also capable of leveraging the stigmergic tightening of the AMD patterns.

In time, the AMD trace is well established and settles into a thin slice (displayed as a dark-orange slice at the center). Once the iterative uncertainty has been removed and the stigmergic wedge well established, a waterfall approach would work just as well. In other words, the complex has now been tamed (at least in part) into the complicated/simple regimes, i.e., good practice and best practice available in the industry (see Cynefin, Fig. 22.7). It is indeed a waste of scarce resources to indiscriminately treat every problem as if it were always attached to the complex regime in each of its decompositional details.

Example 22.8

Discuss practical ways to aid the stigmergic tightening of an ensemble of iterative AMD patterns (as shown in Fig. 22.11f).

Solution: Any form of stigmergic tightening requires the existence and accumulation of a wide variety of stigmergic markings that have been carefully curated across multiple iterations. In the case of software/hardware assets (such as in the case of the cloud), this would imply the capture of succinct documentation of the design as well as the operational logs of the application in use. As shown in Example 22.3, stigmergic tightening occurs (in the local context) between control-point DPs that need to be discerned and explicated. With each such iterative/tightening run, the local context becomes more and more global in scope until the overall contour plot is in play. The key step in the above stigmergic tightening run is the discernment and explicit establishment of successive control-point DPs.

22.11 Non-Functional Requirements from a Complex Adaptive System Perspective

Non-functional requirements (non-FRs) dominate the design of cloud architectures. These include system-wide *-ilities* such as

- scalability;
- adaptability;
- reliability;
- security;
- maintainability;
- availability;
- customizability;
- testability, etc.

But as a term of common usage, the non-FRs are indeed a misnomer; there is nothing non-functional about the concern at hand. Thus, the ability to rapidly scale-up or scale-down a certain website based on the seasonal load at hand is most definitely a FRs—except that instead of it being at a final user level, it is now at a system-wide/population-wide level. It is, therefore, a failure in the design community to understand the functional domain when it asserts that the above list of requirements is somehow non-functional (Thompson 2014; Adams 2016).

The deeper question that, however, needs to be probed is where do these non-FRs come from? To solve the puzzle of the origin of functionally relevant non-FRs, one has to study the requirement formation as an iterative CAS process (Fig. 22.3b). If the regular FRs are to be found in the $\beta 1$ ensemble, the non-FRs are to be found in the β2 ensemble. Thus, the so-called non-FRs are indeed FRs and therefore subject to the standard design approaches. Indeed, it is easy to project a future point where there will be a β3 ensemble one day. It is, therefore, best to acknowledge levels of design in preference to ad hoc terminology (such as non-FR) when dealing with systems that are fundamentally CAS in nature. In other words, the various -*ilities* requirements are likely to adapt and evolve away from the current strictures. Or to put it differently, of all the ilities mentioned above, the adaptability requirement is dominant and overarching over asset/agent/artifact space as well as time. The cloud is fundamentally operating and evolving at a much faster cadence than the systems that are residing in the traditional on-prem ecosystem. Architecting such rapidly evolving systems requires the architect to understand the CAS $\alpha \leftrightarrow \beta$ pattern forming mechanism and consider the problem of design from the highest β-level reached thus far, as well as the projected CAS trajectory. Restating the above in Boydian OODA terms, asymmetric fast transients in the cloud are operating with latency in milliseconds instead of weeks or months. Missteps can be fatal. This is especially true when considering cloud cybersecurity.

Example 22.9

Discuss the possible consequences of treating system-wide FRs as non-FRs.

Solution: When legitimate, system-wide FRs are treated as if they were non-functional stipulations that exist outside the purview of design principles, it effectively results in ad - hoc designs that are fragile, non-holistic, and seldom scale. As they are considered to be non-functional, valuable compositional insights from the AD framework are likely to be ignored. Larger the number of such competing non-FRs, greater is the risk of lack of coherence. In some cases (such as security as a non-FR), such dereliction of the designerly mandate could be fatal.

22.12 Security of Cloud Computing

Once the corporate assets have been migrated (in part or whole) over to the cloud, the legacy threat surface is significantly altered. Depending on the cloud footprint (Sroczkowski 2019) (i.e., IaaS, PaaS, SaaS), the onus of securing the assets is now a joint responsibility. What was previously an in-house responsibility is now a shared undertaking that juxtaposes the evolving footprint and complexity of the vendors' cloud infrastructure and operations (with its global reach and geophysical asset spread) against the cloud maturity of the in-house architects, developers, users, and operators.

Some recent quotes regarding cloud-related security breaches in the news include the following:

- *A group of angry customers filed a lawsuit against Capital One…following the hack that affected more than 106 million people…the group also named Amazon Web Services, Capital One's cloud provider, alleging the tech giant is also culpable for the breach.* (August 9, 2019, (Levy 2019))

- *Unprotected Database Puts 65% of American Households at Risk...data included on the 24 GB database [hosted on Microsoft Azure] is people's full names, full street addresses, marital status, date of birth, income bracket, home ownership status and more.* (April 29, 2019. (Morris 2019))
- *Verizon Partner Exposed Millions of Customer Accounts...a misconfigured cloud-based file repository exposed the names, addresses, account details, and account personal identification numbers (PINs) of as many as 14 million US customers of telecommunications carrier Verizon.* (December 12, 2018. (O'Sullivan 2018))
- *In December [2018], Google revealed the details of...data breach that happened...leaving the data of close to 52.5 million Google + users vulnerable to hackers...Google + is shutting down in 2019.* (Roussey 2019)
- *Between July and September 2018, hackers leveraged the "view as" feature on Facebook to steal tokens for access profiles. This breach compromised the personal details of close to 29 million users across the globe. It divulged personal information including names, phone numbers, email addresses, and other personal details Facebook collected over time. The breach was disclosed to the general users on September 28.* (Roussey 2019)

According to a recent multi-factor industry survey of the leading concerns of 400,000 cloud cybersecurity professionals (Cloud Security Report 2018):

- Biggest threats to cloud security—misconfiguration of cloud platforms (62%).
- Legacy on-prem security tools are ill-designed for the virtual, dynamic, and distributed cloud. Traditional security solutions either don't work at all in cloud environments or have only limited functionality (84%).
- Operationally, the leading security control challenges (SOCs) include (a) poor visibility into infrastructure security (43%); (b) compliance (38%); (c) Setting consistent security policies across cloud and on-premises environments (35%); and (d) security not keeping up with the pace of change in applications (35%).
- Compared to an on-prem deployment, 49% of the respondents believe that the public cloud poses a greater security risk, 30% responded about the same, and only 17% responded in favor of the cloud.

Many cloud-related cyberinsecurities are related to poor design. These design issues could show up as misconfiguration, poor consistency, lack of transparency, inadequate security tools, inability to keep pace with application changes, etc. With the rapid evolution of the threat surface (Thomas and Mantri 2015a, b), it is no wonder that even well-configured systems sprout leaks.

But the greatest cybersecurity vulnerability in cloud computing has to do with a flawed defense-in-depth (DiD) mindset that currently dominates the industry (see Sect. 22.5 for a prior discussion on this topic in connection to knowledge hierarchy/heterarchy). There are two major problems with the DiD posture (Igbe 2017):

- **Technological Exposure:** Rapid evolution of technology exposes interface mismatches across the various onion layers. Ubiquitous and remotely located edge nodes and IoT devices can be compromised. Each system is designed for a certain system range. Swarm attacks can be designed to overwhelm the elasticity of these system ranges. While traditional attacks used to be sequentially directed against any single layer, modern swarm attacks target multiple layers simultaneously. Traditional attacks were directed at the network layer that is easier to detect, while modern attacks target the application layer that is harder to detect.
- **Socio-technical Exposure:** Human cognitive biases and vulnerabilities are constantly being probed via social engineering techniques and strategies such as weak passwords, robocalls, and phishing attacks. The performance overhead from any of the security defenses can reach a point of intolerance for the human agents to become overwhelmed and then switch it off.

In contrast to defense-in-depth, the emerging defense-in-breadth (DiB) approach also considers the wider angle of vulnerabilities. NIST has helped in defining and contrasting the two (Ross et al. 2016):

- **Defense-in-depth:** *Information security strategy integrating people, technology, and operations capabilities to establish variable barriers across multiple layers and missions of the organization.*
- **Defense-in-breadth:** *A planned, systematic set of **multidisciplinary** activities that seek to identify, manage, and reduce risk of exploitable vulnerabilities at every stage of the system, network, or subcomponent life cycle (system, network, or product design and development; manufacturing; packaging; assembly; system integration; distribution; operations; maintenance; and retirement).*

It is the multidisciplinary emphasis in DiB that provides the hint that the underlying system and the concerns thereof are heterarchical in nature (see Fig. 22.12). In contrast to traditional hierarchical systems, the combinatorial space that the architect has to master when dealing with heterarchical systems is vastly more complex and expanded. As shown in Sect. 22.10 (i.e., iterative AMD), such systems may best be designed in a systematic and principled way by leveraging the stigmergic patterns that accrue over time.

Example 22.10

Why is it easier to penetrate heterarchic vulnerabilities of a system as compared to the hierarchical?

Solution: All designs require the basic awareness that a problem exists in the first place. Given the highly specialized training that professionals (such as engineers and scientists) receive, it is far more likely that they are aware of the hierarchical linkages within their areas of specialization as compared to heterarchical linkages between specialties. In other words, heterarchical vulnerabilities are located in the collective blind spot of a hierarchically trained workforce. This is the fundamental reason why it is easier to penetrate heterarchic vulnerabilities of a system as compared to the hierarchical.

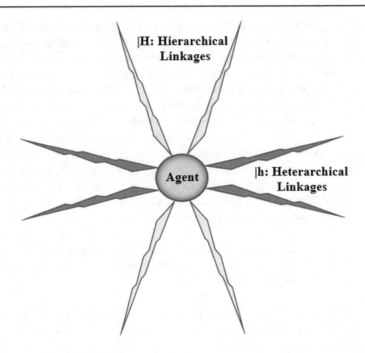

Fig. 22.12 Defense-in-depth/width (hierarchy vs. heterarchy). (Reproduced from Thomas and Mantri (2019), originally published open access under a CC BY 4.0 license: https://doi.org/10. 1051/matecconf/201930100024)

22.13 Econo-Complex Adaptive System Strategy in the Cloud

None of the top four companies by Market Cap from the year 2000 (i.e., General Electric, ExxonMobil, Pfizer, and Citigroup) were able to retain their leadership positions. Instead, it is now Microsoft, Amazon, Apple, and Alphabet (Google). Among these four, three have strong vendor presence in the cloud; only Apple is weak and is dependent on Amazon. As reported in (Statt 2019):

> *Apple is deeply reliant on AWS to operate core parts of its business, even though doing so means working with a soon-to-be-rival in online video and a current competitor in areas like artificial intelligence, streaming music, and smart home products.*

Apple is facing a similar problem as was the case with Borders. Many other major firms (including Netflix) face the same conundrum that Borders faced when dealing with a power-law-driven knowledge economy.

As was mentioned earlier, cloud computing is strategic and needs to be considered in warfare terms. Critical assets deployed on the cloud are no longer business-as-usual, it, in fact, is being positioned on an asymmetric, winner-take-all, fast-transient OODA basis. In such a context, every aspect of the OODA loop needs to be examined for its asymmetry potential.

In order to scale a higher peak, one often has to climb down from the current summit. Traditionally, it is economics that has provided navigational guidance in the summit-to-summit route-finding endeavors. But what if the economic heuristics we have here-to-fore depended on themselves change? What if the governing economic rules are being rewritten to accommodate fat tails even as the corporate econo-strategist tries to navigate across the shifting landscape? It is in this sense that cloud computing is *"both an existential threat and an irresistible opportunity* (Weinman 2012)."

It is indeed an existential threat for those wedded to the status quo, but it is also an opportunity for those willing *"to climb down"* from their current summits and look at the de novo econo-design landscape that is opening up. These include social network economies (Facebook, LinkedIn, Twitter etc.), Big Data plays (Green-Plum, Cloudera/Hortonworks, Palantir, etc.), streaming economies (Netflix, Hulu, Amazon Prime, YouTube TV, etc.), gaming plays (PlayStation Now, Shadow, GeForce NOW, etc.), and others.

As one steps back from the micro-view in order to then take in the big picture/macro-view, it is becoming increasingly clear that the architectural design of the cloud computing play is anything but simple and straightforward. For example, in the context of cybersecurity, the attack surface is the map of all ports of entry/exit whereby an attacker may launch an attack and/or spirit off corporate assets. And as the business grows, the dangers of cyberinsecurity increase as the attack surface proliferates and mutates across pathways and resources that the corporation does not fully command.

Likewise, the economic attack surface for cloud-based corporate ventures is orders of magnitude more complex than the traditional on-prem ventures. Once the corporation establishes key assets in the cloud, it is operating in a shared environment where its business activities leave open and visible stigmergic traces. These include what is openly known about the strengths/weaknesses of the cloud vendor.

Once the business model proves viable in the cloud, the competitive attack surface can bring in a swarm of traditional/non-traditional challengers unconstrained by erstwhile barriers to entry that have either been leveled or rendered irrelevant. The cloud fundamentally lowers many of the traditional barriers to entry. For example, it is true that the Chinese firm Ant-Financial was rebuffed in establishing a FinTech foothold in the U.S. via the purchase of MoneyGram (Roumeliotis 2018). But there are no such barriers for the rapid migration/replication by native agents of a successful business model such as the Ant-Financial. And it is in such a rapidly evolving cloud ecosystem that a well-thought-out adaptive architectural design could take advantage of the new economies-of-scale and elasticity that the cloud makes available. Creating a viable cloud enterprise increasingly involves architecting of a complex adaptive system (Urquhart 2012). The following

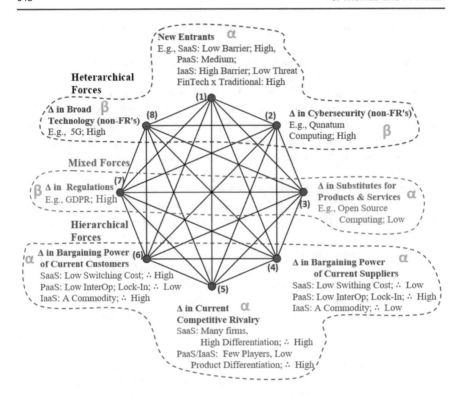

Fig. 22.13 CAS-based extension of Porters 5 α-level competitive cloud forces (Wikipedia 2019j) to include 3 β-level forces. (Reproduced from Thomas and Mantri (2019), originally published open access under a CC BY 4.0 license: https://doi.org/10.1051/matecconf/201930100024)

discussion is a CAS-based extension of Porters original five α-level competitive cloud forces to include three β-level forces for a total of eight (see Fig. 22.13).

The fundamental difference to notice is that all eight competitive forces are at the periphery and jostling with each other for dominance, whereas Porter's framework had centralized on current rivalry as the core node. Also, the forces are characterized using the CAS α-β notation to help identify the level at which agents are forming their strategic intent. Porter's formulation had the original five forces occurring at the inter-agent α-level. The three new entries (i.e., cybersecurity, technological shifts, and global regulations) exist at the β → α level. These additions are just a sampling of the missing entries in the original formulation; there could, of course, be many more than just these three additions.

The set of eight competitive forces is split into three groups: hierarchical, heterarchical, and mixed. Hierarchical forces are incremental, slow-moving, and works within the confines of the current competitive landscape. For example, if there is a PaaS Lock-In (as is at node 6 in Fig. 22.13), it is not easy to shift out of this. Heterarchical forces could also be slow-moving. But a few are strategic, rapid, and works orthogonal to the current competitive landscape (e.g., 5G at node 8, Fig. 22.13). Mixed items have both heterarchical and hierarchical elements within them.

To illustrate the framework, consider the IaaS cloud offering. Here, there is a low threat from new entrants (see node 1, Fig. 22.13) given the sizable upfront Capex outlays that the hosting of a full-stack cloud infrastructure requires. Nevertheless, given the state-level strategic significance of the cloud for any given nation, the above deep-pocket Capex stricture, therefore, does not preclude state-level agents from entering the competitive landscape. Yet given the speed at which the underlying technology shifts (for example, the impending shift from 4G to 5G), any state sponsor faces steep odds in keeping up with the fast-moving heterarchic front. State sponsors tend to be hierarchical in nature; they have yet to master the unwieldy socio-technical heterarchic hierarchies of today. But when cybersecurity issues are raised (see node-2, Fig. 22.13), the state may have a strategic incentive to take on the infrastructural challenge head-on. All three competitive forces as shown in brown (new entrants, technological shifts, and cybersecurity) fall in the heterarchical space as each of these driving forces has the power to shift the competitive landscape from a point of view that is orthogonal to the $\alpha \leftrightarrow \alpha$ focus (in Porter's framework), and that too, potentially overnight.

Now consider the hierarchical tranche. From a consumer's perspective, the shift from Capex to Opex has fundamentally lowered the bargaining power of the IaaS supplier as there is very little lock-in (see node 6, Fig. 22.13). If one of the competitors offers a similar or enhanced set of infrastructural offerings at a sufficiently competitive price (competitive enough to overcome the switching costs), the consumer has every incentive to shift. The real bargaining power of the supplier exists not at the level of any given α-agent-level supplier–consumer contract; instead, it is in successfully leveraging the β-level *-ilities* which the industry mistakenly identifies as the non-FRs (see Sect. 22.11).

The mixed set includes the realm of substitutes that rise up either hierarchically within the current competitive landscape or heterarchically orthogonal to it. The mixed set also includes the shifting regulatory fractal landscape that has a global reach. It is "mixed" in the sense that much of the regulatory landscape is hierarchically constrained by precedent, but occasionally, the regulatory bodies do reach across and claim jurisdiction (especially in uncharted areas that new technological mash-ups have recently opened up). From a regulatory perspective, any of the major state-level agents have the power to overnight shift the competitive landscape with the understanding that when dealing with a CAS, the overall system will react back. In other words, in a CAS system, any unilateral action would face resistance at various levels. This is the reason why all the eight forces (and there may be many more β-level forces) are depicted at the periphery and engaging each other in a complete network. Porter's framework only considered the α-level agents and the direct interplay between them; it is silent about the β-level play wherein much of the competitive landscape has shifted.

Example 22.11

What is the strategic impact of 5G in the context of cloud computing?

Solution: 5G is supposed to be 100 times faster than the prevalent 4G, thus bringing the latency between devices to near-zero levels. This will flatten the current hierarchies such as cloud↔smartphones↔wearables to be just between cloud and wearables. In other words, compute, storage, and networking in the middle layers will face increasing obsolescence. The overall architecture between the cloud and the edge devices will become more and more bipartite with large-scale consolidation in the centralized cloud offerings on account of the aforementioned (see Sect. 22.2) economies of scale and scope. Edge devices will increasingly become highly sensitive and action-oriented agents alongside the begin and end of the OODA loop (observe/act), while the middle two roles (orient/decide) are retained at the centralized cloud.

22.14 Weickian Versus Axiomatic Adaptive Coupling in Complex Adaptive System Architectures

Organizational Psychologist, Karl Weick originated the modern concept of loose- versus tight-coupling in the mid-1970s. Coupling plays a central role in AD. The following discussion frames both the Weickian and the axiomatic approaches on coupling in the CAS framework.

As Prof. Suh noted in (Suh 1990, 2001):

> When the design matrix [A] is diagonal, each of the FRs can be satisfied independently by means of one DP. Such a design is called an uncoupled design. When the matrix is triangular, the independence of FRs can be guaranteed if and only if the DPs are deter- mined in a proper sequence. Such a design is called decoupled design. Any other form of the design matrix is called a full matrix and results in a coupled design.

Likewise, as Prof. Weick noted in (Weick and Orton 1990):

> ...loose coupling is evident when elements affect each other "suddenly (rather than con- tinuously), occasionally (rather than constantly), negligibly (rather than significantly), indirectly (rather than directly), and eventually (rather than immediately).

The dynamics embedded in the Weickian concept of loose-coupling may be best understood using CAS framework that emphasizes levels, temporal spans as well as impact:

- **Levels:** Rejects direct intervention ($\alpha \rightarrow \alpha$) in favor of the indirect ($\alpha \rightarrow \beta \rightarrow \alpha$) (i.e., *"indirectly (rather than directly)"*).
- **Time Delay:** Rejects the chronic and continuous in favor of episodic in the short term or long term (i.e., *"suddenly (rather than continuously), occasionally (rather than constantly), ...eventually (rather than immediately)"*).
- **Impact:** Favors small versus the large impact (i.e., *"negligibly (rather than significantly)"*).

In (Weick 1976), Prof. Weick further notes that:

By loose coupling, the author intends to convey the image that coupled events are responsive, but that each event also preserves its own identity and some evidence of its physical or logical separateness.

Based on the above characteristics, Prof. Weick defines the following types (Weick and Orton 1990):

If there is neither responsiveness nor distinctiveness, the system is not really a system, and it can be defined as a noncoupled system. If there is responsiveness without distinctiveness, the system is tightly coupled. If there is distinctiveness without responsiveness, the system is decoupled. If there is both distinctiveness and responsiveness, the system is loosely coupled.

A system of CAS agents is responsive when sufficient β-level orchestrating patterns have accumulated (within a given iteration) in order to help α-level agents respond in a coordinated fashion to the events at hand. Furthermore, the system is distinctive (within a given iteration) when the α-level agents have retained sufficient degrees of freedom (DOFs) to move orthogonally to the restrictions placed by the previous $\beta \rightarrow \alpha$ coordination.

Based on the above CAS reframing, the four Weickian categories (see Fig. 22.14 above) may be restated as follows:

- **Noncoupled:** No $\alpha \leftrightarrow \alpha$, $\alpha \rightarrow \beta$, No $\beta \rightarrow \alpha$.
- **Tightly coupled:** $\alpha \leftrightarrow \alpha$ & $\beta \rightarrow \alpha$ exists, but no orthogonal $\alpha \rightarrow \beta$ exists in the next iteration (i.e., no degrees of freedom left).

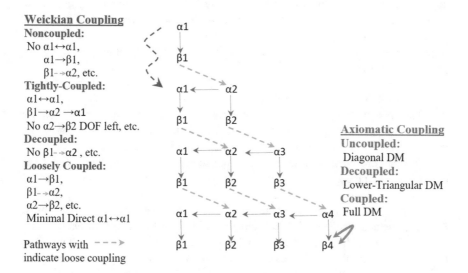

Fig. 22.14 Axiomatic versus Weickian coupling. (Reproduced from Thomas and Mantri (2019), originally published open access under a CC BY 4.0 license: https://doi.org/10.1051/matecconf/201930100024)

- **Decoupled:** $\alpha \to \beta$ exists, but the β-level patterns are either non-existent or not mature enough to provide $\beta \to \alpha$ coordination and control.
- **Loosely coupled:** Minimum $\alpha \leftrightarrow \alpha$; both $\beta \to \alpha$ coordination and control as well as next orthogonal/iterative $\alpha \to \beta$ exists (i.e., remainder degrees of freedom exist even after $\beta \to \alpha$ coordination and control).

Loosely coupled systems are an organizational ideal for social, technical as well as socio-technical systems. They are neither brittle (i.e., they are resilient in the face of change dynamics) nor anarchic (i.e., not lacking in coordination and concerted action). The resilience is because (when faced with novel situations) the agents retain sufficient degrees of freedom to coordinate and self-organize new structures outside the current strictures. But for the most part, the agents are operating within the current strictures. Or as Weick asserts in (Weick 2001), *"the real trick in highly reliable systems is somehow to achieve simultaneous centralization and decentralization."*

Here, the centralization mandate is achieved via $\beta \to \alpha$ coordination (Thomas and Mantri 2018). The α-level decentralization captures the remaining orthogonal degrees of available freedom given the current state of centralization. As the overall system gears across multiple $\alpha \to \beta$ iterations (see Fig. 22.3b), and the agents get more organized, the loose-coupling frontier shifts to the highest iterate. Everything lower down is stable, highly orchestrated, coordinated, waterfallish, and tightly coupled. Since there are no degrees of freedom available at the lower levels, consequently the problem of design itself does not exist. An example of this is assembly programming, i.e., for most higher level programming language cases, there are no degrees of freedom left at this base layer. All the remaining degrees of freedom exist in one of the higher level programming languages. Thus, the problem of design exists only in the outermost iterate where degrees of freedom exist for the respective agents. All the lower levels exist as constraints and context for the problem of design.

The fundamental problem of design only exists where there are degrees of freedom available, which typically exists in the outermost layers of the CAS system. The problem of coupling in AD, therefore, exists at the outermost iterate layer (see bottom-right in Fig. 22.14). Given the symbiotic reach of both of these systems, the AD framework (as well as that for agile) could, therefore, work well with the Weickian loose-coupling framework. Across each iteration (as the system gears up), the axiomatic approach of preferring uncoupled/decoupled in preference to the coupled is, therefore, sound advice.

The question now is how does the above discussion relate to cloud architectures? As we indicated in Sect. 22.9, the cloud is anything but static. Instead, it is a socio-technical CAS system that is rapidly morphing, adapting, and evolving. And it is in this context that the Weickian approach could work symbiotically alongside the axiomatic approaches, i.e., via Weickian loose-coupling at the basal layers alongside AD uncoupling/decoupling at the growing meristem of the CAS edifice. For example, as in (Fehling et al. 2014), by using an intermediary broker mechanism, direct $\alpha \leftrightarrow \alpha$ interactions are streamlined and minimized. Instead, new broker agents are used (under the guidance of $\beta \rightarrow \alpha$ patterns) for indirect information exchange between agents. AD could assist in the establishment of such a CAS scaffold. This would provide for framing the loose-coupling between $\alpha \leftrightarrow \alpha$. Once the α-β architecture of the loosely coupled bipartite CAS framework is established, AD could further be used in designing each of the layers as per the AD coupling/decoupling logic.

Example 22.12

Compare the axiomatic versus Weickian structures to that found in plant biology between meristematic and non-meristematic tissue.

Solution: In plant biology, tissues (such as the shoot and root systems) that engage in cell division and growth are considered as meristematic. After division, a certain number of these daughter cells differentiate and lose their stem-cell-like flexibility to become permanent tissues such as the dermal tissue that functions as the protective skin for the plant. Likewise, the axiomatic versus the Weickian structures have a very similar meristematic versus non-meristematic property in that the growing front affords maximum design flexibility in the form of designerly degrees of freedom, while the Weickian under-structures are well defined and minimally invested in designerly degrees of freedom. But there is a fundamental difference between the two in that the loose-coupling aspect of the underlying Weickian structures helps to retain and exercise all the degrees of freedom that were left unassigned. In other words, there could be valuable stem-cell-like designerly degrees of freedom in the Weickian sub-structures that when resolved may avoid downstream couplings.

22.15 Conclusions

A number of theoretical/practical issues related to an adaptive architectural design surrounding cloud computing were covered in this chapter. Nine mutually supportive decision-making frameworks were formally integrated for the first time in providing a comprehensive, overarching approach to help tackle design problems at large. These included axiomatics, knowledge hierarchy/heterarchy, Cynefin, OODA, stigmergy, CAS, AMD, Non-FRs, and adaptive loose-coupling.

Some of the key findings include the following:

- The cloud is a CAS system. The architectural design of the cloud requires coming to terms with the underlying CAS dynamics and patterns.
- The framework of knowledge hierarchy/heterarchy provides a simple but robust approach to help integrate many orthogonal, but mutually supportive frameworks such as axiomatics, OODA, and Cynefin.
- Time-axis extension of the iterative AMD approach as reported in (Puik and Ceglarek 2018) provides a pragmatic way to bring agility, axiomatics, and the stigmergic-tightening pattern logic together in one place to help bring about principled design, but in an agile fashion.
- Using CAS, the non-FRs have been folded into the standard FR–DP mappings.

- Security of the cloud has been critiqued, both from a design perspective and from a defense-in-depth/defense-in-breadth perspective.
- Using CAS, the fundamental concept of coupling has been broadened to include loose-coupling which powers much of modern technology, including the cloud.

The global economy is facing unprecedented challenges. While cloud computing is not an all-round panacea for alleviating the human condition, it has much to offer in bringing us together in solving the myriad large-scale problems spanning the globe. And as shown, design plays a central role across all levels in this conversation.

Problems

1. Compare and contrast the historical development of space exploration versus cloud computing using the axiomatic framework. Based on your study, what future trends could be projected in each of the above endeavors?
2. Eusocial entities (including humans) fall back on stigmergic techniques when the scale and scope of the problem reach beyond the problem-solving capacity of the individual or the group. Make a case for how stigmergy may have played a role in the creation of each of the seven wonders of the ancient world.
3. Find three examples where complex adaptive systems are operative at the micro, meso, and macro-scales in human biology, sociology, and politics.
4. Create a conceptual trace of the knowledge hierarchy in any two domains of your choice. Then link them up to illustrate the heterarchical connections between the two. Study the historical chronology in the development of the above two conceptual networks.
5. Forensically illustrate the importance of power laws in the modern knowledge economy by studying three cases of the decline and fall of legacy corporations in the face of upstarts.
6. Develop the econo-CAS framework (as shown in Fig. 22.13) to include three more competitive cloud forces from Sect. 22.11 on non-FRs.
7. Investigate the role of design in cloud security.
8. Compare and contrast Weickian loose versus tight-coupling in engineering versus socio-technical systems. Compare and contrast the role of axiomatic decoupling in each of the above cases.

References

Adams KM (2016) Non-functional requirements in systems analysis and design. Springer

Akhtar SMF (2018) Big Data Architect's Handbook: a guide to building proficiency in tools and systems used by leading big data experts. Packt Publishing

Anfodillo T, Carrer M, Simini F, Popa I, Banavar JR, Maritan A (2013) An allometry-based approach for understanding forest structure, predicting tree-size distribution and assessing the degree of disturbance. Royal Society Publishing. https://doi.org/10.1098/rspb.2012.2375

Barabási AL, Albert R (1999) Emergence of scaling in random networks. Science 286:509. https://doi.org/10.1126/science.286.5439.509

Brizard TJ (2015) Broken Agile. Apress

Chellapp R (1997) Intermediaries in cloud-computing: a new computing paradigm. Presented at INFORMS Meeting, Dallas, 1997R. Chellapp, Intermediaries in Cloud-Computing: A New Computing Paradigm, Presented at INFORMS Meeting, Dallas

Cloud Industry Forum (20019). 8 Criteria to ensure you select the right cloud service provider. https://www.cloudindustryforum.org/content/8-criteria-ensure-you-select-right-cloud-service-provider. Accessed 14 July 2019

Schulze H. Cloud Security Report-2018. https://pages.cloudpassage.com/rs/857-FXQ-213/images/2018-Cloud-Security-Report%20%281%29.pdf

Coram R (2002) Boyd: the fighter pilot who changed the art of war. Brown and Company, Little

DevOps@Logicworks (2019) ArchOps vs. DevOps: Foundation and Automation. https://www.logicworks.com/blog/2015/03/aws-devops-archops-automation/. Accessed 14 July 2019

Erl T, Khattak W, Buhler P (2016) Big data fundamentals: concepts, drivers & techniques. Prentice Hall

Erl T, Cope R, Naserpour A (2017) Cloud computing design patterns, 1 edn. Prentice Hall

Fehling C, Leymann F, Retter R, Schupeck W, Arbitter P (2014) Cloud computing patterns: fundamentals to design, build, and manage cloud applications. Springer

Grassé PP (1959) Insectes Sociaux VI 79

Hohpe G (2019) The architect elevator—visiting the upper floors. https://martinfowler.com/articles/architect-elevator.html#ArchopsBuildAVerticalArchitectureTeam. Accessed 14 July 2019

Holland JH (2006) Studying complex adaptive systems. J Syst Sci Complexity 19(1):1–8

Igbe D (2017) Defense in breadth or defense in depth? https://www.cloudtechnologyexperts.com/defense-in-breadth-or-defense-in-depth/. Accessed 14 July 2019

Jansen W, Grance T (2011) Guidelines on security and Privacy in public cloud computing. National Institute of Standards and Technology. Special Publication 800-144. https://nvlpubs.nist.gov/nistpubs/Legacy/SP/nistspecialpublication800-144.pdf. Accessed 14 July 2019

Jastrow (2006) Bust of aristotle. Marble, Roman copy after a Greek bronze original by Lysippos from 330 BC; the alabaster mantle is a modern addition. Wikimedia website. https://commons.wikimedia.org/wiki/File:Aristotle_Altemps_Inv8575.jpg. Accessed May 26 2020. Public domain

Karthikeyan SA (2017) Azure automation using the ARM model: an in-depth guide to automation with Azure resource manager, 1st edn. Apress

Kern J (2018) Agile in the context of a holistic approach. https://www.infoq.com/articles/agile-holistic-approach/. Accessed 14 July 2019

Lee J, Wei T, Mukhiya SK (2018) Hands-on Big Data modeling: effective database design techniques for data architects and business intelligence professionals. Packt Publishing

Levy N (2019) Amazon and Capital One face legal backlash after massive hack affects 106 M customers. https://www.geekwire.com/2019/amazon-capital-one-face-lawsuits-massive-hack-affects-106m-customers/

Loboz CZ (2010) Cloud resource usage—heavy tailed distributions invalidating traditional capacity planning models. J Grid Comput. https://doi.org/10.1145/1996109.1996112

Louridas P, Spinellis D, Vlachos V (2008) Power laws in software. ACM Trans Soft Eng Method 18(1):1–26. Article 2. https://doi.org/10.1145/1391984.1391986

Mell PM, Grance T (2011) The NIST definition of cloud computing. Special Publication (NIST SP)—800-145. September 28, 2011. https://www.nist.gov/publications/nist-definition-cloud-computing

Meyer B (2014) Agile!: The good, the hype and the ugly. Springer

Morris C (2019) A Goldmine for identity thieves: unprotected database puts 65% of American Households at risk. April 29, 2019. http://fortune.com/2019/04/29/security-gap-personal-information-breach/

Newman-Toker D (2013) Diagnostic errors more common, costly and harmful than treatment mistakes. https://www.hopkinsmedicine.org/news/media/releases/diagnostic_errors_more_common_costly_and_harmful_than_treatment_mistakes. Accessed 14 July 2019

Niklas KJ (1994) Plant allometry: the scaling of form and process. University of Chicago Press

O'Sullivan D (2018) Cloud leak: how a Verizon partner exposed millions of customer accounts. https://www.upguard.com/breaches/verizon-cloud-leak

Parunak HVD (2006) A survey of environments and mechanisms for human-human stigmergy. Environ Multi-Agent Syst II: 163–186

Passmore E (2016) Migrating large-scale services to the cloud: a master checklist of everything you need to know to move to the cloud. Apress

Puik E, Ceglarek D (2018) Application of axiomatic design for agile product development. In: MATEC web of conferences 223, 01004 (2018). ICAD 2018. https://doi.org/10.1051/matecconf/201822301004

Richards C (2004) Certain to win: the strategy of John Boyd, applied to business. Xlibris

Ross R, McEvilley M, Oren JC (2016) Systems security engineering considerations for a multidisciplinary approach in the engineering of trustworthy secure systems. NIST Special Publication 800-160. https://doi.org/10.6028/NIST.SP.800-160

Roumeliotis G (2018) U.S. blocks MoneyGram sale to China's ant financial on national security concerns. https://www.reuters.com/article/us-moneygram-intl-m-a-ant-financial/u-s-blocks-moneygram-sale-to-chinas-ant-financial-on-national-security-concerns-idUSKBN1ER1R7. Accessed 14 July 2019

Roussey B (2019) 10 biggest 2018 data breaches—and what they mean for 2019. March 22, 2019. http://techgenix.com/2018-data-breaches/

Siegel E (2013) Predictive analytics: the power to predict who will click, buy, lie, or die. Wiley

Snowden D (2006) Safe-fail or fail-safe. https://cognitive-edge.com/blog/safe-fail-or-fail-safe/. Accessed 14 July 2019

Snowden DJ, Boone ME (2007) A leader's framework for decision making. Harvard Bus Rev. https://hbr.org/2007/11/a-leaders-framework-for-decision-making. Accessed 14 July 2019

Sonmez J (2014) Soft skills: The software developer's life manual. Manning Publications

Sroczkowski P (2019) Cloud: IaaS vs PaaS vs SaaS vs DaaS vs FaaS vs DBaaS. https://brainhub.eu/blog/cloud-architecture-saas-faas-xaas/. Accessed 14 July 2019

Statt N (2019) Apple's cloud business is hugely dependent on Amazon. https://www.theverge.com/2019/4/22/18511148/apple-icloud-cloud-services-amazon-aws-30-million-per-month. Accessed 14 July 2019

Suh NP (1990) The principles of design, 1st edn. Oxford University Press, New York

Suh NP (2001) Axiomatic design–advances and applications. Oxford University Press

Suh NP (2005) Complexity: theory and applications, 1st edn. Oxford University Press, New York

Surowiecki J (2005) The wisdom of crowds. Anchor

The Open Group (2019). Cloud Computing Governance Framework. http://www.opengroup.org/cloud/gov_snapshot/p3.htm. Accessed July 14 2019

Thomas J (1995) Archstand theory of design for innovation. Ph.D. Thesis. http://dspace.mit.edu/handle/1721.1/11722. MIT. Accessed 14 July 2019

Thomas J, Mantri P (2015a) Axiomatic design/design patterns Mashup: part 1. In: 9th International conference on axiomatic design (ICAD), Procedia CIRP 34:269–275. http://www.sciencedirect.com/science/article/pii/S2212827115008501

Thomas J, Mantri P (2015b) Axiomatic design/design patterns Mashup: part 2. In: 9th International conference on axiomatic design (ICAD), Procedia CIRP 34:276–283. https://www.sciencedirect.com/science/article/pii/S2212827115008513

Thomas J, Mantri P (2018) Complex adaptive Blockchain Governance. MATEC Web of Conferences 223, 01010 (2018) https://doi.org/10.1051/matecconf/201822301010

Thomas J, Zaytseva A (2016) Mapping complexity/human knowledge as a complex adaptive system. 2016 Wiley Periodicals, Inc., vol 21, no S2. https://doi.org/10.1002/cplx.21799, https://onlinelibrary.wiley.com/doi/abs/10.1002/cplx.21799

Thomas J, Mantri P (2019) Axiomatic Cloud Computing Architectural Design. In: the 13th International Conference on Axiomatic Design (ICAD 2019). MATEC web of conferences 301, 00024 (2019). https://doi.org/10.1051/matecconf/201930100024

Thompson MK (2014) Where is the 'Why' in axiomatic design? ICAD2014. The Eighth International Conference on Axiomatic Design. Campus de Caparica, September 24–26, 2014

Tollen DW (2016) The tech contracts handbook: cloud computing agreements, software licenses, and other IT contracts for lawyers and businesspeople. Am Bar Assoc

Urquhart J (2012) Cloud is complex—deal with it. Jan 8, 2012. https://gigaom.com/2012/01/08/cloud-is-complex-deal-with-it/. Accessed 14 July 2019

Vleck TV (2019) Project MAC. https://multicians.org/project-mac.html. Accessed 14 July 2019

Ward H (2016) How to hire. https://medium.com/eshares-blog/how-to-hire-34f4ded5f176#.b04yy5bka. Accessed 14 July 2019

Weick KE (1976) Educational organizations as loosely coupled systems. Adm Sci Q 21(1):1–19. Published by: Sage Publications, Inc

Weick KE (2001) Making sense of the organization, Oxford. Blackwell Publishers, England

Weick KE, Orton JD (1990) Loosely coupled systems: a reconceptualization. loosely coupled systems: a reconceptualization. Acad Manage Renew 15(2):203–223

Weinman J (2008) The 10 laws of cloudonomics. https://gigaom.com/2008/09/07/the-10-laws-of-cloudonomics/. Accessed 14 July 2019

Weinman J (2012) Cloudonomics: the business value of cloud computing. Wiley

Wikipedia (2019a) Borders Group. https://en.wikipedia.org/wiki/Borders_Group. Accessed 14 July 2019

Wikipedia (2019b) Power law. https://en.wikipedia.org/wiki/Power_law. Accessed 14 July 2019

Wikipedia (2019c). Intergalactic Computer Network. https://en.wikipedia.org/wiki/Intergalactic_Computer_Network. Accessed 14 July 2019

Wikipedia (2019d). Timeline of virtualization development. https://en.wikipedia.org/wiki/Timeline_of_virtualization_development. Accessed 14July 2019

Wikipedia (2019e). Horizontal gene transfer. https://en.wikipedia.org/wiki/Horizontal_gene_transfer. Accessed 14 July 2019

Wikipedia (2019f) Markov property. https://en.wikipedia.org/wiki/Markov_property. Accessed 14 July 2019

Wikipedia (2019g). Stent. https://en.wikipedia.org/wiki/Stent. Accessed 14 July 2019

Wikipedia (2019h). Ironic process theory. https://en.wikipedia.org/wiki/Ironic_process_theory. Accessed 14 July 2019

Wikipedia (2019i) SWOT analysis. https://en.wikipedia.org/wiki/SWOT_analysis. Accessed 14 July 2019

Wikipedia (2019j). Porter's five forces analysis. https://en.wikipedia.org/wiki/Porter%27s_five_forces_analysis. Accessed 14 July 2019

Wikipedia (2019k). OODA loop. https://en.wikipedia.org/wiki/OODA_loop. Accessed 14 July 2019

Wikipedia (2019l). Matthew 6:3. https://en.wikipedia.org/wiki/Matthew_6:3. Accessed 14 July 2019

Wiktionary (2019). Give a man a fish and you feed him for a day. https://en.wiktionary.org/wiki/give_a_man_a_fish_and_you_feed_him_for_a_day;_teach_a_man_to_fish_and_you_feed_him_for_a_lifetime. Accessed 14 July 2019

Wilensky U (1997). Ants. NetLogo Models Library. http://ccl.northwestern.edu/netlogo/models/Ants

Winters GS (2016) Why Agile is failing at large companies. Ty yn Goch Forrest Publications

Wong G (2011) Jumping the S-curve. https://cognitive-edge.com/blog/jumping-the-s-curve/. Accessed 14 July 2019

Zapf GW (1801) Gallerie der alten Griechen und Roemer. Bürglen, Augsburg, Austria. http://digi.ub.uni-heidelberg.de/diglit/zapf1801/, public domain

Future Design Challenges

23

Nam Pyo Suh

Abstract

One thing that never ends as long as humanity continues to exist: the emergence of new challenging problems that humanity must solve for their posterity through creative design. In the 1950s, few people would have thought that the invention of polymers with amazing properties would someday create new problems for humanity to solve. In the early decades of the twenty-first century, the pollution of the Pacific Ocean by the debris of solid plastics from countries around the Pacific rim is a major catastrophe with significant negative implications for the entire global community, especially for the people living in the nearby islands. Somehow, we must solve this problem without banning the use of plastics in the future, because the appropriate use of plastics fulfills human needs. Similarly, a century ago, few ever thought that the replacement of horse-drawn buggies with automobiles would result in global warming that might change and threaten the future of humankind. In each case, a new innovative technology begat new unanticipated technological or societal problems for future generations to solve or deal with. Therefore, it may be rational and reasonable to assume that current technologies and socio-political norms would someday become the source of new challenges for future generations to solve. In a way, it is the price humanity has to pay to make continuing progress through innovation and discovery. Thus, the saga of humanity continues. The natural progression always leaves new challenges for the next generation to solve—rationally and creatively. Therefore, the need for new knowledge and creative design will always be with humanity as long as humans exist. In the early twenty-first century, humanity is facing a unique set of challenges. Either people solve them in time, or the events will overtake humanity's ability to solve them, leading to instability in human and societal

N. P. Suh (✉)
Cambridge, MA, USA
e-mail: npsuh@mit.edu

© Springer Nature Switzerland AG 2021
N. P. Suh et al. (eds.), *Design Engineering and Science*,
https://doi.org/10.1007/978-3-030-49232-8_23

evolution. Some of these problems are results of the ever-expanding population of the world, which has been increasing at the rate of 1–2% a year and will exceed 8 billion people in the early part of the twenty-first century. An associated problem is a wide variation in the rate of population increase throughout the world, which results in migration and immigration of people from highly populated to less populated, from politically unstable to stable regions, and from poor regions to affluent areas of the world. The problems created by this imbalanced population increase and distribution will lead to many challenging design issues. If we cannot come up with the right design solution, humans might again resort to wars to settle their differences, which should be avoided at all costs. In this sense, the human ability to design will continue to be critical and in high demand. When and if new solutions do not emerge to deal with new problems, Nature may dictate the future of humanity, including a catastrophic demise of the world and humankind.

A partial list of significant design challenges humanity is facing in the early twenty-first century is related to, but not limited to, the following:

Energy needs;

Global warming;

Instability of weather patterns;

Need for portable water;

Pollution-free electric power generation;

Pollution-free transportation systems;

Protection of privacy in the information-intensive technological world;

Preservation of green plants;

Feeding of people,

Control of weather;

Prevention and elimination of contagious diseases;

The ability to maintain free society in a peaceful world;

Supplementary brain; and

Protection of fundamental human rights.

The solution to any one of these problems could consist of different kinds of design solutions—technical, scientific, socio-political, and economic as well as a combination of these fields. There could be more than one solution. Regardless of the specific approach chosen, the method and the process of developing design solutions are ecumenical, as described in Chaps. 1–3.

Furthermore, a solution to one of these problems may generate a set of new issues that the next generation must solve. The responsibility of the current generation is to educate the next generation well. That is the primary guarantee that their posterity can deal with their own set of challenges well.

The human ability to solve many of the above-listed problems are continuously improved because humans continue to invent new tools and advance sciences. Recent advances made in several fields such as artificial intelligence (AI), quantum computing, neuro-biological, brain sciences, nano-scale materials, and other areas of science and technology are most encouraging as well as promising.

Every problem discussed in this book, as well as many that are not addressed, will, ultimately, require "design solutions" similar to those discussed in the previous 22 chapters. The one(s) who create solutions to major challenging problems will richly be rewarded through various recognitions by humanity, which may include financial, intellectual, political, and personal recognition and esteem. Solve them we must, because the other option will only invite demise for humankind.

Often, we do not know which problem will require new designs. Also, at the beginning of the execution of design, one cannot have all the specific knowledge in the relevant field(s) because we may not have the requisite expertise. Once we understand the design task and associated questions (i.e., functional requirement (FRs)), we can acquire the necessary fundamental knowledge of the related fields quickly to develop design solutions in terms of DPs and PVs. Even the most complex problems can be systematically solved through design by following the steps outlined in this book. An exemplary design problem related to water and weather is discussed that can have a significant worldwide impact if a rational design solution can be devised.

23.1   Introduction: Continuing Human "Saga"

"Inputs to an operating system generate outputs, some desired, some unwanted, and some even detrimental. Humanity must deal with the detrimental outputs of the system. They will not disappear by themselves."

When people invented the internal combustion engines near the end of the nineteenth century, they thought that finally, they could have manure-free streets in addition to having faster moving vehicles. Automobiles, with other technologies, indeed led the industrial renaissance of the twentieth century. A century later, however, people are discovering that it is a major source of the environmental problem. The emission of carbon dioxide (CO_2) from these powerful engines, which have served humanity so well, is contributing about 30% of the CO_2 gases that are responsible for greenhouse effects and global warming that are threatening the very survival of human society as we know it.

Similarly, when the electrification of the rural community was finally accomplished in the United States, a new era of modernization came to every corner of the nation. It also enabled the modernization of many other countries. Electrification raised the standard of living, bringing in high quality of life through the replacement of human labor with machines and equipment powered by electricity. Now more than a century later, we are discovering that the generation of electricity through the combustion of fossil fuel is leading the world to global warming, threatening the very existence of the infrastructure of modern society and the habitat of animals and marine life. Similarly, through much research and development, engineers and scientists designed nuclear power plants to replace the fossil-fuel power plants to generate electricity without generating greenhouse gases. However, after accidents at a few of these nuclear power plants, people are abandoning this powerful technology for fear of new nuclear accidents and contamination, taking actions that will accelerate global warming.

These examples illustrate how technologies must continue to evolve to seek the next level of improvement and innovations to satisfy human needs and overcome problems created by past deeds of human beings. The consequence of technological advancement may generate new design problems that require unique solutions. In a larger scheme of things, these by-products of technological progress will always be there. It is a fundamental nature of systems, that is,

$$\text{Old system} + \text{design innovation} \rightarrow \text{new system} + \text{new by-products} \quad (23.1)$$

Equation (23.1) states that there are "new by-products" embedded in techno-logical solutions (i.e., global warming with industrialization and invention of internal engines). Some of these by-products cannot be ignored over a long period, thus creating the need to design a new solution that can overcome the problem created while solving an old problem. Equation (23.1) can be used to achieve many positive results if humanity can deal with undesired by-products, if any, success-fully and well. The conversion process indicated by Eq. (23.1) generates economic activity, creates jobs, and continues to advance knowledge in all spheres of human activity. The shortcomings of horse-drawn buggies created cars with internal combustion engines, which have served humanity well for over 100 years. Still, a new problem in the form of global warming emerged, forcing the creation of new alternative transportation systems. This continuing evolution of human society is part of the natural process.

So far, humanity has managed the process of evolution indicated by Eq. (23.1) well, mostly through the design of the next advanced solutions as well as through finding new solutions. Economic and financial investments in education, research, and development enabled the continuing evolution and advancement of human society since the Industrial Revolution, albeit a few calamitous blow-ups among people. For this process to go on, we need the enlightenment of the large fraction of people who support the dynamics of successful human, social, and economic progress. When this process fails, humanity frequently discovered themselves in ugly conflicts such as the First and Second World Wars. Humanity is often skirting the boundaries of these disasters, a symptom of a poorly designed socioeconomic–political system.

In this chapter, a few of the major problems that may require innovations, solutions, and design will be discussed as examples of future design tasks that may require the attention of the next generations of designers, leaders, and the society at large. Predicting future events and functions is not an easy task—with many risks of being wrong—perhaps best left to those with psychic minds. In the following sections, randomly selected topics are discussed with no assurance that they will indeed be the most important topics. For instance, if nuclear war engulfs the world, many things will change with irrecoverable dramatic ends of the world, which is hard to imagine at this time. In that sense, we should do everything we can to design a system that will prevent events that may culminate in such a disaster.

23.2 A Challenging Design Problem: Creating Forest in North Africa

Living beings such as animals and vegetation cannot survive in the absence of water, as well known. The availability (or scarcity) of water has determined the politics and conflicts among nations, especially in the Middle East. The control of water of the Jordan River (River Jordan) that flows through Jordan, Syria, and Israel is politically and historically significant. In China, there are five or more large deserts. The Gobi Desert, which is between China and Mongolia, is a vast and arid region. The sandstorm from the Gobi desert reaches Korea, Japan, and parts of the northern American continent every spring. People in Korea wear masks, and sometimes, schools close during the peak season of the sandstorm. In North Africa, the vast land area is mostly desert with limited human habitation. The world's largest Sahara desert covers about one-third of the African continent (about 3.5 million square miles) from the Red Sea on the west and the Nile River on the east (extending about 3,000 miles) and from the Atlas Mountains of the south to the Mediterranean sea of the north (about 1,000 miles).

Many theories have been advanced to explain how the deserts in North Africa were created. It appears that the changes in the weather pattern created the North African desert some seven million years ago. One theory is that when the North and the South poles became extremely cold, the moisture condensed at these two poles, thus depriving the moisture condensation in the hot regions near the Equator of Earth, creating the vast desert of North Africa. There is also a theory that when people and animals overglaze a particular area, the region becomes a desert, especially in a hot climate. For example, the urbanization of the suburb near Cairo and the Nile River created a small desert in the adjacent area between Cairo and the Nile River. The population density of these desert areas is very low since the climate is not very hospitable to people and other living beings, including vegetation.

Some of the deserts in the world became habitable through massive irrigation. The southern part of the State of California became thriving urban centers of the United States with extensive agricultural business and high-tech industries thanks to the water diverted from the Colorado River. Many other countries such as Israel, Saudi Arabia, and the United Arab Emirates converted desert into valuable urban centers by securing freshwater either through de-salination or divergence of rivers.

There is also a "theory," cum speculation that the presence of green plants and vegetation near the shore areas changes the weather pattern that brings in moisture to the area, which condensate and rain in the region with forest and vegetation. Assuming that these observations or theories are correct, can we design a solution to convert some parts of the desert areas into habitable land for plants, animals, and people? The first requirement for converting the desert into inhabitable land is to bring more water to the region. In many areas, the de-salination processes, such as the evaporation process or a reverse osmosis (RO) process, are used to generate freshwater. The evaporation process and RO processes of producing freshwater are energy-intensive processes, which are the major processes used for de-salination in many countries in the Middle East, including Saudi Arabia and all neighboring countries. These energy-intensive processes are expensive to operate. We should design a more energy-efficient de-salination process by making use of solar energy or wind power.

The following story illustrates how the desert can be converted into a modern university–city complex with lots of trees and vegetation when sufficient financial resources are available. A design challenge is how a similar transformation of the desert can be achieved at a lower cost of construction and maintenance, using less energy.

The KAUST Story:

About 40 miles north of Jeddah, which is a major city of Saudi Arabia on the Red Sea, there used to be a small town called Thuwal. Its western border is the Red Sea, and the desert surrounds it on the other three sides. Thuwal is also about 87 miles south of Mecca, the holiest city of Muslims—the birthplace of the Prophet Muhammad and the Muslim faith. Thuwal used to be a small fishing village until about 2009. In mere a decade, Thuwal has become a well-known city in the world because it became the home for King Abdulah University of Science and Technology (KAUST). King Abdulah of Saudi Arabia, a visionary and benevolent king, established the university because he wanted to see Saudi Arabia regain its eminence in mathematics and science.

KAUST was established in 2009 at a location that used to be a vast desert. Now its campus consists of 3,600 hectares (8,900 acres) of land with more than 16,000 palm trees, 17,000 other trees, modern research buildings with advanced instruments and equipment, academic buildings, a fire station, apartments for students, faculty housing, movie theatre, restaurants, etc. Its graduate students do not pay any tuition, receives a stipend for living expenses, and have access to some of the best-equipped laboratories. The student body is co-educational, international, and highly selective. The goal of KAUST is to become one of the best university of science and technology in the world. To achieve this goal, it has attracted leading researchers and students from many parts of the world.

KAUST is a private university with the second-largest endowment in the world, next to Harvard University. KAUST is a relatively small graduate school of science and technology with approximately 1,200 graduate students and about 200 faculty in 2020. It may double its size within ten years. Its physical facilities are most impressive. About two-thirds of the students and faculty, both men and women, are from outside of Saudi Arabia. There are many Saudi women students. KAUST is truly co-educational free from many restrictions of Saudi Arabia. In many ways, it is comparable to the leading universities in advanced nations on other continents. About half of the trustees of the university are non-Saudis.

KAUST survives and thrives because of the electric energy supplied by electric power plants that burn oil in Saudi Arabia. All the buildings are air-conditioned with the electrical energy provided by electric powerplants that combust oil. To generate freshwater, KAUST pumps water in from the Red Sea to its de-salination plants on the campus. The de-salinated water is used throughout the entire KAUST community. The water that keeps all the trees and vegetation alive is the re-circulated residual water after its primary use. Its annual water consumption varied from a high of 9 million cubic meters in 2015 to about six million cubic meters in 2019, decreasing every year since 2015. The electric power required for de-salination varied from 51 million kilowatt-hours (kWh) in 2014 to 33.5 million kWh in 2019. The beautifully landscaped green area of KAUST is 1.1 million square meters (m^2). The total number of people that work and live in the KAUST campus is around 7,200. The total power consumption in 2015 was 530 million kilowatt-hours (kWh), decreasing to 509 million kWh. The electric power used at KAUST for de-salination was from 9.6% in 2015 to 6.5% in 2019 of the total electrical energy consumed. On per capita basis, the total power consumption at KAUST was about 73,000 kWh per capita and for de-salination about 4,000 kWh per capita. To put these numbers in a proper context, the electricity consumption per capita of various countries in kWh are as follows: Saudi Arabia (9,400), U.S. (13,000), Sweden (13,000), Korea (10,400), China (3,900), and Norway (23,000). A conclusion from this rough analysis is that to solve the water problem in the North African desert (or any other dessert), we cannot only use the energy-intensive de-salination processes such as evaporation or reverse osmosis (RO) process. These high energy-intensive processes are needed when the rate of de-salination is high. However, in many situations, we may not need such a high rate of de-salination. Thus, we may have the possibility to design a new system of de-salination.

Saudi Arabia is exceptionally fortunate to be sitting on a vast reservoir of clean oil with the least amount sulfur, etc., below the sand, which was discovered in 1938. Its production cost is the lowest in the world, being as low as $3 a barrel of oil, which is only about 7% of the cost of producing oil by fracking of rocks in the United States. The amount of oil reserves in Saudi Arabia is difficult to estimate because of the yet-to-be-discovered fields. It appears to be huge. Just a the Stone Age did not end because the world ran out of stone (a statement made by a previous Oil Minister of KSA), Saudi Arabia may not be able to sustain its economy based on oil. Saudi Arabia will not be running out of oil any time soon. Still, because of global warming, the oil industry may, in the future, have a limited market because the world cannot depend on oil as their primary energy source. Saudi Arabia is well aware of this situation and is planning to change its economic structure to avoid being entirely dependent on the petroleum industry because of limited global demand for oil as the renewable energy sources take over the energy market. They are trying to create new economic engines that can create jobs for a rapidly growing population of the Kingdom, a goal of their 2030 economic plan.

The amazing thing about the modern world's economy is that the value of natural resources is minuscule in comparison to the value-added created by ideas that do not depend on natural resources. For example, the vast annual revenue of the giant oil company, Saudi Aramco, is much less than those of four companies in the United States, i.e., Microsoft, Amazon, Facebook, and Google, that does not depend on natural resources for their revenue. Thus, the need for the Kingdom of Saudi Arabia to restructure its economy is quite apparent, i.e., to go from a nation that depends on natural resources in the ground to an economy that is vastly different from the petroleum-based economy by finding new economic engines.

In the twenty-first century, the irony for Saudi Arabia is facing is the following: it is one of the most energy-rich countries in the world, not because of the oil under the ground, but rather the immense solar energy it gets from the Sun every day of the year! Yet, they are unable to tap into this vast energy source and capitalize on it. The following design task is formulated to solve this problem.

The Design Problem for the Future Well-Being of the People Throughout the World:

Suppose you are a bright graduate student at KAUST, doing design research under the guidance of a globally renowned KAUST professor Sandra Cavique-Foley. The design task is to design de-salination plants to establish "forest" in Saudi Arabia and Egypt along the coast of the Red Sea, using the uninterrupted supply of solar energy (except at night), the availability of the water of the Red Sea, and vast desert area in these two countries.

If the water from the Red Sea can be de-salinated inexpensively using solar energy, it can be used to grow plants in what is now desert. When a forest exists through this process, some claim that the weather may change in these areas because the trees will transform the weather pattern, generating additional condensation. The moist air will condensate, create more rain, and eventually make the current desert area into livable and arable land with trees and other vegetation.

State your FRs and develop ideas that can fulfill this dream. Then state the DPs that can satisfy the FRs. What would be your process variables (PVs)?

As you embark on this design assignment, you should remember that, in general, slow processes that require low levels of energy require larger equipment, which requires more capital investment. This is the case when we try to make use of the tidal wave of the ocean to generate electric power. This argument also applies to the case of electricity generation with windmills. It requires large long blades to be economical. One has to consider the financial viability of your idea as you decide on FRs, design parameters (DPs), and PVs.

23.3 Design Challenges Related to Renewable Energy

1. Issues associated with solar cells

   a. One big problem with the use of solar cells is that the output of electricity cannot be easily controlled or modulated quickly once installed. The output depends primarily on the availability of sunlight, which cannot be regulated. Thus, when the electricity generation by solar cells exceeds consumption, we must store it for future use or dissipate it, neither of which is a trivial task. Some countries may find it cheaper to give it away to their neighboring states if they can use the electricity. We need to design solutions for storing excess energy.

   b. Various electric energy storage schemes have been considered. One idea that has been promoted is to compress CO_2 gas in a closed cavity such as underground salt mine and generate electricity by decompressing CO_2 when electric power is needed. An idea of storing energy that is in use today is to pump water to a reservoir at a higher elevation, e.g., mountains. Then use the power of the waterfall by running a hydropower plant when needed. If such clean electrical energy is abundantly available, we can create hydrogen and oxygen through electrolysis, which can be used to power automobiles without creating CO_2.

c. Another solution is to limit the power generation by solar cells to be always below the demand level. When the demand exceeds the supply, supplementary electric power generation by other means can be used, such as conventional fossil fuel-burning power plants or through activation of nuclear power plants. One of the design issues is the creation of control system that can deal with a continuously varying demand and supply system.

d. The above-mentioned electric power transmission efficiency has other implications. If the electrical power can be transmitted less expensively, then electricity can be generated in hydrocarbon-rich and less densely populated areas. Then the electricity can be transmitted to highly populated urban regions. This transmission of power rather than crude oil will eliminate the oil consumption associated with transportation, which should help in CO_2 emission by ships. This transmission of electric power, especially wireless transmission, is a challenging issue in design.

e. One current popular solution is to put solar cells on top of the roofs of individual houses, which may alleviate the problems related to electricity transmission in addition to creating a distributed power generation system. Still, the electricity generated from the rooftops of these houses may not be sufficient to supply reliable electric power for industrial operations and transportation.

2. Wind Power

a. Wind power is another source of renewable electric energy. Windmills have been installed in many countries, e.g., Denmark, the United States, and many others. The power generation is proportional to the square of the blade length, requiring tall towers for installation.

b. The availability of wind power is often highly location-specific. In some countries, they are installed offshore or on top of mountains away from densely populated areas for noise reduction and safety. It has to be located away from urban areas to prevent the disastrous consequence of accidents due to fatigue of materials and noise. In many countries, they are often installed offshore, which solves many problems if the initial capital cost of installation can be justified and is reasonable.

c. Wind power has the same issue as solar power in terms of the storage of excess electric energy.

3. Nuclear Power

a. The nuclear power plant supplies a significant fraction of electricity in many countries, e.g., France, South Korea, Japan, and China. In many countries, they have operated these power plants for decades without any major accidents.

b. The biggest threat to the use of nuclear power is the fear factor. The past accidents that occurred, for example, in the Soviet Union as well as in Japan, were truly horrendous. There are indications that the accident in Fukushima, Japan, was due to the coupling of FRs at the system level. Building safe electric power plants based on fusion is still a dream that requires creative design for containing energy that is at extremely high temperatures.

c. The design challenge is to develop 100% accident-free nuclear power plants. This means that the design must be thoroughly reviewed for any coupling at the system level, i.e., in physical layout, software design, and operational level.

d. Some countries have considered building small modular nuclear reactors that are safer than large plants.

e. A more serious challenge in the use of nuclear power plants for electricity generation is the disposal of the spent nuclear fuel, which must be stored forever with 100% assurance. One way is to send the spent fuel toward the Sun, which will be a challenging design task.

23.4   Design Problems Related to Transportation

Transportation of goods and people is both a necessity for economic activities and fulfills the basic human desire to expand the sphere of human activities and interactions. As the population continues to grow, both the issues and needs related to transportation will continue to expand. Unfortunately, one major villain for causing global warming is also the transportation of goods and people; the most guilty one being automobiles, followed by airplanes and ocean-going vessels, because ground transportation is the dominant mode of transportation of goods and people. Roughly 30% of the CO_2 emission is from the internal combustion engines of automobiles and airplanes, another 30% coming from electricity generation. Currently, the primary emission that concerns regulators is that of cars. In both cases, alternative power sources consist of batteries, electric motors, and engines.

The most often-cited solution is to use lithium batteries that supply electric power to electric motors. There are three problems associated with this solution: the cost, weight, and safety of batteries. The weight of batteries can be as much as 30% of the total vehicle weight. The other potential issue is the possible explosion of the lithium batteries. As the number of accidents increases, the explosion of these batteries during a collision can have a disastrous effect, especially if water seeps into these batteries. These batteries contain both the oxidizer and the fuel, which can be activated by water.

A successful alternative design is the use of wireless electric power transmission to propel the vehicle. At the Korea Advanced Institute of Science and Technology (KAIST), a university specializing in science and technology, a new of kind electric vehicle was invented. It receives electric power wirelessly from power supply systems embedded under the pavement and stores some of the energy in the on-board batteries to use it to propel vehicles on roads without the embedded power supply system. In 2019, the "On-Line Electric Vehicle (OLEV)" was running in five cities in Korea including at KAIST. The number of batteries on board is small since the bus receives most of its electric power from the electrical power supply system embedded in the underground. The size of the battery depends on the length of the underground power supply system and the speed of the vehicle. The OLEV vehicles are quiet, and the driver does not have to worry about the supply of fuel. The OLEV system has been running in Korea since 2012, very reliably and quietly without any significant issues. It may soon be installed outside of Korea. When the electricity is generated from renewable sources and nuclear power plants, OLEV is entirely emission-free. Its installation is simple and straight forward, especially when installing new roads.

Also, there are possibilities of reducing fuel consumption of jet airplanes through several concurrent means. The problem of current airplane design is that it has to have powerful engines to propel the airplane to "lift-off speeds, about 160 miles an hour" on a fixed-length runway. However, when the airplane reaches the cruising altitude, the engine is too big and generates aerodynamic drag, which in turn consumes more fuel. In other words, the need for "take-off" from ground determines the engine size, which at the cruising speed, is too big and adds to fuel inefficiency.

There are several possibilities of reducing engine size. One is to reduce the mixing section of the engine by coming up with faster means of mixing fuel with oxygen, such as impingement of fuel and oxidizer rather than depending on the slow diffusion process. Another method of reducing the engine size is by assisting the airplane in reaching the lift-off speed by providing an externally assisted take-off force. For instance, an external "train" can pull the plane forward to help the acceleration of the airplane, similar to the way fighter planes take off from the deck of naval carrier ships. The simplest solution is to extend the length of the runways to enable aircraft to reach the take-off speed without having large engines. All of these possibilities offer exciting design tasks.

23.5 Design Problems Related to CO_2 and Methane Gas (CH_4) Emission

There have been many proposals for dealing with CO_2. The most commonly discussed solution is to bury CO_2 in-ground, dissolve in the ocean, or pump liquid CO_2 into ground or under the ground floor of deep sea. Another possibility is to convert CO_2 to other more useful materials. The difficulty is developing technologies that are economical and use less energy to transform. Becasuse CO_2 is one of the most stable forms of carbon products, it isn't straightforward to develop inexpensive and environmentally acceptable conversion technologies. A research center established at KAIST under the joint sponsorship of KAIST and Saudi Aramco has been working on this problem for the past several years.

Methane (CH_4) is another environmentally harmful gas. The primary sources of CH_4 are agricultural processes, degrading plants, and from cracking for oil. The quantity of CH_4 emission is about 9%, which is less than the emission of CO_2. Still, its environmental impact in the atmosphere can be substantial relative to its small quantity. The diffused sources of CH_4 gas are harder to control than the CO_2 emission from internal combustion engines and electric power plants. However, as the CO_2 emission is reduced, the discharge of CH_4 will receive more attention.

The free energy of CH_4 is high, and therefore, it should be easier to convert it into other useful products, the most stable reaction products of CH_4 being is CO_2 and H_2O. Thus, CH_4 can more easily be transformed into other useful materials because CH_4 can be reacted with other substances more efficiently than CO_2.

23.6 Future Roles of Artificial Intelligence (AI) and Quantum Computing in Design

Axiomatic Design (AD) teaches how to create an original design from scratch correctly. Its axioms and theorems also explain how to find design flaws. This process is going to benefit if the database on past designs, constitutive relationships, various FR-DP-PV relationships, and past failures were readily available. A promising approach is to generate plausible concepts by going through vast databases to mine the data in the literature, hoping to find the right design solution. This approach makes use of three development: the ability of computers to store a vast database, process an extensive database rapidly at low cost, and the recent advances in AI with the potential to extract the desired information quickly from the vast database. A promising approach is to generate plausible concepts by going through vast databases to mine the data in the literature, hoping to find the right design solution. This approach makes use of three development: the ability of computers to store a vast database, process an extensive database rapidly at low cost, and the recent advances in AI with the potential to extract the desired information quickly from the vast database.

AI can be used in many designed systems to make better decisions expeditiously and to improve the effectiveness of the decision-making process. This use of AI is possible because of the availability of high-speed computers, the vast memory space available at low cost, and the development of sensors that can monitor the behavior of the system. Already commercial software systems that incorporate AI are being introduced. Such development will need a supervisory AI system that can check for the correctness and accuracy of the AI decisions made.

Like many new technologies, one of the dangers is that AI may be used for unsavory purposes. It can be used to cheat in elections for public offices, oppress less fortunate people, and create systems that favor those with means at the expense of democracy. If the history of technology provides a lesson, humanity eventually finds positive and beneficial applications of technology. However, people were concerned about the possible negative impact of new technologies on human beings, society, and individuals. So far, problems created by new technologies have been solved through technologies, often advancing societal goals in addition to technological advances. As long as we do not let technologies dominate human decisions, we may be in good stead.

Many software and computer companies are active in these fields. Broadcom of the United States (stock listing: AVGO) launched Automation.ai, an AI-based software platform for supporting decision-making processes across different industries. It deals with large volumes of data, which is challenging to do by digital transformation, which can lead to slower decision-making. According to Broadcom, Automation.ai is a platform designed to ease complications stemming from the interference of diverse tools and data, and thereby facilitate informed decision-making. It correlates and examines data to another software called Digital BizOps to analyze the data and combine them to generate solutions to aid decision-making. According to the company's brochure, the technique harnesses the power of machine learning, intelligent automation, and internet-scale open-source frameworks to transform data. It is not clear if Automation.ai can develop design solutions based on an original set of FRs.

Many other companies, such as IBM, have also been exploiting AI and quantum computing, using their ability to store and manipulate vast data to improve decision-making through cloud computing. IBM has been one of the first industrial firms to work on quantum computing from many decades ago. Many of these tools, including those of IBM and Broadcom, are based on their idea that there are vast data available in the literature and companies that can be exploited and recombined to create solutions to existing or new problems. The idea is to do what people can do faster, utilizing the capability of machines to gather and sort out the data quicker and more extensively. Ultimately, the hope is that the machines will also become smarter than people in creating and designing new solutions. If this can be done, the same thing will happen to scientists and engineers that happened to factory workers due to automation using robotic technologies. Then, engineers and scientists must work on a higher intellectual platform to do things that machines cannot do, which will turn out to be a challenge. Computers are getting smarter faster than perhaps an average person!

Some people are concerned that AI, the especially advanced form of AI, will overtake the human ability to solve problems and create new solutions. In other words, machine intelligence will be superior to human intelligence. That has been the case for decades. For some tasks, machines have done a better job than human beings ever since the Industrial Revolution. That is why we use many different kinds of devices and tools. Now the computer can perform better than human beings in some logical reasoning fields. This trend will continue. However, as machine intelligence improves, so will human intelligence, often faster than machines.

23.7   Design and Large Databases

The collection and management of the vast data that exist throughout the world is a significant challenge. Cloud computing has enabled the creation and management of an extensive database. Major corporations have jumped into the business of managing the database and extracting the desired information. For most people, it will soon be reasonable to assume that anyone can obtain personal information and manipulate them by companies, individuals, and the government using facial recognition. Regulating these activities will be extremely difficult. Individuals should assume that it will be challenging to maintain personal secrets confidential because the data have been automatically collected and stored through various means by the government, merchants, schools, hospitals, and the like. Ultimately, the government must regulate the use of these personal data, because no individual can manage, protect, and restrict the use of personal data collected by machines and organizations of various kinds.

The irony of the situation discussed above is that eventually, machines may know more about us than we know ourselves! Under that circumstance, each morning, we should consult the computer what we should do that day. Similarly, in the evening, we should ask the machine to review what we have done during the daytime and assess our performance and effectiveness, hoping that we can improve our performance and efficiency the following day!

23.8   Design Issues Related to De-Salination

Today de-salination has become big business. Most de-salination processes in use today are done using either reverse osmosis (RO) processes or various evaporation processes. These processes are energy-intensive since these processes break the atomic bonds between sodium chloride molecules and water molecules, both of which are energy-intensive. Therefore, these are high-cost processes.

There are other possibilities for de-salination, such as de-salination by phase separation. One of the techniques developed at MIT is to apply an electric potential across the flowing brine water to create two streams: one salt-rich stream and the other with low salt content. Then, the stream with high salt contents was separated continuously from the lower concentration stream by draining off to a sink. By continuing this process, what flows to the end of the stream is the water with low salt concentration. The methods such as this need new design solutions.

Another possibility investigated at MIT and KFUPM is the use of graphene to separate water molecules from other molecules. Making the graphene sheets without flaws such as large holes is a challenging task. However, it is a conceptually promising means of making atomic-scale filters.

There may be other effective designs that are economical and reliable.

23.9 Design of Software

Software is embedded in almost every product, in addition to substantial central computing facilities that are maintained by all major corporations, universities, and government agencies. Many software system developers often start coding their software without first designing the software system, which may result in coupled systems, requiring extensive revisions and testing.

One of the problems many software developers are facing is that they often build new software systems on existing legacy software codes and policies. It isn't very easy to know the intention of the designer of the original software unless they have made thorough documentation on the system.

When large software systems are being developed, the design matrix must be concurrently constructed to be sure that there is no coupling of FRs in the software system. The current practice is to develop software codes and test before designing the software system.

23.10 Control of the Weather Pattern

If we can control weather patterns, we can change the world for the better. Then, we can improve many things such as agriculture, quality of life, prevention of forest fire, conversion of dessert to useful land, low consumption of energy to heat houses and factories, and many other beneficial things. Now unstable weather patterns are causing significant problems in many parts of the world. For instance, a hurricane that begins off the east coast of northern Africa due to high water temperature and wind patterns creates vortices above the warm water. The vortices move toward the southeastern area of the United States, where the temperature is lower, creating hurricanes in the fall of every year and causing human tragedy as well as a lot of economic losses. With global warming, the problem is going to get worse, more tropical storms, the creation of more dessert, higher water levels, and unpredictable weather patterns.

Hurricanes are caused by instability. When hot air forms a vortex motion on top of the surface of the warm ocean water, it sucks up the water vapor, which strengthens the vortex motion as it continues to move on top of the warm water. This vortex motion generates strong wind as it grows. When the vortex moves toward the colder surface of the land and the moisture condenses, it can unleash rains with strong wind on the cold land surface. The damage done by these hurricanes, wind, rain, surging ocean waves causes tremendous damage every year.

On the other hand, the weather pattern in Saudi Arabia and northern Africa is the opposite. The whole region is hot throughout the year, and the Red Sea is relatively small to develop unstable air-motion and create vortices. Therefore, the hot vapor of the sea cannot be picked up and dumped on the top of the tropical land. Thus, the region around Saudi Arabia is arid and became a dessert.

The design question is the following: Can we create and control vortices using the instability phenomena of the circular motion of atmosphere by creating a large number of small vortices artificially at different parts of the ocean surfaces to control the weather pattern of Earth. If we can do that, we can change Earth to make it more habitable, useful, and productive. The author of this chapter believes it can and should be done.

23.11 Design of a Better Educational System

Human beings are created equal. However, the quality of education often ruptures this "god-endowed" equality. The secondary variables such as family background, financial resources, family stability, neighborhood, quality of education, and early childhood education have deterministic effects on the well-being of the individual as well as their society. Often, education has created a demarcation line between those who will do well in society and those who would have problems in a merit-based society. Therefore, parents in all countries are concerned about the education of their children.

Similarly, the future development of a nation depends on the quality and effectiveness of its educational system. Yet the educational system in many countries is not effective and efficient for a variety of different reasons. In fact, in many countries, educational systems are the primary reason for the lack of advancement in the country. Ultimately, the educational system of most countries is determined by design. In most nations, the emphasis is on teaching rather than learning, i.e., *teaching methods, teaching materials, teaching techniques,* and less on *learning methods, learning efficiency,* etc.

Many of these nations should redesign their educational systems. It should be designed to bring out the best in their young people, must be rational, and must be merit-based. It must emphasize ethical behavior, the concept of equality, the importance of guarding justice, and doing one's best in their profession. All these features must be designed in the curriculum, institutional culture, and reward systems. The future of a nation depends primarily on its educational system, because other socioeconomic-political factors are more difficult to change without improving educational systems.

23.12 Design of a Democratic and Transparent Government

Eventually, most nations will have a democratic form of government as a consequence of significant advances in telecommunications, computers, and sensors that can record most transactions and documents. It will be challenging to hide corruptive practices, illegal activities, dictatorial practices, and unsavory acts.

Technologies will make it increasingly difficult to lie to the public for too long! When technology is appropriately used, it will make society, politics, and government more transparent.

Recently, one of the most advanced democracies in the world has gone through significant debates about the effectiveness, adequacy, and reliability of its election system, which is the underlying lynchpin of democracy. Even after so many decades and centuries of maintaining effective democracy, people are finding that modern technology can undermine the election system, especially when foreign adversaries are interested in disrupting the system to bias the outcome in their favor. In addition to the external interference, governments in many countries are tilted in favor of those governing the nation. Such corrupt practices lead to both unfair and undemocratic practices. We need an improved system for transparency in governments, an effective governing structure, and a reliable election system to sustain democracy. Truly democratic and fair practices can exist only with the citizens are well educated, and laws and democratic principles rule governments. We will also need continuous improvement in protecting the election system and in preventing unlawful practices.

Democracy is a way of governing by following the majority opinion for a fixed period and then reset the rule the group must adopt until the next period, i.e., *functional periodicity*. As Churchill said in 1947 in the House of Commons, "No one pretends that democracy is perfect or all-wise. Indeed it has been said that democracy is the worst form of government except for all those other forms that have been tried from time to time...." It took about two thousand years from Aristotle to the first English democracy. It changed the question from "who must rule?" to "how to rule?" and "what to achieve?" To achieve this goal of a democratic nation, FRs must be established for the government and society through free and democratic means based on fundamental governing rules and principles. FRs are typically related to security, prosperity, welfare, health, aspiration, and freedom of the people. Corrupting democracy leads to unpeaceful and conflicted societies.

23.13 Design of Improved Health Delivery Systems

The quality and cost of healthcare are two major issues that concern average citizens in most countries. Gradually, every country is moving toward some form of universal healthcare for all its citizens that can deliver the best care at the lowest cost, which may be an oxymoron.

Many things must be done right to enact and maintain an affordable and effective healthcare system. We need to design a healthcare system that has the following qualities:

(a) High-quality hospitals with best trained medical staff, the right equipment, and facilities,
(b) Efficient medical and pharmaceutical systems,

(c) Incentive system that rewards the medical skill, knowledge, efficiency and dedicated work, and minimum bureaucracy.

Many countries have done much to improve their system, but none seem to satisfy all these criteria.

23.14 Design of a Peaceful World

Almost everyone is seeking to live in a peaceful world. Yet, it has eluded humankind for centuries. There are many reasons for it. Perhaps the most prominent causes are human greed, a fundamental desire to protect one's tribe and family, even at the expense of others. Sometimes, national and regional interests, different religious beliefs, limited resources to share, creeping dictatorship, and others tend to override democratic tenents and a sense of justice. People have attempted to create a peaceful and prosperous world through the establishment of the United Nations (UN), the Worlds Health Organizations (WHO), the World Bank, and others. Their effectiveness of these world organizations was checked by bureaucracy, lack of real power to implement the best practices, limited incentives for good work, and financial dependence on the member nations.

One significant danger is that many unstable people may have access to weapons of mass destruction such as nuclear bombs, biochemical agents, disruption of the electric power grid, and spreading of false information. We need to design means of controlling and safeguarding these weapons of mass destruction.

23.15 Design of Better Drugs for Brains

We have many brain-related illnesses such as Alzheimer's disease, autism, and others. Yet, one of the least developed fields of medicine is those related to the human brain. We have limited knowledge of the details of brain functions. Consequently, we do not have a systematic means of diagnosis and fundamental expertise in developing new pharmaceutical medicine that can deal with human memory, enhanced brain functions, and the like. Can we design a system that can assist brain functions through the use of embedded electronic microchips and the like rather than depending on medication?

23.16 Design of Computer Assisted Brains (I.E., Supplementary Brain)

The brain is the most complicated and complex organ in human beings. The brain performs various functions. Many of the workings of these functions of the brain are yet to be fully understood.

The brain retains information and analyzes them. It assembles and synthesizes new information to create new ideas. Its logic circuits deduce conclusions from a random set of data. Many other characteristics and functions of the brain we do not yet fully understand. Some people retain and perform more of these capabilities than others, e.g., Albert Einstein, Ludwig van Beethoven, Thomas Edison, Abraham Lincoln, and others. We do not know whether these exceptional people had more powerful brains or had used their brainpower more wisely and cleverly.

If we assume that human brainpower can be supplemented and complemented through external means by attaching human-made nano-devices to human neuron cells in the brain, we may be able to make "super-human beings." The goal is not only to provide more memory and logic capabilities to the brain but also to give higher and faster reasoning and synthesis power to the person with this "supplementary brainpower." Then, human beings must make sure that the person with such power does not become abusive to harm other people. Morality and ethics must be built in such devices to be sure that we do not create a monster. Human record on morality and ethics is not particularly reassuring.

Physiological functions of humans are affected by *human thought processes*, although some people tend to minimize the effect. Human thought processes must affect biological processes. The following true story supports this view:

Why Do People Sweat when They Eat Spicy Food?

In many countries, especially in the United States, the human palate has changed during the past 50 years. More people eat spicy, hot food more than ever before. The meat and potato culture of Americans has given away to spicy Mexican, Korean, Chinese, and Indian food in major metropolitan areas of the United States. The massive immigration of people from these countries has changed the palate of Americans gradually. Now the minorities in the United States constitute a significant fraction of Americans, which is more multi-racial and cross-cultural than ever before.

One of these hot dishes that have become very popular in the United States is "Kimchi," a Korean fermented cabbage, famous for its hot spice and garlic. Many people sweat when they eat kimchi for the first time, especially if they have not had spicy food before. What is interesting is that once people start eating this dish, they can no longer do without eating it once in a while. Koreans eat kimchi almost every day with their main meals. Most people have attributed their sweat when they eat kimchi to hot spices (primarily hot pepper, garlic, salt) that somehow affected their biological and physiological systems.

One day an engineer who had researched mass production technologies was watching a television program on mass production of kimchi in factories. He was fascinated to learn that they were using a mass-production system similar to those used in making automobiles to make kimchi. It was astonishing and interesting to learn that kimchi is no longer produced by housewives sitting around a table, which used to be the case it was made in Korean households.

After watching the kimchi-manufacturing program for 20–30 min, he was surprised to realize that he was sweating heavily. His shirts got wet, wiping away the sweat from his face with paper towels, although he has not eaten anything spicy that morning! He called his wife to see him sweating so heavily. She was surprised as well. This sweat was purely psychosomatic. When learning of this experience, most people cannot quite believe what they have heard. Some might have tried to replicate the experience.

It is abundantly clear that we have a lot to learn about the brain. What we know and what we need to know are separated by a wall of missing information and knowledge. Much investment will be required to close the gap. Future research should seek a better balance between molecular-level scientific research and hypothesis-based research to solve some of the urgent human sufferings such as autism soon. These two different approaches will reinforce and complement each other for faster advancement in this remaining frontier of human knowledge and technologies.

23.17 Recycling of Materials

The world is rapidly becoming inundated with junk, toxic, and harmful materials. When scientists first invented polymeric materials by creating long-chained molecules, the resulting high molecular materials solved many problems that were impeding the progress of societal functions. Only 70 years later, after the invention of high molecular materials, the world is running out of space to store these materials after using them because human beings consume so much of these non-degradable materials. We need to design solutions for this waste disposal problem. There may be several approaches: first, rapidly degrading these materials to convert them to the original elements without harming nature. Second, recycle waste into useful products. Third, levy enough taxes to finance recycling efforts. Forth, forbid the use of some of these materials through international agreements and legislation, and finally, incorporate, during the design stage, a life cycle scenario to have a net-zero impact on the environment.

23.18 Design Problems Related to Self-Driving Cars

Many companies are developing self-driving automobiles. Their goals are admirable, but there will be many accidents and fatalities before a reliable system can be installed unless they are correctly and adequately designed. Problems will arise in the least expected situations, where machines are not pre-equipped to deal with for lack of a database. Keeping everything else the same and only equipping cars with sensors of many different kinds may be a wrong approach. We need to consider all the issues of such a system and developing a systems solution involving "smart cars," intelligent roads, design of decision-making systems for a group of automobiles nearby, etc. We need to construct FRs, DPs, and the design matrix, considering the interaction of multiple vehicles, conflicting requirements of the vehicle in the proximity, etc. The issues involved are not confined to the car, but the entire system comprising a group of the vehicle with different goals and needs.

23.19 Concluding Remarks

This chapter dealt with the challenging design problems of the future. The preceding chapters showed that if people can identify the problem, they can come up with design solutions, following the steps outlined in this book. There may be exceptions when the underlying science base is absent.

In many fields, humans have designed many incredible things. Various designs and advanced technologies created since the Industrial Revolution attest to the human ability to develop artifacts based on needs and goals. They invented things to solve problems they identified to achieve specific goals. Chapter 1, through Chap. 3, attempted to provide a logical structure for these designs to enhance, expedite, and provide an intellectual framework for creating these designs. We showed how to identify and define the problems, which were then transformed into a set of FRs, followed by the development of DPs to satisfy the FRs. If some of the early pioneers had known AD, they might have done a much better job of synthesizing solutions more quickly! What people have achieved during the past four centuries, at an ever increasingly faster rate, gives us confidence in what humans can do to deal with future challenges.

The purpose of this last chapter is to speculate and consider what kinds of future problems people will be called upon to solve through design. Some may be difficult to address through design. However, what may be surprising to some is that the basic AD methodology presented in this book will be equally applicable to all future design problems. What would be equally remarkable to those learning design for the first time is that the thought processes are similar, i.e., the same thinking process and structure regardless of what we have to design. What was different in designing the OLEV and the laminated coffee cup was the specific basic knowledge involved in each field, such as physics of electromagnetic fields, materials behavior, mechanics, thermodynamics, the need for relevant data, etc. That is why designers need to learn the fundamentals of physics, chemistry, mathematics, and other related subjects as much as possible. The same person who designed OLEV had designed the coffee cup manufacturing systems and organizations in diverse fields using the same process of design outlined in this book.

What the designer must know is the basic principles covered in this book and ask questions to be able to define the design goals to proceed with the design task. One can learn what one does not know to complete a design task. When one does not have the necessary knowledge and cannot answer basic questions, then one should acquire the required knowledge from appropriate books and colleagues, and proceed to design. The person who knows the "question to ask" can develop design solutions! One should not be afraid of tackling a new problem, provided that we are willing to acquire the missing knowledge to be able to ask field-specific questions relevant to a given design task. As one executes more and more design tasks, it becomes easier to be an ecumenical designer, who can function in many different areas. It isn't straightforward to know everything from the beginning, but one can always learn.

The preceding statements apply in many fields. The power of AD enables to organize one's thought, quickly identify what needs to be done, identify the missing knowledge, facilitate the quick acquisition of the tasks involved, and come up with a conceptual design. When the design goals are clear, the designer can acquire the necessary knowledge quickly. These steps are discussed and illustrated in the preceding chapters. If one knows what one ought to know but does not have detailed knowledge, the learning efficiency improves a great deal. Many students spend a great deal of time to learn new subject matters. The effectiveness of learning can be low when one does not know what the question is and what one wants to achieve by learning the subject. To paraphrase it, "when people do not know the question, they cannot find answers." What AD enables the designer to do is quick identification of missing knowledge when attempting to define the FRs, DPs, and PVs.

There are two kinds of design tasks that are challenging and uniquely suited for human designers. The first is the ability to define the design problem, for which only human beings are uniquely qualified. The second is the ability to design logically and rationally, following the steps outlined in this book. The cost of creating something new based purely on experience and trial-and-error methods may be too high with the uncertain and precarious outcome. (Question: Was the failure of Boeing 737 MAX due to a coupling of FRs?) Creative solutions often follow the identification of the most important and critical problem, followed by the development of an uncoupled design.

Among the most critical problems, humanity must solve in the early twenty-first century through design is global warming. Yet, the response of most nations to this existential threat is so slow that we may not solve it in time. In comparison to what many countries spend on defense, hardly any money is spent on global warming. If all nations spend one-tenth of what they are spending on military defense to solve the global warming problem, we may have a chance of preventing this impending disaster before it is too late. The development of practical solutions to global warming problems will require the human ability to design rationally, logically, and without committing significant errors.

Another equally important issue that also requires "design thinking" is the re-orientation of our thinking on "world peace" and "human prosperity and advancement of human habitat." Since the end of the Second World War in 1945, many nations spent more financial resources to develop weapons and in defense because of perceived external threats to their existence. Although many useful technologies resulted from defense research (e.g., GPS, the Internet, new materials, and many others), the world is yet to find peace. In retrospect, it is clear that if leading nations had spent 50% of its defense-related resources for the "peace dividend" for economic and educational development of developing countries, the world today might be more secure, peaceful, productive, healthy, and more prosperous.

Index

© Springer Nature Switzerland AG 2021
N. P. Suh et al. (eds.), *Design Engineering and Science*,
https://doi.org/10.1007/978-3-030-49232-8

Printed in the United States
by Baker & Taylor Publisher Services